Micl

Clinical Manual of Psychopharmacology in the Medically Ill

Second Edition

10/24/16

Clinical Manual of Psychopharmacology in the Medically Ill

Second Edition

Edited by

James L. Levenson, M.D.
Stephen J. Ferrando, M.D.

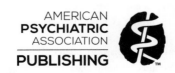

AMERICAN
PSYCHIATRIC
ASSOCIATION
PUBLISHING

If you wish to buy 50 or more copies of the same title, please go to www.appi.org/specialdiscounts for more information.

Copyright © 2017 American Psychiatric Association Publishing
ALL RIGHTS RESERVED
Second Edition
Manufactured in the United States of America on acid-free paper
20   19   18   17   16   5   4   3   2   1
American Psychiatric Association Publishing
1000 Wilson Boulevard
Arlington, VA 22209-3901
www.appi.org

Library of Congress Cataloging-in-Publication Data
Names: Levenson, James L., editor. | Ferrando, Stephen J., editor. | American Psychiatric Association, issuing body.
Title: Clinical manual of psychopharmacology in the medically ill / edited by James L. Levenson, Stephen J. Ferrando.
Description: Second edition. | Arlington, Virginia : American Psychiatric Association Publishing, [2017] | Includes bibliographical references and index.
Identifiers: LCCN 2016026422 (print) | LCCN 2016027149 (ebook) | ISBN 9781585625017 (pb : alk. paper) | ISBN 9781615371075 ()
Subjects: | MESH: Psychotropic Drugs—pharmacokinetics | Psychotropic Drugs—adverse effects | Drug Interactions | Comorbidity
Classification: LCC RM315 (print) | LCC RM315 (ebook) | NLM QV 77.2 | DDC 615/.78—dc23
LC record available at https://lccn.loc.gov/2016026422
British Library Cataloguing in Publication Data
A CIP record is available from the British Library.

Contents

James L. Levenson, M.D.
Stephen J. Ferrando, M.D.

Part I
General Principles

James A. Owen, Ph.D.
Ericka L. Crouse, Pharm.D.

E. Cabrina Campbell, M.D.
Stanley N. Caroff, M.D.
Stephan C. Mann, M.D.
Robert M. Weinrieb, M.D.
Rosalind M. Berkowitz, M.D.
Kimberly N. Olson, CRNP

Part II
Psychopharmacology in Organ System Disorders and Specialty Areas

9 Central Nervous System Disorders 341

Adam P. Pendleton, M.D., M.B.A.
Jason P. Caplan, M.D.

10 Endocrine and Metabolic Disorders 389

Stephen J. Ferrando, M.D.
Sahil Munjal, M.D.
Jennifer Kraker, M.D., M.S.

Contributors

Margaret Altemus, M.D.
Associate Professor, Department of Psychiatry, Yale University School of Medicine, and VA Connecticut Health Care System, West Haven, Connecticut

Rosalind M. Berkowitz, M.D.
Private Practice, Hematology and Oncology, Moorestown, New Jersey

Philip A. Bialer, M.D.
Attending Psychiatrist, Memorial Sloan Kettering Cancer Center; Associate Professor of Clinical Psychiatry, Weill Cornell Medical College, New York, New York

Jozef Bledowski, M.D.
Assistant Professor of Psychiatry and Director, STAT/Crisis Stabilization Service, Virginia Commonwealth University Health System, Richmond, Virginia

E. Cabrina Campbell, M.D.
Director, Inpatient Psychiatry, Corporal Michael J. Crescenz Veterans Affairs Medical Center; Associate Professor of Psychiatry, Perelman School of Medicine at the University of Pennsylvania, Philadelphia, Pennsylvania

Jason P. Caplan, M.D.
Professor and Chair of Psychiatry, Creighton University School of Medicine–Phoenix Campus, Phoenix, Arizona

Stanley N. Caroff, M.D.
Emeritus Professor of Psychiatry, Perelman School of Medicine at the University of Pennsylvania, Philadelphia, Pennsylvania

Michael R. Clark, M.D., M.P.H., M.B.A.
Vice Chair, Clinical Affairs, and Director, Adolf Meyer Chronic Pain Treatment Programs, Department of Psychiatry and Behavioral Sciences, The Johns Hopkins Medical Institutions, Baltimore, Maryland

Catherine C. Crone, M.D.
Associate Professor of Psychiatry, George Washington University Medical Center, Washington, D.C.; Vice Chair, Department of Psychiatry, Inova Fairfax Hospital, Falls Church, Virginia; Clinical Professor of Psychiatry, Virginia Commonwealth University School of Medicine, Northern Virginia Branch, Fairfax, Virginia

Ericka L. Crouse, Pharm.D.
Clinical Pharmacy Specialist—Psychiatry; Clinical Associate Professor, Departments of Pharmacy and Psychiatry; Director, PGY2 Psychiatric Pharmacy Residency, Virginia Commonwealth University Medical Center, Richmond, Virginia

Catherine Daniels-Brady, M.D.
Assistant Clinical Professor, Department of Psychiatry and Behavioral Science, New York Medical College at Westchester Medical Center, Valhalla, New York

Andrea F. DiMartini, M.D.
Professor of Psychiatry and Professor of Surgery, Western Psychiatric Institute; Consultation Liaison to the Liver Transplant Program, Starzl Transplant Institute, University of Pittsburgh Medical Center, Pittsburgh, Pennsylvania

Stephen J. Ferrando, M.D.
Professor and Chairman, Department of Psychiatry, Westchester Medical Center Health Network, New York Medical College, Valhalla, New York

Marian Fireman, M.D.
Clinical Professor of Psychiatry, Oregon Health & Science University, Portland, Oregon

Madhulika A. Gupta, M.D., FRCPC
Professor, Department of Psychiatry, Schulich School of Medicine and Dentistry, University of Western Ontario, London, Ontario, Canada

J. Greg Hobelmann, M.D., M.P.H.
Chief Resident, Department of Psychiatry and Behavioral Sciences, The Johns Hopkins Medical Institutions, Baltimore, Maryland

Christopher P. Kogut, M.D.
Assistant Professor, Department of Psychiatry, Virginia Commonwealth University, Richmond, Virginia

Jennifer Kraker, M.D., M.S.
Private Practice in Psychiatry, New York, New York

Jeanne Lackamp, M.D.
Assistant Professor, Department of Psychiatry, and Director, Division of Psychiatry and Medicine, University Hospitals Case Medical Center, Cleveland, Ohio

James L. Levenson, M.D.
Rhona Arenstein Professor of Psychiatry and Professor of Medicine and Surgery and Vice-Chair of Psychiatry, Virginia Commonwealth University School of Medicine, Richmond, Virginia

Stephan C. Mann, M.D.
Lenape Valley Foundation, Doylestown, Pennsylvania

Michael Marcangelo, M.D.
Associate Professor, Department of Psychiatry and Behavioral Neuroscience, and Director of Medical Student Education in Psychiatry, Pritzker School of Medicine, University of Chicago, Chicago, Illinois

Sahil Munjal, M.D.
Resident in Psychiatry, New York Medical College, Valhalla, New York

Mallay Occhiogrosso, M.D.
Clinical Assistant Professor, Department of Psychiatry, Weill Cornell Medical College, New York, New York

Kimberly N. Olson, CRNP
PENN Rodebaugh Diabetes Center, Clinical Practices of the University of Pennsylvania, Philadelphia, Pennsylvania

James A. Owen, Ph.D. (deceased)
Associate Professor, Department of Psychiatry and Department of Pharmacology and Toxicology, Queen's University; Director of Psychopharmacology, Providence Care Mental Health Services, Kingston, Ontario, Canada

Adam P. Pendleton, M.D., M.B.A.
Chief Resident for Inpatient Services, Department of Psychiatry, Vanderbilt University School of Medicine, Nashville, Tennessee

Peter A. Shapiro, M.D.
Professor of Psychiatry at Columbia University Medical Center, Columbia University; Director, Fellowship Training Program in Psychosomatic Medicine; Associate Director, Consultation-Liaison Psychiatry Service, New York Presbyterian Hospital–Columbia University Medical Center, New York, New York

Yvette L. Smolin, M.D.
Director, Psychosomatic Medicine Service and Fellowship, Department of Psychiatry and Behavioral Science, New York Medical College at Westchester Medical Center, Valhalla, New York

Wendy Thompson, M.D.
Clinical Professor, Department of Family and Community Medicine, New York Medical College at Westchester Medical Center, Valhalla, New York

Robert M. Weinrieb, M.D.
Director, Psychosomatic Medicine and Psychosomatic Medicine Fellowship Program, and Associate Professor of Psychiatry, Perelman School of Medicine at the University of Pennsylvania, Philadelphia, Pennsylvania

Shirley Qiong Yan, Pharm.D., BCOP
Pediatric Hematology/Oncology Clinical Pharmacy Specialist, Department of Pharmacy, Memorial Sloan Kettering Cancer Center, New York, New York

Disclosure of Interests

The following contributors to this book have indicated a financial interest in or other affiliation with a commercial supporter, a manufacturer of a commercial product, a provider of a commercial service, a nongovernmental organization, and/or a government agency, as listed below:

E. Cabrina Campbell, M.D.   *Grant:* Sunovion.
Stanley N. Caroff, M.D.   *Research Grant:* Sunovion. *Consultant:* Auspex.

The following contributors to this book have no competing interests to report:

Rosalind M. Berkowitz, M.D.; Jozef Bledowski, M.D.; Catherine C. Crone, M.D.; Stephen J. Ferrando, M.D.; Marian Fireman, M.D.; Madhulika A. Gupta, M.D., FRCPC; James L. Levenson, M.D.; Stephan C. Mann, M.D.; Kimberly N. Olson, CRNP; Wendy L. Thompson, M.D; Robert M. Weinrieb, M.D.; Shirley Qiong Yan, Pharm.D., BCOP

Dedication

The editors would like to dedicate this edition of the manual to James Owen, Ph.D., our former coeditor and friend. Jim was diagnosed with a severe cardiomyopathy shortly after the publication of the first edition and passed away prematurely on November 7, 2013. As was always our experience of Jim, he dealt with his illness in a steadfast and calm manner. Jim was the consummate gentleman and scholar. He was instrumental not only in providing the highest-quality information on psychopharmacology but also in cementing and motivating our editorial team, always with energy and enthusiasm. The pleasure he took in the academic aspects of psychopharmacology was infectious, with a lasting impact on both of us, as was his dedication to the highest quality and safety of patient care. We have missed him greatly in the preparation of this edition of the manual, although his presence continues to be felt both in content and in spirit.

James L. Levenson, M.D.

Stephen J. Ferrando, M.D.

Acknowledgments

The editors would collectively like to acknowledge multiple individuals for their support, encouragement, and thoughtful input during the preparation of this book. We thank our original contributors, who have undertaken to update their original contributions, and welcome our newest authors for their high-quality contributions. We continue to appreciate the wisdom and dedication of Dr. Robert E. Hales, Editor-in-Chief of American Psychiatric Association (APA) Publishing, as well as John McDuffie and the editorial staff of APA Publishing, for their enthusiastic encouragement to produce a second edition.

Dr. Levenson would like to thank his wife and family for their support and his father, Milton Levenson, whose lifelong dedication to his profession has been an inspiration throughout his own.

Dr. Ferrando would like to thank his wife, Maria, and his children, Luke, Nicole, Marco, and David, for all of their support.

Introduction

James L. Levenson, M.D.
Stephen J. Ferrando, M.D.

The mission of this second edition is the very same as the first: to serve as a clinical manual and educational tool for specialist and nonspecialist clinicians for the psychopharmacological treatment of patients with medical illness. There was great interest in the first edition, with the first printing selling out in less than a year. We are pleased that many fellowship programs approved by the Accreditation Council for Graduate Medical Education have adopted this book as a core reference and text for teaching the principles and practice of prescribing psychotropic medication to psychiatrically and medically ill patients. Further, physicians in other specialties of medicine, including primary care specialties, have found the manual to be useful.

Since the publication of the first edition, the importance of the co-occurrence of psychiatric and medical illness has become even more evident. There is increasing recognition that patients with medical and psychiatric comorbidity have more functional impairment, disability days, emergency department use, rehospitalization, and other medical care costs than do those without such comorbidity (Druss and Reisinger Walker 2011). Government-based reform efforts, such as the Delivery System Reform Incentive Payment Program (New York State Department of Health 2016) in New York State, have begun to incentivize health care systems to develop new and innovative models of population-based care that integrate medical and psychiatric care in an effort to increase quality and prevention while decreasing use of expensive services such as emergency department visits and hospitalizations. In this context, a broader array of physician and nonphysician practitioners will be called on to prescribe psychiatric medications to individuals with medical illness, taking into account neuropsychiatric, metabolic, and other side effects as well as drug-drug and drug-disease interactions. Of further importance is the fact that outpatient practitioners will be called on to take care of sicker patients more than ever before, making issues of safe prescribing even more critical. It is our hope that this manual will continue to fill a key need for up-to-date and practical information.

How to Use This Manual

The organization of the second edition is the same as the first. We aim to provide clinically relevant information regarding psychopharmacology in patients who are medically ill, including pharmacokinetic and pharmacodynamic principles, drug-drug interactions, and organ system disease–specific issues. Chapters are authored and updated by experts in the field, with editorial input to maintain consistency of format and style.

The manual has two sections. Part I, "General Principles," provides fundamental background information for prescribing psychotropic drugs across medical disease states and is suggested reading prior to advancing to the disease-specific information in the second section. Part I includes discussion of pharmacodynamics and pharmacokinetics, principles of drug-drug interactions, major systemic adverse effects of psychotropic drugs, and alternative routes of psychotropic drug administration.

Part II, "Psychopharmacology in Organ System Disorders and Specialty Areas," includes chapters on psychopharmacological treatment in specific organ system diseases, such as renal and cardiovascular disease, as well as other relevant subspecialty areas, such as critical care, organ transplantation, pain, and substance use disorders. With some variation, chapters are structured to include the following elements: key differential diagnostic considerations, including adverse neuropsychiatric side effects of disease-specific medications; disease-specific pharmacokinetic principles in drug prescribing; review of evidence for psychotropic drug treatment of psychiatric disorders in the specific disease state or specialty area; disease-specific adverse psychotropic drug side effects; and interactions between psychotropic drugs and disease-specific drugs. Each chapter has tables that summarize information on adverse neuropsychiatric side effects of disease-specific medications, adverse disease-specific side effects of psychotropic drugs, and drug-drug interactions. Chapters are heavily referenced with source information should readers wish to expand their knowledge in a specific area. Finally, each chapter ends with a list of key summary points pertaining to psychotropic prescribing in the specific medical disease(s) or specialty area covered in the chapter.

With this structure, we hope that we have contributed a comprehensive yet practical guide for psychotropic prescribing for patients who are medically ill. We will consider this manual a success if it proves useful for a broad range of specialists, such as the psychosomatic medicine specialist caring for a delirious patient with cancer, the general psychiatrist in the community mental health clinic whose patient with schizophrenia develops liver disease in the setting of alcohol dependence and hepatitis C infection, and the general medical practitioner prescribing an antidepressant to a diabetic patient who recently had a myocardial infarction. We hope that this manual, beyond serving as a clinical guide, will also become a mainstay of curricula in general psychiatric residency programs, in psychosomatic medicine fellowships, and in nonpsychiatric residency training programs that seek to provide training in psychopharmacology for medically ill patients.

References

Druss BG, Reisinger Walker R: Mental Disorders and Medical Comorbidity. Research Synthesis Report No 21. Princeton, NJ, The Synthesis Project, Robert Wood Johnson Foundation, February 2011. Available at: www.integration.samhsa.gov/workforce/mental_disorders_and_medical_comorbidity.pdf. Accessed February 21, 2016.

New York State Department of Health: Delivery System Reform Incentive Payment (DSRIP) Program. Available at: www.health.ny.gov/health_care/medicaid/redesign/dsrip/. Accessed February 21, 2016.

PART I

General Principles

1

Pharmacokinetics, Pharmacodynamics, and Principles of Drug-Drug Interactions

James A. Owen, Ph.D.
Ericka L. Crouse, Pharm.D.

Psychotropic drugs are commonly employed in the management of patients who are medically ill. At least 35% of psychiatric consultations include recommendations for medication (Bronheim et al. 1998). The appropriate use of psychopharmacology in medically ill patients requires careful consideration of the underlying medical illness, potential alterations to pharmacokinetics, drug-drug interactions, and contraindications. In this chapter, we review drug action, drug pharmacokinetics, and drug interactions to provide

3

a basis for drug-drug and drug-disease interactions presented in later disease-specific chapters.

The effects of a drug—that is, the magnitude and duration of its therapeutic and adverse effects—are determined by the drug's pharmacodynamic and pharmacokinetic characteristics. *Pharmacodynamics* describes the effects of a drug on the body. Pharmacodynamic processes determine the relationship between drug concentration and response for both therapeutic and adverse effects. *Pharmacokinetics* describes what the body does to the drug. It characterizes the rate and extent of drug absorption, distribution, metabolism, and excretion. These pharmacokinetic processes determine the rate of drug delivery to and the drug's concentration at the sites of action. The relationship between pharmacokinetics and pharmacodynamics is diagrammed in Figure 1–1.

Pharmacodynamics

For most drugs, the pharmacological effect is the result of a complex chain of events, beginning with the interaction of drug with receptor. Pharmacodynamic response is further modified—enhanced or diminished—by disease states, aging, and other drugs. For example, the presence of Parkinson's disease increases the incidence of movement disorders induced by selective serotonin reuptake inhibitors. Pharmacodynamic disease-drug interactions are reviewed in the relevant chapters; pharmacodynamic drug-drug interactions are discussed later in this chapter in the subsection "Pharmacodynamic Drug Interactions."

A drug's spectrum of therapeutic and adverse effects is due to its interaction with multiple receptor sites. The effects produced depend on which receptor populations are occupied by the drug; some receptor populations are readily occupied at low drug concentrations, whereas other receptor sites require high drug levels for interaction. In this way, different responses are recruited in a stepwise manner with increasing drug concentration. As drug levels increase, each effect will reach a maximum as all active receptors responsible for that effect are occupied by the drug. Further increases in drug concentration cannot increase this response but may elicit other effects. Figure 1–2 illustrates three pharmacological effects produced by a drug in a concentration-dependent

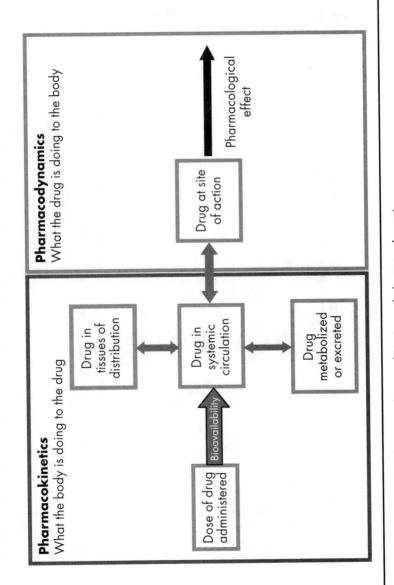

Figure 1–1.   Relationship between pharmacokinetics and pharmacodynamics.

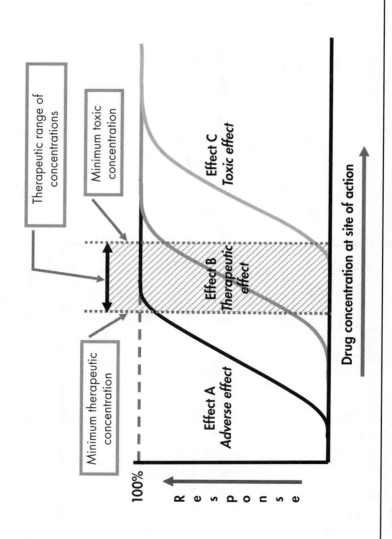

Figure 1–2.   Concentration-response relationship (see text for details).

manner. In this example, *Effect B* is the primary therapeutic effect, *Effect A* is a minor adverse effect, and *Effect C* is a significant toxic effect. Low drug concentrations recruit only Effect A; the patient experiences a nuisance side effect without any therapeutic gain. As drug concentration increases, Effect B is engaged, and Effect A is maximized. Clearly, for this drug, except in the rare situation where Effect B antagonizes Effect A (e.g., where the initial sedating effect of a drug is counteracted by stimulating effects recruited at a higher concentration), Effect A will always accompany a therapeutically effective dose because it is recruited at a lower concentration than that required for the therapeutic effect. Further increases in drug concentration improve the therapeutic effect until reaching its maximum, but these increases also introduce toxic Effect C.

Optimum therapy requires that drug concentrations be confined to a therapeutic range to maximize the therapeutic effect and minimize any adverse and/or toxic effects. Developing a dosage regimen to maintain drug levels within this therapeutic range requires consideration of pharmacokinetic processes.

Drug-receptor interactions produce effects on several timescales. Immediate effects are the result of a direct receptor interaction. Several psychoactive drugs, including benzodiazepines, have immediate therapeutic effects and therefore are useful on an acute or as-needed basis. However, many psychoactive drugs, such as antidepressant and antipsychotic agents, require chronic dosing over several weeks for a significant therapeutic response. These drugs appear to alter neuronal responsiveness by modifying slowly adapting cellular processes. Unfortunately, many adverse effects appear immediately—the result of a direct receptor interaction. Medication adherence may be eroded when adverse effects are experienced before therapeutic effects are realized. Table 1–1 lists strategies to maximize medication adherence.

Pharmacokinetics

Drug response, including the magnitude and duration of the drug's therapeutic and adverse effects, is significantly influenced by the drug's pharmacokinetics (absorption from administration sites, distribution throughout the body, and metabolism and excretion). Individual differences in constitutional

Table 1–1.   Strategies to maximize medication adherence

Provide patient education

Inform the patient about potential adverse effects, their speed of onset, and whether tolerance will develop over time.

Indicate the time for onset of the therapeutic effect. Many psychotropic drugs have a considerable delay (weeks) before the appearance of significant therapeutic effects yet give rise to adverse effects immediately. Patients not aware of this temporal disconnect between adverse and therapeutic effects may consider the medication a failure and discontinue the drug if only adverse effects and no therapeutic effects are initially experienced.

Select drugs with a convenient dosing schedule

Select drugs with once-daily dosing (i.e., those with a suitably long half-life or available in an extended-release formulation) to maximize adherence.

Consider the use of long-acting injectable formulations for antipsychotic agents. Depending on the agent, they may be dosed every 2 or 4 weeks. A new formulation of paliperidone palmitate is available as a once every 3 months injection. Adherence can be confirmed from administration records. However, the patient must have undergone a successful trial of the equivalent oral formulation to verify therapeutic response and tolerance to adverse effects and to establish the appropriate dose.

Minimize adverse effects

Select drugs with minimal pharmacokinetic interaction where possible (e.g., avoid cytochrome P450 inhibitors or inducers).

Gradually increase drug dosage to therapeutic levels over several days or weeks ("start low, go slow") so that patients experience minimal adverse effects while gradually developing tolerance.

Use the minimum effective dose.

Select a drug with an adverse-effect profile the patient can best tolerate. Drugs within a class may be similar therapeutically but differ in their adverse-effect profile. Patients may vary in their tolerance of a particular effect.

Reduce peak drug levels following absorption of oral medications. Many adverse effects are concentration dependent and are exacerbated as drug levels peak following oral dosing. Consider administering the drug with food or using divided doses or extended-release formulations to reduce and delay peak drug levels and diminish adverse effects.

Table 1–1.   Strategies to maximize medication
adherence *(continued)*

Minimize adverse effects *(continued)*

Schedule the dose so the side effect is less bothersome. If possible, prescribe activating
drugs in the morning and sedating drugs or those that cause gastrointestinal distress
in the evening.

Utilize therapeutic drug monitoring

Keep in mind that therapeutic drug monitoring is available for many psychotropic
drugs. This is valuable for monitoring adherence and ensuring that drug levels are
within the therapeutic range.

Check for patient adherence

Schedule office or telephone visits to discuss adherence and adverse effects for newly
prescribed drugs.

factors, compromised organ function, and disease states and the effects of
other drugs and food all contribute to the high variability in drug response observed across patients. Understanding the impact of these factors on a drug's
pharmacokinetics will aid in drug selection and dosage adjustment in a therapeutic environment complicated by polypharmacy and medical illness.

Absorption and Bioavailability

The speed of onset and, to a certain extent, the duration of the pharmacological effects of a drug are determined by the route of administration. *Bioavailability* of a drug formulation describes the rate and extent of drug delivery to
the systemic circulation from the formulation. Intravenous or intra-arterial
administration delivers 100% of the drug dose to the systemic circulation
(100% bioavailability) at a rate that can be controlled if necessary. For drugs
delivered by other routes, bioavailability is typically less than 100%, often
much less.

   Drug absorption is influenced by the characteristics of the absorption site
and the physiochemical properties of a drug. Specific site properties affecting
absorption include surface area, ambient pH, mucosal integrity and function,
and local blood flow, all of which may be altered by, for example, peptic ulcer
disease or inflammatory bowel disease and the drugs used to treat the disease.

Orally administered drugs face several pharmacokinetic barriers that limit drug delivery to the systemic circulation. Drugs must dissolve in gastric fluids to be absorbed, and drug dissolution in the stomach and gut may be incomplete (e.g., after gastric bypass surgery). Drugs may be acid labile and degrade in the acidic stomach environment, or they may be partially metabolized by gut flora. Some medications require food to enhance absorption. For example, the bioavailability of ziprasidone is enhanced almost twofold with food, and lurasidone exposure (area under the curve [AUC]) is doubled in the presence of food. Drugs absorbed through the gastrointestinal tract may be extensively altered by first-pass metabolism before entering the systemic circulation (see Figure 1–3). *First-pass metabolism* refers to the transport and metabolism of drugs from the gut lumen to the systemic circulation via the portal vein and liver. Drug passage from the gut lumen to the portal circulation may be limited by two processes: 1) a P-glycoprotein (P-gp) efflux transport pump, which serves to reduce the absorption of many compounds (some P-gp substrates are listed in the appendix to this chapter) by countertransporting them back into the intestinal lumen, and 2) metabolism within the gut wall by cytochrome P450 3A4 (CYP3A4) enzymes. Because P-gp is co-localized with and shares similar substrate affinity with CYP3A4, drug substrates of CYP3A4 typically have poor bioavailability. Bioavailability may be further decreased by hepatic extraction of drugs as they pass through the liver before gaining access to the systemic circulation. Sublingual and topical drug administration minimizes this first-pass effect, and rectal delivery, although often resulting in erratic absorption, may reduce first-pass effect by 50%.

Bioavailability can be markedly altered by disease states and drugs that alter gut and hepatic function. As with the CYP and uridine 5′-diphosphate glucuronosyltransferase (UGT) enzyme systems involved in drug metabolism, drugs can also inhibit or induce the P-gp transporter. Common P-gp inhibitors include paroxetine, sertraline, trifluoperazine, verapamil, and proton pump inhibitors. Because intestinal P-gps serve to block absorption in the gut, inhibition of these transporters can dramatically increase the bioavailability of poorly bioavailable drugs. For example, oral fentanyl absorption in humans is increased 2.7-fold when the drug is administered with quinidine, a known intestinal P-gp inhibitor (Kharasch et al. 2004). P-gp inhibitors are listed in the appendix to this chapter. For drugs administered chronically, the *extent* of drug absorption is the key factor in maintaining drug levels within the thera-

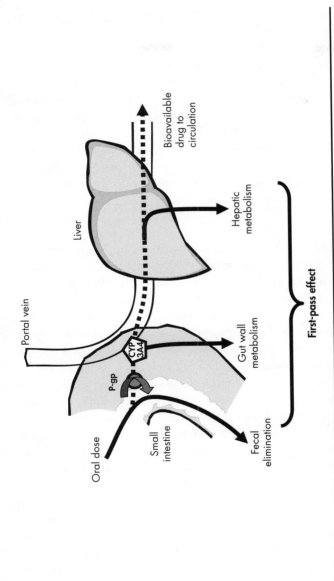

Figure 1–3.   First-pass metabolism of orally administered drugs.

Many drugs undergo a first-pass effect as they are absorbed from the intestinal lumen before they are delivered to the systemic circulation. The first-pass effect limits oral bioavailability through countertransport by P-glycoprotein (P-gp) back into the intestinal lumen and by gut wall (mainly cytochrome P450 3A4 [CYP3A4]) and hepatic metabolism.

peutic range. In situations where bioavailability may be significantly altered, parenteral administration of drugs may be preferable.

Drug formulation, drug interactions, gastric motility, and the characteristics of the absorptive surface all influence the *rate* of absorption, a key factor when rapid onset is desired. Oral medications are absorbed primarily in the small intestine because of its large surface area. Delayed gastric emptying or drug dissolution will slow absorption and therefore blunt the rise in drug levels following an oral dose. In this way, the occurrence of transient concentration-related adverse effects following an oral dose may be reduced by administering a drug with food, whereas the common practice of dissolving medications in juice may produce higher peak levels and exacerbate these transient adverse reactions.

Distribution

Following absorption into the systemic circulation, the drug is distributed throughout the body in accordance with its physiochemical properties and the extent of protein binding. *Volume of distribution* describes the relationship between the bioavailable dose and the plasma concentration. Lipophilic drugs, including most psychotropic medications, are sequestered into lipid compartments of the body. Because of their low plasma concentrations relative to dose, these drugs appear to have a large volume of distribution. In contrast, hydrophilic drugs (e.g., lithium, oxazepam, valproate), being confined mainly to the vascular volume and other aqueous compartments, have a high plasma concentration relative to dose, suggesting a small volume of distribution. Volume of distribution is often unpredictably altered by disease-related changes in organ and tissue perfusion or body composition. Edema (e.g., in congestive heart failure, cirrhosis, nephrotic syndrome) causes expansion of the extracellular fluid volume and may significantly increase the volume of distribution for hydrophilic drugs. Lipophilic drugs experience an increase in volume of distribution with obesity, which is sometimes iatrogenic (e.g., with corticosteroids or antipsychotics), and age-related increases in body fat. P-gp, a major component of the blood-brain barrier, may limit entry of drugs into the central nervous system (CNS). Many antiretroviral agents have limited CNS penetration because they are P-gp substrates (see the appendix to this chapter). Besides the P-gp efflux transport pump, the blood-brain barrier itself presents a physical barrier through tight junctions that limits the movement of agents into the CNS.

Most drugs bind, to varying degrees, to the plasma proteins albumin or α_1 acid glycoprotein. Acidic drugs (e.g., valproic acid, barbiturates) bind mostly to albumin, and more basic drugs (e.g., phenothiazines, tricyclic antidepressants, amphetamines, most benzodiazepines) bind to globulins.

Drug in plasma circulates in both bound and free (unbound to plasma proteins) forms. Generally, only free drug is pharmacologically active. The amount of drug bound to plasma proteins is dependent on the presence of other compounds that displace the drug from its protein binding sites (a protein-binding drug interaction) and the plasma concentration of albumin and α_1 acid glycoprotein. Medical conditions may alter plasma concentrations of albumin or α_1 acid glycoprotein (see Table 1–2) or increase the levels of endogenous displacing compounds. For example, uremia, chronic liver disease, and hypoalbuminemia may significantly increase the proportion of free drug relative to total drug in circulation (Dasgupta 2007).

Changes in drug protein binding, either disease induced or the result of a protein-binding drug interaction, were once considered a common cause of drug toxicity because therapeutic and toxic effects increase with increasing concentrations of free drug. These interactions are now seen as clinically significant only in very limited cases involving rapidly acting, highly protein bound (>80%), narrow therapeutic index drugs with high hepatic extraction (propafenone, verapamil, and intravenous lidocaine) (Benet and Hoener 2002; Rolan 1994). For drugs with low hepatic extraction, such as warfarin (Greenblatt and von Moltke 2005) and phenytoin (Tsanaclis et al. 1984) (see Table 1–3 later in this chapter), metabolism is not limited by hepatic blood flow, and a reduction in protein binding serves to increase the amount of free drug available for metabolism and excretion. Consequently, hypoalbuminemia or the presence of a displacing drug enhances drug elimination, which generally limits changes in circulating unbound drug levels to only a transient, and clinically insignificant, increase. (Many warfarin drug interactions previously thought to be protein-binding interactions are now recognized as pharmacodynamic and CYP2C9 and CYP1A2 metabolic interactions.) However, although free drug levels may remain unchanged, changes in protein binding will reduce plasma levels of total drug (free+bound fractions). Although of no consequence therapeutically, therapeutic drug monitoring procedures that measure total drug levels could mislead the clinician by suggesting lower, possibly subtherapeutic, levels and might prompt a dosage increase with possible toxic

Table 1–2.   Conditions that alter plasma levels of albumin and α_1 acid glycoprotein

Decrease albumin

Surgery

Burns

Trauma

Pregnancy

Alcoholism

Sepsis

Bacterial pneumonia

Acute pancreatitis

Uncontrolled diabetes

Hepatic cirrhosis

Nephritis, nephrotic syndrome, and renal failure

Malnutrition

Increase albumin

Hypothyroidism

Decrease α_1 acid glycoprotein

Pancreatic cancer

Pregnancy

Uremia

Hepatitis, cirrhosis

Cachexia

Increase α_1 acid glycoprotein

Stress response to disease states

Inflammatory bowel disease

Table 1–2.   Conditions that alter plasma levels of albumin and
α_1 acid glycoprotein *(continued)*

Increase α_1 acid glycoprotein *(continued)*

Acute myocardial infarction

Trauma

Epilepsy

Stroke

Surgery

Burns

Cancer (except pancreatic)

Acute nephritic syndrome, renal failure

Rheumatoid arthritis and systemic lupus erythematosus

Source.   Compiled in part from Dasgupta 2007; Israili and Dayton 2001.

effects. For this reason, in patients with uremia, chronic hepatic disease, hypo-albuminemia, or a protein-binding drug interaction, the use of therapeutic drug monitoring for dose adjustment requires caution; clinical response to the drug (e.g., international normalized ratio for warfarin), rather than laboratory-determined drug levels, should guide dosage (Nadkarni et al. 2011). Where therapeutic drug monitoring is employed, methods selective for unbound drug should be used, if available, for phenytoin, valproate, tacrolimus, cyclosporine, amitriptyline, haloperidol, and possibly carbamazepine (Dasgupta 2007). Clinically free phenytoin levels are the most widely utilized, especially in the elderly and malnourished populations.

Disease-related changes to a drug's protein binding have little effect on steady-state plasma concentrations of free drug as long as the disease does not affect metabolic and excretory processes (Benet and Hoener 2002). However, most diseases that affect protein binding also affect metabolism and excretion, with clinically significant consequences, especially for drugs with a low therapeutic index.

Drug Elimination: Metabolism and Excretion

The kidney is the primary organ of drug excretion, with fecal and pulmonary excretion being of less importance. Hydrophilic compounds are removed from the body through excretion into the aqueous environment of urine and feces. In contrast, lipophilic drugs, including most psychoactive medications, are readily reabsorbed through the intestinal mucosa (enterohepatic recirculation) and renal tubules, which limits their excretion. Because all drugs undergo glomerular filtration, lipophilic drugs would experience significant renal elimination were it not for renal resorption. Renal resorption, and thus the elimination, of several drugs, including amphetamines, meperidine, and methadone, can be significantly changed by altering urine pH (discussed later in the subsection "Pharmacokinetic Drug Interactions").

The general function of metabolism is to convert lipophilic molecules into more polar water-soluble compounds that can be readily excreted. Although biotransformation often results in less active or inactive metabolites, this is not always true. For some drugs, metabolites have pharmacological activities similar to, or even greater than, the parent compound, and thus contribute to the therapeutic effect. Indeed, some metabolites are separately marketed, including paliperidone (principal active metabolite of risperidone) and temazepam and oxazepam (both metabolites of diazepam). Some drugs are administered as prodrugs—inactive compounds requiring metabolic activation—including lisdexamfetamine (metabolized to dextroamphetamine), tramadol, codeine (metabolized to morphine), clopidogrel, fosphenytoin, primidone (metabolized to phenobarbital), and tamoxifen (metabolized to endoxifen). Other drug metabolites may have pharmacological effects considerably different from those of the parent drug and may cause unique toxicities (e.g., the meperidine metabolite normeperidine has proconvulsant activity, and carbamzepine 10, 11 epoxide is a toxic metabolite of carbamazepine).

Metabolism

Biotransformation occurs throughout the body, with the greatest activity in the liver and gut wall. Most psychotropic drugs are eliminated by hepatic metabolism followed by renal excretion. Hepatic biotransformation processes are of two types, identified as Phase I and Phase II reactions. Phase I reactions typically convert the parent drug into a more polar metabolite by introducing or unmasking a polar functional group in preparation for excretion or further metabolism by Phase II pathways. Phase II metabolism conjugates the drug or Phase I metabolite with an endogenous acid such as glucuronate, acetate, or sulfate. The resulting highly polar conjugates are usually inactive and are rapidly excreted in urine and feces (see Figure 1–4).

Phase I metabolism. Phase I reactions include oxidation, reduction, and hydrolysis. Most Phase I oxidation reactions are carried out by the hepatic CYP system, with a lesser contribution from the monoamine oxidases (MAOs). CYP enzymes exist in a variety of body tissues, including the gastrointestinal tract, liver, lung, and brain. Approximately 12 enzymes within three main families, CYP1, CYP2, and CYP3, are responsible for the majority of drug metabolism (Zanger and Schwab 2013). These families are divided into subfamilies identified by a capital letter (e.g., CYP3A). Subfamilies are further subdivided into isozymes on the basis of the homology between subfamily proteins. Isozymes are denoted by a number following the subfamily letter (e.g., CYP3A4, CYP2J2).

In humans, CYP1A2, CYP2C9, CYP2C19, CYP2D6, and CYP3A4 are the most important enzymes for drug metabolism. These enzymes exhibit substrate specificity. Functional deficiencies in one CYP enzyme will impact the metabolism of only those compounds that are substrates for that enzyme. Because some of these enzymes exist in a polymorphic form, a small percentage of the population, varying with ethnicity, has one or more CYP enzymes with significantly altered activity. For example, polymorphisms of the 2D6 gene give rise to populations with the capacity to metabolize CYP2D6 substrates extensively (normal condition), poorly (5%–14% of whites, ~1% of Asians), or ultraextensively (1%–3% of the population) (Zanger and Schwab 2013; Zanger et al. 2004). CYP enzyme activity can also be altered (inhibited or enhanced through induction) by environmental compounds or drugs, giving rise to many drug-drug interactions (discussed in the section "Drug-Drug Interactions" later in this chapter).

Phase II metabolism. Phase II conjugation reactions mainly involve enzymes belonging to the superfamily of UGTs. UGT enzymes are located hepatically (primarily centrizonal) (Debinski et al. 1995) and in the kidney and small intestine (Fisher et al. 2001). The UGT enzyme superfamily is classified

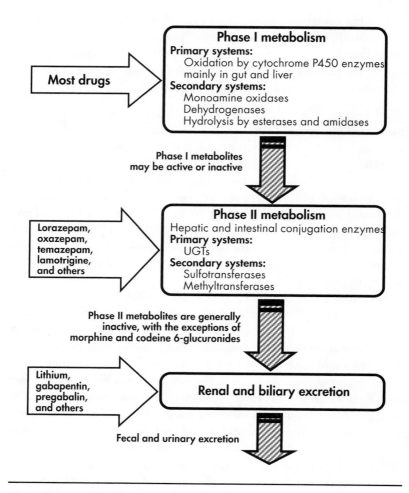

Figure 1–4.   General pathways of metabolism and excretion.
UGTs=uridine 5'-diphosphate glucuronosyltranferases.

in a manner similar to the CYP system. There are two clinically significant UGT subfamilies: 1A and 2B. As with the CYP system, there can be substrates, inhibitors, and inducers of UGT enzymes. For example, those benzodiazepines that are primarily metabolized by conjugation (oxazepam, lorazepam, and temazepam) are glucuronidated by UGT2B7. Valproic acid, tacrolimus, cyclosporine, and a number of nonsteroidal anti-inflammatory drugs (NSAIDs), including diclofenac, flurbiprofen, and naproxen, are competitive inhibitors of UGT2B7. Carbamazepine, phenytoin, rifampin (rifampicin), phenobarbital, and oral contraceptives are general inducers of UGTs (Kiang et al. 2005).

Drug interactions involving Phase II UGT-mediated conjugation reactions are increasingly becoming recognized. These interactions between critical substrates, inducers, and inhibitors follow the same rationale as for CYP interactions (discussed later in the section "Drug-Drug Interactions").

Effect of disease on metabolism.   Hepatic clearance of a drug may be limited by either the rate of delivery of the drug to the hepatic metabolizing enzymes (i.e., hepatic blood flow) or the intrinsic capacity of these enzymes to metabolize the substrate. Reduced hepatic blood flow impairs the clearance of drugs with high hepatic extraction (>6 mL/min/kg; flow-limited drugs) but has little effect on drugs with low hepatic extraction (<3 mL/min/kg; capacity-limited drugs), whose clearance depends primarily on hepatic function. Table 1–3 lists psychotropic drugs according to their degree of hepatic extraction.

Clinically significant decreases in hepatic blood flow, which occur in severe cardiovascular disease, chronic pulmonary disease, and severe cirrhosis, impair the clearance of flow-limited drugs. A reduction in the metabolic capacity of hepatic enzymes, as often accompanies congestive heart failure, renal disease, or hepatic disease, mainly impairs the clearance of capacity-limited drugs. Renal disease can significantly reduce hepatic Phase I and Phase II metabolism and increase intestinal bioavailability by reducing metabolic enzyme and P-gp gene expression (Pichette and Leblond 2003). Hepatic disease may preferentially affect anatomic regions of the liver, thereby altering specific metabolic processes. For example, oxidative metabolic reactions are more concentrated in the pericentral regions affected by acute viral hepatitis or alcoholic liver disease. Disease affecting the periportal regions, such as chronic hepatitis (in the absence of cirrhosis), may spare some hepatic oxidative func-

Table 1–3.   Systemic clearance of hepatically metabolized psychotropic drugs

High extraction ratio (clearance > 6 mL/min/kg)

Amitriptyline	Flumazenil	Olanzapine
Asenapine	Fluoxetine	Paroxetine
Bupropion	Fluvoxamine	Quetiapine
Buspirone	Haloperidol	Rizatriptan
Chlorpromazine	Hydrocodone	Ropinirole
Clozapine	Hydromorphone	Sertraline
Codeine	Imipramine	Sumatriptan
Desipramine	Meperidine	Venlafaxine
Diphenhydramine	Midazolam	Zaleplon
Doxepin	Morphine	Zolmitriptan
Fentanyl	Nortriptyline	

Intermediate extraction ratio (clearance 3–6 mL/min/kg)

Bromocriptine	Flunitrazepam	Risperidone
Citalopram	Flurazepam	Triazolam
Clonidine	Protriptyline	Zolpidem

Low extraction ratio (clearance < 3 mL/min/kg)

Alprazolam	Lamotrigine	Paliperidone
Carbamazepine	Levetiracetam	Phenytoin
Chlordiazepoxide	Lorazepam	Temazepam
Clonazepam	Methadone	Tiagabine
Clorazepate	Modafinil	Topiramate
Diazepam	Nitrazepam	Trazodone
Donepezil	Oxazepam	Valproate
Ethosuximide	Oxcarbazepine	Vilazodone

Source.   Compiled from Physicians' Desk Reference 2009; Thummel et al. 2005.

tion. Acute and chronic liver diseases generally do not impair glucuronide conjugation reactions.

Severity of hepatic disease may be calculated with the Child-Pugh score. Five markers are used to calculate the score: serum bilirubin, serum albumin, prothrombin time, presence of encephalopathy, and the presence of ascites, with 5–6 considered mild and 10–15 considered severe hepatic dysfunction. Some psychotropic medications with dosage adjustment recommendations based on Child-Pugh score include eszopiclone, venlafaxine, galantamine, and atomoxetine (Spray et al. 2007).

Excretion

The kidney's primary pharmacokinetic role is drug excretion. However, renal disease may also affect drug absorption, distribution, and metabolism. Reduced renal function, due to age or disease, results in the accumulation of drugs and active metabolites predominantly cleared by renal elimination. Dosage reduction may be required for narrow therapeutic index drugs that undergo significant renal excretion.

For renally eliminated drugs, a 24-hour urine creatinine clearance determination is a more useful indicator of renal function than is serum creatinine. In elderly patients, reduced creatinine production because of decreased muscle mass and possibly reduced exercise and dietary meat intake causes the calculation of creatinine clearance from serum creatinine levels by the commonly used Cockcroft-Gault formula to overestimate glomerular filtration rate (GFR; Sokoll et al. 1994). Creatinine clearance is sufficiently accurate for dosage adjustment of renally eliminated drugs in this population (Baracskay et al. 1997). In patients with severe liver disease, estimates of GFR must be interpreted with caution. The reduced muscle mass and impaired metabolism of creatine associated with severe liver disease often results in inaccurate estimates of GFR when based on either serum creatinine levels (Cockcroft-Gault method) or creatinine clearance (Papadakis and Arieff 1987).

Drug-Drug Interactions

Polypharmacy is common in medically ill patients and frequently leads to clinically significant pharmacokinetic or pharmacodynamic drug-drug interactions. Pharmacokinetic interactions alter drug absorption, distribution, metabolism, or excretion and change the drug concentration in tissues. These interactions are most likely to be clinically meaningful when the drug involved has a low therapeutic index. Pharmacodynamic interactions alter the pharmacological response to a drug. These interactions may be additive, synergistic, or antagonistic. Pharmacodynamic interactions may occur directly by altering drug binding to the receptor site or indirectly through other mechanisms.

Pharmacokinetic Drug Interactions

The majority of drugs are substrates for metabolism by one or more CYP enzymes. The most common pharmacokinetic drug-drug interaction involves changes in the CYP-mediated metabolism of the substrate drug by an interacting drug. The interacting drug may be either an inducer or an inhibitor of the specific CYP enzymes involved in the substrate drug's metabolism. In the presence of an *inducer*, CYP enzyme activity and the rate of metabolism of the substrate are increased. Enzyme induction is not an immediate process but occurs over several weeks. Induction will decrease the amount of circulating parent drug and may cause a decrease or loss of therapeutic efficacy. Consider a patient, stabilized on olanzapine (a CYP1A2 substrate), who begins to smoke (a CYP1A2 inducer). Smoking will increase olanzapine metabolism, and, unless drug dosage is suitably adjusted, olanzapine levels will fall and psychotic symptoms may worsen. If the interacting drug is a metabolic *inhibitor* (e.g., fluvoxamine, a potent CYP1A2 inhibitor), drug metabolism mediated through the inhibited CYP isozyme will be impaired. The resulting rise in substrate drug levels may increase drug toxicity and prolong the pharmacological effect. Although enzyme inhibition is a rapid process, substrate drug levels respond more slowly, taking five half-lives to restabilize.

Not all combinations of substrate drug and interacting drug will result in clinically significant drug-drug interactions. For a drug eliminated by several mechanisms, including multiple CYP enzymes or non-CYP routes (e.g., UGTs, renal elimination), the inhibition of a single CYP isozyme serves only to divert elimination to other pathways, with little change in overall elimination rate. For these interactions to be clinically relevant, a critical substrate drug must have a narrow therapeutic index and one primary CYP isozyme mediating its metabolism. For example, aripiprazole is metabolized primarily by the CYP3A4 and CYP2D6 isozymes. The addition of a potent CYP3A4 inhibitor, such as voriconazole or ritonavir, will inhibit aripiprazole's metabolism. Without a compensatory reduction in aripiprazole dose, aripiprazole levels will rise and toxicity may result. Aripiprazole, brexpiprazole, and iloperidone require dosage adjustment with concurrent CYP2D6 or CYP3A4 inhibitors. When prescribing in a polypharmacy environment, the clinician should minimize use of medications that significantly inhibit or induce CYP enzymes and should prefer those that are eliminated by multiple pathways and have a wide safety margin. Attention to drug interactions should occur in the polypharmacy environment of HIV because many protease inhibitors (e.g., ritonavir, darunavir) are potent CYP3A4 inducers. Drugs that are significant CYP isozyme inhibitors, inducers, and critical substrates are listed in the appendix to this chapter.

The abundance of clinically significant pharmacokinetic interactions involving monoamine oxidase inhibitors (MAOIs), especially inhibitors of MAO-A, has limited their therapeutic use. Many of these interactions involve foods containing high levels of tyramine, a pressor amine metabolized by gut MAO-A. Several drugs, including some sympathomimetics and triptan antimigraine medications, are also metabolized by MAO (Eadie 2001). Drugs and foods associated with MAO-related interactions are listed in the appendix to this chapter. Linezolid and tedizolid are antibiotics with MAOI properties and carry a potential risk for serotonin syndrome if combined with serotonergic antidepressants (Flanagan et al. 2013; Woytowish and Maynor 2013).

Although the role of Phase II UGT-mediated conjugation is being increasingly recognized in clinical pharmacology, surprisingly few clinically significant drug interactions are known to involve UGTs. The clinically significant interaction between valproate and lamotrigine is considered a consequence of valproate inhibition of lamotrigine glucuronidation. In patients taking lamotrigine, the addition of valproate resulted in a dose-dependent increase in systemic exposure (AUC) to lamotrigine ranging from 84% at a valproate dose of 200 mg/day to 160% at 1,000 mg/day. Correspondingly, lamotrigine half-life increased from pre-valproate values by 2.5-fold in the presence of 1,000 mg/day valproate (Morris et al. 2000). In human subjects, the addition of the UGT inducer rifampicin (600 mg/day) produced the opposite effect on lamotrigine levels. In comparison to the pre-rifampicin condition, lamotrigine half-life declined by more than 40%, accompanied by a similar decrease in AUC (Ebert et al. 2000). Another potentially UGT-mediated interaction is between carbapenem antibiotics and valproate. Case reports of seizures have been described when a carbapenem antibiotic was added in stable patients treated with valproate because of reduced plasma valproate levels (Mori et al. 2007).

Only those drugs dependent on UGT biotransformation for their elimination and having no other significant metabolic or excretory routes are candidates for clinically important UGT-based drug interactions. Most drugs undergoing conjugation by UGTs are also substrates for Phase I metabolism and other metabolic and excretory processes and therefore are little affected by the addition of UGT inhibitors or inducers. Some UGT substrates, inducers, and inhibitors are listed in the appendix to this chapter.

Metabolic drug interactions are most likely to occur in three situations: when an interacting drug (inhibitor or inducer) is added to an existing critical substrate drug, when an interacting drug is withdrawn from a dosing regimen containing a substrate drug, or when a substrate drug is added to an existing regimen containing an interacting drug. The addition of an interacting drug to a medication regimen containing a substrate drug at steady-state levels will dramatically alter substrate drug levels, possibly resulting in toxicity (addition of an inhibitor) or loss of therapeutic effect (addition of an inducer).

A much overlooked interaction involves the withdrawal of an interacting drug from a drug regimen that includes a critical substrate drug. Previously, the substrate drug dosage will have been titrated, in the presence of the interacting drug, to optimize therapeutic effect and minimize adverse effects. Withdrawal of an enzyme inhibitor will allow metabolism to return (increase) to normal levels. This increased metabolism of the substrate drug will lower its levels and decrease therapeutic effect. In contrast, removal of an enzyme inducer will result in an increase in substrate drug levels and drug toxicity as metabolism of the drug decreases to the normal rate over a period of several days to weeks. For example, discontinuation of carbamazepine can result in increased sedation with diazepam if the diazepam dose is not reduced.

The addition of a critical substrate drug to an established drug regimen containing an interacting drug can result in a clinically significant interaction if the substrate is dosed according to established guidelines. Dosing guidelines do not account for the presence of a metabolic inhibitor or inducer and thus may lead to substrate concentrations that are toxic or subtherapeutic, respectively.

Metabolic drug interactions can be minimized by avoiding drugs that are known critical substrates or potent inhibitors or inducers. Although avoiding these drugs is not always possible, adverse effects of these metabolic interactions can be reduced by identifying potentially problematic medications, making appropriate dosage adjustments, and monitoring drug levels (where possible).

An appreciation of drug interactions with the P-gp efflux transporter system is now emerging. P-gps influence the distribution and elimination of many clinically important hydrophobic compounds by transporting them out of the brain (P-gps are a major component of the blood-brain barrier), gonads, and other organs and into urine, bile, and the gut. Inhibition of P-gps can lead to drug toxicity due to dramatic increases in the oral bioavailability of poorly bioavailable drugs and to increased drug access to the CNS. Itraconazole, a CYP3A4 and P-gp inhibitor, has been demonstrated to increase the bioavailability of paroxetine, a P-gp substrate, in human subjects. The addition of itraconazole to an existing paroxetine regimen increased paroxetine AUC by 1.5-fold and peak blood levels by 1.3-fold in spite of only a 10% increase in half-life (Yasui-Furukori et al. 2007). Other psychotropic drugs transported by P-gp include opiates, risperidone, paliperidone, olanzapine, nortriptyline, imipramine, citalopram, escitalopram, and fluvoxamine (Moons et al. 2011). Some drug interactions with P-gp are listed in the appendix to this chapter. Rodent models are exploring the role of verapamil (a P-gp inhibitor) in increasing antidepressant (imipramine and escitalopram) levels in the brain to enhance antidepressant effects (Clarke et al. 2009; O'Brien et al. 2013).

Drug interactions that affect renal drug elimination are clinically significant only if the parent drug or its active metabolite undergoes appreciable renal excretion. By reducing renal blood flow, some drugs, including many NSAIDs, decrease GFR and impair renal elimination. This interaction is often responsible for lithium toxicity. Other drug interactions that increase lithium levels include thiazide diuretics, angiotensin-converting enzyme inhibitors, and angiotensin receptor blockers (Finley et al. 1995).

Changes in urine pH can modify the elimination of those compounds whose ratio of ionized to un-ionized forms is dramatically altered across the physiological range of urine pH (4.6–8.2) (i.e., the compound has a pK_a within this pH range). Common drugs that alkalinize urine include antacids and carbonic anhydrase inhibitor diuretics. Un-ionized forms of drugs undergo greater glomerular resorption, whereas ionized drug forms have less resorption and greater urinary excretion. For a basic drug, such as amphetamine, alkalinization of urine increases the un-ionized fraction, enhancing resorption and prolonging activity. Other basic drugs, such as amitriptyline, imipramine, meperidine, methadone (Nilsson et al. 1982), memantine (Freudenthaler et al. 1998), and flecainide, may be similarly affected (Cadwallader 1983).

Pharmacodynamic Drug Interactions

Pharmacodynamic interactions occur when drugs with similar or opposing effects are combined. The nature of the interaction relates to the addition or antagonism of the pharmacological and toxic effects of each drug. Generally, pharmacodynamic interactions are most apparent in individuals who have compromised physiological function, such as cardiovascular disease, or who are elderly.

For example, drugs with anticholinergic activity cause a degree of cognitive impairment, an effect that is exacerbated when several anticholinergic agents are combined (Tune et al. 1992). Unfortunately, anticholinergic activity is an often unrecognized property of many common drugs, such as diphenhydramine, loperamide, olanzapine, or paroxetine (for a listing, see American Geriatrics Society 2015 Beers Criteria Update Expert Panel 2015; Chew et al. 2008; Durán et al. 2013; Owen 2011; Rudolph et al. 2008). This additive interaction is most disruptive in patients with cognitive impairment, such as those who are elderly or who have Alzheimer's disease, and forms the basis for many cases of delirium. Often, additive pharmacodynamic interactions are employed therapeutically to enhance a drug response—this is the use of adjunctive medications. Antagonistic pharmacodynamic interactions are sometimes used deliberately to diminish a particular adverse effect. In the treatment of chronic pain syndromes, psychostimulants, such as amphetamine or methylphenidate, may be combined with morphine or other opiates to reduce opiate sedation (Dalal and Melzack 1998). Unintentional antagonistic interactions may be countertherapeutic, as with the erosion of asthma control in a patient who has successfully employed a β agonist inhaler and is recently prescribed a β-blocker or the negation of any cognitive benefit from a cholinesterase inhibitor when taken with an anticholinergic drug such as diphenhydramine or oxybutynin. Knowledge of a drug's therapeutic and adverse effects is essential to avoid unwanted pharmacodynamic drug interactions, such as additive or synergistic toxicities, or countertherapeutic effects.

Drug Interactions of Psychotropic Agents

Pharmacodynamic interactions between psychoactive drugs and drugs used to treat medical disorders are common and are discussed in the respective medical disorder chapters. Psychotropic drugs frequently contribute to or precipitate pharmacodynamic interactions. Excessive sedation or delirium frequently results from the combination of psychotropic drugs that have sedating properties. Psychotropic polypharmacy can also precipitate severe adverse reactions, such as serotonin syndrome or cardiac arrhythmias due to prolonged QT interval (see Chapter 2, "Severe Drug Reactions").

Any psychotropic drug can be the recipient of a pharmacokinetic interaction, but only a few psychotropic drugs commonly precipitate a pharmacokinetic interaction. Fluoxetine, paroxetine, fluvoxamine, duloxetine, bupropion, modafinil, armodafinil, and atomoxetine significantly inhibit one or more CYP isozymes. The MAOIs block metabolism of some sympathomimetics and several triptan antimigraine medications. The mood stabilizer anticonvulsants carbamazepine and valproate induce one or more CYP isozymes (see the appendix to this chapter). Preference should be given to psychotropic medications with little ability to precipitate a pharmacokinetic interaction (see Table 1–4), especially when used in a polypharmacy situation. However, even though many psychotropic agents do not precipitate pharmacokinetic interactions, they can still be the subject of a pharmacokinetic interaction. For example, neither ziprasidone nor aripiprazole affects the pharmacokinetics of other drugs, but carbamazepine reduces the AUC of ziprasidone by 35% and aripiprazole by 70%.

Table 1–4.   Psychotropic drugs that cause few pharmacokinetic interactions

Antidepressants

SSRIs/SNRIs

　　Citalopram

　　Desvenlafaxine

　　Escitalopram

　　Levomilnacipran

　　Sertraline (CYP2D6 inhibition at >200 mg/day)

　　Venlafaxine

TCAs

　　Amitriptyline

　　Clomipramine (slight CYP2D6 inhibition)

　　Desipramine (slight CYP2D6 inhibition)

　　Doxepin

　　Imipramine

　　Maprotiline

　　Nortriptyline

　　Protriptyline

　　Trimipramine

Mixed serotonin agents

　　Trazodone

　　Vilazodone

　　Vortioxetine

Novel action agents

　　Amoxapine

　　Mirtazapine

Table 1–4.   Psychotropic drugs that cause few pharmacokinetic
interactions *(continued)*

Antipsychotics

All antipsychotics

Agents for drug-induced extrapyramidal symptoms

Benztropine

Biperiden

Ethopropazine

Trihexyphenidyl

Anxiolytics/sedative-hypnotics

All benzodiazepines

Nonbenzodiazepines

  Buspirone

  Eszopiclone

  Zaleplon

  Zolpidem

  Zopiclone

Cognitive enhancers

Donepezil

Galantamine

Memantine

Rivastigmine

Opiate analgesics

All opiate analgesics

Psychostimulants

Amphetamine

Dextroamphetamine

Table 1–4.   Psychotropic drugs that cause few pharmacokinetic interactions *(continued)*

Psychostimulants *(continued)*

Lisdexamfetamine

Methamphetamine

Methylphenidate

Note.   CYP2D6 = cytochrome P450 2D6 isoenzyme; SNRIs = serotonin-norepinephrine reuptake inhibitors; SSRIs = selective serotonin reuptake inhibitors; TCAs = tricyclic antidepressants.

Key Clinical Points

- Maintaining drug levels within the therapeutic range maximizes beneficial effects and minimizes adverse effects. Drug pharmacokinetics must be considered when developing a dosage regimen to achieve drug levels within this therapeutic range.
- When prescribing in a polypharmacy environment, it is best to minimize use of medications that significantly inhibit or induce cytochrome P450 enzymes and to prefer those eliminated by multiple pathways and with a wide safety margin.
- Over-the-counter drugs, herbal and complementary medicines, and certain foods can all affect drug pharmacokinetics.
- For a drug administered on an acute basis, the magnitude of the therapeutic effect is a function of peak drug levels, which are determined mainly by dose and the rate of drug absorption.
- For a drug administered chronically, the therapeutic effect is a function of the extent of absorption, not the speed of absorption. Rapid absorption is likely to cause transient, concentration-dependent adverse effects.
- Therapeutic drug monitoring should employ methods selective for free (unbound) drug.

References

American Geriatrics Society 2015 Beers Criteria Update Expert Panel: American Geriatrics Society 2015 updated Beers criteria for potentially inappropriate medication use in older adults. J Am Geriatr Soc 63(11):2227–2246, 2015 26446832

Armstrong SC, Cozza KL: Triptans. Psychosomatics 43(6):502–504, 2002 12444236

Balayssac D, Authier N, Cayre A, Coudore F: Does inhibition of P-glycoprotein lead to drug-drug interactions? Toxicol Lett 156(3):319–329, 2005 15763631

Baracskay D, Jarjoura D, Cugino A, et al: Geriatric renal function: estimating glomerular filtration in an ambulatory elderly population. Clin Nephrol 47(4):222–228, 1997 9128788

Benet LZ, Hoener BA: Changes in plasma protein binding have little clinical relevance. Clin Pharmacol Ther 71(3):115–121, 2002 11907485

Bristol-Myers Squibb (Otsuka): Abilify (aripiprazole) prescribing information, updated December 2014. Available at: http://www.abilify.com/. Accessed April 11, 2016.

Bronheim HE, Fulop G, Kunkel EJ, et al; Academy of Psychosomatic Medicine: The Academy of Psychosomatic Medicine practice guidelines for psychiatric consultation in the general medical setting. Psychosomatics 39(4):S8–S30, 1998 9691717

Cadwallader DE: Biopharmaceutics and Drug Interactions. New York, Raven, 1983

Chew ML, Mulsant BH, Pollock BG, et al: Anticholinergic activity of 107 medications commonly used by older adults. J Am Geriatr Soc 56(7):1333–1341, 2008 18510583

Clarke G, O'Mahony SM, Cryan JF, Dinan TG: Verapamil in treatment resistant depression: a role for the P-glycoprotein transporter? Hum Psychopharmacol 24(3):217–223, 2009 19212940

Cozza KL, Armstrong SC, Oesterheld JR: Concise Guide to Drug Interaction Principles for Medical Practice: Cytochrome P450s, UGTs, P-Glycoproteins. Washington, DC, American Psychiatric Publishing, 2003

Dalal S, Melzack R: Potentiation of opioid analgesia by psychostimulant drugs: a review. J Pain Symptom Manage 16(4):245–253, 1998 9803052

Dasgupta A: Usefulness of monitoring free (unbound) concentrations of therapeutic drugs in patient management. Clin Chim Acta 377(1–2):1–13, 2007 17026974

Debinski HS, Lee CS, Danks JA, et al: Localization of uridine 5'-diphosphate-glucuronosyltransferase in human liver injury. Gastroenterology 108(5):1464–1469, 1995 7729639

DeVane CL, Nemeroff CB: 2002 Guide to psychotropic drug interactions. Prim psychiatry 9:28–57, 2002

Durán CE, Azermai M, Vander Stichele RH: Systematic review of anticholinergic risk scales in older adults. Eur J Clin Pharmacol 69(7):1485–1496, 2013 23529548

Eadie MJ: Clinically significant drug interactions with agents specific for migraine attacks. CNS Drugs 15(2):105–118, 2001 11460889

Ebert U, Thong NQ, Oertel R, Kirch W: Effects of rifampicin and cimetidine on pharmacokinetics and pharmacodynamics of lamotrigine in healthy subjects. Eur J Clin Pharmacol 56(4):299–304, 2000 10954343

Eli Lilly: Strattera (atomoxetine) prescribing information, updated April 6, 2015. Available at: http://pi.lilly.com/us/strattera-pi.pdf. Accessed April 11, 2016.

Finley PR, Warner MD, Peabody CA: Clinical relevance of drug interactions with lithium. Clin Pharmacokinet 29(3):172–191, 1995 8521679

Fisher MB, Paine MF, Strelevitz TJ, Wrighton SA: The role of hepatic and extrahepatic UDP-glucuronosyltransferases in human drug metabolism. Drug Metab Rev 33(3–4):273–297, 2001 11768770

Flanagan S, Bartizal K, Minassian SL, et al: In vitro, in vivo, and clinical studies of tedizolid to assess the potential for peripheral or central monoamine oxidase interactions. Antimicrob Agents Chemother 57(7):3060–3066, 2013 23612197

Freudenthaler S, Meineke I, Schreeb KH, et al: Influence of urine pH and urinary flow on the renal excretion of memantine. Br J Clin Pharmacol 46(6):541–546, 1998 9862242

Gardner DM, Shulman KI, Walker SE, Tailor SA: The making of a user friendly MAOI diet. J Clin Psychiatry 57(3):99–104, 1996 8617704

Gillman PK: Monoamine oxidase inhibitors, opioid analgesics and serotonin toxicity. Br J Anaesth 95(4):434–441, 2005 16051647

Greenblatt DJ, von Moltke LL: Interaction of warfarin with drugs, natural substances, and foods. J Clin Pharmacol 45(2):127–132, 2005 15647404

Guédon-Moreau L, Ducrocq D, Duc MF, et al: Absolute contraindications in relation to potential drug interactions in outpatient prescriptions: analysis of the first five million prescriptions in 1999. Eur J Clin Pharmacol 59(8–9):689–695, 2003 14557905

Israili ZH, Dayton PG: Human alpha-1-glycoprotein and its interactions with drugs. Drug Metab Rev 33(2):161–235, 2001 11495502

Kharasch ED, Hoffer C, Altuntas TG, Whittington D: Quinidine as a probe for the role of p-glycoprotein in the intestinal absorption and clinical effects of fentanyl. J Clin Pharmacol 44(3):224–233, 2004 14973303

Kiang TK, Ensom MH, Chang TK: UDP-glucuronosyltransferases and clinical drug-drug interactions. Pharmacol Ther 106(1):97–132, 2005 15781124

Lexicomp Inc: Lexicomp Online. Hudson, OH, Lexi-Comp Inc, 2015. Available at: http://online.lexi.com/lco/action/home. Accessed April 11, 2016.

McEvoy G (ed): American Hospital Formulary Service (AHFS) Drug Information 2015. Bethesda, MD, American Society of Health-System Pharmacists, 2015

Michalets EL: Update: clinically significant cytochrome P-450 drug interactions. Pharmacotherapy 18(1):84–112, 1998 9469685

Moons T, de Roo M, Claes S, Dom G: Relationship between P-glycoprotein and second-generation antipsychotics. Pharmacogenomics 12(8):1193–1211, 2011 21843066

Mori H, Takahashi K, Mizutani T: Interaction between valproic acid and carbapenem antibiotics. Drug Metab Rev 39(4):647–657, 2007 18058328

Morris RG, Black AB, Lam E, Westley IS: Clinical study of lamotrigine and valproic acid in patients with epilepsy: using a drug interaction to advantage? Ther Drug Monit 22(6):656–660, 2000 11128232

Nadkarni A, Oldham M, Howard M, et al: Detrimental effects of divalproex on warfarin therapy following mechanical valve replacement. J Card Surg 26(5):492–494, 2011 21859435

Nilsson MI, Widerlöv E, Meresaar U, Anggård E: Effect of urinary pH on the disposition of methadone in man. Eur J Clin Pharmacol 22(4):337–342, 1982 6286317

O'Brien FE, O'Connor RM, Clarke G, et al: P-glycoprotein inhibition increases the brain distribution and antidepressant-like activity of escitalopram in rodents. Neuropsychopharmacology 38(11):2209–2219, 2013 23670590

Owen JA: Psychopharmacology, in The American Psychiatric Publishing Textbook of Psychosomatic Medicine: Psychiatric Care of the Medically Ill, 2nd Edition. Edited by Levenson JL. Arlington, VA, American Psychiatric Publishing, 2011, pp 957–1019

Pal D, Mitra AK: MDR- and CYP3A4-mediated drug-drug interactions. J Neuroimmune Pharmacol 1(3):323–339, 2006 18040809

Papadakis MA, Arieff AI: Unpredictability of clinical evaluation of renal function in cirrhosis: prospective study. Am J Med 82(5):945–952, 1987 3578363

Physicians' Desk Reference 2009, 63rd Edition. Montvale, NJ, Thomson Reuters, 2009

Pichette V, Leblond FA: Drug metabolism in chronic renal failure. Curr Drug Metab 4(2):91–103, 2003 12678690

Procyshyn RM, Bezchlibnyk-Butler KZ, Jeffries JJ: Clinical Handbook of Psychotropic Drugs, 21st Revised Edition. Ashland, OH, Hogrefe, 2015

Repchinsky C (ed): CPS 2008: Compendium of Pharmaceuticals and Specialties: The Canadian Drug Reference for Health Professionals. Ottawa, ON, Canadian Pharmacists Association, 2008

Rolan PE: Plasma protein binding displacement interactions—why are they still regarded as clinically important? Br J Clin Pharmacol 37(2):125–128, 1994 8186058

Rudolph JL, Salow MJ, Angelini MC, McGlinchey RE: The Anticholinergic Risk Scale and anticholinergic adverse effects in older persons. Arch Intern Med 168(5):508–513, 2008 18332297

Sokoll LJ, Russell RM, Sadowski JA, Morrow FD: Establishment of creatinine clearance reference values for older women. Clin Chem 40(12):2276–2281, 1994 7988015

Spray JW, Willett K, Chase D, et al: Dosage adjustment for hepatic dysfunction based on Child-Pugh scores. Am J Health Syst Pharm 64(7):690–693, 692–693, 2007 17384352

Thummel KE, Shen DD, Isoherranen N, et al: Appendix II, Design and optimization of dosage regimens: pharmacokinetic data, in Goodman and Gilman's The Pharmacological Basis of Therapeutics, 11th Edition. Edited by Brunton LL, Lazo JS, Parker KL. New York, McGraw-Hill, 2005, pp 1787–1888

Tsanaclis LM, Allen J, Perucca E, et al: Effect of valproate on free plasma phenytoin concentrations. Br J Clin Pharmacol 18(1):17–20, 1984 6430316

Tune L, Carr S, Hoag E, Cooper T: Anticholinergic effects of drugs commonly prescribed for the elderly: potential means for assessing risk of delirium. Am J Psychiatry 149(10):1393–1394, 1992 1530077

USP DI Editorial Board (ed): United States Pharmacopeia Dispensing Information, Volume 1: Drug Information for the Health Care Professional, 27th Edition. Greenwood Village, CO, Thomson Micromedex, 2007

Woytowish MR, Maynor LM: Clinical relevance of linezolid-associated serotonin toxicity. Ann Pharmacother 47(3):388–397, 2013 23424229

Yasui-Furukori N, Saito M, Niioka T, et al: Effect of itraconazole on pharmacokinetics of paroxetine: the role of gut transporters. Ther Drug Monit 29(1):45–48, 2007 17304149

Zanger UM, Schwab M: Cytochrome P450 enzymes in drug metabolism: regulation of gene expression, enzyme activities, and impact of genetic variation. Pharmacol Ther 138(1):103–141, 2013 23333322

Zanger UM, Raimundo S, Eichelbaum M: Cytochrome P450 2D6: overview and update on pharmacology, genetics, biochemistry. Naunyn Schmiedebergs Arch Pharmacol 369(1):23–37, 2004 14618296

Appendix

Drugs With Clinically Significant Pharmacokinetic Interactions

Drug	Cytochrome P450 isozyme						
	1A2	2C[a]	2D6	3A4	MAO-A	UGT	P-gp
ACE inhibitor							
Captopril							X
Antianginal							
Ranolazine				S, X			S, X
Antiarrhythmics							
Amiodarone	X	S, X	X	S, X			X
Disopyramide				S			
Flecainide			S				
Lidocaine	S, X			S			X
Mexiletine	X		S				
Propafenone	X		S, X	S		S	X
Quinidine			X	S			S, X
Anticoagulants and antiplatelet agents							
Apixaban				S			S
Clopidogrel		S					
Dabigatran							S
Rivaroxaban				S			S
R-warfarin	S	S		S			
S-warfarin		S					
Ticagrelor				S			
Ticlopidine		X					
Anticonvulsants and mood stabilizers							
Carbamazepine	I	I		S, I		S, I	S
Ethosuximide				S, I			
Felbamate							S
Lamotrigine						S	S
Phenytoin	I	S, I		I		I	S
Tiagabine		S	S	S			
Valproate		I				S, X	

Drug	Cytochrome P450 isozyme						
	1A2	2C[a]	2D6	3A4	MAO-A	UGT	P-gp
Antidepressants							
Amitriptyline	S	S	S	S			S, X
Bupropion			X	S			
Citalopram		S					
Clomipramine	S	S	S, X	S			
Desipramine			S, X				X
Desvenlafaxine						S	
Doxepin			S				
Duloxetine	S		S, X				
Escitalopram		S					S
Fluoxetine	X	X	S, X	S, X			
Fluvoxamine	S, X	X		X			S
Gepirone				S			
Imipramine	S	S	S	S			S, X
Levomilnacipran				S			
Maprotiline			S				X
Milnacipran							
Mirtazapine			S	S			
Moclobemide		S	X		X		
Nefazodone				S, X			
Nortriptyline			S				S
Paroxetine			S, X				S, X
Phenelzine					X		
Sertraline							X
Tranylcypromine		X			X		
Trazodone			S	S			I
Trimipramine			S				
Venlafaxine			S	S			S
Vilazodone				S			
Vortioxetine			S	S			
Antidiarrheal agent							
Loperamide							S

| Drug | Cytochrome P450 isozyme | | | | | UGT | P-gp |
	1A2	2C[a]	2D6	3A4	MAO-A		
Antiemetic							
Ondansetron							S
Antihyperlipidemics							
Atorvastatin				S			X
Fenofibrate							X
Fluvastatin		X		S			
Gemfibrozil		X					
Lovastatin		X		S			S, X
Pravastatin				S			
Simvastatin		X		S			X
Antihyponatremic							
Conivaptan				S, X			X
Antimicrobials							
Chloramphenicol		X					
Ciprofloxacin	X			X			S
Clarithromycin	X			S, X			X
Co-trimoxazole		X					
Enoxacin	X						S
Erythromycin	X			S, X			S, X
Fluconazole		X		X			
Grepafloxacin							S
Griseofulvin	I						
Isoniazid	X			I	X		
Itraconazole				S, X			S, X
Ketoconazole	X			S, X			X
Levofloxacin	X						
Linezolid					X		
Metronidazole				X			
Miconazole		S, X		S, X			
Nafcillin				S, I			
Norfloxacin	X			X			
Ofloxacin	X						X
Posaconazole				X		S	S

Drug	Cytochrome P450 isozyme				MAO-A	UGT	P-gp
	1A2	2C[a]	2D6	3A4			
Antimicrobials *(continued)*							
Rifabutin				I			
Rifampin (rifampicin)	I	I		S, I		I	S, I
Roxithromycin				X			
Sulfaphenazole		X					
Sulfonamides		X					
Tedizolid					X		
Troleandomycin	X			S, X			
Valinomycin							S
Antimigraine							
Almotriptan				S	S		
Eletriptan	S			S			S
Ergotamine				S			
Frovatriptan	S						
Rizatriptan					S		
Sumatriptan					S		
Zolmitriptan	S				S		
Antineoplastic agents							
Dactinomycin							S, X
Dasatinib				S, X			
Docetaxel				S			S
Doxorubicin							S, X
Etoposide				S			S
Gefitinib				S			
Ifosfamide				S			
Imatinib			X	S, X			S
Irinotecan				S		S	S
Lapatinib				S, X			S, X
Methotrexate							S
Nilotinib		X	X	S, X		X	S, X
Paclitaxel		S		S			S

Drug	Cytochrome P450 isozyme				MAO-A	UGT	P-gp
	1A2	2C[a]	2D6	3A4			
Antineoplastic agents *(continued)*							
Procarbazine					X		
Sorafenib		X		S		S, X	
Sunitinib				S			
Tamoxifen			S	S			S, X
Tegafur (ftorafur)	S, I			I			
Teniposide				S			S
Topotecan							S
Vinblastine				S			S, X
Vincristine				S			S
Vinorelbine				S			S
Antiparkinsonian agents							
Rasagiline	S						
Selegiline					X		
Antipsychotics							
Aripiprazole			S	S			S
Asenapine	S					S	
Brexpiprazole			S	S			
Cariprazine			S	S			
Chlorpromazine	S		S				X
Clozapine	S		S	S			
Fluphenazine			S				X
Haloperidol	S		S, X				X
Iloperidone			S	S			
Lurasidone				S			
Molindone			S				
Olanzapine	S		S			S	S
Perphenazine			S				
Pimavanserin				S			
Pimozide				S			X
Quetiapine				S			S
Risperidone			S				S, X
Thioridazine	S	S	S				

Drug	Cytochrome P450 isozyme				MAO-A	UGT	P-gp
	1A2	2C[a]	2D6	3A4			
Antipsychotics *(continued)*							
Trifluoperazine							X
Ziprasidone				S			
Antiretroviral agents							
Amprenavir				S			S, I
Atazanavir		X		S, X		X	X
Cobicistat				S, X			
Darunavir				S, X			
Delavirdine		X		S, X			
Efavirenz		X		S, X			
Indinavir				S, X			S
Lopinavir				S			S
Maraviroc				S			S
Nelfinavir				S, X			S, X
Nevirapine				S, I			
Raltegravir						S	
Ritonavir	I	X	X	S, X			S, X
Saquinavir				S, X			S, X
Tipranavir/ritonavir			X	S, X			S, I
Zidovudine						S	
Anxiolytics and sedative-hypnotics							
Alprazolam				S			
Bromazepam				S			
Buspirone				S			
Clonazepam				S			
Diazepam		S		S			
Hexobarbital		S					
Lorazepam						S	
Midazolam				S			X
Oxazepam						S	
Phenobarbital	I	I		I			
Ramelteon	S						

Drug	Cytochrome P450 isozyme				MAO-A	UGT	P-gp
	1A2	2C[a]	2D6	3A4			
Anxiolytics and sedative-hypnotics *(continued)*							
Suvorexant				S			
Tasimelteon	S						
Temazepam						S	
Triazolam				S			
β-Blockers							
Alprenolol			S				
Bisoprolol			S				
Bufuralol			S				
Labetalol			S				
Metoprolol			S				
Pindolol			S				
Propranolol	S	S	S, X				X
Talinolol							S, X
Timolol		S	S				
Bronchodilator							
Theophylline	S			S			
Calcium channel blockers							
Amlodipine				S			
Diltiazem				S, X			S, X
Felodipine				S			X
Isradipine				S			
Nicardipine				S			X
Nifedipine				S			
Nimodipine				S			
Nisoldipine				S			
Verapamil	S			S			S, X
Cardiac glycoside							
Digoxin							S
Cognitive enhancer							
Tacrine	S						
Gastrointestinal motility modifier							
Domperidone							S

Drug	Cytochrome P450 isozyme					UGT	P-gp
	1A2	2C[a]	2D6	3A4	MAO-A		
Gout therapy							
Colchicine							S, X
Probenecid						X	
Sulfinpyrazone		X					
Histamine H$_2$-receptor antagonists							
Cimetidine	X	X	X	X			S
Ranitidine						X	S
Immunosuppressive agents							
Cyclosporine				S, X			S, X
Sirolimus				S			
Tacrolimus				S			S
Muscle relaxant							
Cyclobenzaprine	S		S	S			
Nonsteroidal anti-inflammatory drugs and analgesic agents							
Acetaminophen						S	
Diclofenac		X					X
Flurbiprofen		X					X
Naproxen							X
Phenylbutazone		S, X					
Opiate analgesics							
Alfentanil				S			
Codeine			S	S		S	
Fentanyl				S			X
Hydrocodone			S				
Meperidine			S				
Methadone			S	S			X
Morphine						S	S
Oxycodone			S				
Tramadol			S				
Oral hypoglycemics							
Chlorpropamide		S					
Glimepiride		S					

Drug	Cytochrome P450 isozyme						
	1A2	2C[a]	2D6	3A4	MAO-A	UGT	P-gp
Oral hypoglycemics *(continued)*							
Glipizide		S					
Glyburide		S					
Pioglitazone		S					
Tolbutamide		S, X					
Proton pump inhibitors							
Esomeprazole							X
Lansoprazole	I	S					S, X
Omeprazole	I	S, X		S			S, X
Pantoprazole							S, X
Psychostimulants							
Armodafinil	I	X		S, I			
Atomoxetine			S, X				
Modafinil	I	X		S, I			
Steroids							
Aldosterone							S
Cortisol				S			S
Dexamethasone				I			S, I
Estradiol				S			S
Estrogen				S		I	
Ethinyl estradiol				S, X			
Hydrocortisone							S, X
Prednisolone				S			S
Prednisone				S			S
Progesterone				S			X
Testosterone				S			
Triamcinolone							S
Foods and herbal medicines							
Caffeine	S			S			
Cannabinoids		S		S, X			
Cruciferous vegetables[b]	I						
Grapefruit juice				X			X

Drug	Cytochrome P450 isozyme				MAO-A	UGT	P-gp
	1A2	2C[a]	2D6	3A4			
Foods and herbal medicines *(continued)*							
Smoking (tobacco, etc.)	I				S		
St. John's wort			I				I
Tyramine-containing foods[c]					S		

Note. Pharmacokinetic drug interactions: I, inducer; S, substrate; X, inhibitor. Only significant interactions are listed.

ACE = angiotensin-converting enzyme; MAO-A = monoamine oxidase type A; P-gp = P-glycoprotein efflux transporter; UGT = uridine 5′-diphosphate glucuronosyltransferase.

[a]Combined properties on 2C8/9/10 and 2C19 cytochrome P450 isozymes.

[b]Cruciferous vegetables include cabbage, cauliflower, broccoli, brussels sprouts, and kale.

[c]Tyramine-containing foods include banana peel, beer (all tap, "self-brew," and nonalcoholic), broad bean pods (not beans), fava beans, aged cheese (tyramine content increases with age), sauerkraut, sausage (fermented or dry), soy sauce and soy condiments, and concentrated yeast extract (Marmite).

Source. Compiled in part from Armstrong and Cozza 2002; Balayssac et al. 2005; Bristol-Myers Squibb (Otsuka) 2014; Cozza et al. 2003; DeVane and Nemeroff 2002; Eli Lilly 2015; Flanagan et al. 2013; Gardner et al. 1996; Gillman 2005; Guédon-Moreau et al. 2003; Kiang et al. 2005; Lexicomp Inc 2015; McEvoy 2015; Michalets 1998; Pal and Mitra 2006; Procyshyn et al. 2015; Repchinsky 2008; USP DI Editorial Board 2007.

2

Severe Drug Reactions

E. Cabrina Campbell, M.D.

Stanley N. Caroff, M.D.

Stephan C. Mann, M.D.

Robert M. Weinrieb, M.D.

Rosalind M. Berkowitz, M.D.

Kimberly N. Olson, CRNP

This chapter diverges from others by reviewing not how psychotropic drugs are used in treating patients with medical illnesses but, conversely, how psychotropic drugs occasionally cause medical disorders. Although many important common side effects are associated with psychotropic drugs, the discussion in this chapter is limited to selected rare, severe, and potentially life-threatening drug reactions that occur at therapeutic doses and may require emergency medical treatment. Mirroring the book as a whole, the discussion is organized by specific organ systems. Severe drug-induced dermatological reactions are covered in Chapter 13, "Dermatological Disorders."

In reading this chapter, clinicians should keep in mind that psychotropic drugs, when indicated and used properly, are potentially beneficial for the majority of patients and should not be withheld because of the risk of these rare reactions. Instead, the best defense against adverse reactions consists of careful monitoring of patients, informed by familiarity with adverse signs and symptoms to allow prompt recognition, rapid drug discontinuation, and supportive treatment.

Central Nervous System Reactions

Although psychotropic drugs are developed for their therapeutic effects on specific neurotransmitter pathways in the brain, several severe and life-threatening drug reactions have been reported stemming either from a toxic exaggeration of the desired effect on a single neurotransmitter system (e.g., neuroleptic malignant syndrome) or from an unexpected action on systemic or other central nervous system mechanisms that affect brain function (e.g., seizures) (Table 2–1).

Neuroleptic Malignant Syndrome

Neuroleptic malignant syndrome (NMS) has been the subject of numerous clinical reviews (Caroff 2003a; Strawn et al. 2007). The incidence of NMS is about 0.02% among patients treated with antipsychotic drugs (Spivak et al. 2000; Stübner et al. 2004). Newer antipsychotics have also been implicated in cases of NMS, but they may result in milder symptoms with a better prognosis (Ananth et al. 2004; Nakamura et al. 2012; Picard et al. 2008). NMS may also result from treatment with other dopamine-blocking drugs, such as the phenothiazine antiemetics (promethazine, prochlorperazine) and metoclopramide used in medical settings. Risk factors include dehydration, exhaustion, agitation, catatonia, previous episodes, and large doses of high-potency drugs given parenterally at a rapid rate of titration. The effect of concurrent administration of multiple antipsychotics and other drugs, including lithium and selective serotonin reuptake inhibitors (SSRIs) or serotonin-norepinephrine

Table 2–1. Central nervous system drug reactions

Disorders	Implicated drugs	Risk factors	Signs and symptoms	Diagnostic studies[a]	Management[b]
Neuroleptic malignant syndrome (NMS)	Dopamine antagonists (antipsychotics, antiemetics)	Dehydration, exhaustion, agitation, catatonia, prior episodes, dose and parenteral route	Hyperthermia, rigidity, mental status changes, dysautonomia	Enzyme elevations (CPK), ↑WBCs, acidosis, ↓iron, hypoxia	Specific agents (lorazepam, dopamine agonists, dantrolene, ECT)?
Hyperthermia-parkinsonian syndrome	Dopamine withdrawal	Parkinson's disease Reduced CSF HVA	Hyperthermia, rigidity, mental status changes, dysautonomia		Dopaminergic therapy
Neuroleptic sensitivity syndrome	Antipsychotics	Lewy body dementia	Confusion, immobility, rigidity, postural instability, falls, fixed-flexion posture, poor oral intake		

Table 2–1. Central nervous system drug reactions (*continued*)

Disorders	Implicated drugs	Risk factors	Signs and symptoms	Diagnostic studies[a]	Management[b]
Lithium-neuroleptic encephalopathy	Antipsychotics plus lithium	Same as for NMS plus lithium toxicity	Same as for NMS plus lithium toxicity (ataxia, dysarthria, myoclonus, seizures)	Lithium level	
Serotonin syndrome	Antidepressants (TCAs, MAOIs, SSRIs, SNRIs) Triptans Linezolid Methylene blue Some opiates (meperidine, tramadol, dextromethorphan, fentanyl) Herbals (St. John's wort) Drugs of abuse (MDMA)	Overdose, polypharmacy	Behavioral (delirium, agitation, restlessness) Neuromotor (tremor, myoclonus, hyperreflexia, ataxia, rigidity, shivering) Dysautonomia (tachycardia, tachypnea, hyperthermia, mydriasis, blood pressure lability) Gastrointestinal (diarrhea, nausea, vomiting, incontinence)		Serotonin antagonists (cyproheptadine)? Benzodiazepines? Dantrolene (hyperthermia)?

Table 2–1. Central nervous system drug reactions *(continued)*

Disorders	Implicated drugs	Risk factors	Signs and symptoms	Diagnostic studies[a]	Management[b]
Mortality in dementia-related psychosis	Antipsychotics	Elderly	Cerebrovascular events Cardiovascular (heart failure, sudden death) Infections (pneumonia)		
Seizures	Antipsychotics (clozapine, chlorpromazine) Antidepressants (clomipramine, bupropion) Lithium (toxicity) Withdrawal of benzodiazepines, anticonvulsants Flumazenil	Epilepsy, substance abuse, brain damage, overdose, drug interactions, dose and rate of titration			

Note. CPK=creatine phosphokinase; CSF HVA=cerebrospinal fluid homovanillic acid; ECT=electroconvulsive therapy; EEG=electroencephalogram; MAOIs=monoamine oxidase inhibitors; MDMA=3,4-methylenedioxymethamphetamine; SNRIs=serotonin–norepinephrine reuptake inhibitors; SSRIs=selective serotonin reuptake inhibitors; TCAs=tricyclic antidepressants; WBC=white blood cell count.
[a]Standard imaging and laboratory studies to rule out other conditions in the differential diagnosis or complications are assumed. Only studies associated with or specific to each reaction are listed.
[b]Mainstay of management in all reactions includes careful monitoring, prompt recognition, rapid cessation of the offending drug, and supportive medical care. Only specific therapies that have been reported are listed. A question mark indicates lack of evidence of safety and efficacy.

reuptake inhibitors (SNRIs), in enhancing the risk of NMS has been suggested but is unproven (Stevens 2008).

NMS is an idiosyncratic drug reaction that occurs at therapeutic doses and may develop within hours but usually evolves over days. About two-thirds of cases occur during the first 1–2 weeks after drug initiation. Classic signs are elevated temperatures (from minimal to life-threatening hyperthermia), generalized rigidity with tremors, altered consciousness with catatonia, and autonomic instability (Caroff 2003a; Gurrera et al. 2011). Laboratory findings are not specific or pathognomonic but commonly include muscle enzyme elevations (primarily creatine phosphokinase [CPK], median elevations 800 IU/L) (Meltzer et al. 1996), myoglobinuria, leukocytosis, metabolic acidosis, hypoxia, elevated serum catecholamines, and low serum iron levels (Rosebush and Mazurek 1991). Neuroimaging findings in NMS are nonspecific, except for generalized slowing reported on electroencephalogram (EEG). However, a recent report described nearly complete loss of striatal dopamine transporter binding on single-photon emission computed tomography in patients with NMS or akinetic crises (Martino et al. 2015).

The differential diagnosis of NMS is complex, including other disorders in which patients present with elevated temperatures and encephalopathy, including malignant catatonia due to psychosis (Mann et al. 1986); central nervous system infections and autoimmune disorders (Caroff and Campbell 2015; Caroff et al. 2001a); benign extrapyramidal side effects; agitated delirium of diverse causes; heatstroke; serotonin syndrome; malignant hyperthermia associated with anesthesia (Caroff et al. 2001b); and withdrawal from dopamine agonists, sedatives, or alcohol. Although no single laboratory test is diagnostic for NMS, a thorough laboratory assessment and neuroimaging studies are essential for excluding other serious medical conditions. Several lines of evidence strongly implicate drug-induced dopamine blockade as the primary triggering mechanism in the pathogenesis of NMS (Mann et al. 2000). Efforts at identifying underlying genetic vulnerabilities, focusing on mutations in neurotransmitter, ryanodine receptor, and cytochrome enzyme genes, have been inconclusive to date.

Once dopamine-blocking drugs are withheld, two-thirds of NMS cases resolve within 1–2 weeks, with an average duration of 7–10 days (Caroff 2003a). Patients may experience prolonged symptoms if injectable long-acting drugs are implicated. Occasionally, patients develop a residual catatonic and parkinsonian state that can last for weeks but may be responsive to administration of electroconvulsive therapy (ECT; Caroff et al. 2000). Despite advances in recognition and treatment, NMS is still potentially fatal in approximately 5%–10% of cases because of renal failure, cardiorespiratory arrest, disseminated intravascular coagulation, pulmonary emboli, or aspiration pneumonia (Nakamura et al. 2012).

The mainstay of treatment consists of early diagnosis, discontinuation of dopamine antagonists, and supportive medical care. Benzodiazepines, dopamine agonists, dantrolene, and ECT have been advocated in clinical reports, but randomized controlled trials comparing these agents with supportive care may not be feasible because NMS is rare; often self-limited after drug discontinuation; and heterogeneous in presentation, course, and outcome. We have proposed that these agents may be considered empirically in individual cases on the basis of symptoms, severity, and duration of the episode (Strawn et al. 2007). For additional information about the diagnosis and management of NMS, the Neuroleptic Malignant Syndrome Information Service offers a list of volunteer consultants and provides educational material and e-mail access through its Web site (www.nmsis.org).

Parkinsonian-Hyperthermia Syndromes in Lewy Body Disorders

In view of the underlying nigrostriatal dopamine deficiency in Parkinson's disease and Lewy body dementia, patients with these disorders are at risk for severe exacerbations of motor symptoms progressing to NMS-like akinetic crises in relation to drug-induced changes in dopamine activity. In Parkinson's disease there are few reports of NMS attributable to antipsychotics alone without concomitant withdrawal of dopamine agonists (Lertxundi et al. 2015) or without the addition of cholinesterase inhibitors (Grace and Thompson 2006; Matsumoto et al. 2004). However, following discontinuation or loss of efficacy of dopaminergic drugs, following spontaneous "off" episodes, or following malfunction of deep brain stimulation devices, patients with Parkinson's disease may develop a parkinsonian-hyperthermia syndrome that is indistinguishable from NMS, which provides direct evidence of the pivotal role of acute dopamine deficiency in the pathophysiology of both disorders (Harada et al. 2003; Poston and Frucht 2008). Further support for hypodopaminergia is provided by Ueda et al. (2001), who showed that patients with Parkinson's disease who had low concentrations of homovanillic acid, a dopamine metabolite, in cerebrospinal fluid were more likely to develop the syndrome after drug withdrawal. Reports suggest an incidence of parkinsonian-hyperthermia syndrome of about 2%–3% among patients treated for Parkinson's disease, including several deaths (Factor and Santiago 2005; Harada et al. 2003).

Most patients who develop parkinsonian-hyperthermia syndrome are male, with a duration of preexisting Parkinson's disease ranging from 2 to 16 years. Apart from lower concentrations of cerebrospinal fluid homovanillic acid reported by Ueda et al. (2001), other risk factors proposed for developing the syndrome have included more severe preexisting parkinsonism; higher daily doses of levodopa; and the presence of motor fluctuations, psychosis, or dehydration (Factor and Santiago 2005). The clinical features of the syndrome closely resemble NMS and range in onset from 18 hours to 7 days after changes in dopaminergic therapy. However, Serrano-Dueñas (2003) reported finding that parkinsonian-hyperthermia developed more slowly, resulted in less robust laboratory abnormalities, resolved more quickly, and had a better prognosis than NMS. The mainstay of treatment is rapid reintroduction of dopaminergic medications, as well as aggressive medical support, with reversal of symptoms occurring in 10 hours to 7 days (Factor and Santiago 2005). In a unique randomized trial, Sato et al. (2003) reported that the addition of methylprednisolone to a combination of levodopa, bromocriptine, and dantrolene significantly reduced the severity and duration of symptoms compared with placebo in patients with parkinsonian-hyperthermia syndrome.

Neuroleptic sensitivity syndrome, considered a supporting criterion in the diagnosis of Lewy body dementia, is a potentially fatal complication of treatment with antipsychotic drugs that may affect up to 50% of patients with Lewy body dementia (Baskys 2004; McKeith et al. 1992, 2005). McKeith et al. (1992) reported that 4 (29%) of 14 patients receiving antipsychotics showed mild extrapyramidal symptoms, but 8 (57%) showed severe symptoms with half the survival of untreated patients. Neuroleptic (or antipsychotic) sensitivity is characterized by the acute onset or exacerbation of parkinsonism and impaired consciousness, with sedation followed by rigidity, postural instability, and falls. Rapid deterioration with increased confusion, immobility, rigidity, fixed-flexion posture, and decreased food and fluid intake is not reversed by anticholinergic medications and has even resulted in misdiagnosis of Lewy body dementia as the more fulminant Creutzfeldt-Jakob dementia (Lemstra et al. 2006). Aarsland et al. (2005) reported that patients with Lewy body dementia, Parkinson's disease with dementia, or Parkinson's disease alone had high frequencies of severe neuroleptic sensitivity (53%, 39%, and 27%, respectively), which distinguished them from patients with Alzheimer's disease who had no instances of this reaction. A positive history of severe neuroleptic sensitivity is therefore strongly suggestive of Lewy body disorders. Death results usually from complications of immobility and/or reduced food and fluid intake and may occur within days to weeks. As a substitute for neuroleptics, cholinesterase inhibitors have been recommended as the first-line treatment for neuropsychiatric symptoms in Lewy body dementia (despite occasional reports of NMS in patients with Parkinson's disease cited earlier), but if they are ineffective, clozapine or quetiapine may be used cautiously; however, patients should be carefully monitored for worsening motor symptoms and mental status changes (Baskys 2004; McKeith et al. 2005; Weintraub and Hurtig 2007) (see also Chapter 9, "Central Nervous System Disorders").

Lithium-Neuroleptic Encephalopathy

In 1974, a severe encephalopathic syndrome, characterized by neuromuscular symptoms, hyperthermia, and impairment of consciousness, was reported in four patients treated with lithium and haloperidol, suggesting synergistic toxic effects between these two drugs (Cohen and Cohen 1974). This report was both alarming and highly controversial and was met with disbelief as to the iatrogenic nature of the syndrome, but similar cases continued to be reported. For example, Miller and Menninger (1987) reported neurotoxicity consisting of delirium, extrapyramidal symptoms, and ataxia in 8 (19.5%) of 41 patients receiving concurrent treatment with lithium and antipsychotics. Similar cases, most often associated with haloperidol and lithium but implicating newer antipsychotics as well (Boora et al. 2008; Swartz 2001), have continued to be reported (Caroff 2003b).

The manifestations of neurotoxicity in these cases may include stupor, delirium, catatonia, rigidity, ataxia, dysarthria, myoclonus, seizures, and fever. EEG findings of diffuse slowing or triphasic waves have been suggested as a useful method in these cases for differentiating lithium-associated toxic encephalopathy from purely psychiatric changes in mental status and from nonconvulsive status (Kaplan and Birbeck 2006).

Spring and Frankel (1981) proposed two types of combined lithium-antipsychotic drug toxicity: an NMS-like reaction associated with haloperidol and other high-potency antipsychotics and a separate reaction associated with phenothiazines, especially thioridazine, resulting in lithium toxicity. Goldman (1996) reviewed 237 cases of neurotoxicity ascribed to lithium with or without antipsychotics and found support for Spring and Frankel's bipartite concept. However, the heterogeneity of cases led Goldman to suggest that adverse reactions to combination therapy form a continuum ranging from predominantly antipsychotic induced (NMS) to largely lithium induced. The mechanism for possible toxic synergy remains unknown.

Lithium-neuroleptic encephalopathy is extremely rare and does not outweigh the potential benefit and tolerance of this drug combination in the vast majority of patients presenting with mania and psychosis. Rather, the clinician is obligated to carefully monitor the response to treatment, including lithium levels, and to promptly recognize this reaction in order to rapidly discontinue medications and institute supportive medical care.

Serotonin Syndrome

Serotonin syndrome generally results when two or more serotonergic drugs are taken concurrently, but it also occurs following overdose and during single-drug exposure. Nearly all serotonergic drugs have been implicated in the syndrome, the occurrence of which appears to be primarily dose related or resulting from toxic levels of serotonin in the brain. Agents associated with severe or fatal cases typically include monoamine oxidase inhibitors (MAOIs) when combined with other antidepressants or with certain opioids that potentiate serotonergic activity (meperidine, tramadol, dextromethorphan, or fentanyl) (Boyer and Shannon 2005). Morphine has not been implicated in this interaction and is a reasonable choice for pain control in the context of concurrent serotonergic treatment, provided an allowance is made for possible potentiation of its depressive narcotic effect (Browne and Linter 1987). Some nonpsychiatric drugs that increase serotonergic activity, including triptans used for treating migraines, also have been implicated in serotonin syndrome. Certain drugs used in medical settings (e.g., linezolid, methylene blue) (Gillman 2011) or derived from herbal products (e.g., St. John's wort) have clandestine MAOI activity and may produce severe instances of serotonin syndrome when used inadvertently in combination with serotonergic drugs.

Use of illicit drugs (e.g., cocaine, synthetic cathinone derivatives ["bath salts"]) has been associated with hyperthermic states (Hohmann et al. 2014), and serotonergic mechanisms have been specifically implicated in toxic reactions following abuse of 3,4-methylenedioxymethamphetamine (MDMA or Ecstasy) (Armenian et al. 2013).

The incidence of serotonin syndrome among patients on SSRI) monotherapy has been estimated in the range of 0.5–0.9 cases per 1,000 patient-months of treatment (Mackay et al. 1999), increasing to 14%–16% in persons who overdose on SSRIs (Boyer and Shannon 2005). In a recent analysis of both a Department of Veterans Affairs database and a commercial insurance database, Nguyen et al. (2015) reported that the incidence of reported claims for serotonin syndrome in 2012 among patients prescribed serotonergic agents was 0.07% and 0.09%, respectively, and that the incidence had declined by about half since 2009. In addition, they found that the highest relative risk for developing the syndrome was observed in patients prescribed MAOIs in combination with other agents and in patients prescribed five or more non-MAOI serotonergic agents. Abadie et al. (2015) reviewed cases of serotonin syndrome reported to a pharmacovigilance database between the years 1985 and 2013 and found 125 cases that met standard criteria. The syndrome was caused by a single serotonergic drug in 40.8% of these cases, most often at therapeutic doses, whereas 59.2% resulted from combined use of a serotonin reuptake inhibitor with either an opioid or an MAOI. Although 86.9% of patients recovered without sequelae, 6 cases were fatal, and the more severe cases were associated with use of a serotonin reuptake inhibitor in combination with an MAOI.

Although serotonin syndrome has been known for decades (Oates and Sjoerdsma 1960), Sternbach (1991) is credited with developing operational diagnostic criteria on the basis of a triad of cognitive-behavioral, neuromuscular, and autonomic abnormalities. These criteria were later revised by Radomski et al. (2000). The onset of symptoms is usually abrupt, and clinical manifestations range from mild to fatal. Presentation of serotonin syndrome reflects a spectrum of concentration-dependent toxicity, ranging in severity from a transient agitated delirium to a full-blown hypermetabolic syndrome that is indistinguishable from NMS.

Behavioral symptoms of serotonin syndrome include alterations in consciousness and mood and restlessness and agitation. Autonomic disturbances include tachycardia, labile blood pressure, diaphoresis, shivering, tachypnea, mydriasis, sialorrhea, and hyperthermia. Neuromuscular signs include tremor, myoclonus, ankle clonus, hyperreflexia, ataxia, incoordination, and muscular rigidity. Gastrointestinal symptoms, including diarrhea, incontinence, nausea, and vomiting, may also occur. In a review of cases of overdose on SSRIs alone, Dunkley et al. (2003) derived the Hunter serotonin toxicity criteria. They proposed that these criteria are simpler and more sensitive and specific for serotonin toxicity than Sternbach's criteria and involve the use of only a few well-defined clinical features (clonus, agitation, diaphoresis, tremor, hyperreflexia, hypertonia, and elevated temperature).

The differential diagnosis of serotonin syndrome includes anticholinergic toxicity, heatstroke, carcinoid syndrome, infection, drug or alcohol withdrawal, lithium toxicity, and SSRI withdrawal. In more severe cases, it may be difficult to differentiate serotonin syndrome from NMS, especially in patients receiving serotonergic drugs in combination with antipsychotics. This latter conundrum prompted inclusion of warnings in product labeling of serotonergic antidepressants, cautioning against precipitation of NMS-like reactions when these two drug classes are prescribed simultaneously.

Management of serotonin syndrome entails recognition of the syndrome, cessation of serotonergic medications, and provision of supportive care. Serotonin syndrome is usually self-limited and resolves rapidly, but it can be sustained and fatal in severe cases of hyperthermia, associated most often with the use of MAOIs (Abadie et al. 2015). Sedation with benzodiazepines may be useful for controlling agitation and for correcting mild increases in heart rate and blood pressure. On the basis of anecdotal clinical reports, moderate cases appear to benefit from administration of 5-hydroxytryptamine type 2A receptor (5-HT$_{2A}$) antagonists such as cyproheptadine (Boyer and Shannon 2005). Antipsychotics with serotonergic antagonist properties have been suggested as well, but they may add the confounding autonomic, neurologic, and thermoregulatory effects of dopamine blockade. Dantrolene has been used in cases of serotonin syndrome with extreme hyperthermia.

Cerebrovascular Events and Mortality Associated With Antipsychotics in Elderly Patients With Dementia-Related Psychosis

In 2003, the U.S. Food and Drug Administration (FDA) issued an advisory that the incidence of cerebrovascular adverse events, including fatalities, was significantly higher in elderly patients with dementia-related psychosis treated with atypical antipsychotics. Collectively, 11 risperidone and olanzapine trials indicated that 2.2% of drug-treated subjects experienced cerebrovascular adverse events compared with 0.8% of those taking placebo, indicating a relative risk of 2.8 versus placebo but an absolute risk of only 1.4% when these drugs are prescribed (Jeste et al. 2008). Subsequent database studies have indeed confirmed an approximately twofold increase in risk of cerebrovascular events in elderly patients receiving antipsychotics (Hsieh et al. 2013; Prior et al. 2014; Wang et al. 2012). However, results from studies comparing atypical versus typical antipsychotics have been inconsistent, with the studies finding greater risk with atypicals (Prior et al. 2014), greater risk with typicals (Hsieh et al. 2013), or no significant difference in risk of cerebrovascular events (Gill et al. 2005; Herrmann et al. 2004; Smith et al. 2008). Moreover, risk of cerebrovascular events is not limited to antipsychotics; recent evidence indicates a significant association between serotonin reuptake inhibitors and cerebral vasoconstriction (Call-Fleming syndrome) and ischemic and hemorrhagic stroke (adjusted odds ratio of approximately 1.4–2.7) (Hung et al. 2013; Noskin et al. 2006; Shin et al. 2014; Singhal et al. 2002).

In 2005, the FDA analyzed 17 placebo-controlled trials and followed with a black box warning of increased mortality (relative risk 1.6–1.7 vs. placebo), primarily due to cardiovascular (heart failure, sudden death) or infectious (pneumonia) causes, associated with atypical antipsychotics in elderly patients with dementia-related psychosis (U.S. Food and Drug Administration 2005). Although these data implicated newer drugs, higher mortality with typical than with atypical antipsychotics among older adults was reported in retrospective analyses of large health system databases (Kales et al. 2007; Schneeweiss et al. 2007; Wang et al. 2005). In a community sample, Rochon et al. (2008) reported that compared with control subjects, older adults who received atypical antipsychotics were three times more likely and those who received typical antipsychotics were almost four times more likely to experience a serious adverse event within 30 days of starting therapy. More recently, Kales et al. (2012) conducted a retrospective cohort study examining the mortality risk in a large national sample of veterans with dementia during the 6 months after the start of risperidone, olanzapine, quetiapine, haloperidol, or valproic acid. Mortality was highest for those receiving haloperidol (relative risk 1.54), followed by risperidone (1.00), olanzapine (0.99), and quetiapine (0.73). Relative risk for patients treated with valproic acid was 0.91. These findings of relative risk were recently replicated and confirmed by the same group in another database analysis of veterans (Maust et al. 2015). This latter study also showed a greater risk of mortality from antipsychotics in comparison with antidepressants in this population and suggested a dose-response relationship between atypical antipsychotics and risk of mortality.

The use of antipsychotic drugs to treat psychosis, aggression, and agitation in elderly patients with dementia is a standard off-label practice. Data from randomized controlled trials are inconclusive on the risk-benefit ratio of these drugs in elderly patients (Schneider et al. 2006; Sink et al. 2005; Sultzer et al. 2008). However, given the lack of evidence to support the efficacy and safety of other agents or psychosocial treatments, the use of antipsychotics after informed discussion with patients and caregivers and with careful clinical monitoring is reasonable (Jeste et al. 2008).

Several mechanisms may be suggested for antipsychotic-associated cerebrovascular adverse events and death, including cardiac conduction disturbances, sedation leading to venous stasis or aspiration pneumonia, metabolic disturbances, orthostatic hypotension, tachycardia, and increased platelet aggregation. These risk factors underscore the need for thorough medical evaluation pretreatment and ongoing monitoring of elderly patients receiving antipsychotics.

Seizures

The risk of drug-induced seizures is difficult to estimate because of predisposing factors, such as epilepsy, drug interactions, or substance abuse, which are infrequently cited in clinical trials (Alper et al. 2007; Montgomery 2005; Stimmel and Dopheide 1996). Thus, if a seizure occurs in a given patient, a thorough history and neurological investigation are necessary to identify underlying risk factors. Patients with epilepsy are at risk of drug-induced seizures; however, psychotropic drugs are not contraindicated but require more careful monitoring of anticonvulsant therapy and actually have been shown to improve seizure control once psychiatric symptoms are controlled (Alper et al. 2007; Stimmel and Dopheide 1996). As a rule, seizures correlate with drug dose and rate of titration and are more likely to be observed after an overdose.

Clozapine is associated with the highest rate of seizures among antipsychotics, followed by chlorpromazine (Stimmel and Dopheide 1996; Wong and Delva 2007). Olanzapine and quetiapine may have pro-convulsant effects compared with other atypical drugs (Alper et al. 2007). Because clozapine is most often indicated and most effective for treatment-refractory schizophrenia patients, lowering the dose or adding valproic acid may be worthwhile prior to switching to a different antipsychotic if a seizure occurs.

Among antidepressants, tricyclic drugs at therapeutic doses were associated with an incidence of seizures of about 0.4%–2.0% and are particularly hazardous in overdose (Montgomery 2005). Clomipramine is considered most likely to be associated with seizures. MAOIs are considered to have low risk for seizures. Bupropion has a tenfold increase in seizure risk in dosages over 600 mg/day relative to patients on 450 mg/day or less, and it is relatively contraindicated in patients with epilepsy or severe eating disorders, or at least requires careful documentation and monitoring in these patients (Alper et al. 2007). The SSRIs and SNRIs have a low risk of seizures, except in large overdoses, and have been associated with reduction in seizure frequency compared with placebo (Alper et al. 2007; Cardamone et al. 2013). However, some SSRIs and SNRIs can increase plasma levels of other drugs, with potential for secondarily increasing seizure activity.

Among mood stabilizers, lithium is associated with seizures only during intoxication. Carbamazepine has been associated with seizures after overdose and can increase the risk of seizures during withdrawal; as a rule, the risk of withdrawal seizures can be minimized by not abruptly stopping carbamazepine, valproic acid, or any anticonvulsant and by slowly tapering the drug over a 2-week period (Stimmel and Dopheide 1996). Short- and intermediate-acting benzodiazepines, especially alprazolam, have been associated with withdrawal seizures. Finally, seizure induction is a serious complication of the benzodiazepine receptor antagonist flumazenil, with fatal cases of status epilepticus having been reported.

Cardiovascular Reactions

Severe adverse cardiovascular reactions in association with sudden death are often the most unexpected and catastrophic reactions to psychotropic drugs (Table 2–2). Cardiac reactions are observed primarily with antipsychotic drugs, especially clozapine, and with tricyclic antidepressants, whereas hypertensive crises are associated with nonselective and irreversible MAOIs.

Table 2–2. Cardiovascular drug reactions

Disorders	Implicated drugs	Risk factors	Signs and symptoms	Diagnostic studies[a]	Management[b]
Ventricular arrhythmias and sudden death					
QTc prolongation and torsades de pointes	Antipsychotics (thioridazine, mesoridazine, clozapine, chlorpromazine, haloperidol, droperidol, pimozide, sulpiride, ziprasidone)	Long QT syndrome; cardiac, renal, or hepatic disease; family history; syncope; drug history; electrolytes; drug interactions; abnormal ECG; QTc>500 ms	Palpitations, syncope, chest pain	ECGs in at-risk patients	
Brugada syndrome	Antipsychotics, antidepressants	Genetic predisposition, overdose, drug combinations	ECG (RBBB, ST elevations)	ECGs in at-risk patients	
Heart block	TCAs	Intraventricular conduction defects	Heart block	ECGs in at-risk patients	

Table 2–2. Cardiovascular drug reactions *(continued)*

Disorders	Implicated drugs	Risk factors	Signs and symptoms	Diagnostic studies[a]	Management[b]
Hypertensive crisis	MAOIs	Tyramine-containing food Sympathomimetic drugs	Hypertension, stiff neck, nausea, palpitations, diaphoresis, confusion, seizures, arrhythmias, headache, stroke	Blood pressure monitoring	Phentolamine iv; nifedipine for headache
Myocarditis, pericarditis, and cardiomyopathy	Antipsychotics (clozapine)	Cardiovascular disease, pulmonary disease	Fever, dyspnea, flu-like symptoms, chest pain, fatigue	Echocardiography (reduced ejection fraction, ventricular dysfunction), ECG (T wave changes), leukocytosis, eosinophilia, cardiac enzyme elevations	

Note. ECG = electrocardiogram; iv = intravenous; MAOIs = monoamine oxidase inhibitors; RBBB = right bundle branch block; TCAs = tricyclic antidepressants.

[a]Standard imaging and laboratory studies to rule out other conditions in the differential diagnosis or complications are assumed. Only studies associated with or specific for each reaction are listed.

[b]Mainstay of management in all reactions includes careful monitoring, prompt recognition, rapid cessation of the offending drug, and supportive medical care. Only specific therapies that have been reported are listed.

Ventricular Arrhythmias and Sudden Cardiac Death

Reports of sudden death in patients receiving antipsychotic drugs emerged soon after introduction of the drugs. Several studies have confirmed a twofold to five-fold increased risk of sudden cardiac death in patients receiving antipsychotics (Hennessy et al. 2002; Liperoti et al. 2005; Mehtonen et al. 1991; Modai et al. 2000; Ray et al. 2001; Reilly et al. 2002; Straus et al. 2004). The risk is dose related and is heightened by preexisting cardiovascular disease and use of some first-generation drugs. Implicated drugs include thioridazine, mesoridazine, pimozide, sertindole, sulpiride, clozapine, and low-potency phenothiazines, whereas other atypical drugs appear to have reduced risk. Butyrophenones, including haloperidol and droperidol used parenterally, have also been implicated.

The increased risk of arrhythmias and sudden death has been attributed to specific drug effects on cardiac conduction (Glassman and Bigger 2001; Sicouri and Antzelevitch 2008). QTc prolongation predicts risk of torsades de pointes, ventricular fibrillation, syncope, and death. Although QTc is the best available predictor, it is imperfect; the threshold for increased risk is usually set at 500 ms, but other risk factors (see below) may determine occurrence of torsades (De Ponti et al. 2001; Glassman and Bigger 2001). Among psychotropic drugs, the antipsychotic drugs, particularly thioridazine, have the highest potential for QTc prolongation and resulting arrhythmias. Although ziprasidone has not been associated with torsades, this drug does prolong the QTc interval and is considered to be contraindicated in patients with a history of QTc prolongation, recent myocardial infarction, or uncompensated heart failure.

A second mechanism for sudden death may be Brugada syndrome, which is characterized by right bundle branch block and ST elevation in right precordial leads but relatively normal QTc intervals. This syndrome has been associated with genetic predisposition, as well as with the use of antipsychotic and antidepressant drugs, mostly in the context of overdose or use of drug combinations.

Early concerns over cardiac effects of tricyclic antidepressants derived primarily from the occurrence of heart block and arrhythmias observed after drug overdoses. However, subsequent studies suggested that risk of conduction disturbances also existed when therapeutic doses were used (Roose et al. 1989). QTc prolongation and torsades de pointes have been reported with tri-

cyclics, but far less often than with antipsychotics (Sala et al. 2006). QTc prolongation with tricyclics is primarily due to prolonged QRS conduction,
which, along with increased PR intervals, reflects delays in the intraventricular
His-Purkinje conduction system involved in depolarization. Tricyclics proved
to be effective Type 1A quinidine-like antiarrhythmics, capable of suppressing
ventricular ectopy. Although tricyclic-induced suppression of conduction at
therapeutic doses is of no consequence in patients with normal hearts, there is
a tenfold risk of significant atrioventricular block in patients with preexisting
intraventricular conduction defects (Roose et al. 1989). Newer antidepressants have less risk of arrhythmias and sudden death (Feinstein et al. 2002;
Sala et al. 2006); however, there have been isolated reports of torsades following SSRI overdose (Lherm et al. 2000; Tarabar et al. 2008).

Patients who are considered for antipsychotic and antidepressant treatment should be screened for heart disease, congenital long QT and Brugada
syndromes, family history of sudden death, syncope, prior drug history of adverse cardiac effects, electrolyte imbalance (especially hypokalemia, hypocal-
cemia, or hypomagnesemia), and renal or hepatic disease. The list of drugs
implicated in QTc prolongation and torsades de pointes when used concurrently can be divided into the following: drugs that directly prolong QTc, including antiarrhythmics (quinidine, procainamide, sotalol, amiodarone),
antihistamines (diphenhydramine), antibiotics (erythromycin, clarithromycin, amantadine), and others (cisapride, methadone); drugs and substances
that interfere with metabolism of agents associated with torsades, including
antifungals (ketoconazole), antivirals (indinavar, ritonavir), calcium antagonists (diltiazem, verapamil), antibiotics (erythromycin, clarithromycin), and
grapefruit juice; and drugs that may affect electrolytes or other risk factors (diuretics) (Kao and Furbee 2005). An electrocardiogram (ECG) should be obtained at baseline and after drug administration in patients with any of these
risk factors. Conservative doses of psychotropic drugs should be prescribed
and polypharmacy minimized, with close clinical monitoring and warnings
for patients to report promptly any new symptoms such as palpitations or near
syncope as well as the prescription of new medications. Cessation and change
of medication should be considered if the ECG shows significant prolongation of the QTc, a QTc interval greater than 500 ms, new T wave abnormalities, marked bradycardia, or a Brugada phenotype.

Hypertensive Crises Due to Monoamine Oxidase Inhibitors

Hypertension is a known side effect of several psychotropic drugs, including venlafaxine, bupropion, and stimulants (Smith et al. 2008). This is usually mild and can be detected by routine blood pressure measurements. In contrast, MAOIs may produce a potentially fatal hypertensive crisis. Symptoms include throbbing headaches with marked blood pressure elevations, nausea, neck stiffness, palpitations, diaphoresis, and confusion, sometimes complicated by seizures, cardiac arrhythmias, myocardial infarction, intracerebral hemorrhage, and death. Episodes follow ingestion of sympathomimetic drugs or foods containing high concentrations of tyramine (Rapaport 2007). Prior to recognition of the need for dietary restrictions, rates of hypertensive reactions were estimated to range from 2.4% to 25% (Krishnan 2007). Previous MAOI diets were probably overly conservative, and more recent dietary restrictions are less daunting (Gardner et al. 1996). Sympathomimetic drugs also may cause a hypertensive crisis in MAOI-treated patients.

Monoamine oxidase (MAO) is the principal enzyme responsible for the oxidative deamination of monoamines. There are two subtypes of MAO isozymes: MAO-A and MAO-B. MAO-A occurs primarily in the brain, where its primary substrates are epinephrine, norepinephrine, dopamine, and serotonin, and in the intestine and liver, where it plays a critical role in the catabolism of dietary tyramine. Inhibition of MAO-A by MAOIs permits absorption of tyramine into the systemic circulation, triggering a significant release of norepinephrine from sympathetic nerve terminals, with resultant hypertensive crisis.

Extreme blood pressure elevations constitute a medical emergency and incur the risk of intracranial hemorrhage or myocardial infarction unless treated quickly with α-adrenergic antagonists. Intravenous phentolamine is the preferred treatment to reverse the acute rise in blood pressure in hypertensive crisis. In the event of a severe headache that may reflect elevated blood pressures, patients may be provided with nifedipine to take by mouth until they can be seen by a clinician.

Several selective and reversible inhibitors of MAO-A that do not require dietary restrictions have been developed but are not currently marketed in the United States. Selegiline, a selective but irreversible inhibitor of MAO-B at dosages used to increase dopaminergic activity in Parkinson's disease, becomes an inhibitor of both MAO-A and MAO-B at higher dosages needed to treat depression. A transdermal delivery system has become available that allows selegiline to be directly absorbed into the systemic circulation, bypassing the gastrointestinal tract and avoiding the need for dietary restrictions (see Chapter 3, "Alternative Routes of Drug Administration"). However, dietary restrictions are still required at higher dosages. A number of authorities argue that transdermal selegiline has been markedly underutilized in treatment-resistant depression (Asnis and Henderson 2014; Culpepper 2013). Rasagiline is an orally administered selective but irreversible inhibitor of MAO-B. However, it contains the tyramine warning even at the recommended dosages of 0.5 mg/day or 1 mg/day.

Myocarditis, Cardiomyopathy, and Pericarditis

Disorders of the myocardium and pericardium are associated primarily with clozapine (Alawami et al. 2014; Haas et al. 2007; Merrill et al. 2005). The risk of myocarditis from clozapine ranges from 0.015% to 1.2%, with a mortality rate of 10%–51%. The median age of affected patients is 30–36 years. Myocarditis occurs at therapeutic doses, and the median time of onset is less than 3 weeks after initiation of treatment. Symptoms can be diverse and nonspecific, such as fever, dyspnea, flu-like illness, chest discomfort, and fatigue. Diagnostic studies may reveal ventricular dysfunction and reduced ejection fraction on echocardiography; ECG abnormalities, particularly T wave changes; leukocytosis and eosinophilia; and elevations in cardiac enzymes. Symptoms may improve following discontinuation of clozapine, but several recurrences on rechallenge have been reported. The exact pathophysiology has yet to be determined but is thought to reflect an acute hypersensitivity reaction to the drug.

Dilated or congestive cardiomyopathy characterized by ventricular dilatation, contractile dysfunction, and congestive heart failure has also been associated with clozapine (Alawami et al. 2014; Merrill et al. 2005). Symptoms reflective of heart failure include dyspnea, palpitations or tachycardia, pedal edema, chest pain, and fatigue. Nonspecific ECG changes may occur, but reduced ejection fraction on echocardiogram can confirm the diagnosis. The incidence of clozapine-induced cardiomyopathy has been estimated at 0.01%–0.02%. As with myocarditis, the median age of patients with clozapine-related cardiomyopathy is in the 30s, and it does not appear to be dose related; doses among reported cases ranged from 125 mg to 700 mg. The duration of treatment with clozapine before cardiomyopathy onset ranges from weeks to years, with a median duration of 6–9 months. Improvement after clozapine discontinuation has been described depending on severity; patients with ejection fractions below 25% have a poorer prognosis. Rechallenge is generally discouraged. The mortality rate has been estimated between 15% and 25%. Cardiomyopathy could represent a direct cardiotoxic effect of clozapine, but more likely it evolves from clozapine-induced myocarditis.

Pericarditis and polyserositis (involving the pleura as well) have also been described in association with clozapine (Merrill et al. 2005; Wehmeier et al. 2005). These inflammatory disorders occur within the first few weeks after drug initiation and appear to resolve after drug discontinuation.

Clozapine should be used cautiously in patients with cardiovascular and pulmonary disease. Patients and families should be informed of symptoms and questioned for any signs of cardiac dysfunction. A baseline ECG should be obtained prior to starting clozapine and repeated 2–4 weeks afterward. The value of repeat ECGs, echocardiography, magnetic resonance imaging, and monitoring of serum cardiac enzymes and eosinophilia has not been substantiated but should be considered together with cardiology consultation if new symptoms of cardiovascular disease develop. In elderly patients, an echocardiogram is recommended every 6 months to monitor for myocarditis (Gareri et al. 2008). If myocarditis, pericarditis, or cardiomyopathy is suspected, clozapine should be discontinued immediately and should not be reinstituted if the diagnosis is confirmed.

Gastrointestinal Reactions

Although mild gastrointestinal upset is not uncommon as a side effect associated with several psychotropic drug classes (e.g., SSRIs, lithium), severe hepatic and pancreatic toxicity may occur rarely (Table 2–3). The goal of this section is to provide the reader with a summary of the current literature regarding the association between psychiatric medications and drug-induced liver and pancreatic injury.

Table 2–3. Gastrointestinal drug reactions

Disorders	Implicated drugs	Risk factors	Signs and symptoms	Diagnostic studies[a]	Management[b]
Hepatotoxicity	Anticonvulsants (valproic acid, carbamazepine, lamotrigine, topiramate) Antipsychotics (phenothiazines)	Children, multiple anticonvulsants	Lethargy, jaundice, nausea, vomiting, anorexia, hemorrhages, seizures, fever, facial edema	Transaminitis, hyperbilirubinemia	L-Carnitine (for valproate toxicity?)
Hyperammonemic encephalopathy	Valproic acid		Decreased consciousness, focal deficits, impaired cognition, lethargy, vomiting, seizures	Serum ammonia, EEG	L-Carnitine (valproate toxicity?)
Acute pancreatitis	Valproic acid	Children, multiple anticonvulsants	Abdominal pain, nausea, vomiting, anorexia, fever	Serum amylase, lipase	

Note. EEG = electrocardiogram.

[a]Standard imaging and laboratory studies to rule out other conditions in the differential diagnosis or complications are assumed. Only studies associated with or specific to each reaction are listed.

[b]Mainstay of management in all reactions includes careful monitoring, prompt recognition, rapid cessation of the offending drug, and supportive medical care. Only specific therapies that have been reported are listed. A question mark indicates lack of evidence of safety and efficacy.

Drug-Induced Liver Injury

Prescribers of psychotropic medications must be mindful of the potential for idiosyncratic drug-induced liver injury (DILI), which, in a worst-case scenario, can cause chronic liver injury or death or require liver transplantation. Although the symptoms and signs of hepatotoxicity are nonspecific when considered individually, a clustering of symptoms that includes some or all of the following should assist the clinician in a diagnostic formulation: weakness, anorexia, fever, lethargy, jaundice, nausea, vomiting, hemorrhages, confusion, asterixis, seizures, and facial edema. Furthermore, liver chemistry results are variable; for example, transaminases and bilirubin can range from mild to extreme elevations and do not reliably predict progression to fatal hepatotoxicity. Thus, regular clinical monitoring for prodromal symptoms is essential, followed by withholding of the suspected drug if symptoms emerge or enzyme elevations are found.

The best available evidence from population-based studies indicates that the annual incidence of idiosyncratic, all-cause DILI in the general population is between approximately 14 and 19 events per 100,000 (Björnsson et al. 2013; Sgro et al. 2002). Varying degrees of liver injury will occur in up to 27% of cases of DILI, and of those, nearly 1 in 5 will develop chronic liver injury within 6 months and 1 in 10 will die or require liver transplantation to survive (Fontana et al. 2014).

The Drug-Induced Liver Injury Network (DILIN), funded by the National Institutes of Health, is a multisite observational study of DILI in children and adults in the United States for which data collection began in 2004. In the DILIN's latest report, characteristics and subgroup analysis from the first 1,257 enrolled patients found that 899 had definite, highly likely, or probable DILI (Chalasani et al. 2015). The investigators reported that central nervous system (CNS) agents are the fourth most likely class of drugs linked to a DILI and accounted for 9% of 190 different causative agents identified in their study. The DILIN study found that of the CNS drugs associated with DILIs, anticonvulsants and antipsychotics were the two most common agents resulting in liver injury, and they were most likely to affect younger subjects with organic brain disease, developmental delay, congenital metabolic disorders, or malnutrition (Chalasani et al. 2015).

In terms of the histopathology of liver injury associated with the psychotropic drugs, Voican et al. (2014) classified DILI as either hepatocellular, cholestatic, or mixed, depending on the presence or absence of an underlying liver injury. Hepatocellular injury was identified as having abnormally high serum alanine transaminase (ALT) levels with small or no increase in titers of alkaline phosphatase (ALP). If bilirubin levels are also elevated, this suggests that severe hepatocellular damage has occurred and is a marker of a poor prognosis. Cholestatic injury to the liver is characterized by high serum ALP levels with only slightly elevated levels of ALT and sometimes with elevated bilirubin. In mixed injuries, both ALT and ALP titers are high. The authors reported that because serum transaminase levels less than three times the upper limit of normal (ULM) were found in 1%–5% of the general population, ALT levels greater than three times the ULM or ALP titers greater than two times the ULM are strongly suggestive of DILI.

Drug-Induced Liver Injury and Antiepileptic Drugs

In a thorough review of the literature, Devarbhavi and Andrade (2014) reported that the majority of antiepileptic drug (AED)–induced DILIs are more likely to be associated with the older AEDs, such as carbamazepine, valproate, or phenobarbital. These injuries are associated with development of the potentially fatal drug rash (or reaction) with eosinophilia and systemic symptoms (DRESS). In the DILIN study, nine patients (1%) had severe skin reactions in addition to their liver injury, and of those, four died; however, the AED drugs most often implicated were lamotrigine and carbamazepine (Chalasani et al. 2015).

Carbamazepine is associated with liver injury in all age groups but with no gender specificity (Devarbhavi and Andrade 2014). The clinical picture can range from an asymptomatic rise in liver chemistries to acute liver failure. Carbamazepine can also cause isolated asymptomatic elevations in γ-glutamyltransferase (GGT). These GGT elevations do not warrant stopping the medication as long as bilirubin levels do not increase as well. This is also true for mild elevations in transaminases. When bilirubin levels do increase, carbamazepine must be stopped immediately because mortality or the need for liver transplantation has been estimated to be as high as 17% in such cases, especially in children under the age of 10 or when the patient has developed hepatocellular injury and DILI after several weeks of drug exposure. The typical latency period is 6–12 weeks.

Results from the DILIN study indicate that valproic acid is the most frequently implicated AED associated with drug-induced hepatotoxicity, affecting an age range of 2–47 years (median 27 years) (Devarbhavi and Andrade 2014). Valproic acid typically causes one of two types of liver injury. The more common type is characterized by a reversible relatively mild elevation in transaminases (ALT, ALP) and usually presents without clinical symptoms. This reaction is dose dependent, typically occurs during initiation of treatment, and can occur in up to 44% of patients (Lopez and Hendrickson 2014). The second type of DILI associated with valproic acid is less common, but it is irreversible, idiosyncratic, and potentially fatal. Children younger than 2 years taking multiple AEDs are at greatest risk, but fatal outcomes in adults may be underestimated. The incidence is estimated to be 1 per 550 patients if valproic acid is used with other antiepileptic mediations and 1 per 8,000 if it is used as a single agent (Lopez and Hendrickson 2014).

The putative mechanism for hepatotoxicity from valproic acid is related to its inhibition of fatty acid transport and mitochondrial β-oxidation (Devarbhavi and Andrade 2014). A deficiency in coenzyme A is thought to impair the mitochondrial enzymes responsible for breaking down fatty acids, which then results in a shift of the metabolism to a different type of oxidation reaction, thus generating hepatotoxic metabolites (Voican et al. 2014).

One such hepatotoxic metabolite is called 4-en-valproic acid, which can elevate serum ammonia levels by inhibiting urea production. Although hyperammonemia occurs in nearly 50% of patients receiving valproic acid, it remains asymptomatic in most cases (Lheureux et al. 2005). Rarely, patients taking valproic acid can develop a severe form of hyperammonemic encephalopathy characterized by decreased consciousness, focal neurological deficits, asterixis, cognitive slowing, vomiting, lethargy, and increased seizure frequency (Segura-Bruna et al. 2006). These symptoms should prompt immediate discontinuation of the drug and screening for serum ammonia levels, which can be elevated despite normal liver chemistry results. Signs of severe hyperammonemic encephalopathy, which are evident on EEG, can be reversed once valproic acid is discontinued. Another proposed mechanism for hyperammonemia is that valproic acid decreases serum levels and body stores of carnitine, an amino acid derivative that facilitates mitochondrial metabolism of ammonia. A deficiency of carnitine can therefore result in the accumulation of ammonia (Lheureux et al. 2005).

Elevations in levels of ammonia have been implicated more broadly in the development of hepatic encephalopathy due to hepatic failure in general. A review by Malaguarnera (2013) described the results of six randomized controlled studies of acetyl-L-carnitine (ALC) in the treatment of hepatic encephalopathy associated with hyperammonemia. In this review, Malaguarnera provided evidence suggesting that supplementation with 4 g daily of ALC improved physical and mental fatigue in patients who developed mild to moderate hepatic encephalopathy and significantly improved EEG, cognitive and memory functions, and visual scanning and tracking in patients with severe hyperammonemic encephalopathy. Lopez and Hendrickson (2014) also reported that ALC benefited patients whose serum ammonia levels were greater than 450 mg/mL by facilitating fatty acid transport and regulating the ratio of coenzyme A into mitochondria. In cases where serum ammonia levels were between 850 and 1,000 mg/mL in patients who also had hemodynamic instability or significant metabolic derangements or were in a coma, hemodialysis was shown to be beneficial.

Hepatotoxicity from lamotrigine is typically seen in the setting of rash and severe hypersensitivity reactions (Devarbhavi and Andrade 2014). Most symptoms will subside with discontinuation of the drug, but some cases will progress to Stevens-Johnson syndrome and toxic epidermal necrolysis. Younger age and rapid titration of the medicine can increase the risk of a DILI, and because valproic acid increases the serum lamotrigine concentration by more than 200%, giving both drugs simultaneously should be avoided whenever possible.

Drug-Induced Liver Injury and Antidepressant Drugs

A recent review of DILI and antidepressants reported that mild liver chemistry elevations were found in 0.5%–1% of patients treated with second-generation antidepressants such as SSRIs and SNRIs and in up to 3% of patients taking MAOIs, tricyclics, or tetracyclic antidepressants (Voican et al. 2014). The overall incidence of antidepressant-induced liver injury resulting in hospitalization is between 1.28 and 4 cases per 100,000 patient-years, with the exception of nefazodone, which was estimated to be 29 cases per 100,000 patient-years.

The mechanism of antidepressant-associated hepatic injury is usually hepatocellular and is thought to be metabolic or immunoallergic (Voican et al. 2014). As with the AEDs, patients with antidepressant-associated hepatic injury can present with a hypersensitivity syndrome of fever, rash, eosinophilia, auto-antibodies, and a short latency period of between 1 and 6 weeks. When the latency period is longer (1 month to 1 year), the metabolic mechanism of heptotoxicity is more likely to be idiosyncratic. Furthermore, Chen et al. (2013) found that high daily doses and high lipophilicity of an antidepressant are more predictive of liver injury. Interestingly, preexisting liver disease is not usually associated with a greater risk of antidepressant-associated DILI. However, duloxetine is known to pose a greater risk of DILI in people at risk of liver disease or in those with cirrhosis or chronic liver disease. Cases of acute liver failure leading to liver transplantation or death have been reported for the following antidepressants: phenelzine, imipramine, amitriptyline, venlafaxine, sertraline, bupropion, trazodone, and, in Europe, agomelatine (Voican et al. 2014).

Drug-Induced Liver Injury and Antipsychotic Drugs

Marwick et al. (2012) reviewed the literature concerning the association between regular antipsychotic use and abnormal liver function in adults and found that a median of 32% (5%–78%) of patients had abnormal liver chemistries while taking antipsychotics, and 4% (0%–15%) had clinically significant elevations in liver chemistries. Transaminases were the most likely liver enzymes to be elevated. Most cases were asymptomatic, arose within 6 weeks of starting the drug, and either resolved with ongoing treatment or stably persisted (Marwick et al. 2012).

Although there are case reports of multiple different antipsychotics associated with fatalities due to drug-induced heptotoxicity, Marwick et al. (2012) found that chlorpromazine was the antipsychotic most commonly associated with acute liver injury. The mechanism of liver injury is thought to be due to the drug or its metabolites causing impairment of bile secretions, leading to cholestasis via immune-mediated mechanisms. A primary care database study in the United Kingdom was referenced that reported an incidence rate of chlorpromazine-associated liver injury of approximately 1.3 per 1,000 patients, which was more likely to affect patients older than 70 years. Marwick et al. (2012) advised that patients with preexisting liver disease not be prescribed chlorpromazine. They also noted that because of the potential for patients with serious mental illness to develop antipsychotic-associated metabolic syndrome, patients taking antipsychotics long term may also be at increased risk for the development of nonalcoholic steatohepatitis, which can eventually lead to cirrhosis.

Valproic Acid and Acute Pancreatitis

Acute pancreatitis has been reported as an idiosyncratic reaction to therapeutic dosages of valproic acid in 1 per 40,000 treated patients (Gerstner et al. 2007). When valproic acid–induced pancreatitis does occur, it is most common in children, especially if they are being treated with multiple anticonvulsants. The onset is variable and ranges from drug initiation to several years after treatment initiation. The causative mechanisms are currently unknown. Diagnosis is based on the presence of abdominal pain, nausea, vomiting, anorexia, and fever and is associated with elevations in amylase and lipase. Mortality can reach 15%–20%, and treatment is supportive after discontinuation of valproic acid. Transient asymptomatic hyperamylasemia occurs in 20% of adult patients taking valproate but is unrelated to risk of pancreatitis (Gerstner et al. 2007). Drug-induced pancreatitis has been reported less often with other anticonvulsants (carbamazepine, lamotrigine, topiramate, levetiracetam, vigabatrin) (Zaccara et al. 2007), antipsychotics (clozapine, olanzapine, risperidone, haloperidol) (Koller et al. 2003), and antidepressants (mirtazapine, bupropion, venlafaxine, SSRIs) (Hussain and Burke 2008; Spigset et al. 2003). Alcohol use disorder increases the risk for drug-induced pancreatitis. Following recovery, the offending drug should not be reinstated; use of a drug from a different class is preferred (Dhir et al. 2007).

Renal Reactions

Severe renal toxicity, including renal insufficiency and nephrogenic diabetes insipidus (NDI), has been associated primarily with lithium administration (Table 2–4). However, the syndrome of inappropriate antidiuretic hormone secretion (SIADH) leading to hyponatremia has been associated with several drug classes. These disorders necessitate careful clinical and laboratory monitoring to prevent irreversible kidney damage.

Chronic Renal Insufficiency

Lithium has been implicated in several disorders of kidney function, including renal tubular acidosis, interstitial nephritis, proteinuria with nephrotic syndrome, acute renal failure after intoxication, NDI, and chronic renal insufficiency progressing to end-stage renal disease (Boton et al. 1987; Oliveira

Table 2–4.   Renal drug reactions

Disorders	Implicated drugs	Risk factors	Signs and symptoms	Diagnostic studies[a]	Management[b]
Chronic renal insufficiency	Lithium	Elderly, duration of treatment, concomitant drugs (NSAIDs), lithium toxicity		Creatinine, creatinine clearance (at least every 3–6 months)	
Nephrogenic diabetes insipidus	Lithium, pimozide, alcohol		Excessive urine volume→dehydration, encephalopathy, lithium toxicity	Water deprivation Serum vasopressin Response to exogenous vasopressin	Monitor urinary output Specific agents (amiloride, thiazides, NSAIDs)?
Acute hyponatremia (SIADH)	Antipsychotics Antidepressants (tricyclics, SSRIs, SNRIs) Opiates		Nausea, vomiting, anorexia, dysgeusia, disorientation, confusion, fatigue, headaches, weakness, irritability, lethargy, muscle cramps→delirium, hallucinations, diminished consciousness, seizures, coma, respiratory arrest	Hyponatremia Elevated urine, reduced plasma osmolality	Hyponatremic encephalopathy; hypertonic fluids[c]

Table 2–4. Renal drug reactions *(continued)*

Disorders	Implicated drugs	Risk factors	Signs and symptoms	Diagnostic studies[a]	Management[b]
Chronic hyponatremia (SIADH)	Antipsychotics Antidepressants (tricyclics, SSRIs, SNRIs) Opiates		Impaired cognition, falls, mood change		Fluid restriction[c] Specific agents (clozapine, demeclocycline, conivaptan, tolvaptan)?

Note. NSAIDs=nonsteroidal anti-inflammatory drugs; SIADH=syndrome of inappropriate antidiuretic hormone secretion; SNRIs=serotonin-norepinephrine reuptake inhibitors; SSRIs=selective serotonin reuptake inhibitors.

[a]Standard imaging and laboratory studies to rule our other conditions in the differential diagnosis or complications are assumed. Only studies associated with or specific to each reaction are listed.

[b]Mainstay of management in all reactions includes careful monitoring, prompt recognition, rapid cessation of the offending drug, and supportive medical care. Only specific therapies that have been reported are listed. Only specific therapies that have been reported are listed. A question mark indicates lack of evidence of safety and efficacy.

[c]Risk of central pontine or extrapontine myelinolysis (mood changes, lethargy, mutism, dysarthria, pseudobulbar palsy, and quadriplegia) if serum sodium corrected at >8 mMol/L over 24-hour period.

et al. 2010; Raedler and Wiedemann 2007). Histopathological studies reveal that about 10%–20% of patients receiving long-term lithium therapy demonstrate changes including tubular atrophy, interstitial fibrosis, cysts, and glomerular sclerosis.

Evidence supports an association between long-term lithium treatment and progressive renal insufficiency (Raedler and Wiedemann 2007). Studies have shown that about 15%–20% of patients show evidence of reduced renal function after 10 years of taking lithium. Abnormalities may develop as early as 1 year after beginning treatment. Kidney dysfunction is related to duration of lithium treatment and is progressive, even after lithium is discontinued in some cases. The rate of progression is variable; although many patients show a decreased filtration rate, few develop renal insufficiency, and frank renal failure is rare. In a study among dialysis patients, 0.22% had lithium-induced nephropathy (Presne et al. 2003). No reliable risk factors predict renal failure, but decreased renal function has been associated with duration of treatment, age, concomitant medications (e.g., NSAIDs, especially indomethacin), and episodes of lithium toxicity.

Management focuses on prevention by screening patients for underlying kidney disease, discussing risks and benefits of treatment, using lowest effective doses, avoiding lithium intoxication, carefully monitoring lithium levels, measuring kidney function every 3–6 months or as indicated by the patient's condition, and reassessing risks of continuing lithium if renal function declines. Useful measures to follow include serum creatinine, glomerular filtration rate, and urinalyses (Jefferson 2010). Imaging studies of the kidneys have recently been studied as well (Karaosmanoglu et al. 2013). Withdrawal of lithium after prolonged treatment may not result in reversal of kidney dysfunction; rather, kidney function may continue to decline and, conversely, may increase the risk of psychiatric relapse with associated risk of suicide (Rej et al. 2012; Werneke et al. 2012).

Nephrogenic Diabetes Insipidus

In early studies, impairment in urine concentration with resulting polyuria, which was observed in 20%–30% of patients receiving lithium, was considered benign (Khanna 2006). However, lithium is the most common cause of acquired NDI. NDI is defined as the inability of the kidneys to concentrate urine, resulting in excessive volumes of dilute urine due to the insensitivity of the distal nephron to the antidiuretic hormone, vasopressin. Although mild cases, which may occur within a few weeks of initiating treatment, can be compensated by increased fluid intake, severe cases can result in dehydration, neurological symptoms, encephalopathy, and lithium intoxication. NDI can be congenital or acquired from drugs, including pimozide and alcohol in addition to lithium (Moeller et al. 2013).

The diagnosis of NDI can be confirmed and distinguished from primary psychogenic polydipsia by comparing urine and plasma osmolality during a water deprivation or dehydration test (Garofeanu et al. 2005; Khanna 2006; Moeller et al. 2013). In primary polydipsia, patients will show concentration of urine (osmolality > 500 mOsmol/kg with plasma osmolality > 295 mOsmol/kg) after water deprivation, whereas patients with NDI will continue to show dilute urine (< 300 mOsmol/kg). To distinguish NDI from central diabetes insipidus (CDI), plasma vasopressin is measured after dehydration. In NDI, plasma vasopressin exceeds 5 ng/L, whereas in CDI, vasopressin will be reduced or negligible. After exogenous vasopressin, patients with CDI will increase urine osmolality, whereas patients with NDI will experience little or no change (Khanna 2006).

Although the mechanism of lithium-induced NDI has been attributed to the effects of lithium on aquaporin-2, probably through interference in the adenylate cyclase system, more recent evidence suggests multifactorial effects on signaling pathways and cellular organization of the tubular system (Khanna 2006; Moeller et al. 2013). Aquaporin-2 is the primary target for vasopressin regulation of collecting duct water permeability. Downregulation of aquaporin-2 expression is only partially reversed after lithium discontinuation, which is consistent with findings suggesting that NDI can become irreversible even after lithium discontinuation, depending on the duration of treatment. Although impaired concentration is usually reversible within 1–2 years of treatment, concentrating capacity may not improve at all after 10–20 years of lithium treatment (Garofeanu et al. 2005).

Management of NDI consists of regular monitoring of urinary symptoms and output, with testing of urine osmolality and electrolytes as necessary, followed by discontinuation of lithium. Current evidence supports the use of amiloride as treatment for NDI, but thiazide diuretics and NSAIDs have been suggested as well, although close monitoring of lithium levels, which can be raised by these agents, is required (Moeller et al. 2013; Rej et al. 2012).

Syndrome of Inappropriate Antidiuretic Hormone Secretion

The converse of diabetes insipidus is the retention of water resulting in hyponatremia. Hyponatremia may occur in 5%–15% of chronic psychiatric patients (Siegel 2008; Sterns 2015). Severity of symptoms is related to the rate of onset as well as the absolute serum sodium. In acute-onset hyponatremia, patients may first develop nausea, vomiting, anorexia, dysgeusia, disorientation, headache, fatigue, weakness, irritability, lethargy, confusion, and muscle cramps, with progression to hypotonic encephalopathy characterized by impaired responsiveness, delirium, and hallucinations. If not corrected, the resulting cerebral edema may result in seizures, coma, and death from cerebral herniation, brain stem compression, and respiratory arrest (Ellison and Berl 2007; Siegel 2008). Patients with slow-onset or chronic hyponatremia may be asymptomatic or may present with impaired cognition, frequent falls, anxiety, and depression, after an adaptive response to hypotonicity restores brain volume.

SIADH is the most frequent cause of hyponatremia (Ellison and Berl 2007). SIADH is diagnosed in patients with normal renal, thyroid, and adrenal function who develop hyponatremia with reduced plasma osmolality, reduced renal excretion of sodium, absence of volume depletion or overload, and elevated urine osmolality despite plasma hypotonicity. Phenothiazines, tricyclics, anticonvulsants (carbamazepine and oxcarbazepine), atypical antipsychotics (except for clozapine, which has shown positive results, correcting idiopathic hyponatremia in schizophrenia patients) (Canuso and Goldman 1999), opiates, and SSRIs and SNRIs have been implicated in causing SIADH from stimulating release of or enhancing renal sensitivity to vasopressin. The incidence of hyponatremia with SSRIs has been reported to range from 0.5% to 32% of patients, with elderly patients at highest risk (Siegel 2008). SIADH associated with psychotropic drugs usually has a slow onset and reverses within 24–48 hours after the drugs are discontinued. However, if the hyponatremia is asymptomatic and undetected, sodium levels can decrease to dangerous levels, resulting in acute encephalopathy.

Treatment depends on the severity and duration of the hyponatremia and neuropsychiatric symptoms. Definitive treatment consists of discontinuing the causative drug. Acute, life-threatening hyponatremic encephalopathy is a medical emergency, dictating the need for treatment with hypertonic solutions to reverse cerebral edema. Management of patients with chronic hyponatremia with uncertain onset or absence of symptoms is less clear. With a lower risk of neurological sequelae of hyponatremia, patients with longer durations of hyponatremia are paradoxically at higher risk for osmotic demyelination if the serum sodium is corrected by more than 8 mMol/L over a 24-hour period (Ellison and Berl 2007; Sterns 2015). Osmotic demyelination, resulting in central pontine or extrapontine myelinolysis, begins with affective changes and lethargy, progressing to mutism, dysarthria, spastic quadriplegia, and pseudobulbar palsy. For chronic patients, fluid restriction is the critical intervention, but salt tablets and slow infusion of 3% saline or administration of furosemide or urea have been tried. Several drugs have been used as well (e.g., demeclocycline, which inhibits vasopressin), but recently developed vasopressin-receptor antagonists (e.g., conivaptan, tolvaptan) offer a promising treatment for hyponatremia resulting from drug-induced SIADH (Berl 2015; Josiassen et al. 2008). However, the effects of vasopressin antagonists on serum sodium are delayed, and they may increase the risk of osmotic demyelination, such that these agents are not useful in patients with acute CNS symptoms. Their use in patients with chronic hyponatremia, who may require maintenance treatment with antipsychotics, for example, has yet to be established.

Hematological Reactions

Essentially all classes of psychotropic drugs have been associated with blood dyscrasias (Table 2–5) (Flanagan and Dunk 2008). Serious hematological toxicity is rare, with an annual incidence of only 1–2 per 100,000 population. The white blood cells are affected most commonly, resulting in neutropenia (neutrophils < 1,500/mm^3) or agranulocytosis (neutrophils < 500/mm^3). Blood dyscrasias may result from a direct toxic effect on the bone marrow, peripheral destruction, or formation of antibodies that target the hematopoietic cells or their precursors. Antipsychotics are most likely to cause neutropenia or agranulocytosis (Nooijen et al. 2011). Among patients beginning therapy with clozapine, 3% may develop neutropenia and 0.8% may develop agranulocytosis, usually in the first year of treatment (Alvir et al. 1993). The risk of neutropenia in patients taking phenothiazines may be 1 per 10,000, and for patients taking chlorpromazine the risk of agranulocytosis is 0.13% (Flanagan and Dunk 2008). Tohen et al. (1995) reported that 2.1% of 977 patients given carbamazepine developed mild ($3{,}000{-}4{,}000/mm^3$) or moderate ($<3{,}000/mm^3$) neutropenia, about six to seven times higher in rate than with valproic acid or antidepressants.

Clinically, drug-induced neutropenia will become evident after 1–2 weeks of therapy; the degree of the neutropenia is related to the dose and duration of exposure. Recovery can be expected within 3–4 weeks after stopping the causative drug. Agranulocytosis can take longer to appear, up to 3–4 weeks after starting treatment. With clozapine, the risk is greatest during the first 6–18 weeks of treatment, and agranulocytosis is more frequent in females and more frequent and more severe in the elderly (Alvir et al. 1993). After 6 months of treatment, the risk with clozapine may be similar to the risk with other antipsychotics (Nooijen et al. 2011).

For patients taking drugs known to cause neutropenia or agranulocytosis, proper management involves obtaining a complete blood count (CBC) with differential initially and periodically. A strict protocol of monitoring in patients taking clozapine, along with treatment including broad-spectrum antibiotics, supportive care, and agents to stimulate the production of granulocytes, has resulted in a decrease in the mortality from clozapine-induced agranulocytosis from 3%–4% to 0.01% (Meltzer et al. 2002; Nooijen et al. 2011). Fever or infection, particularly pharyngitis, may be the only symptom of neutropenia or agranulocytosis and is an indication for withholding the drugs until a CBC with differential can be performed.

Although they occur less frequently than problems with white blood cells, platelet abnormalities have been associated with psychotropic drugs. SSRIs decrease platelet serotonin, which may cause a decrease in platelet function and prolongation of bleeding time. Patients with known coagulation disorders or von Willebrand disease and those taking NSAIDs and coumarins should be monitored if SSRIs are prescribed (Halperin and Reber 2007). There is some evidence that serotonergic antidepressants and antipsychotics may be associated with increased risk of hospitalization for bleeding, especially in new users of the drugs, probably as a result of decreased platelet aggregation (Verdel et al. 2011). Previous work by this same group showed an association between serotonergic antidepressant drugs and the need for perioperative blood transfusion in orthopedic surgery, whereas nonserotonergic

Table 2–5. Hematological drug reactions

Disorders	Implicated drugs	Risk factors	Signs and symptoms	Diagnostic studies[a]	Management[b]
Neutropenia and agranulocytosis	Antipsychotics (clozapine, chlorpromazine) Anticonvulsants (carbamazepine)		Fever, infection	CBC with differential	
Thrombocytopenia	Antipsychotics Antidepressants (SSRI effects on platelet function) Benzodiazepines	Existing coagulopathies	Hemorrhages	Platelet count	
Anemia	Antipsychotics (chlorpromazine, clozapine, risperidone) Antidepressants (MAOIs, SSRIs) Anticonvulsants (valproic acid, oxcarbazepine) Benzodiazepines		Weakness, fatigue	CBC	

Note. CBC=complete blood count; MAOIs=monoamine oxidase inhibitors; SSRIs=selective serotonin reuptake inhibitors.
[a]Standard imaging and laboratory studies to rule out other conditions in the differential diagnosis or complications are assumed. Only studies associated with or specific to each reaction are listed.
[b]Mainstay of management in all reactions includes careful monitoring, prompt recognition, rapid cessation of the offending drug, and supportive medical care. Only specific therapies that have been reported are listed.

drugs showed no such association (Movig et al. 2003). Clinicians and patients should be aware of the potential for bleeding during procedures.

Most of the typical and atypical antipsychotics have been reported to cause thrombocytopenia. Clozapine has also been reported to cause thrombocytosis, and there are case reports of quetiapine-induced thrombotic thrombocytopenic purpura. Valproate monotherapy has been associated with thrombocytopenia and rare bleeding complications, with potential risk factors being increasing serum levels, female sex, and lower baseline platelet count (Nasreddine and Beydoun 2008). Thrombocytopenia has also been reported with tricyclic antidepressants, MAOIs, and benzodiazepines.

Chlorpromazine, clozapine, risperidone, and sertraline have also been associated with anemia. There are case reports of valproic acid causing pure red cell aplasia, which resolves when the drug is discontinued (Bartakke et al. 2008). Oxcarbazepine was reported to cause hemolytic anemia in an elderly man, which resolved after discontinuation of the drug (Chaudhry et al. 2008). Lithium has been well known to cause leukocytosis and thrombocytosis. Pancytopenia has been reported with fluphenazine and lamotrigine.

Discontinuation of the offending drug is usually followed by hematological recovery. If the patient cannot be treated with a different class of drug, hematology consultation should be obtained regarding appropriate monitoring of hematological parameters.

Metabolic Reactions and Body as a Whole

Antipsychotic-Induced Heatstroke

Patients with serious mental illness have an increased risk of heatstroke (Bark 1998; Page et al. 2012), related to behavioral and environmental factors. For example, Page et al. (2012), in a primary care cohort study, found that patients with psychosis, dementia, or substance abuse and those prescribed sedatives or antipsychotics had more than twice the risk of heat-related mortality compared with controls subject. Antipsychotic drugs can promote heatstroke by impairing heat loss (Mann and Boger 1978) (see Table 2–6). Substantial evidence supports a key role for dopamine in preoptic anterior hypothalamic thermoregulatory heat loss mechanisms (Lee et al. 1985). All typical antipsychotics promote hyperthermia by blocking dopamine receptors. The role of

Table 2–6. Metabolic drug reactions and body as a whole

Disorders	Implicated drugs	Risk factors	Signs and symptoms	Diagnostic studies[a]	Management[b]
Drug-induced heatstroke					
Classic heatstroke	Antipsychotics Anticholinergics	Heat waves, systemic illness, elderly age	Hyperthermia, anhidrosis, confusion→multiorgan failure, delirium, coma, seizures		Rapid cooling measures
Exertional heatstroke	Antipsychotics Anticholinergics	Exertion, heat waves	Hyperthermia, rhabdomyolysis, confusion, metabolic acidosis→multiorgan failure, delirium, coma, seizures		Rapid cooling measures
Diabetic ketoacidosis	Antipsychotics (clozapine, olanzapine)	African Americans, younger age	Anorexia, nausea, vomiting, polydipsia, polyuria→altered mental status, coma	Urine ketones	
Rhabdomyolysis	Antipsychotics	Agitation, trauma, substance abuse, injections, restraints, dystonia	Weakness, myalgias, edema, dark urine→compartment syndromes, DIC, renal failure, hyperkalemia and arrhythmias	Serum CPK, urine myoglobin	

Note. CPK=creatine phosphokinase; DIC=disseminated intravascular coagulation.

[a]Standard imaging and laboratory studies to rule out other conditions in the differential diagnosis or complications are assumed. Only studies associated with or specific to each reaction are listed.

[b]Mainstay of management in all reactions includes careful monitoring, prompt recognition, rapid cessation of the offending drug, and supportive medical care. Only specific therapies that have been reported are listed.

atypical antipsychotics in suppressing heat loss appears less clear. Although atypicals block dopamine receptors, they also block 5-hydroxytryptamine type 2C ($5\text{-}HT_{2C}$) and postsynaptic $5\text{-}HT_{1A}$ receptors, which participate in heat-loss mechanisms, suggesting that atypicals could further promote hyperthermia in a hot environment (Mann 2003).

In most cases, anticholinergic-induced inhibition of sweating appears to contribute significantly to the development of antipsychotic-induced heatstroke. Low-potency typical antipsychotic drugs having marked anticholinergic activity are frequent offenders, whereas heatstroke associated with high-potency typical antipsychotics often involves concurrent treatment with anticholinergic drugs (Clark and Lipton 1984). In addition, some atypical antipsychotics (clozapine, quetiapine, and olanzapine) possess anticholinergic activity. Comorbid medical illnesses, especially cardiovascular disease, which necessitates treatment with drugs such as diuretics that may also impair thermoregulation, and substance abuse further increase the risk of heatstroke.

Clark and Lipton (1984) reviewed 45 cases of antipsychotic-induced heatstroke and concluded that the majority of cases resembled classic environmental heatstroke. Classic heatstroke is characterized by body temperature above 40.6°C, anhidrosis, and profound CNS dysfunction, typically occurring during summer heat waves in elderly and medically compromised patients. Other cases associated with antipsychotics, however, resembled exertional heatstroke, which occurs primarily in young, healthy people with normal thermoregulatory capacity in whom muscular work in a hot environment exceeds the body's capacity for heat loss. Both forms of heatstroke may result in multiorgan failure, with lactic acidosis, rhabdomyolysis, coagulopathy, and renal failure occurring more commonly in exertional heatstroke. CNS manifestations include delirium, stupor, coma, seizures, pupillary dysfunction, and cerebellar symptoms. Rising temperatures due to climate change are increasing the risk of heatstroke, particularly in urban areas (Martinez et al. 2011).

Antipsychotic-induced heatstroke is a preventable condition. During summer heat waves, psychiatric patients must be warned to avoid excessive heat, sunlight, and exertion and should be urged to drink fluids. Air-conditioning probably represents the most effective way of preventing heatstroke, with even an hour a day helpful. Heatstroke is a medical emergency and may be fatal in up to 50% of cases. All forms of treatment aim at rapid cooling, fluid and electrolyte support, and management of seizures.

Diabetic Ketoacidosis

A serious life-threatening complication of diabetes mellitus is diabetic keto-acidosis (DKA). Having schizophrenia doubles the rate of diabetes, and the added risk with typical and atypical antipsychotics prompted development of guidelines for monitoring glucose given the gravity of this chronic illness and the potential lethality of DKA (American Diabetes Association et al. 2004).

DKA occurs in patients requiring exogenous insulin and can be the first indication that diabetes has developed. DKA most often occurs in type 1 diabetes, but it can occur in type 2 diabetes mellitus. DKA results from persistent hyperglycemia, increased concentration of ketones, and metabolic acidosis. It occurs when insulin is no longer present and glucose cannot be transported into the cells. Hence, fatty acids are broken down for energy, creating an acidotic state. The clinical manifestations are anorexia, nausea, vomiting, polydipsia, and polyuria. One of the first-line laboratory assessments to determine DKA is to test urine for ketones. If DKA is untreated, an altered mental status ensues and eventually coma. The mortality rate is approximately 5% (Umpierrez and Kitabchi 2003).

The most common factor leading to DKA is underlying infection, such as pneumonia or urinary tract infection, which should be investigated. However, psychological stress, pancreatitis, surgery, or myocardial ischemia may also precipitate an episode of DKA. These physiological antecedent stressors are less evident in drug-induced DKA cases (Ely et al. 2013).

In a study comparing typical and atypical antipsychotics in patients with schizophrenia in the Department of Veterans Affairs health care system (Leslie and Rosenheck 2004), 0.2% of all patients on antipsychotic medications required hospitalization for DKA. Hazard ratios for DKA were significant only for clozapine and olanzapine. In addition, the risk plateaued at 90 days for risperidone versus 360 days for olanzapine. Among atypical antipsychotics, quetiapine and risperidone have less risk of diabetes and DKA, whereas ziprasidone and aripiprazole are infrequently associated with DKA, although all have a class black box warning in their package labeling (Guo et al. 2006).

Apart from treatment with clozapine or olanzapine, risk factors for DKA in patients receiving antipsychotics include African American descent, younger age, and schizophrenia (Ramaswamy et al. 2007). The risk is not dose dependent and continues with extended treatment. In patients taking atypical antipsychotics, it is imperative to monitor weight, fasting lipids, and glucose. If hyperglycemia develops, changing to a metabolically neutral agent may reverse glucose elevation. Glucose should be carefully monitored and hypoglycemic agents adjusted accordingly when changing antipsychotic agents in patients with diabetes.

Rhabdomyolysis

Rhabdomyolysis results from injury to skeletal muscle cells, with leakage of myoglobin, aldolase, potassium, lactate dehydrogenase, aspartate transaminase, CPK, and phosphate into the extracellular space and general circulation (Cervellin et al. 2010; Khan 2009). The classic triad of clinical symptoms consists of weakness; muscle pain; and dark, cola-colored urine if myoglobinuria occurs. However, rhabdomyolysis may be detected coincidentally on laboratory examination in patients who are otherwise asymptomatic (Masi et al. 2014). Serious complications include compartment syndromes; arrhythmias from hyperkalemia; disseminated intravascular coagulation; and acute tubular necrosis with renal failure, which occurs in up to 16.5% of patients with myoglobinuria (David 2000). The estimated risk of mortality associated with rhabdomyolysis is 8% (Cervellin et al. 2010).

Diagnosis of rhabdomyolysis can be confirmed by the CPK level, which is the most sensitive indicator of muscle damage and correlates with degree of muscle necrosis. Most authorities agree that a fivefold increase in CPK is consistent with the diagnosis (Walter and Catenacci 2008). Myoglobin is released and cleared earlier than CPK and is therefore less reliable in diagnosing muscle breakdown, and it is not predicted by a specific CPK level. Patients with unexplained elevations of muscle enzymes should be referred for thorough diagnostic evaluation, which includes workup for underlying neuromuscular genetic diseases, infections, hypothyroidism, and trauma (Cervellin et al. 2010; Khan 2009).

Elevations of CPK are often observed in psychiatric patients, who are at risk for several reasons, such as agitation, physical trauma, use of restraints, substance abuse (especially alcohol, cocaine, amphetamines, and phencyclidine), intramuscular injections, prolonged immobility, and dystonia (Melkersson 2006; Meltzer et al. 1996). CPK elevations may occur in association with other disorders (e.g., NMS, heatstroke, serotonin syndrome, seizures) but may be observed independently. For example, Star et al. (2012) found 26 cases of rhabdomyolysis in children and adolescents treated with antipsychotics among reports of adverse reactions in a World Health Organization database; 6 of these cases were associated with NMS, but the other 20 occurred without evidence of NMS. Most symptomatic patients presented with muscle and abdominal pain and dark urine, which usually developed within 2 months of drug initiation or dosage changes (Star et al. 2012).

Among psychotropic drugs, antipsychotics are most often implicated in causing increases in CPK, occasionally resulting in clinical signs of rhabdomyolysis. A review of published cases (Laoutidis and Kioulos 2014) reported a prevalence of significant CPK elevations in 2%–7% of antipsychotic-treated patients. Meltzer et al. (1996) found significant increases in CPK levels in 11 of 121 patients (10%) who received antipsychotic drugs. Peak levels ranged from 1,591 to 177,363 IU/L (median 11,004 IU/L), with only 1 patient developing myoglobinuria. Onset ranged from 5 days to 2 years after initiation of drug treatment, and elevations lasted from 4 to 28 days. Most patients were asymptomatic without complications. CPK elevations were more common with atypical antipsychotics. Similarly, Melkersson (2006) studied 49 patients receiving clozapine (median 66 IU/L, range 30–299 IU/L), olanzapine (median 81 IU/L, range 30–713 IU/L), or typical antipsychotics (median 48 IU/L, range 17–102 IU/L) and found that CPK levels were higher and more often elevated in patients receiving the atypical drugs, although reported increases were minimal in comparison with the findings of Meltzer et al. Laoutidis et al. (2015) found 4 cases of patients treated with amisulpride in a pharmacovigilance database who developed myalgias and elevated CPK concentrations ranging from 1,498 IU/L to 21,018 IU/L. The reasons for overrepresentation of atypical drugs is unclear, but it may be an artifact of increased recognition and reporting in the years since introduction of these drugs (Laoutidis and Kioulos 2014).

Management of frank rhabdomyolysis rests on monitoring to detect clinical signs, including checking CPK levels and myoglobinuria in symptomatic patients. Discontinuation of suspected drugs with correction of any predisposing risk factors and preventing complications are essential. It is important to remember that prescription drugs apart from psychotropics (e.g., statins, antiretrovirals) are also associated with rhabdomyolysis (Klopstock 2008). General supportive measures include aggressive volume and fluid repletion, correction of electrolyte abnormalities, and use of mannitol or alkalinization of the urine to prevent renal failure; hemodialysis may become necessary in some cases. In contrast, the clinical significance of mild or asymptomatic CPK elevations during pharmacotherapy is unclear (Masi et al. 2014). A careful differential diagnosis of CPK elevations should be considered. Although patients with pronounced elevations should be followed and managed to prevent progression to rhabdomyolysis and renal failure and risk factors should be identified and corrected (by holding or switching suspected drugs such as antipsychotics), only limited data suggest that mild asymptomatic CPK elevations correlate with risk of developing NMS or other acute or chronic complications (Hermesh et al. 2002a, 2002b). In most asymptomatic cases of CPK elevation, stopping or switching the antipsychotic drug may be sufficient. Laoutidis and Kioulos (2014) proposed a reasonable management algorithm for detecting, diagnosing, and treating patients who have CPK elevations.

Key Clinical Points

- Severe psychotropic drug reactions are best managed by careful monitoring, familiarity with adverse symptoms, prompt recognition, rapid drug discontinuation, and supportive treatment.
- Adverse central nervous system syndromes are diverse and are associated mostly with antipsychotic and antidepressant drugs.
- Antipsychotic drugs have been associated with arrhythmias and sudden death.
- Severe hepatic toxicity is mostly associated with antiepileptic drugs.
- Severe renal syndromes are primarily associated with lithium, but SIADH is associated with several drug classes.
- Several psychotropic drug classes are associated with hematological toxicity.
- Lives can be saved by maintaining awareness of and a high index of suspicion for potentially lethal iatrogenic drug reactions.
- Severe drug reactions provide evidence for the importance of careful postmarketing surveillance measures to detect rare serious drug reactions.

References

Aarsland D, Perry R, Larsen JP, et al: Neuroleptic sensitivity in Parkinson's disease and parkinsonian dementias. J Clin Psychiatry 66(5):633–637, 2005 15889951

Abadie D, Rousseau V, Logerot S, et al: Serotonin syndrome: analysis of cases registered in the French Pharmacovigilance Database. J Clin Psychopharmacol 35(4):382–388, 2015 26082973

Alawami M, Wasywich C, Cicovic A, Kenedi C: A systematic review of clozapine induced cardiomyopathy. Int J Cardiol 176(2):315–320, 2014 25131906

Alper K, Schwartz KA, Kolts RL, Khan A: Seizure incidence in psychopharmacological clinical trials: an analysis of Food and Drug Administration (FDA) summary basis of approval reports. Biol Psychiatry 62(4):345–354, 2007 17223086

Alvir JM, Lieberman JA, Safferman AZ, et al: Clozapine-induced agranulocytosis: incidence and risk factors in the United States. N Engl J Med 329(3):162–167, 1993 8515788

American Diabetes Association, American Psychiatric Association, American Association of Clinical Endocrinologists, North American Association for the Study of Obesity: Consensus development conference on antipsychotic drugs and obesity and diabetes. J Clin Psychiatry 65(2):267–272, 2004 15003083

Ananth J, Parameswaran S, Gunatilake S, et al: Neuroleptic malignant syndrome and atypical antipsychotic drugs. J Clin Psychiatry 65(4):464–470, 2004 15119907

Armenian P, Mamantov TM, Tsutaoka BT, et al: Multiple MDMA (Ecstasy) overdoses at a rave event: a case series. J Intensive Care Med 28(4):252–258, 2013 22640978

Asnis GM, Henderson MA: EMSAM (deprenyl patch): how a promising antidepressant was underutilized. Neuropsychiatr Dis Treat 10:1911–1923, 2014 25336957

Bark N: Deaths of psychiatric patients during heat waves. Psychiatr Serv 49(8):1088–1090, 1998 9712220

Bartakke S, Abdelhaleem M, Carcao M: Valproate-induced pure red cell aplasia and megakaryocyte dysplasia. Br J Haematol 141(2):133, 2008 18353161

Baskys A: Lewy body dementia: the litmus test for neuroleptic sensitivity and extrapyramidal symptoms. J Clin Psychiatry 65 (suppl 11):16–22, 2004 15264967

Berl T: Vasopressin antagonists. N Engl J Med 372(23):2207–2216, 2015 26039601

Björnsson ES, Bergmann OM, Björnsson HK, et al: Incidence, presentation, and outcomes in patients with drug-induced liver injury in the general population of Iceland. Gastroenterology 144:1419–1425, 2013 23419359

Boora K, Xu J, Hyatt J: Encephalopathy with combined lithium-risperidone administration. Acta Psychiatr Scand 117(5):394–395, discussion 396, 2008 18331580

Boton R, Gaviria M, Batlle DC: Prevalence, pathogenesis, and treatment of renal dysfunction associated with chronic lithium therapy. Am J Kidney Dis 10(5):329–345, 1987 3314489

Boyer EW, Shannon M: The serotonin syndrome. N Engl J Med 352(11):1112–1120, 2005 15784664

Browne B, Linter S: Monoamine oxidase inhibitors and narcotic analgesics: a critical review of the implications for treatment. Br J Psychiatry 151:210–212, 1987 2891392

Canuso CM, Goldman MB: Clozapine restores water balance in schizophrenic patients with polydipsia-hyponatremia syndrome. J Neuropsychiatry Clin Neurosci 11(1):86–90, 1999 9990561

Cardamone L, Salzberg MR, O'Brien TJ, Jones NC: Antidepressant therapy in epilepsy: can treating the comorbidities affect the underlying disorder? Br J Pharmacol 168(7):1531–1554, 2013 23146067

Caroff S: Neuroleptic malignant syndrome, in Neuroleptic Malignant Syndrome and Related Conditions, 2nd Edition. Edited by Mann S, Caroff S, Keck PE Jr, Lazarus A. Arlington, VA, American Psychiatric Publishing, 2003a, pp 1–44

Caroff SN: Hyperthermia associated with other neurpsychiatric drugs, in Neuroleptic Malignant Syndrome and Related Conditions, 2nd Edition. Edited by Mann S, Caroff S, Keck PE Jr, Lazarus A. Arlington, VA, American Psychiatric Publishing, 2003b, pp 93–120

Caroff SN, Campbell EC: Risk of neuroleptic malignant syndrome in patients with NMDAR encephalitis. Neurol Sci 36:479–480, 2015

Caroff SN, Mann SC, Keck PE Jr, Francis A: Residual catatonic state following neuroleptic malignant syndrome. J Clin Psychopharmacol 20(2):257–259, 2000 10770467

Caroff SN, Mann SC, Gliatto MF, et al: Psychiatric manifestations of acute viral encephalitis. Psychiatr Ann 31:193–204, 2001a

Caroff SN, Rosenberg H, Mann SC, et al: Neuroleptic malignant syndrome in the perioperative setting. Am J Anesthesiol 28:387–393, 2001b

Cervellin G, Comelli I, Lippi G: Rhabdomyolysis: historical background, clinical, diagnostic and therapeutic features. Clin Chem Lab Med 48:749–756, 2010 20298139

Chalasani N, Bonkovsky HL, Fontana R, et al: Features and outcomes of 899 patients with drug-induced liver injury: the DILIN Prospective Study. Gastroenterology.148(7):1340–1352.e7, 2015 25754159

Chaudhry MM, Abrar M, Mutahir K, Mendoza C: Oxcarbazepine-induced hemolytic anemia in a geriatric patient. Am J Ther 15(2):187–189, 2008 18356642

Chen M, Borlak J, Tong W: High lipophilicity and high daily dose of oral medications are associated with significant risk for drug-induced liver injury. Hepatology 58(1):388–396, 2013 23258593

Clark WG, Lipton JM: Drug-related heatstroke. Pharmacol Ther 26(3):345–388, 1984 6152566

Cohen WJ, Cohen NH: Lithium carbonate, haloperidol, and irreversible brain damage. JAMA 230(9):1283–1287, 1974 4479505

Culpepper L: Reducing the burden of difficult-to-treat major depressive disorder: revisiting monoamine oxidase inhibitor therapy. Prim Care Companion CNS Disord 15(5):15, 2013 24511450

David WS: Myoglobinuria. Neurol Clin 18(1):215–243, 2000 10658177

De Ponti F, Poluzzi E, Montanaro N: Organising evidence on QT prolongation and occurrence of torsades de pointes with non-antiarrhythmic drugs: a call for consensus. Eur J Clin Pharmacol 57(3):185–209, 2001 11497335

Devarbhavi H, Andrade RJ: Drug-induced liver injury due to antimicrobials, central nervous system agents, and nonsteroidal anti-inflammatory drugs. Semin Liver Dis 34(2):145–161, 2014 24879980

Dhir R, Brown DK, Olden KW: Drug-induced pancreatitis: a practical review. Drugs Today (Barc) 43(7):499–507, 2007 17728850

Dunkley EJ, Isbister GK, Sibbritt D, et al: The Hunter Serotonin Toxicity Criteria: simple and accurate diagnostic decision rules for serotonin toxicity. QJM 96:635–642, 2003 12925718

Ellison DH, Berl T: Clinical practice: the syndrome of inappropriate antidiuresis. N Engl J Med 356(20):2064–2072, 2007 17507705

Ely SF, Neitzel AR, Gill JR: Fatal diabetic ketoacidosis and antipsychotic medication. J Forensic Sci 58(2):398–403, 2013 23278567

Factor SA, Santiago A: Parkinsonism-hyperpyrexia syndrome in Parkinson's disease, in Movement Disorder Emergencies: Diagnosis and Treatment. Edited by Frucht SJ, Fahn S. Totowa, NJ, Humana Press, 2005, pp 29–40

Feinstein RE, Khawaja IS, Nurenberg JR, Frishman WH: Cardiovascular effects of psychotropic drugs. Curr Probl Cardiol 27(5):190–240, 2002 12060825

Flanagan RJ, Dunk L: Haematological toxicity of drugs used in psychiatry. Hum Psychopharmacol 23 (suppl 1):27–41, 2008 18098216

Fontana RJ, Hayashi PH, Gu J, et al: Idiosyncratic drug-induced liver injury is associated with substantial morbidity and mortality within 6 months from onset. Gastroenterology 147:96–108, 2014 24681128

Gardner DM, Shulman KI, Walker SE, Tailor SA: The making of a user friendly MAOI diet. J Clin Psychiatry 57(3):99–104, 1996 8617704

Gareri P, De Fazio P, Russo E, et al: The safety of clozapine in the elderly. Expert Opin Drug Saf 7(5):525–538, 2008 18759705

Garofeanu CG, Weir M, Rosas-Arellano MP, et al: Causes of reversible nephrogenic diabetes insipidus: a systematic review. Am J Kidney Dis 45(4):626–637, 2005 15806465

Gerstner T, Büsing D, Bell N, et al: Valproic acid–induced pancreatitis: 16 new cases and a review of the literature. J Gastroenterol 42(1):39–48, 2007 17322992

Gill SS, Rochon PA, Herrmann N, et al: Atypical antipsychotic drugs and risk of ischaemic stroke: population based retrospective cohort study. BMJ 330(7489):445, 2005 15668211

Gillman PK: CNS toxicity involving methylene blue: the exemplar for understanding and predicting drug interactions that precipitate serotonin toxicity. J Psychopharmacol 25(3):429–436, 2011 20142303

Glassman AH, Bigger JT Jr: Antipsychotic drugs: prolonged QTc interval, torsade de pointes, and sudden death. Am J Psychiatry 158(11):1774–1782, 2001 11691681

Goldman SA: Lithium and neuroleptics in combination: the spectrum of neurotoxicity [corrected]. Psychopharmacol Bull 32(3):299–309, 1996 8961772

Grace JB, Thompson P: Neuroleptic malignant like syndrome in two patients on cholinesterase inhibitors. Int J Geriatr Psychiatry 21(2):193–194, 2006 16440373

Guo JJ, Keck PE Jr, Corey-Lisle PK, et al: Risk of diabetes mellitus associated with atypical antipsychotic use among patients with bipolar disorder: a retrospective, population-based, case-control study. J Clin Psychiatry 67(7):1055–1061, 2006 16889448

Gurrera RJ, Caroff SN, Cohen A, et al: An international consensus study of neuroleptic malignant syndrome diagnostic criteria using the Delphi method. J Clin Psychiatry 72(9):1222–1228, 2011 21733489

Haas SJ, Hill R, Krum H, et al: Clozapine-associated myocarditis: a review of 116 cases of suspected myocarditis associated with the use of clozapine in Australia during 1993–2003. Drug Saf 30(1):47–57, 2007 17194170

Halperin D, Reber G: Influence of antidepressants on hemostasis. Dialogues Clin Neurosci 9(1):47–59, 2007 17506225

Harada T, Mitsuoka K, Kumagai R, et al: Clinical features of malignant syndrome in Parkinson's disease and related neurological disorders. Parkinsonism Relat Disord 9 (suppl 1):S15–S23, 2003 12735911

Hennessy S, Bilker WB, Knauss JS, et al: Cardiac arrest and ventricular arrhythmia in patients taking antipsychotic drugs: cohort study using administrative data. BMJ 325(7372):1070, 2002 12424166

Hermesh H, Manor I, Shiloh R, et al: High serum creatinine kinase level: possible risk factor for neuroleptic malignant syndrome. J Clin Psychopharmacol 22(3):252–256, 2002a 12006894

Hermesh H, Stein D, Manor I, et al: Serum creatine kinase levels in untreated hospitalized adolescents during acute psychosis. J Am Acad Child Adolesc Psychiatry 41(9):1045–1053, 2002b 12218425

Herrmann N, Mamdani M, Lanctôt KL: Atypical antipsychotics and risk of cerebrovascular accidents. Am J Psychiatry 161(6):1113–1115, 2004 15169702

Hohmann N, Mikus G, Czock D: Effects and risks associated with novel psychoactive substances: mislabeling and sale as bath salts, spice, and research chemicals. Dtsch Arztebl Int 111(9):139–147, 2014 24661585

Hsieh PH, Hsiao FY, Gau SS, Gau CS: Use of antipsychotics and risk of cerebrovascular events in schizophrenic patients: a nested case-control study. J Clin Psychopharmacol 33(3):299–305, 2013 23609396

Hung CC, Lin CH, Lan TH, Chan CH: The association of selective serotonin reuptake inhibitors use and stroke in geriatric population. Am J Geriatr Psychiatry 21:811–815, 2013 23567390

Hussain A, Burke J: Mirtazapine associated with recurrent pancreatitis—a case report. J Psychopharmacol 22(3):336–337, 2008 18208920

Jefferson JW: A clinician's guide to monitoring kidney function in lithium-treated patients. J Clin Psychiatry 71(9):1153–1157, 2010 20923621

Jeste DV, Blazer D, Casey D, et al: ACNP White Paper: update on use of antipsychotic drugs in elderly persons with dementia. Neuropsychopharmacology 33(5):957–970, 2008 17637610

Josiassen RC, Goldman M, Jessani M, et al: Double-blind, placebo-controlled, multicenter trial of a vasopressin V2-receptor antagonist in patients with schizophrenia and hyponatremia. Biol Psychiatry 64(12):1097–1100, 2008 18692175

Kales HC, Valenstein M, Kim HM, et al: Mortality risk in patients with dementia treated with antipsychotics versus other psychiatric medications. Am J Psychiatry 164(10):1568–1576, quiz 1623, 2007 17898349

Kales HC, Kim HM, Zivin K, et al: Risk of mortality among individual antipsychotics in patients with dementia. Am J Psychiatry 169(1):71–79, 2012 22193526

Kao LW, Furbee RB: Drug-induced q-T prolongation. Med Clin North Am 89(6):1125–1144, x, 2005 16227057

Kaplan PW, Birbeck G: Lithium-induced confusional states: nonconvulsive status epilepticus or triphasic encephalopathy? Epilepsia 47(12):2071–2074, 2006 17201705

Karaosmanoglu AD, Butros SR, Arellano R: Imaging findings of renal toxicity in patients on chronic lithium therapy. Diagn Interv Radiol 19(4):299–303, 2013 23439253

Khan FY: Rhabdomyolysis: a review of the literature. Neth J Med 67(9):272–283, 2009 19841484

Khanna A: Acquired nephrogenic diabetes insipidus. Semin Nephrol 26(3):244–248, 2006 16713497

Klopstock T: Drug-induced myopathies. Curr Opin Neurol 21(5):590–595, 2008 18769254

Koller EA, Cross JT, Doraiswamy PM, Malozowski SN: Pancreatitis associated with atypical antipsychotics: from the Food and Drug Administration's MedWatch surveillance system and published reports. Pharmacotherapy 23(9):1123–1130, 2003 14524644

Krishnan KR: Revisiting monoamine oxidase inhibitors. J Clin Psychiatry 68 (suppl 8):35–41, 2007 17640156

Laoutidis ZG, Kioulos KT: Antipsychotic-induced elevation of creatine kinase: a systematic review of the literature and recommendations for the clinical practice. Psychopharmacology (Berl) 231(22):4255–4270, 2014 25319963

Laoutidis ZG, Konstantinidis A, Grohmann R, et al: Reversible amisulpride-induced elevation of creatine kinase (CK): a case series from the German AMSP Pharmacovigilance Project. Pharmacopsychiatry 48(4–5):178–181, 2015 25984709

Lee TF, Mora F, Myers RD: Dopamine and thermoregulation: an evaluation with special reference to dopaminergic pathways. Neurosci Biobehav Rev 9(4):589–598, 1985 3001601

Lemstra AW, Schoenmaker N, Rozemuller-Kwakkel AJ, van Gool WA: The association of neuroleptic sensitivity in Lewy body disease with a false positive clinical diagnosis of Creutzfeldt-Jakob disease. Int J Geriatr Psychiatry 21(11):1031–1035, 2006 16955430

Lertxundi U, Ruiz AI, Aspiazu MA, et al: Adverse reactions to antipsychotics in Parkinson disease: an analysis of the Spanish pharmacovigilance database. Clin Neuropharmacol 38(3):69–84, 2015 25970275

Leslie DL, Rosenheck RA: Incidence of newly diagnosed diabetes attributable to atypical antipsychotic medications. Am J Psychiatry 161(9):1709–1711, 2004 15337666

Lherm T, Lottin F, Larbi D, et al: Torsade de pointes after poisoning with fluoxetine alone [in French]. Presse Med 29(6):306–307, 2000 10719447

Lheureux PE, Penaloza A, Zahir S, Gris M: Science review: carnitine in the treatment of valproic acid–induced toxicity—what is the evidence? Crit Care 9(5):431–440, 2005 16277730

Liperoti R, Gambassi G, Lapane KL, et al: Conventional and atypical antipsychotics and the risk of hospitalization for ventricular arrhythmias or cardiac arrest. Arch Intern Med 165(6):696–701, 2005 15795349

Lopez AM, Hendrickson RG: Toxin-induced hepatic injury. Emerg Med Clin North Am 32(1):103–125, 2014 24275171

Mackay FJ, Dunn NR, Mann RD: Antidepressants and the serotonin syndrome in general practice. Br J Gen Pract 49(448):871–874, 1999 10818650

Malaguarnera M: Acetyl-L-carnitine in hepatic encephalopathy. Metab Brain Dis 28(2):193–199, 2013 23389620

Mann SC: Thermoregulatory mechanisms and antipsychotic drug–related heatstroke, in Neuroleptic Malignant Syndrome and Related Conditions, 2nd Edition. Edited by Mann SC, Caroff SN, Keck PE Jr, Lazarus A. Arlington, VA, American Psychiatric Publishing, 2003, pp 45–74

Mann SC, Boger WP: Psychotropic drugs, summer heat and humidity, and hyperpyrexia: a danger restated. Am J Psychiatry 135(9):1097–1100, 1978 29501

Mann SC, Caroff SN, Bleier HR, et al: Lethal catatonia. Am J Psychiatry 143(11):1374–1381, 1986 3777225

Mann SC, Caroff SN, Fricchione G, Campbell EC: Central dopamine hypoactivity and the pathogenesis of neuroleptic malignant syndrome. Psychiatr Ann 30:363–374, 2000

Martinez GS, Imai C, Masumo K: Local heat stroke prevention plans in Japan: characteristics and elements for public health adaptation to climate change. Int J Environ Res Public Health 8(12):4563–4581, 2011 22408589

Martino G, Capasso M, Nasuti M, et al: Dopamine transporter single-photon emission computerized tomography supports diagnosis of akinetic crisis of parkinsonism and of neuroleptic malignant syndrome. Medicine (Baltimore) 94(13):e649, 2015 25837755

Marwick KF, Taylor M, Walker SW: Antipsychotics and abnormal liver function tests: systematic review. Clin Neuropharmacol 35(5):244–253, 2012 22986798

Masi G, Milone A, Viglione V, et al: Massive asymptomatic creatine kinase elevation in youth during antipsychotic drug treatment: case reports and critical review of the literature. J Child Adolesc Psychopharmacol 24(10):536–542, 2014 25387323

Matsumoto T, Kawanishi C, Isojima D, et al: Neuroleptic malignant syndrome induced by donepezil. Int J Neuropsychopharmacol 7(1):101–103, 2004 14731314

Maust DT, Kim HM, Seyfried LS, et al: Antipsychotics, other psychotropics, and the risk of death in patients with dementia: number needed to harm. JAMA Psychiatry 72(5):438–445, 2015 25786075

McKeith IG, Perry RH, Fairbairn AF, et al: Operational criteria for senile dementia of Lewy body type (SDLT). Psychol Med 22(4):911–922, 1992 1362617

McKeith IG, Dickson DW, Lowe J, et al; Consortium on DLB: Diagnosis and management of dementia with Lewy bodies: third report of the DLB Consortium. Neurology 65(12):1863–1872, 2005 16237129

Mehtonen OP, Aranko K, Mälkonen L, Vapaatalo H: A survey of sudden death associated with the use of antipsychotic or antidepressant drugs: 49 cases in Finland. Acta Psychiatr Scand 84(1):58–64, 1991 1681681

Melkersson K: Serum creatine kinase levels in chronic psychosis patients—a comparison between atypical and conventional antipsychotics. Prog Neuropsychopharmacol Biol Psychiatry 30(7):1277–1282, 2006 16806625

Meltzer HY, Cola PA, Parsa M: Marked elevations of serum creatine kinase activity associated with antipsychotic drug treatment. Neuropsychopharmacology 15(4):395–405, 1996 8887994

Meltzer HY, Davidson M, Glassman AH, Vieweg WV: Assessing cardiovascular risks versus clinical benefits of atypical antipsychotic drug treatment. J Clin Psychiatry 63 (suppl 9):25–29, 2002 12088173

Merrill DB, Dec GW, Goff DC: Adverse cardiac effects associated with clozapine. J Clin Psychopharmacol 25(1):32–41, 2005 15643098

Miller F, Menninger J: Correlation of neuroleptic dose and neurotoxicity in patients given lithium and a neuroleptic. Hosp Community Psychiatry 38(11):1219–1221, 1987 2889659

Modai I, Hirschmann S, Rava A, et al: Sudden death in patients receiving clozapine treatment: a preliminary investigation. J Clin Psychopharmacol 20(3):325–327, 2000 10831019

Moeller HB, Rittig S, Fenton RA: Nephrogenic diabetes insipidus: essential insights into the molecular background and potential therapies for treatment. Endocr Rev 34(2):278–301, 2013 23360744

Montgomery SA: Antidepressants and seizures: emphasis on newer agents and clinical implications. Int J Clin Pract 59(12):1435–1440, 2005 16351676

Movig KL, Janssen MW, de Waal Malefijt J, et al: Relationship of serotonergic antidepressants and need for blood transfusion in orthopedic surgical patients. Arch Intern Med 163(19):2354–2358, 2003 14581256

Nakamura M, Yasunaga H, Miyata H, et al: Mortality of neuroleptic malignant syndrome induced by typical and atypical antipsychotic drugs: a propensity-matched analysis from the Japanese Diagnosis Procedure Combination database. J Clin Psychiatry 73(4):427–430, 2012 22154901

Nasreddine W, Beydoun A: Valproate-induced thrombocytopenia: a prospective monotherapy study. Epilepsia 49(3):438–445, 2008 18031547

Nguyen C, Xie L, Alley S, et al: Epidemiology and economic burden of serotonin syndrome with concomitant use of serotonergic agents in the U.S. clinical practice. Poster presented at the 2015 American Society of Clinical Psychopharmacology Annual Meeting, Miami, FL, June 22–25, 2015

Nooijen PM, Carvalho F, Flanagan RJ: Haematological toxicity of clozapine and some other drugs used in psychiatry. Hum Psychopharmacol 26(2):112–119, 2011 21416507

Noskin O, Jafarimojarrad E, Libman RB, Nelson JL: Diffuse cerebral vasoconstriction (Call-Fleming syndrome) and stroke associated with antidepressants. Neurology 67(1):159–160, 2006 16832100

Oates JA, Sjoerdsma A: Neurologic effects of tryptophan in patients receiving a monoamine oxidase inhibitor. Neurology 10:1076–1078, 1960 13730138

Oliveira JL, Silva Júnior GB, Abreu KL, et al: Lithium nephrotoxicity. Rev Assoc Med Bras 56(5):600–606, 2010 21152836

Page LA, Hajat S, Kovats RS, Howard LM: Temperature-related deaths in people with psychosis, dementia and substance misuse. Br J Psychiatry 200(6):485–490, 2012 22661680

Picard LS, Lindsay S, Strawn JR, et al: Atypical neuroleptic malignant syndrome: diagnostic controversies and considerations. Pharmacotherapy 28(4):530–535, 2008 18363536

Poston KL, Frucht SJ: Movement disorder emergencies. J Neurol 255 (suppl 4):2–13, 2008 18821080

Presne C, Fakhouri F, Noël LH, et al: Lithium-induced nephropathy: rate of progression and prognostic factors. Kidney Int 64(2):585–592, 2003 12846754

Prior A, Laursen TM, Larsen KK, et al: Post-stroke mortality, stroke severity, and preadmission antipsychotic medicine use—a population-based cohort study. PLoS One 9(1):e84103, 2014 24416196

Radomski JW, Dursun SM, Reveley MA, Kutcher SP: An exploratory approach to the serotonin syndrome: an update of clinical phenomenology and revised diagnostic criteria. Med Hypotheses 55(3):218–224, 2000 10985912

Raedler TJ, Wiedemann K: Lithium-induced nephropathies. Psychopharmacol Bull 40(2):134–149, 2007 17514192

Ramaswamy K, Kozma CM, Nasrallah H: Risk of diabetic ketoacidosis after exposure to risperidone or olanzapine. Drug Saf 30(7):589–599, 2007 17604410

Rapaport MH: Dietary restrictions and drug interactions with monoamine oxidase inhibitors: the state of the art. J Clin Psychiatry 68 (suppl 8):42–46, 2007 17640157

Ray WA, Meredith S, Thapa PB, et al: Antipsychotics and the risk of sudden cardiac death. Arch Gen Psychiatry 58(12):1161–1167, 2001 11735845

Reilly JG, Ayis SA, Ferrier IN, et al: Thioridazine and sudden unexplained death in psychiatric inpatients. Br J Psychiatry 180:515–522, 2002 12042230

Rej S, Herrmann N, Shulman K: The effects of lithium on renal function in older adults—a systematic review. J Geriatr Psychiatry Neurol 25(1):51–61, 2012 22467847

Rochon PA, Normand SL, Gomes T, et al: Antipsychotic therapy and short-term serious events in older adults with dementia. Arch Intern Med 168(10):1090–1096, 2008 18504337

Roose SP, Glassman AH, Dalack GW: Depression, heart disease, and tricyclic antidepressants. J Clin Psychiatry 50(suppl):12–16, discussion 17, 1989 2661547

Rosebush PI, Mazurek MF: Serum iron and neuroleptic malignant syndrome. Lancet 338(8760):149–151, 1991 1677067

Sala M, Coppa F, Cappucciati C, et al: Antidepressants: their effects on cardiac channels, QT prolongation and torsade de pointes. Curr Opin Investig Drugs 7(3):256–263, 2006 16555686

Sato Y, Asoh T, Metoki N, Satoh K: Efficacy of methylprednisolone pulse therapy on neuroleptic malignant syndrome in Parkinson's disease. J Neurol Neurosurg Psychiatry 74(5):574–576, 2003 12700295

Schneeweiss S, Setoguchi S, Brookhart A, et al: Risk of death associated with the use of conventional versus atypical antipsychotic drugs among elderly patients. CMAJ 176(5):627–632, 2007 17325327

Schneider LS, Tariot PN, Dagerman KS, et al; CATIE-AD Study Group: Effectiveness of atypical antipsychotic drugs in patients with Alzheimer's disease. N Engl J Med 355(15):1525–1538, 2006 17035647

Segura-Bruna N, Rodriguez-Campello A, Puente V, Roquer J: Valproate-induced hyperammonemic encephalopathy. Acta Neurol Scand 114(1):1–7, 2006 16774619

Serrano-Dueñas M: Neuroleptic malignant syndrome-like, or—dopaminergic malignant syndrome—due to levodopa therapy withdrawal: clinical features in 11 patients. Parkinsonism Relat Disord 9(3):175–178, 2003 12573874

Sgro C, Clinard F, Ouazir K, et al: Incidence of drug-induced hepatic injuries: a French population-based study. Hepatology 36(2):451–455, 2002 12143055

Shin D, Oh YH, Eom CS, Park SM: Use of selective serotonin reuptake inhibitors and risk of stroke: a systematic review and meta-analysis. J Neurol 261(4):686–695, 2014 24477492

Sicouri S, Antzelevitch C: Sudden cardiac death secondary to antidepressant and antipsychotic drugs. Expert Opin Drug Saf 7(2):181–194, 2008 18324881

Siegel AJ: Hyponatremia in psychiatric patients: update on evaluation and management. Harv Rev Psychiatry 16(1):13–24, 2008 18306096

Singhal AB, Caviness VS, Begleiter AF, et al: Cerebral vasoconstriction and stroke after use of serotonergic drugs. Neurology 58(1):130–133, 2002 11781419

Sink KM, Holden KF, Yaffe K: Pharmacological treatment of neuropsychiatric symptoms of dementia: a review of the evidence. JAMA 293(5):596–608, 2005 15687315

Smith FA, Wittmann CW, Stern TA: Medical complications of psychiatric treatment. Crit Care Clin 24(4):635–656, vii, 2008 18929938

Spigset O, Hägg S, Bate A: Hepatic injury and pancreatitis during treatment with serotonin reuptake inhibitors: data from the World Health Organization (WHO) database of adverse drug reactions. Int Clin Psychopharmacol 18(3):157–161, 2003 12702895

Spivak B, Maline DI, Kozyrev VN, et al: Frequency of neuroleptic malignant syndrome in a large psychiatric hospital in Moscow. Eur Psychiatry 15(5):330–333, 2000 10954877

Spring G, Frankel M: New data on lithium and haloperidol incompatibility. Am J Psychiatry 138(6):818–821, 1981 6113770

Star K, Iessa N, Almandil NB, et al: Rhabdomyolysis reported for children and adolescents treated with antipsychotic medicines: a case series analysis. J Child Adolesc Psychopharmacol 22(6):440–451, 2012 23234587

Sternbach H: The serotonin syndrome. Am J Psychiatry 148(6):705–713, 1991 2035713

Sterns RH: Disorders of plasma sodium—causes, consequences, and correction. N Engl J Med 372(1):55–65, 2015 25551526

Stevens DL: Association between selective serotonin-reuptake inhibitors, second-generation antipsychotics, and neuroleptic malignant syndrome. Ann Pharmacother 42(9):1290–1297, 2008 18628446

Stimmel GL, Dopheide JA: Psychotropic drug–induced reductions in seizure threshold: incidence and consequences. CNS Drugs 5:37–50, 1996

Straus SM, Bleumink GS, Dieleman JP, et al: Antipsychotics and the risk of sudden cardiac death. Arch Intern Med 164(12):1293–1297, 2004 15226162

Strawn JR, Keck PE Jr, Caroff SN: Neuroleptic malignant syndrome. Am J Psychiatry 164(6):870–876, 2007 17541044

Stübner S, Rustenbeck E, Grohmann R, et al: Severe and uncommon involuntary movement disorders due to psychotropic drugs. Pharmacopsychiatry 37 (suppl 1):S54–S64, 2004 15052515

Sultzer DL, Davis SM, Tariot PN, et al; CATIE-AD Study Group: Clinical symptom responses to atypical antipsychotic medications in Alzheimer's disease: phase 1 outcomes from the CATIE-AD effectiveness trial. Am J Psychiatry 165(7):844–854, 2008 18519523

Swartz CM: Olanzapine-lithium encephalopathy (letter). Psychosomatics 42(4):370, 2001 11496035

Tarabar AF, Hoffman RS, Nelson L: Citalopram overdose: late presentation of torsades de pointes (TdP) with cardiac arrest. J Med Toxicol 4(2):101–105, 2008 18570170

Tohen M, Castillo J, Baldessarini RJ, et al: Blood dyscrasias with carbamazepine and valproate: a pharmacoepidemiological study of 2,228 patients at risk. Am J Psychiatry 152(3):413–418, 1995 7864268

Ueda M, Hamamoto M, Nagayama H, et al: Biochemical alterations during medication withdrawal in Parkinson's disease with and without neuroleptic malignant-like syndrome. J Neurol Neurosurg Psychiatry 71(1):111–113, 2001 11413275

Umpierrez GE, Kitabchi AE: Diabetic ketoacidosis: risk factors and management strategies. Treat Endocrinol 2(2):95–108, 2003 15871546

U.S. Food and Drug Administration: Public health advisory: deaths with antipsychotics in elderly patients with behavioral disturbances. Washington, DC, U.S. Food and Drug Administration, April 11, 2005. Available at: http://www.fda.gov/drugs/drugsafety/postmarketdrugsafetyinformationforpatientsandproviders/ucm053171. Accessed March 30, 2016.

Verdel BM, Souverein PC, Meenks SD, et al: Use of serotonergic drugs and the risk of bleeding. Clin Pharmacol Ther 89(1):89–96, 2011 21107313

Voican CS, Corruble E, Naveau S, Perlemuter G: Antidepressant-induced liver injury: a review for clinicians. Am J Psychiatry 171(4):404–415, 2014 24362450

Walter LA, Catenacci MH: Rhabdomyolysis. Hosp Physician 44:25–31, 2008

Wang PS, Schneeweiss S, Avorn J, et al: Risk of death in elderly users of conventional vs. atypical antipsychotic medications. N Engl J Med 353(22):2335–2341, 2005 16319382

Wang S, Linkletter C, Dore D, et al: Age, antipsychotics, and the risk of ischemic stroke in the Veterans Health Administration. Stroke 43(1):28–31, 2012 22033997

Wehmeier PM, Heiser P, Remschmidt H: Myocarditis, pericarditis and cardiomyopathy in patients treated with clozapine. J Clin Pharm Ther 30(1):91–96, 2005 15659009

Weintraub D, Hurtig HI: Presentation and management of psychosis in Parkinson's disease and dementia with Lewy bodies. Am J Psychiatry 164(10):1491–1498, 2007 17898337

Werneke U, Ott M, Renberg ES, et al: A decision analysis of long-term lithium treatment and the risk of renal failure. Acta Psychiatr Scand 126(3):186–197, 2012 22404233

Wong J, Delva N: Clozapine-induced seizures: recognition and treatment. Can J Psychiatry 52(7):457–463, 2007 17688010

Zaccara G, Franciotta D, Perucca E: Idiosyncratic adverse reactions to antiepileptic drugs. Epilepsia 48(7):1223–1244, 2007 17386054

3

Alternative Routes of Drug Administration

James A. Owen, Ph.D.

Ericka L. Crouse, Pharm.D.

Psychotropic medications are usually delivered orally, but this administration route may not be the best or may not even be possible for many patients. Oral administration of medications may be difficult in patients who are medically compromised, including patients with severe nausea or vomiting, dysphagia, or severe malabsorption; unconscious or uncooperative patients; and patients who are unable or unwilling to take medications by mouth (see Table 3–1). In such situations, a non-oral route is preferred or necessary.

Medication administration is especially problematic with patients who are cognitively impaired and acutely psychotic. With an alternative delivery route, adherence may be more easily verified and may improve if the route is perceived as being more convenient. Non-oral routes of administration in-

Table 3–1.   Situations potentially requiring alternative routes of administration

Severe nausea and vomiting

Cancer chemotherapy

Severe gastroparesis

Gastric outlet obstruction

Intestinal obstruction

Esophageal disorders

Severe gastroesophageal reflux disease

Carcinoma

Severe dysphagia (e.g., poststroke)

Severe malabsorption

Short gut syndrome

Inflammatory bowel disease

Pancreatic insufficiency

Dysphagia

Parkinson's disease

Amyotrophic lateral sclerosis

Delirium, stupor, or coma

Patient's refusal of oral medication

NPO (nothing per oral) orders in effect

Perioperative period

Intra-abdominal abscesses or fistulae

clude intravenous, intramuscular, subcutaneous, sublingual or buccal, rectal, topical or transdermal, and intranasal.

In this chapter, we review the availability of non-oral formulations of anxiolytics and sedative-hypnotics, antidepressants, antipsychotics, mood stabilizers, psychostimulants, and cognitive enhancers. Many formulations discussed are commercially available, although not necessarily in the United States or Canada (see Table 3–2). We also report customized formulations for a few agents. Caution is indicated when using a formulation for unapproved purposes and for which adequate studies of safety and efficacy are lacking.

Properties of Specific Routes of Administration

Intravenous Administration

Intravenous administration delivers drug directly into the patient's circulation and avoids first-pass metabolism. It provides rapid drug distribution with 100% bioavailability and ensures compliance. The rate of drug delivery can be controlled from very rapid to slow infusion. Potential complications include difficulty with venous access, infiltration, and infection. Intravenous forms of several benzodiazepines (in the United States and Canada) and valproate (in the United States) are available. Intravenous administration of short-acting intramuscular forms of some typical antipsychotics is a common clinical practice.

Intramuscular Administration

Fast absorption, avoidance of first-pass metabolism, and ensured compliance are advantages of intramuscular administration, but bioavailability is often less than 100% because of drug retention or metabolism by local tissues. Intramuscular injections should be avoided in cachectic patients and those with poor muscle perfusion, such as cardiac insufficiency. Repeated injections of some drugs may cause muscle irritation, necrosis, or abscesses.

Sublingual or Buccal Administration

The rapid sublingual absorption and good bioavailability of small lipid–soluble drugs suggest that many psychotropic medications could be administered sublingually. Drugs absorbed sublingually avoid first-pass metabolism and may

Table 3–2. Non-oral preparations of psychotropic medications

Medication	Route of administration						
	IV	IM	Sublingual	Rectal	Transdermal	Intranasal	Oral inhalation
Anxiolytics							
Alprazolam			n				
Clonazepam			n	n			
Diazepam	US, C	US, C[a]	n	US, C			
Flunitrazepam	O		n				
Lorazepam	US, C	US, C	C	n		n	
Lormetazepam			n				
Midazolam	US, C	US, C	n	n		n	
Prazepam			n				
Temazepam			O				
Triazolam			n	n			
Hypnotics							
Zolpidem			US				US
Antidepressants							
Amitriptyline	O			n			
Citalopram	O						
Clomipramine	O			n			

Table 3–2. Non-oral preparations of psychotropic medications (*continued*)

Medication		Route of administration					
	IV	IM	Sublingual	Rectal	Transdermal	Intranasal	Oral inhalation
Antidepressants (*continued*)							
Doxepin	O			n			
Fluoxetine				n			
Imipramine	O			n			
Maprotiline	O						
Mirtazapine	n						
Selegiline			US[b]		US		
Trazodone	O			n			
Viloxazine	O						
Antipsychotics, atypical							
Aripiprazole		US					
Asenapine			US				
Olanzapine		US, C					
		Depot: US					
Paliperidone		Depot: US					
Risperidone		Depot: US, C					
Ziprasidone		US					

Table 3–2.   Non-oral preparations of psychotropic medications *(continued)*

Medication	IV	IM	Sublingual	Rectal	Transdermal	Intranasal	Oral inhalation
Antipsychotics, typical							
Chlorpromazine		US, C					
Droperidol	US, C	US, C					
Flupenthixol		Depot: C					
Fluphenazine		US, C					
		SubQ: C					
		Depot: US, C					
Haloperidol		US, C					
		Depot: US, C					
Loxapine		C					US
Methotrimeprazine		C					
Pipotiazine		Depot: C					
Prochlorperazine		US, C		US, C			
Promazine		C					
Thiothixene		US					
Zuclopenthixol		C					
		Depot: C					

Table 3–2. Non-oral preparations of psychotropic medications (*continued*)

Medication	Route of administration						
	IV	IM	Sublingual	Rectal	Transdermal	Intranasal	Oral inhalation
Mood stabilizers							
Carbamazepine				n			
Lamotrigine				n			
Topiramate				n			
Valproate	US			n			
Psychostimulants							
Dextroamphetamine				n			
Methamphetamine						n	
Methylphenidate					US		
Cognitive enhancers							
Galantamine						n	
Rivastigmine					US, C		

Note.   Depot=long-acting depot formulation; IM=intramuscular; IV=intravenous; n=noncommercial formulation; SubQ=subcutaneous. Approved formulations; C=Canada; O=country other than United States or Canada; US=United States. Noncommercial formulations may be available in Europe but not in the United States. For these formulations, intranasal and sublingual formulations may be administered from injectable formulations; sublingual formulation may also be a tablet administered sublingually; rectal dosage forms are often compounded.

[a]But not advised because of erratic absorption.

[b]Buccal administration. (See text for details.)

Source.   Compiled in part from Gopalakrishna et al. 2013; Kaminsky et al. 2015; Lexicomp Inc. 2015; Thompson and DiMartini 1999.

have fewer gastrointestinal adverse effects. Sublingual delivery can be used in patients who are fasting, have difficulty swallowing, or are unable to absorb medication from the gastrointestinal tract. Sublingual administration may not be practical in patients with severe nausea or who cannot tolerate the taste of some medications.

A few psychotropics are available in a sublingual or buccal form, including the anxiolytic lorazepam (in Canada), the hypnotic zolpidem, the monoamine oxidase B (MAO-B) inhibitor selegiline, and the atypical antipsychotic asenapine. Asenapine is available only sublingually because its bioavailability when administered orally is less than 2%. Sublingual or buccal absorption of many drugs can occur for tablets, orally disintegrating tablets (ODTs), or oral solutions when held under the tongue or in the mouth.

Midazolam solution for injection has been administered sublingually and buccally. Changes in electroencephalogram were seen as early as 5–10 minutes after buccal administration of midazolam. If the solution is swallowed, it is less effective.

Orally Disintegrating Tablets

Many antipsychotics are available in ODTs, which disintegrate quickly when exposed to saliva. The saliva containing medication should be swallowed, and absorption occurs in the esophageal and gastric mucosa (Nordstrom and Allen 2013). This dosage form is thought to improve compliance by reducing the ability to "cheek" medications and may be beneficial in patients with dysphagia. The antipsychotics aripiprazole, clozapine, olanzapine, and risperidone; the antidepressant mirtazapine; the mood stabilizer lamotrigine; and the anxiolytic clonazepam are available as ODTs. Do not administer ODTs to phenylketonurics because the tablets contain phenylalanine.

Although ODTs dissolve in the mouth, time to peak plasma concentrations is similar to that of standard tablet formulations (U.S. Food and Drug Administration 1999). However, absorption may occur earlier within the gastrointestinal tract (i.e., pharynx or esophagus). When olanzapine ODTs were administered buccally, there were no measurable concentrations at 5 minutes (U.S. Food and Drug Administration 1999). Conversely, a small study in 11 healthy volunteers found both sublingual administration (held under tongue for 15 minutes) and oral administration of olanzapine ODTs resulted in earlier plasma concentrations (15 minutes) than regular tablets administered orally (30 minutes) (Markowitz et al. 2006). It is unknown if most ODTs have significant buccal or sublingual absorption.

Rectal Administration

Rectal administration of medications can be used in patients with severe nausea, in those who cannot tolerate any gastric stimulation (including sublingual administration), and for drugs for which a parenteral form is unavailable or not tolerated. Drug absorption is often incomplete and erratic because the rectal mucosa lacks the extensive microvilli and surface area of the small intestine. Because a substantial portion of rectal venous drainage bypasses the portal circulation, first-pass metabolism is about 50% of oral administration. Bioavailability increases when enema volume is increased because the mucosa surface in contact with drug expands; however, increasing the enema volume may cause discomfort, and suppositories may be preferred to enemas.

Diazepam and prochlorperazine are the only psychotropic drugs available in rectal forms. However, rectal administration of many drugs, including lorazepam, dextroamphetamine, anticonvulsants, and antidepressants (primarily tricyclic antidepressants and trazodone), has been reported. Parenteral formulations and oral solutions have been administered as enemas, and rectal insertion of oral capsules has delivered acceptable bioavailability. Suppositories may be compounded from tablets or capsules. Where possible, therapeutic serum level monitoring is recommended.

Topical or Transdermal Administration

Continuous drug delivery from a transdermal patch reduces the peak-to-trough fluctuation of drug levels produced by oral dosing and provides near-constant plasma drug levels, even for drugs with a short half-life, over longer dosing intervals. Transdermal drug delivery bypasses the gut, avoids first-pass metabolism, reduces gastrointestinal adverse effects, and is unaffected by food intake. Local irritation can be avoided by varying the administration site. Transdermal preparations of psychotropics are now approved for depression (selegiline), attention-deficit/hyperactivity disorder (methylphenidate), and Alzheimer's disease (rivastigmine). A topical cream is available for doxepin; however, this medication is indicated for pruritus and not the management of depression. Some compounding pharmacies make an off-label topical formulation of quetiapine for use in agitation, but currently there is no published literature to support this route of administration.

Intranasal Administration

Intranasal administration has been suggested as the best alternative to parenteral injection for rapid systemic drug delivery. However, there are no approved intranasal formulations of psychotropic medications. Custom formulations are reported for anxiolytics (midazolam and lorazepam), psychostimulants (methamphetamine), antipsychotics (haloperidol), and cognitive enhancers (galantamine), and Phase II trials of intranasal midazolam are ongoing. Intranasal midazolam has a faster onset of action than the sublingual route but is similar to intramuscular administration (Nordstrom and Allen 2013). Several devices to atomize drug solutions for intranasal delivery are available (Wolfe and Bernstone 2004).

Oral Inhalation

Administration by oral inhalation has been suggested to be less invasive than intramuscular injection. Zolpidem and loxapine are the only two psychotropic medications available via oral inhalation. Loxapine is used for acute agitation and is contraindicated in persons with pulmonary disorders such as asthma or chronic obstructive pulmonary disease.

Administration via Tube

Many patients in a critical care setting receive medications via nasogastric (NG) tube or percutaneous endoscopic gastrostomy (PEG) tube. Medications available in a liquid form provide easy administration via NG or PEG tube. The antidepressants citalopram, doxepin, escitalopram, fluoxetine, nortriptyline, paroxetine, and sertraline are available as oral liquids. The antipsychotics aripiprazole, clozapine, fluphenazine, haloperidol, risperidone, and ziprasidone are available as oral liquids. Mood stabilizers carbamazepine, lithium, and valproic acid are available as oral liquids. Some tablet forms may be crushed and administered via NG or PEG tube. Some ODT formulations may be dispersed in water or another suitable beverage prior to NG or PEG administration. Olanzapine ODTs can be dispersed in water, juice, milk, or coffee.

Tablets that come as extended-release or sustained-release formulations (e.g., bupropion XL) should not be crushed. Many capsules, such as duloxetine or levomilnacipran, should not be opened (Bostwick and Demehri 2014).

Psychotropic Medications

Anxiolytics and Sedative-Hypnotics

Internationally, many benzodiazepines are available in intravenous, intramuscular, rectal, sublingual, and intranasal preparations. Injectable forms of diazepam, lorazepam, and midazolam are marketed in the United States and Canada; diazepam rectal gel is also available in both countries. Sublingual lorazepam is available in Canada. Lorazepam for injection and midazolam for injection have been used off-label sublingually. Buspirone and the nonbenzodiazepine hypnotics eszopiclone, zopiclone, zaleplon, melatonin, and ramelteon are available only in oral forms. A sublingual preparation and an oral inhalation preparation of zolpidem are available in the United States.

Intravenous benzodiazepines are commonly used to treat status epilepticus and severe alcohol or sedative withdrawal and to calm severely agitated patients. Intravenous lorazepam is preferred because of its more favorable and predictable pharmacokinetics. In patients with status epilepticus, intravenous lorazepam controlled seizures within 3 minutes and for more than 12 hours in adults (Griffith and Karp 1980) and within 6 minutes and for at least 3 hours in children and adolescents (Lacey et al. 1986). Because intravenous lorazepam redistributes more slowly from the central nervous system to peripheral tissues than does diazepam or midazolam, it has a longer duration of effect after a single dose. Midazolam is a rapid-acting short-duration benzodiazepine frequently used in preoperative sedation, induction and maintenance of anesthesia, and treatment of status epilepticus. The effects of intravenous midazolam begin within minutes but last for less than 2 hours (Rey et al. 1999). Intravenous flunitrazepam, available in Europe and Japan, has been used for severe insomnia (Matsuo and Morita 2007) and for the treatment and prevention of alcohol withdrawal (Pycha et al. 1993). Because severe respiratory depression may accompany intravenous benzodiazepine administration, facilities for respiratory resuscitation should always be available when using this route.

Injectable forms of lorazepam, midazolam, and diazepam are available for intramuscular delivery. For behavioral emergencies, lorazepam is preferred because it is readily absorbed and has no active metabolites. Midazolam is also rapidly absorbed after intramuscular administration, with an onset of action between 5 and 15 minutes. Intramuscular diazepam is not recommended because of its erratic absorption (Rey et al. 1999).

Rectal administration of benzodiazepines is useful for the acute management of seizures in children. Diazepam is available as a rectal gel for use when other delivery routes are not readily available. A pharmacokinetic study of a parenteral solution of lorazepam administered rectally to healthy adults found average bioavailability of 80% but with considerable variation in the rate and extent of absorption. Peak concentrations were considerably lower and later than the equivalent intravenous dose. The authors suggested that to achieve rapid therapeutic effect, rectal doses may need to be two to four times the intravenous dose and that these higher doses may cause prolonged toxicity (Graves et al. 1987). Other benzodiazepines, such as clonazepam, triazolam, and midazolam (Aydintug et al. 2004; Leppik and Patel 2015), have also been administered rectally. Although rectal benzodiazepine absorption is rapid, it is not always reliable because rectal bioavailability is highly variable and the onset of action is delayed (Rey et al. 1999).

Sublingual benzodiazepines are often used to control anxiety in patients undergoing dental procedures. Only lorazepam in Canada and temazepam in Europe (Russell et al. 1988) are marketed in a sublingual form, although several benzodiazepines, including alprazolam, clonazepam, diazepam, flunitrazepam, lormetazepam, midazolam, prazepam, and triazolam, have been administered sublingually using commercial nonsublingual formulations or custom preparations. Pharmacokinetic studies comparing sublingual administration of oral tablets against intramuscular administration suggest slightly slower sublingual drug absorption but similar bioavailability.

The pharmacokinetics of a sublingual form of lorazepam has been compared with that of an intramuscular injection or a sublingual dosage of an oral tablet in 10 fasting subjects. Lorazepam blood levels peaked more rapidly with intramuscular injection (1.15 hours postdose) than with sublingual oral tablets (2.35 hours) or the sublingual lozenge (2.25 hours), but these differences were not significant. Bioavailability for all preparations was indistinguishable from 100% (Greenblatt et al. 1982). Midazolam administered buccally for seizures was found to be at least as effective (75% seizure control) as rectal diazepam (59% seizure control) in a case series of 28 children (Sánchez Fernández and Loddenkemper 2015).

The pharmacokinetics of alprazolam oral tablets administered either sublingually or orally has been studied in 13 fasting volunteers. Although not significantly different, plasma drug levels peaked faster and higher following sublingual administration. Sublingual administration of oral tablets may be an alternative for patients with panic disorder who are unable to swallow tablets (Scavone et al. 1987).

Although no benzodiazepines are available in approved intranasal formulations, intranasal formulations of midazolam and lorazepam sprays have been reported to be effective (Anderson and Saneto 2012). Intranasal midazolam produces peak plasma levels within 14 minutes and much higher bioavailability (83%) than the oral form (approximately 20%) (Björkman et al. 1997). In a prospective study of 92 children, seizure cessation with intranasal midazolam was achieved in a mean of 3 minutes versus 4.3 minutes with rectal diazepam (Sánchez Fernández and Loddenkemper 2015). Intranasal lorazepam has similar bioavailability (78%) to intramuscular (100%) or oral (93%) administration but with more rapid absorption (0.5 hours) than the intramuscular route (3 hours) (Wermeling et al. 2001).

Intrathecal administration of a buffered, preservative-free midazolam solution is a safe and effective adjunctive treatment for postoperative pain management in a variety of settings (Duncan et al. 2007).

A sublingual formulation of zolpidem, a nonbenzodiazepine hypnotic, is available in the United States. In a clinical study, the sublingual form produced a significantly earlier sleep initiation than the oral preparation (Staner et al. 2009). Standard dosages are taken at bedtime to improve sleep latency, and lower dosages (1.75 mg and 3.5 mg) are available for middle of the night awakening (Pergolizzi et al. 2014)

Antidepressants

The monoamine oxidase inhibitor (MAOI) selegiline, available in a transdermal patch, is the only non-oral antidepressant formulation approved in the United States. The antidepressant dosage of oral selegiline requires dietary tyramine restriction because of clinically significant inhibition of intestinal MAO-A. By avoiding intestinal exposure to selegiline, transdermal administration reduces intestinal MAO-A inhibition and the need for dietary tyramine restrictions at dosages of 6 mg/day or less, as well as circumventing first-pass metabolism to provide higher plasma levels and reduced metabolite formation. Short-term (8-week; Feiger et al. 2006) and long-term (52-week; Amsterdam and Bodkin 2006) placebo-controlled double-blind clinical trials have demonstrated antidepressant efficacy with similar adverse effects to placebo, except for application site reactions and insomnia. An ODT of selegiline, designed for buccal absorption, is approved in the United States for Parkinson's disease (Valeant Pharmaceuticals International 2009). There are no reports of its use for the treatment of depression.

Transdermal amitriptyline was reported to be well absorbed and effective in a case report (Scott et al. 1999) but to have no significant systemic absorption in a small open trial (Lynch et al. 2005). The variability may be due to different transdermal formulations. This product is not commercially available.

Injectable preparations of amitriptyline, citalopram, clomipramine, doxepin, imipramine, maprotiline, trazodone, and viloxazine are available in Europe and are sometimes used for the initial treatment of hospitalized, severely depressed patients. However, the safety and efficacy of intravenous antidepressants in medically ill patients are uncertain because studies to date have been performed only in medically healthy patients.

No injectable antidepressants are currently available in the United States or Canada. It has been suggested that antidepressants with extensive first-pass metabolism act more rapidly if given intravenously rather than orally, but superior efficacy has not been demonstrated (Moukaddam and Hirschfeld 2004).

Intravenous mirtazapine (15 mg/day) was well tolerated and effective in two small uncontrolled trials (Konstantinidis et al. 2002; Mühlbacher et al. 2006). Citalopram is the only selective serotonin reuptake inhibitor available in an intravenous formulation. To date, open and double-blind controlled clinical studies have shown citalopram infusion followed by oral citalopram (Kasper and Müller-Spahn 2002) or escitalopram (Schmitt et al. 2006) to be effective and well tolerated for severe depression.

Several antidepressants, including amitriptyline, clomipramine, imipramine, and trazodone, have been compounded as rectal suppositories, with anecdotal reports of success in depression (Koelle and Dimsdale 1998; Mirassou 1998). Therapeutic serum levels of doxepin were produced in three of four cancer patients following rectal insertion of oral capsules (Storey and Trumble 1992). The rectal bioavailability of fluoxetine oral capsules, administered rectally, was only 15% that of oral administration, but rectal administration of oral capsules was reasonably well tolerated in seven healthy subjects (Teter et al. 2005). With an appropriate dosage adjustment, rectal administration of antidepressants may be feasible in patients who cannot take oral medications. Serum drug levels (if available) and clinical response should guide dosage.

Sublingual administration of fluoxetine oral solution has been studied in two medically compromised patients with depression. After 4 weeks of 20 mg/day dosing, plasma levels of fluoxetine plus norfluoxetine were in the low therapeutic range, and depressive symptoms had improved in both patients (Pakyurek and Pasol 1999).

Mirtazapine is available in an ODT for gastrointestinal absorption, but the extent of sublingual or buccal absorption from this formulation is unknown.

Antipsychotics

The atypical antipsychotics aripiprazole, olanzapine, and ziprasidone, as well as many typical agents, are available as short-acting intramuscular preparations. Long-acting intramuscular depot formulations of aripiprazole, risperidone, paliperidone, olanzapine, fluphenazine, and haloperidol are available in the United States (Gopalakrishna et al. 2013). In Canada, long-acting intramuscular depot formulations of risperidone, fluphenazine, haloperidol, flupenthixol, pipotiazine, and zuclopenthixol are approved. The olanzapine pamoate long-acting injection requires additional monitoring postinjection to evaluate for postinjection delirium sedation syndrome. Aripiprazole and olanzapine are the only atypical antipsychotics available in oral, short-acting intramuscular and depot intramuscular formulations.

Antipsychotic agents are not approved by the U.S. Food and Drug Administration (FDA) or Health Canada for intravenous use in psychiatric conditions. The short-acting injectable atypical antipsychotics aripiprazole, olanzapine, and ziprasidone have been studied only for intramuscular administration and should not be given intravenously. However, typical antipsychotics, primarily haloperidol, are often administered off-label intravenously in medical inpatient settings, especially for delirium. Exercise caution when administering haloperidol intravenously because this route of administration and higher than recommended doses are considered risk factors for prolonging the QTc interval (Ortho-McNeill 2009).

Intravenous droperidol has been used for rapid tranquilization even though it is approved only as an anesthetic adjunct. Droperidol causes dosage-dependent prolongation of the QTc interval and has been associated with torsades de pointes, although this association is controversial (Nuttall et al. 2007). As a result, droperidol has been withdrawn from the United Kingdom and contains a black box warning in North America.

Intramuscular forms of atypical antipsychotics are less likely than haloperidol to cause acute dystonia and akathisia (Currier and Medori 2006; Zimbroff 2008), but there has been less experience using them in medically ill patients. Haloperidol can be mixed with a benzodiazepine in the same syringe but should not be mixed with diphenhydramine. Ziprasidone and aripiprazole were studied as monotherapy, but they can be administered in conjunction with an intramuscular benzodiazepine. Aripiprazole was shown to be compatible with lorazepam for 30 minutes in the same syringe (Kovalick et al. 2008). Concurrent intramuscular olanzapine within 1 hour of a parenteral benzodiazepine is not recommended because of excessive sedation and cardiorespiratory depression (Wilson et al. 2012b). Intramuscular olanzapine should also be used cautiously in alcohol-intoxicated patients because it may reduce oxygen saturations (Wilson et al. 2012a). Secondary to its potential to cause QTc prolongation, intramuscular ziprasidone is contraindicated in patients with a recent acute myocardial infarction or uncompensated heart failure (Pfizer 2015).

Subcutaneous administration of haloperidol, methotrimeprazine (available in Canada and Europe), and fluphenazine (Health Canada approved for subcutaneous administration) can be used to manage terminal restlessness and nausea or vomiting in palliative care patients (Fonzo-Christe et al. 2005). Most other phenothiazines are too irritating for subcutaneous injection.

Intranasal delivery of antipsychotics is the subject of patent applications, and reports of intranasal quetiapine abuse suggest the feasibility of antipsychotic delivery by this route (Morin 2007). In a small trial, an intranasal haloperidol preparation was more rapidly absorbed and had greater bioavailability than the intramuscular form (Miller et al. 2008).

A transdermal haloperidol patch has been developed and tested in animals, but no human trials have been reported (Samanta et al. 2003). Prochlorperazine is the only phenothiazine currently available in the United States and Canada as a rectal suppository; chlorpromazine suppositories were discontinued in 2002. An off-label topical cream formulation of quetiapine has been compounded and utilized in the long-term-care setting for agitation, and a topical gel haloperidol has been used for chemotherapy-induced nausea and vomiting (Bleicher et al. 2008).

Asenapine is the first and only antipsychotic available in a sublingual preparation. It is not available in other delivery forms at this time.

ODTs, designed to deliver drug for intestinal absorption, are available for most atypical agents. Sublingual absorption of olanzapine ODTs has been studied in healthy volunteers (Markowitz et al. 2006). Sublingual administration resulted in a similar extent and rate of drug absorption compared with regular administration of the ODT and faster absorption than the standard oral tablet. Sublingual or buccal absorption of ODTs for other antipsychotics has not been reported.

Mood Stabilizers

Lithium is marketed in the United States and Canada in an oral form only, but intravenous, intraperitoneal, and sublingual forms of lithium administration have been reported. Non-oral administration of lithium is not approved by the FDA, and insufficient clinical experience or data are available to recommend non-oral routes. Because lithium is not metabolized, parenteral administration has fewer pharmacokinetic advantages than for other psychotropic drugs.

Intravenous valproic acid has been available in Europe for more than 18 years and in the United States since 1997. (It was discontinued in Canada in 2004.) Valproate is the only mood stabilizer, apart from several atypical antipsychotics, with an approved parenteral formulation for which case reports exist describing its use in psychiatric conditions (Grunze et al. 1999; Norton and Quarles 2000; Regenold and Prasad 2001). The infusion does not require cardiac monitoring and causes no significant orthostatic hypotension (Norton 2001).

Rapid systemic loading of valproate with the intravenous formulation has been proposed to accelerate its antimanic effect, but two small case series found no such advantage over orally administered valproate (Jagadheesan et al. 2003; Phrolov et al. 2004). A small study ($n=90$) comparing initial dose of oral loading (20 mg/kg) to intravenous loading (20 mg/kg) to traditional dosing found oral and intravenous loading led to more efficient improvement; similar improvement was seen with oral versus intravenous loading (Ghaleiha et al. 2014).

Findings from several studies indicate that rectal administration of carbamazepine, lamotrigine, and topiramate provides acceptable bioavailability and tolerability. Carbamazepine has been rectally administered as a solution (Neuvonen and Tokola 1987; Leppik and Patel 2015) and as a crushed tablet in a gelatin capsule (Storey and Trumble 1992), attaining therapeutic blood levels in some but not all patients. Rectal preparations of lamotrigine and topiramate have been prepared from oral formulations. Compared with oral dosing, rectal lamotrigine had reduced bioavailability (approximately 50%), leading to lower drug levels and slower absorption (Birnbaum et al. 2001), whereas blood levels were identical after rectally and orally administered topiramate (Conway et al. 2003). Provided relative bioavailability is considered, rectal administration of an aqueous suspension of these tablets may be acceptable.

Rectal absorption of other anticonvulsants, including felbamate, gabapentin, oxcarbazepine, and phenytoin, is not reliable (Clemens et al. 2007; Leppik and Patel 2015). Oxcarbazepine is available as an oral suspension, but its rectal administration achieved only 10% of the oral bioavailability for the parent drug or active metabolite (Clemens et al. 2007). Thus, rectal delivery is not an appropriate route for oxcarbazepine.

Psychostimulants

Transdermal methylphenidate was approved for children in 2006 in the United States. The patch is worn for 9 hours but provides therapeutic effect through 12 hours. Several patch doses are available, and the duration of effect can be modified by early removal of the patch (Manos et al. 2007). In children with attention-deficit/hyperactivity disorder, the adverse-effect profile is similar to that of a placebo patch (McGough et al. 2006). No clinical trial comparing oral and transdermal methylphenidate has been published, let alone a trial in adults with serious medical illness.

Although no other non-oral forms of psychostimulants are available, custom preparations are described. Dextroamphetamine has been administered intravenously to human subjects in research but not clinically (Ernst and Goldberg 2002). There is one published case report of 5-mg dextroamphetamine suppositories compounded by a pharmacy that significantly improved depressed mood in a woman with gastrointestinal obstruction (Holmes et al. 1994).

Cognitive Enhancers

The only cognitive enhancer available in a non-oral formulation is rivastigmine as a transdermal patch. The rivastigmine patch is dosed daily and provides less fluctuating plasma levels than the twice-daily oral capsules or solution. The patch provides greater bioavailability but with slower absorption, which reduces peak drug levels by 20%. This more consistent drug exposure might improve efficacy, but this possibility remains to be investigated. The incidence of nausea and vomiting declined from 33% with the oral form to 20% with the patch (Lefèvre et al. 2008).

Conclusion

Non-oral formulations are now approved in the United States for at least one agent in each psychotropic drug class, and several others are routinely prepared by compounding pharmacies. There is no single best administration route for all patients. In addition to the availability of dosing forms, administrative and pharmacokinetic concerns govern formulation choice. In this regard, non-oral routes of drug delivery have several advantages over oral administration. Medication compliance may improve if the delivery route is perceived as more convenient, and compliance is more easily verified with certain routes. Preparations can be selected to provide rapid drug delivery for acute treatment or more continuous drug absorption for chronic therapy. By decreasing the variation in plasma drug levels, continuous drug delivery reduces adverse effects, improves tolerability and patient compliance, and enhances therapeutic effect. Drugs delivered by a non-oral route at least partly bypass the gastrointestinal tract and avoid first-pass metabolism. Bioavailability is often improved, and metabolite formation, a potential source of adverse effects, is reduced. Also, by avoiding the high gut concentration of drug following oral administration, gastrointestinal adverse effects are lessened.

The recent trend in the development of intranasal and transdermal psychotropic drug delivery systems realizes many of these advantages of non-oral preparations. However, there remains a need for drug forms that are easier, less expensive, and less invasive to administer, especially in situations where medical resources are limited.

Key Clinical Points

- Drug delivery by non-oral routes may improve medication administration in patients with severe nausea or vomiting, dysphagia, or severe malabsorption; unconscious or uncooperative patients; and patients unable or unwilling to take medications by mouth.

- In comparison with oral drug delivery, drugs delivered by a non-oral route may have fewer gastrointestinal adverse effects.

- Bioavailability of medications can vary considerably between different routes of administration. Literature recommendations, therapeutic drug monitoring, and clinical response should be used to guide dosing.

- Oral tablets of many benzodiazepines achieve faster absorption when administered sublingually.

- Short-acting injectable atypical antipsychotics should be administered only intramuscularly.

- Transdermal drug delivery reduces the peak-to-trough fluctuation of drug levels produced by oral dosing and provides near-constant plasma drug levels, even for short-half-life drugs, over longer dosing intervals.

- Transdermal formulations are available for antidepressant, cognitive enhancer, and psychostimulant medications.

- Sublingual or buccal formulations are available for antipsychotic, anxiolytic (lorazepam: Canada only), and hypnotic medications. The MAO-B inhibitor selegiline is available in a sublingual preparation for use in Parkinson's disease.

References

Amsterdam JD, Bodkin JA: Selegiline transdermal system in the prevention of relapse of major depressive disorder: a 52-week, double-blind, placebo-substitution, parallel-group clinical trial. J Clin Psychopharmacol 26(6):579–586, 2006 17110814

Anderson GD, Saneto RP: Current oral and non-oral routes of antiepileptic drug delivery. Adv Drug Deliv Rev 64(10):911–918, 2012 22326840

Aydintug YS, Okcu KM, Guner Y, et al: Evaluation of oral or rectal midazolam as conscious sedation for pediatric patients in oral surgery. Mil Med 169(4):270–273, 2004 15132227

Birnbaum AK, Kriel RL, Im Y, Remmel RP: Relative bioavailability of lamotrigine chewable dispersible tablets administered rectally. Pharmacotherapy 21(2):158–162, 2001 11213851

Björkman S, Rigemar G, Idvall J: Pharmacokinetics of midazolam given as an intranasal spray to adult surgical patients. Br J Anaesth 79(5):575–580, 1997 9422893

Bleicher J, Bhaskara A, Huyck T, et al: Lorazepam, diphenhydramine and haloperidol transdermal gel for rescue from chemotherapy-induced nausea/vomiting: results of two pilot trials. J Support Oncol 6:27–32, 2008

Bostwick JR, Demehri A: Pills to powder: A clinician's reference for crushable psychotropic medications. Curr Psychiatr 13:e1–e34, 2014

Clemens PL, Cloyd JC, Kriel RL, Remmel RP: Relative bioavailability, metabolism and tolerability of rectally administered oxcarbazepine suspension. Clin Drug Investig 27(4):243–250, 2007 17358096

Conway JM, Birnbaum AK, Kriel RL, Cloyd JC: Relative bioavailability of topiramate administered rectally. Epilepsy Res 54(2–3):91–96, 2003 12837560

Currier GW, Medori R: Orally versus intramuscularly administered antipsychotic drugs in psychiatric emergencies. J Psychiatr Pract 12(1):30–40, 2006 16432443

Duncan MA, Savage J, Tucker AP: Prospective audit comparing intrathecal analgesia (incorporating midazolam) with epidural and intravenous analgesia after major open abdominal surgery. Anaesth Intensive Care 35(4):558–562, 2007 18020075

Ernst CL, Goldberg JF: The reproductive safety profile of mood stabilizers, atypical antipsychotics, and broad-spectrum psychotropics. J Clin Psychiatry 63 (suppl 4):42–55, 2002 11913676

Feiger AD, Rickels K, Rynn MA, et al: Selegiline transdermal system for the treatment of major depressive disorder: an 8-week, double-blind, placebo-controlled, flexible-dose titration trial. J Clin Psychiatry 67(9):1354–1361, 2006 17017821

Fonzo-Christe C, Vukasovic C, Wasilewski-Rasca AF, Bonnabry P: Subcutaneous administration of drugs in the elderly: survey of practice and systematic literature review. Palliat Med 19(3):208–219, 2005 15920935

Ghaleiha A, Haghighi M, Sharifmehr M, et al: Oral loading of sodium valproate compared to intravenous loading and oral maintenance in acutely manic bipolar patients. Neuropsychobiology 70(1):29–35, 2014 25171133

Gopalakrishna G, Aggarwal A, Lauriello J: Long-acting injectable aripiprazole: how might it fit in our tool box? Clin Schizophr Relat Psychoses 7(2):87–92, 2013 23644169

Graves NM, Kriel RL, Jones-Saete C: Bioavailability of rectally administered lorazepam. Clin Neuropharmacol 10(6):555–559, 1987 3427562

Greenblatt DJ, Divoll M, Harmatz JS, Shader RI: Pharmacokinetic comparison of sublingual lorazepam with intravenous, intramuscular, and oral lorazepam. J Pharm Sci 71(2):248–252, 1982 6121043

Griffith PA, Karp HR: Lorazepam in therapy for status epilepticus. Ann Neurol 7(5):493, 1980 6104942

Grunze H, Erfurth A, Amann B, et al: Intravenous valproate loading in acutely manic and depressed bipolar I patients. J Clin Psychopharmacol 19(4):303–309, 1999 10440456

Holmes TF, Sabaawi M, Fragala MR: Psychostimulant suppository treatment for depression in the gravely ill. J Clin Psychiatry 55(6):265–266, 1994 8071285

Jagadheesan K, Duggal H, Gupta S, et al: Acute antimanic efficacy and safety of intravenous valproate loading therapy: an open-label study. Neuropsychobiology 47(2):90–93, 2003 12707491

Kaminsky BM, Bostwick JR, Guthrie SK: Alternate routes of administration of antidepressant and antipsychotic medications. Ann Pharmacother 49(7):808–817, 2015 25907529

Kasper S, Müller-Spahn F: Intravenous antidepressant treatment: focus on citalopram. Eur Arch Psychiatry Clin Neurosci 252(3):105–109, 2002 12192466

Koelle JS, Dimsdale JE: Antidepressants for the virtually eviscerated patient: options instead of oral dosing. Psychosom Med 60(6):723–725, 1998 9847031

Konstantinidis A, Stastny J, Ptak-Butta J, et al: Intravenous mirtazapine in the treatment of depressed inpatients. Eur Neuropsychopharmacol 12(1):57–60, 2002 11788241

Kovalick LJ, Pikalov AA III, Ni N, et al: Short-term physical compatibility of intramuscular aripiprazole with intramuscular lorazepam. Am J Health Syst Pharm 65(21):2007–2008, 2008 18945855

Lacey DJ, Singer WD, Horwitz SJ, Gilmore H: Lorazepam therapy of status epilepticus in children and adolescents. J Pediatr 108(5 Pt 1):771–774, 1986 3084747

Lefèvre G, Pommier F, Sedek G, et al: Pharmacokinetics and bioavailability of the novel rivastigmine transdermal patch versus rivastigmine oral solution in healthy elderly subjects. J Clin Pharmacol 48(2):246–252, 2008 18199897

Leppik IE, Patel SI: Intramuscular and rectal therapies of acute seizures. Epilepsy Behav 49:307–312, 2015 26071998

Lexicomp Inc.: Lexicomp Online, Hudson, OH, Lexi-Comp, 2015. Available at: http://online.lexi.com/lco/action/home. Accessed April 11, 2016.

Lynch ME, Clark AJ, Sawynok J, Sullivan MJ: Topical amitriptyline and ketamine in neuropathic pain syndromes: an open-label study. J Pain 6(10):644–649, 2005 16202956

Manos MJ, Tom-Revzon C, Bukstein OG, Crismon ML: Changes and challenges: managing ADHD in a fast-paced world. J Manag Care Pharm 13(9) (suppl B):S2–S13, quiz S14–S16, 2007 18062734

Markowitz JS, DeVane CL, Malcolm RJ, et al: Pharmacokinetics of olanzapine after single-dose oral administration of standard tablet versus normal and sublingual administration of an orally disintegrating tablet in normal volunteers. J Clin Pharmacol 46(2):164–171, 2006 16432268

Matsuo N, Morita T: Efficacy, safety, and cost effectiveness of intravenous midazolam and flunitrazepam for primary insomnia in terminally ill patients with cancer: a retrospective multicenter audit study. J Palliat Med 10(5):1054–1062, 2007 17985961

McGough JJ, Wigal SB, Abikoff H, et al: A randomized, double-blind, placebo-controlled, laboratory classroom assessment of methylphenidate transdermal system in children with ADHD. J Atten Disord 9(3):476–485, 2006 16481664

Miller JL, Ashford JW, Archer SM, et al: Comparison of intranasal administration of haloperidol with intravenous and intramuscular administration: a pilot pharmacokinetic study. Pharmacotherapy 28(7):875–882, 2008 18576902

Mirassou MM: Rectal antidepressant medication in the treatment of depression (letter). J Clin Psychiatry 59(1):29, 1998 9491063

Morin AK: Possible intranasal quetiapine misuse. Am J Health Syst Pharm 64(7):723–725, 2007 17384357

Moukaddam NJ, Hirschfeld RM: Intravenous antidepressants: a review. Depress Anxiety 19(1):1–9, 2004 14978779

Mühlbacher M, Konstantinidis A, Kasper S, et al: Intravenous mirtazapine is safe and effective in the treatment of depressed inpatients. Neuropsychobiology 53(2):83–87, 2006 16511339

Neuvonen PJ, Tokola O: Bioavailability of rectally administered carbamazepine mixture. Br J Clin Pharmacol 24(6):839–841, 1987 3440107

Nordstrom K, Allen MH: Alternative delivery systems for agents to treat acute agitation: progress to date. Drugs 73(16):1783–1792, 2013 24151084

Norton J: The use of intravenous valproate in psychiatry. Can J Psychiatry 46(4):371–372, 2001 11387798

Norton JW, Quarles E: Intravenous valproate in neuropsychiatry. Pharmacotherapy 20(1):88–92, 2000 10641979

Nuttall GA, Eckerman KM, Jacob KA, et al: Does low-dose droperidol administration increase the risk of drug-induced QT prolongation and torsade de pointes in the general surgical population? Anesthesiology 107(4):531–536, 2007 17893447

Ortho-McNeil: Haloperidol injection prescribing information, 2009. Available at: http://www.accessdata.fda.gov/drugsatfda_docs/label/2009/018701s059lbl.pdf. Accessed April 11, 2016.

Pakyurek M, Pasol E: Sublingually administered fluoxetine for major depression in medically compromised patients. Am J Psychiatry 156(11):1833–1834, 1999 10553754

Pergolizzi JV Jr, Taylor R Jr, Raffa RB, et al: Fast-acting sublingual zolpidem for middle-of-the-night wakefulness. Sleep Disord 2014:527109, 2014 24649369

Pfizer: Ziprasidone prescribing information, 2015. Available at: http://labeling.pfizer.com/ShowLabeling.aspx?id=584. Accessed April 11, 2016.

Phrolov K, Applebaum J, Levine J, et al: Single-dose intravenous valproate in acute mania. J Clin Psychiatry 65(1):68–70, 2004 14744171

Pycha R, Miller C, Barnas C, et al: Intravenous flunitrazepam in the treatment of alcohol withdrawal delirium. Alcohol Clin Exp Res 17(4):753–757, 1993 8214408

Regenold WT, Prasad M: Uses of intravenous valproate in geriatric psychiatry. Am J Geriatr Psychiatry 9(3):306–308, 2001 11481141

Rey E, Tréluyer JM, Pons G: Pharmacokinetic optimization of benzodiazepine therapy for acute seizures: focus on delivery routes. Clin Pharmacokinet 36(6):409–424, 1999 10427466

Russell WJ, Badcock NR, Frewin DB, Sansom LN: Pharmacokinetics of a new sublingual formulation of temazepam. Eur J Clin Pharmacol 35(4):437–439, 1988 2904371

Samanta MK, Dube R, Suresh B: Transdermal drug delivery system of haloperidol to overcome self-induced extrapyramidal syndrome. Drug Dev Ind Pharm 29(4):405–415, 2003 12737534

Sánchez Fernández I, Loddenkemper T: Therapeutic choices in convulsive status epilepticus. Expert Opin Pharmacother 16(4):487–500, 2015 25626010

Scavone JM, Greenblatt DJ, Shader RI: Alprazolam kinetics following sublingual and oral administration. J Clin Psychopharmacol 7(5):332–334, 1987 3680603

Schmitt L, Tonnoir B, Arbus C: Safety and efficacy of oral escitalopram as continuation treatment of intravenous citalopram in patients with major depressive disorder. Neuropsychobiology 54(4):201–207, 2006 17337913

Scott MA, Letrent KJ, Hager KL, Burch JL: Use of transdermal amitriptyline gel in a patient with chronic pain and depression. Pharmacotherapy 19(2):236–239, 1999 10030776

Staner L, Eriksson M, Cornette F, et al: Sublingual zolpidem is more effective than oral zolpidem in initiating early onset of sleep in the post-nap model of transient insomnia: a polysomnographic study. Sleep Med 10(6):616–620, 2009 18996742

Storey P, Trumble M: Rectal doxepin and carbamazepine therapy in patients with cancer. N Engl J Med 327(18):1318–1319, 1992 1406828

Teter CJ, Phan KL, Cameron OG, Guthrie SK: Relative rectal bioavailability of fluoxetine in normal volunteers. J Clin Psychopharmacol 25(1):74–78, 2005 15643102

Thompson D, DiMartini A: Nonenteral routes of administration for psychiatric medications: a literature review. Psychosomatics 40(3):185–192, 1999 10341530

U.S. Food and Drug Administration: Clinical pharmacology and biopharmaceutics review for olanzapine (Zyprexa Zydis). Silver Spring, MD, Center for Drug Evaluation and Research, 1999. Available at: http://www.accessdata.fda.gov/drugsatfda_docs/nda/2000/21-086_Zyprexa%20Zydis_biopharmr.pdf. Accessed August 6, 2015.

Valeant Pharmaceuticals International: Zelapar (selegiline oral disintegrating tablets) prescribing information, 2009. Available at: http://valeant.com/Portals/25/Pdf/PI/Zelapar-PI.pdf. Accessed June 28, 2016.

Wermeling DP, Miller JL, Archer SM, et al: Bioavailability and pharmacokinetics of lorazepam after intranasal, intravenous, and intramuscular administration. J Clin Pharmacol 41(11):1225–1231, 2001 11697755

Wilson MP, Chen N, Vilke GM, et al: Olanzapine in ED patients: differential effects on oxygenation in patients with alcohol intoxication. Am J Emerg Med 30(7):1196–1201, 2012a 22633728

Wilson MP, MacDonald K, Vilke GM, Feifel D: A comparison of the safety of olanzapine and haloperidol in combination with benzodiazepines in emergency department patients with acute agitation. J Emerg Med 43(5):790–797, 2012b 21601409

Wolfe TR, Bernstone T: Intranasal drug delivery: an alternative to intravenous administration in selected emergency cases. J Emerg Nurs 30(2):141–147, 2004 15039670

Zimbroff DL: Pharmacological control of acute agitation: focus on intramuscular preparations. CNS Drugs 22(3):199–212, 2008 18278976

PART II

Psychopharmacology in Organ System Disorders and Specialty Areas

4

Gastrointestinal Disorders

Catherine C. Crone, M.D.

Michael Marcangelo, M.D.

Jeanne Lackamp, M.D.

Andrea F. DiMartini, M.D.

James A. Owen, Ph.D.

Diseases of the gastrointestinal (GI) system are prevalent and are frequently associated with emotional distress and psychiatric disorders, which may cause, exacerbate, or be a reaction to these disorders (Jones et al. 2007; Peery et al. 2012). In this chapter, we review the use of psychotropic medications in the treatment of GI disorder symptoms and comorbid psychopathology, potential interactions between GI medications and psychotropic agents, risks of prescribing psychiatric medications in the presence of particular GI disorders, and alterations in the pharmacokinetics of psychotropic drugs induced by GI disorders (e.g., hepatic failure, short bowel syndrome). The chapter is organized first by organ system and then by specific GI disorders.

Oropharyngeal Disorders

Burning Mouth Syndrome

Primary burning mouth syndrome (BMS) is a clinical syndrome characterized by chronic persistent intraoral pain unaccompanied by evidence of oral mucosal changes (Ducasse et al. 2013). BMS typically involves the tongue, lips, and/or hard palate and primarily occurs in perimenopausal or postmenopausal women. The pain is usually sudden in onset and described as burning, tingling, or numbness (Charleston 2013). Dysgeusia and xerostomia often accompany BMS, which may be triggered by dental work, physical illness, or stress (Thoppay et al. 2013). Primary BMS is considered a neuropathic pain disorder whose underlying pathophysiology is not fully understood and is a diagnosis of exclusion (Ducasse et al. 2013). Secondary BMS arises from a variety of causative factors, including autoimmune disorders (e.g., Sjögren's syndrome), endocrine abnormalities (e.g., diabetes), infections, nutritional deficiencies, and medications (e.g., selective serotonin reuptake inhibitors [SSRIs], antiretrovirals, angiotensin II receptor blockers) (Charleston 2013; Ducasse et al. 2013). Psychiatric comorbidity is common among BMS patients, particularly major depressive disorder, generalized anxiety disorder, and illness anxiety disorder (de Souza et al. 2012).

Treatment of BMS is challenging because of the lack of a definitive approach. Evidence from clinical trials is hampered by small sample sizes, short treatment periods, lack of long-term follow-up, and differences in study design. However, results from double-blind randomized controlled trials demonstrate benefits from clonazepam, α-lipoic acid combined with gabapentin, catuama (an herbal supplement), tongue protectors with aloe vera, and capsaicin rinse (Charleston 2013; Gremeau-Richard et al. 2004; Heckmann et al. 2012; López-D'alessandro and Escovich 2011). α-Lipoic acid alone has demonstrated inconsistent therapeutic effects (Charleston 2013). Further findings from randomized clinical trials and pilot studies demonstrate that clonazepam may be used orally, topically, or in a combined manner to reduce pain scores (Amos et al. 2011). Sertraline, paroxetine, and amisulpride (atypical antipsychotic, not available in the United States) were helpful in an earlier 8-week single-blind study; amisulpride also reduced BMS symptoms in a more recent 24-week open trial, as did paroxetine in a 12-week open-label dose escalation study (Maina et al. 2002; Rodriguez-Cerdeira and Sanchez-Blanco 2012; Yamazaki et al. 2009). A 12-week flexible dose study involving duloxetine 20–40 mg/day for patients with orofacial pain including BMS yielded a significant reduction in pain scores (Nagashima et al. 2012).

Xerostomia

Xerostomia is a subjective complaint of dry mouth that may be accompanied by decreased saliva production (Villa et al. 2014). Adequate saliva production is necessary for swallowing, speech, dental health, and the protection of mucous membranes in the upper GI tract. Xerostomia may be due to a number of conditions, including connective tissue disorders, radiation therapy, anxiety, and depression (Han et al. 2015; Villa et al. 2014). Psychotropic agents are a common contributor to xerostomia. All antidepressants, benzodiazepines, typical and atypical antipsychotics, lithium, and carbamazepine cause xerostomia (Fratto and Manzon 2014). This may be particularly problematic for patients who are also taking other medications that produce xerostomia (e.g., antihypertensives, diuretics, opioids, anticholinergics). Management of symptoms may require medication changes or dosage reductions, avoidance of caffeine and alcohol, sips of water, sugarless gum or candies, Xylitol-containing lozenges, saliva substitutes, topical fluoride, and cholinergic agents such as pilocarpine or cevimeline (Han et al. 2015; Masters 2005; Villa et al. 2014).

Dysphagia

Dysphagia is a highly prevalent problem affecting up to 50% of adults older than age 50 and 50% of patients with neurological disorders (Clavé and Shaker 2015). Malnutrition, esophageal rupture, aspiration, and aspiration pneumonia are serious complications of dysphagia (Spieker 2000). Neurological disorders, such as cerebrovascular accidents, multiple sclerosis, myasthenia gravis, and Parkinson's disease, often produce incoordination of swallowing efforts. Case reports frequently cite psychotropic medications as a cause of dysphagia (Logemann 1988). This is especially true with typical or atypical antipsychotics secondary to acute dystonia, parkinsonism, or tardive dyskinesia/dystonia, often occurring in the absence of other movement disorder symptoms (Duggal and Mendhekar 2008; Dziewas et al. 2007; Kohen and Lester 2009; Lin et al. 2012; Nieves et al. 2007; Sico and Patwa 2011). Xerostomia, sedation, or pharyngeal weakness secondary to antidepressants, benzodiazepines, and other psychotropic medications can also produce dysphagia (Dantas and Nobre Souza 1997; Spieker 2000). Last, dysphagia can be caused by muscular rigidity in neuroleptic malignant syndrome and rarely in serotonin syndrome (Passmore et al. 2004; Shamash et al. 1994).

Acute dystonia responds to intravenous diphenhydramine or benztropine. Dysphagia due to drug-induced parkinsonism is not responsive to anticholinergic agents and responds to reduced dosing of antipsychotic medications, switching agents, or discontinuation of therapy (Nieves et al. 2007; O'Neill and Remington 2003). Tardive dyskinesia/dystonia–associated dysphagia may respond to similar measures, with additional benefits from clonazepam, although caution is recommended with sedating medications because of risk of aspiration (Nieves et al. 2007; O'Neill and Remington 2003). For patients whose dysphagia prevents swallowing medications, see Chapter 3, "Alternative Routes of Drug Administration."

Esophageal and Gastric Disorders

Nomenclature and treatment options for esophageal disorders have become increasingly complicated over the past decade. Diagnostic terms in the literature include gastroesophageal reflux disease (GERD), nonerosive reflux disease (NERD), heartburn, esophageal chest pain, esophageal dysmotility, esophageal hypersensitivity, noncardiac chest pain (NCCP), and functional heartburn. In functional GI illnesses, several common physiological elements have been identified. These include dysmotility, visceral hypersensitivity, disturbed central perception of peripheral visceral events, and a predilection for symptoms to worsen under stress (Quigley and Lacy 2013). Patients also may share demographic similarities, including female gender, comorbid anxiety and depression, and decreased quality of life (Quigley and Lacy 2013). Finally, treatment strategies can be quite similar. As one reviews the literature, the overlap among functional GI illnesses is striking.

Reflux Disease and Noncardiac Chest Pain

Presenting symptoms of "chest pain" are a significant burden both on patients and on the medical system. Of roughly 6 million patients who present annually to U.S. emergency departments with chest pain, it is estimated that up to 90% of complaints may be noncardiac in origin (Burgstaller et al. 2014). NCCP may be caused by esophageal pathology in 30%–50% of cases (Coss-Adame et al. 2014; Nguyen and Eslick 2012). GERD is a label routinely used by clinicians and patients alike to define the "heartburn" sensation accompanying re-entry of stomach contents back into the esophagus. Symptomatic reflux continues to be a significant health issue in Western countries, where upward of 20%–40% of people report reflux symptoms (Bashashati et al. 2014; Brahm and Kelly-Rehm 2011; van Soest et al. 2007; Weijenborg et al. 2015).

For patients who have endoscopically identified cellular changes in their esophagus, the label GERD is appropriate. For patients who have no cellular changes noted (upward of 70% of patients with GERD symptoms), the label NERD has been adopted (Quigley and Lacy 2013). These patients may experience similar physical sensations as do patients with GERD, but they are considered to have lower risk of developing Barrett's esophagus or adenocarcinoma. Notably, reflux is a normal occurrence, so it is the decrease of lower esophageal sphincter (LES) pressure and/or the increased number of LES relaxations (transient lower esophageal sphincter relaxations) that is thought to contribute to symptoms (Nwokediuko 2012; van Soest et al. 2007). GERD-related NCCP is commonly treated with histamine H_2-receptor antagonist and proton pump inhibitor medications (Hershcovici et al. 2012). Dysmotility NCCP can be treated with smooth muscle relaxants, including nitrates, nitric oxide donors, phosphodiesterase type 5 inhibitors, anticholinergics, and calcium channel blockers (Hershcovici et al. 2012).

It is thought that visceral hypersensitivity plays a role in GERD/NCCP, as well as other functional GI disorders (Weijenborg et al. 2015). Some authors postulate that up to 80% of patients with unexplained NCCP have lower esophageal sensory thresholds versus those of control peers (Bashashati et al. 2014; Remes-Troche 2010). NCCP related to esophageal hypersensitivity may be best addressed with antidepressants, as well as cognitive-behavioral therapy, biofeedback, and hypnotherapy (Coss-Adame et al. 2014; Hershcovici et al. 2012; Nwokediuko 2012; Remes-Troche 2010). In studies focusing on NCCP and/or esophageal sensitivity, various antidepressant classes such as SSRIs, tricyclic antidepressants (TCAs), trazodone, and serotonin-norepinephrine reuptake inhibitors (SNRIs) have been found to reduce patients' perceptions of the frequency and intensity of chest pain (Coss-Adame et al. 2014; Nguyen and Eslick 2012; Nwokediuko 2012; Remes-Troche 2010; Viazis et al. 2012; Weijenborg et al. 2015). Psychological symptoms such as anxiety, depression, and neurosis are common in upward of one-third of patients with GERD, and psychological stress may worsen GERD in more than half of all cases (Ciovica et al. 2009). Positive effects of antidepressants in GERD/NCCP patients have been noted despite a lack of appreciable improvement in anxiety or depression scores, thus implying that there is a mechanism responsible for improvement aside from amelioration of underlying psychiatric disorders (Bashashati et al. 2014; Nguyen and Eslick 2012; Weijenborg et al. 2015).

Although TCAs and SSRIs may show benefits for esophageal nociception and NCCP, highly anticholinergic medications should be avoided in patients with symptoms of reflux. Anticholinergic medications are thought to decrease LES pressure, leading to an increase in number of reflux episodes (Bashashati et al. 2014; Martín-Merino et al. 2010; van Soest et al. 2007). These medications also may prolong orocecal transit times, leading to an extended time that gastric contents remain in the stomach and giving more opportunity for reflux to occur (van Veggel et al. 2013; Weijenborg et al. 2015). They also may inhibit esophageal peristalsis and salivary secretions, which are needed to clear refluxed material (van Soest et al. 2007). Indeed, some investigators have found that depressed patients treated with TCAs had an increased risk of being diagnosed with GERD as compared with those who were not taking TCAs (Martín-Merino et al. 2010). Similar research on patients taking antipsychotics found that patients taking clozapine had a higher rate of reflux than patients taking other atypical antipsychotics, presumably attributable to the robust anticholinergic properties of clozapine (van Veggel et al. 2013). Benzodiazepines also are associated with GERD exacerbation, possibly related to their muscle-relaxing effect on the LES (Martín-Merino et al. 2010). This, in addition to addiction potential, should lead clinicians to exercise caution in using benzodiazepines for these patients, despite some positive case reports in the past.

Non-ulcer (Functional) Dyspepsia

Of Western patients who report reflux symptoms, 10%–20% may meet criteria for functional heartburn (Weijenborg et al. 2015). Functional esophageal disorders are "disorders presenting with symptoms assumed to originate from the esophagus without a structural or anatomic explanation" (Weijenborg et al.

2015, p. 251). According to the Rome III diagnostic criteria, there are four key functional esophageal disorders: functional heartburn, functional chest pain of presumed esophageal origin, functional dysphagia, and globus (Viazis et al. 2012; Weijenborg et al. 2015).

Functional dyspepsia is thought to affect fewer people than does reflux disease, but it still accounts for annual costs of nearly $1 billion in the United States (Camilleri and Stanghellini 2013). It is estimated that out of all dyspepsia patients, up to 75% may have no identified cause for their symptoms and thus will be labeled with *functional dyspepsia* (Ford and Moayyedi 2013). The four core symptoms of functional dyspepsia include bloating (postprandial fullness), early satiety, epigastric pain, and epigastric burning (Camilleri and Stanghellini 2013; Oustamanolakis and Tack 2012), and symptoms may be worsened by food.

Patients with functional dyspepsia have high rates of comorbid psychopathology, including neuroticism, anxiety, depression, hostility, tension, posttraumatic stress disorder, and somatization (Faramarzi et al. 2014; Ford and Moayyedi 2013; Levy et al. 2006; North et al. 2007; Oustamanolakis and Tack 2012; Piacentino et al. 2011). A history of physical, sexual, and emotional abuse also may be more prevalent in patients with functional GI disorders. However, the role of psychological factors may be better regarded as influencing how GI illnesses are experienced and expressed, rather than as underlying causes of functional dyspepsia (Piacentino et al. 2011). Traditional treatment often includes proton pump inhibitors, H_2 blockers, and prokinetic agents (Oustamanolakis and Tack 2012; Quigley and Lacy 2013).

As in GERD, psychotropic medications are also used in functional dyspepsia. Antidepressants and anxiolytics may have particular benefits for pain reduction in functional dyspepsia (Overland 2014). Although antidepressants may offer symptomatic relief and analgesia, more data support use of TCAs (such as amitriptyline) than SSRIs (Braak et al. 2011; Camilleri and Stanghellini 2013; Overland 2014; Stein et al. 2014). After a relatively weak performance of venlafaxine in a placebo-controlled trial in patients with functional dyspepsia, SNRIs are not recommended (Camilleri and Stanghellini 2013; Oustamanolakis and Tack 2012). The evidence for SSRIs, including paroxetine and escitalopram, is limited, although studies of SSRIs continue (Camilleri and Stanghellini 2013; Stein et al. 2014). Notably, buspirone, a 5-hydroxytryptamine type 1A receptor (5-HT_{1A}) agonist, seemed to have appreciable benefit for patients with functional dyspepsia when compared with placebo in a double-blind, randomized, controlled crossover trial (Camilleri and Stanghellini 2013; Overland 2014; Tack et al. 2012). Patients took buspirone 15 minutes prior to meals and noted overall reduction in functional dyspepsia symptoms (with accompanying increased gastric accommodation but not altered gastric emptying time) (Overland 2014; Tack et al. 2012).

Peptic Ulcer Disease

Found in both the stomach and duodenum, peptic ulcers have been commonly linked to infection with *Helicobacter pylori* and chronic use of nonsteroidal anti-inflammatory medications (NSAIDs). Patients report a gnawing sensation in the abdomen, and this sensation often improves with food, as opposed to functional dyspepsia, which may worsen with food. In addition to *H. pylori* and NSAIDs, alternative etiologies may include other infections (cytomegalovirus, herpes simplex virus, tuberculosis, syphilis) and substances (potassium chloride, bisphosphonates, crack cocaine, amphetamines) (Jones 2006). Some authors note that peptic ulcer disease has long been regarded as a "psychosomatic disease" (Faramarzi et al. 2014). Indeed, one study noted that a high stress index more than doubled the chances of developing an ulcer (Levenstein et al. 2015).

Patients with peptic ulcer disease are often started on multiple medications, including antibiotics, antacids, proton pump inhibitors, and/or H_2 blockers in varying therapeutic regimens (den Hollander and Kuipers 2012). Several small randomized controlled trials in the 1980s demonstrated benefits of TCAs (doxepin, trimipramine) in the treatment and prevention of duodenal ulcers, perhaps via antihistaminic and anticholinergic effects (Mackay et al. 1984; Shrivastava et al. 1985). It is now known that SSRIs have been associated with a hemorrhagic tendency resulting from their effects on platelet aggregation, particularly with respect to GI bleeding (Hallbäck et al. 2012; Oka et al. 2014), and some authors even wonder if SSRIs are directly ulcerogenic (Dall et al. 2010). This may prompt clinicians to use alternative medications, rather than SSRIs, in this population. Interestingly, melatonin and/or its precursor, L-tryptophan, may enhance healing in patients with gastroduodenal ulcer and thus may be worthwhile additions to current treatment regimens (Celinski et al. 2011).

Gastroparesis

GI motility and functional disorders account for roughly 40% of referrals to gastroenterologists (Camilleri 2013). Gastroparesis is characterized by abnormal gastric motility and delayed gastric emptying without identifiable obstruction. Symptoms include abdominal pain, nausea and/or vomiting, bloating, and early satiety (Bielefeldt 2012; Camilleri 2013; Enweluzo and Aziz 2013; Oh and Pasricha 2013; Patrick et al. 2008; Yin et al. 2014). The most common etiologies of gastroparesis are diabetes mellitus, postsurgical complications, iatrogenic causes (medication side effects), and idiopathic causes (Oh and Pasricha 2013). Anxiety, depression, and somatization are common, although it is difficult to tell if they are precursors or sequelae of gastroparesis. Other complications of gastroparesis include esophagitis, Mallory-Weiss tears, and severe peptic ulcer disease (Enweluzo and Aziz 2013).

Advising patients to eat multiple low-fat small meals, encouraging more liquids than solids, and ensuring tight glucose control in patients with diabetes are dietary changes that can be helpful (Bielefeldt 2012; Enweluzo and Aziz 2013; Patrick et al. 2008). A nonpharmacological intervention, gastric electrical stimulation, has been approved, with variable success (and with reported complications including lead perforations in the stomach and bowel obstruction) (Bielefeldt 2012; Enweluzo and Aziz 2013; Kashyap and Farrugia 2010; Oh and Pasricha 2013). Pharmacological treatments include prokinetic medications, such as metoclopramide, erythromycin, bethanechol, and possibly pyridostigmine; other classes include motilin receptor agonists, 5-HT_4 agonists, and botulinum toxin (Bielefeldt 2012; Enweluzo and Aziz 2013; Kashyap and Farrugia 2010; Oh and Pasricha 2013). Metoclopramide, a dopamine D_2 receptor–blocking antiemetic agent, can produce extrapyramidal symptoms, somnolence, anxiety, depression, and decreased mental acuity (Enweluzo and Aziz 2013). Tardive dyskinesia is a risk with chronic use of metoclopramide.

Antidepressants (largely TCAs) may be another treatment option, although it is unclear if they confer prokinetic effects, assist with pain or nausea/vomiting, or simply alleviate distress associated with gastroparesis (Bielefeldt 2012). Many authors cite mirtazapine as beneficial even for patients whose conditions have been treatment resistant to conventional therapies (Oh and Pasricha 2013; Yin et al. 2014). It is possible that mirtazapine acts by virtue of its effects on serotonin and norepinephrine, along with its ability to block 5-HT_3 receptors (Kim et al.

2006). Although other psychotropic drugs (e.g., phenothiazines, benzodiaze-pines) were previously used for their antiemetic properties (Park and Camilleri 2006), these seem to have fallen out of favor in recent years. As noted in the sub-section "Reflux Disease and Noncardiac Chest Pain," anticholinergic psychiatric drugs can worsen GI symptoms, including gastroparesis, and should be avoided.

Nausea and Vomiting

Vomiting of unknown origin was traditionally attributed to psychological stress (so-called psychogenic vomiting), particularly anxiety and panic (Kirk-caldy et al. 2004; Kumar et al. 2012). A history of physical and/or sexual abuse is common in patients with idiopathic nausea and vomiting. Specific syn-dromes of nausea and vomiting include cyclic vomiting syndrome, hypereme-sis gravidarum, cancer-related nausea and vomiting, and cannabinoid hyperemesis syndrome. In patients without evident cause of vomiting, disor-dered eating behaviors should not be overlooked.

Cyclic vomiting syndrome (CVS) is more commonly reported in children but occurs in adults as well (Drossman 2006; Kumar et al. 2012; Olden and Crowell 2005). This syndrome is characterized by episodes of vomiting, sep-arated by prolonged periods without vomiting. These vomiting episodes may have triggers (e.g., migraine headaches, seizures, menstrual cycles, sleep depri-vation, stress, certain foods) or may be unrelated to any triggers or environ-mental cues (Chepyala et al. 2007; Drossman 2006). Some authors report that in both pediatric and adult populations, migraine, anxiety, depression, and irritable bowel syndrome (IBS) are common personal and family comor-bidities (Drossman 2006). Although there is no clear consensus on the most effective treatments for CVS, treatment modalities include prokinetics, anti-emetics, erythromycin, sumatriptan, TCAs, benzodiazepines, anticonvul-sants, and antipsychotics such as chlorpromazine (Chepyala et al. 2007; Clouse et al. 2007; Drossman 2006; Ozdemir et al. 2014; Prakash et al. 2001). Notably, TCAs appear to be particularly effective in reducing the fre-quency and duration of CVS episodes when used at full antidepressant dos-ages (Hejazi and McCallum 2014; Hejazi et al. 2010; Lee et al. 2012).

Upward of 80% of women experience transient nausea and vomiting dur-ing the early stages of pregnancy (McCarthy et al. 2014). Hyperemesis gravi-darum is defined as "persistent and excessive vomiting starting before the end of the 22nd week of gestation," which can lead to nutritional problems, fluid and electrolyte imbalance, weight loss, and possible hospitalization (McCarthy et al. 2014, p. 719). This condition affects between 0.3% and 10% of pregnant women and is one of the most common causes of hospitalization during pregnancy (Hejazi and McCallum 2014; Hejazi et al. 2010; Lee et al. 2012). Hyperemesis gravidarum was previously attributed to maternal psychological distress and has been associated with multiparity and other conditions in which hormonal shifts are thought to be extreme (Aksoy et al. 2015). Drawing connections to depression or anxiety in a patient with hyperemesis gravidarum is still considered controversial. The belief that hyperemesis gravidarum was a physical manifestation of ambivalence about being pregnant has been discredited. More recent reviews have found that psychological distress is a result of, not a cause of, hyperemesis gravidarum (Aksoy et al. 2015; Spiegel and Webb 2012), thus encouraging clinicians to carefully screen patients with hyperemesis gravidarum to ensure that incident depression is not missed.

Many medications have been proposed for the treatment of hyperemesis gravidarum, including GI medications (e.g., metoclopramide, ondansetron, prochlorperazine, promethazine), antiepileptics, corticosteroids, and nontraditional treatments (e.g., acupuncture, pyridoxine [vitamin B_6], ginger root powder) (Einarson et al. 2007; McCarthy et al. 2014; Spiegel and Webb 2012; Wright 2007). Acting on central brain chemoreceptors, first-generation antipsychotics (particularly chlorpromazine) also have been used in hyperemesis gravidarum, postoperative nausea and/or vomiting, and cancer-related nausea and/or vomiting (Lohr 2008; Wright 2007). Mirtazapine has also been found helpful in hyperemesis gravidarum, although clinicians should be aware of potential withdrawal symptoms in the neonate (Abdulkader et al. 2013; Schwarzer et al. 2008). Despite the relative safety of these medications in pregnancy, clinicians should remain vigilant for adverse effects, particularly extrapyramidal symptoms (acute dystonia, akathisia) when using dopamine antagonists.

Cancer patients experience nausea and vomiting for many reasons, including the cancer and its complications (tumor location and metastases, medication effects, metabolic problems, pain, anxiety, impaired gastric emptying), as well as its treatment with chemotherapy and radiation (Warr 2008). These symptoms have negative effects on patients' overall function and quality of life and may deter some patients from continuing in treatment (Badar et al. 2015; Jordan et al. 2014). The prevalence of chemotherapy-induced nausea and vomiting has improved with the use of corticosteroids plus 5-HT$_3$ receptor blockers, and further progress was made by adding aprepitant, a neurokinin-1 receptor antagonist (Jordan et al. 2014; Lohr 2008). Classes of medications used to treat cancer-related nausea and vomiting include typical antipsychotics, 5-HT$_3$ receptor antagonists, neurokinin receptor antagonists, anticholinergics, antihistamines, cannabinoids, and corticosteroids (Jordan et al. 2014; Lohr 2008; Warr 2008). Benzodiazepines also have been cited as helpful in refractory or breakthrough symptoms (Jordan et al. 2014). Mirtazapine, as noted previously, has robust antiemetic properties (Abdulkader et al. 2013); it has been found helpful for both depression and nausea in cancer patients (Kim et al. 2008). Olanzapine has somewhat less empirical support but may prove helpful, perhaps through its blockade of multiple neurotransmitter receptors (Jordan et al. 2014; Srivastava et al. 2003; Wang et al. 2014).

An increasingly recognized clinical entity is cannabinoid hyperemesis syndrome (CHS; Cha et al. 2014; Galli et al. 2011; Iacopetti and Packer 2014; Simonetto et al. 2012; Sun and Zimmermann 2013). This syndrome is sometimes mistaken for CVS, and inaccurate diagnosis can delay appropriate treatment and management. Traditionally, cannabinoids had been thought of as beneficial for nausea, and they are used in conditions such as chemotherapy-induced nausea or vomiting (Parker et al. 2011). However, in cases of regular heavy usage, there appear to be paradoxical effects on the endogenous cannabinoid system. Extreme nausea and vomiting (upward of five to six times per hour), as well as abdominal pain, are accompanied by stereotyped learned behaviors: patients may take repeated hot baths or showers in an effort to relieve the nausea and vomiting (Cha et al. 2014; Galli et al. 2011; Iacopetti and Packer 2014; Simonetto et al. 2012; Sun and Zimmermann 2013). Cessation of cannabis use leads to resolution of GI symptoms. Patients may be resistant to the suggestion of cannabinoid abstinence, but in numerous case reports, abstinence results in complete cessation of symptoms. Although there is no consensus regarding psychopharmacology for CHS, referral to appropriate chemical dependency services may be the most appropriate and effective treatment strategy.

Intestinal Disorders

Bariatric Surgery

Bariatric surgery, including restrictive procedures such as gastric banding and malabsorptive procedures such as the Roux-en-Y gastric bypass, has become a first-line therapy for morbid obesity. The procedures have the potential to significantly impact the absorption of medications by decreasing the time they are subject to gastric breakdown and by decreasing the area across which they are absorbed by the mucosal walls of the intestine (Padwal et al. 2010). This is of particular importance for medications that are encapsulated for extended release and may not have sufficient time in the postbypass gastrum for the capsule to break down. In general, switching back to immediate-release formulations after bariatric surgery is recommended.

Following surgery, patients are at risk of developing dumping syndrome. Nausea, vomiting, diarrhea, palpitations, and flushing can all manifest as part of dumping syndrome, which is most commonly caused by rapid gastric emptying (Titus et al. 2013). Medications that are immediately regurgitated or that pass so quickly through the stomach and small intestine as to not be absorbed will be ineffective. Alternative delivery methods of medications, such as using long-acting intramuscular formulations of antipsychotics (Brietzke and Lafer 2011) or liquid formulations, such as those available for a number of SSRIs, may be necessary in the setting of dumping syndrome. Orally disintegrating formulations of psychiatric medications (e.g., risperidone, olanzapine, aripiprazole, clozapine, mirtazapine, asenapine) may provide more reliable serum levels (see also Chapter 3).

Some medications may actually have higher levels of absorption after bariatric surgery. Medications that undergo cytochrome P450 3A (CYP3A) metabolism may be more highly absorbed in bariatric surgery patients because CYP3A is present in the proximal small bowel, which is shortened by the surgical procedure, thus leading to less of the drug being metabolized prior to absorption (Canaparo et al. 2007). The liver may increase CYP3A activity over time to compensate for the loss of CYP3A function in the gut (Tandra et al. 2013), so checking serum levels of medications that undergo CYP3A metabolism may be advisable following bariatric surgery.

A comparison of duloxetine serum levels after single-dose administration found that patients who had undergone bariatric surgery had levels only 58% as high as control subjects who had not had surgery (Roerig et al. 2013). Sertraline levels were also more than 50% lower after a single administration (Roerig et al. 2012), suggesting that the effects extend across multiple medication classes. Over time, however, serum levels may normalize; in one study, levels returned to normal at 6 months for the majority of patients taking antidepressants (Hamad et al. 2012). There is a case report of lithium toxicity after gastric bypass surgery, thought to be primarily due to dehydration (Tripp 2011).

Overall, it is difficult to predict what will happen to serum levels of psychotropic medications after bariatric surgery because of significant interindividual differences and limited data. Most medications appear to have reduced absorption after gastric bypass surgery when compared with control subjects, with the exceptions of bupropion and lithium (Table 4–1) (Seaman et al. 2005).

Celiac Disease and Microscopic Colitis

Celiac disease is an autoimmune process that impairs intestinal absorption of nutrients. Patients often present with diarrhea, steatorrhea, flatulence, and weight loss (Martucci et al. 2002). Gluten, found in wheat, rye, barley, and oats, worsens the disease; withdrawal of these grains improves symptoms. Mild impairments in cognition ("brain fog") are often reported by patients with untreated celiac disease and can affect performance of daily tasks. Cognitive performance improves with adherence to a gluten-free diet (Lichtwark et al. 2014).

Microscopic colitis, a common cause of diarrhea in the elderly, is found histologically in 33% of patients with celiac disease (Pardi 2014). Although genetic and infectious etiologies have been proposed for microscopic colitis, medication effects have also been implicated. Carbamazepine, sertraline, bupropion, valproic acid, amitriptyline, and duloxetine have been linked to the condition (Fernández-Bañares et al. 2013; Gwillim and Bowyer 2012; Mahajan et al. 1997; Pardi et al. 2002). In patients with chronic diarrhea who are taking psychotropic medications, especially those with celiac disease, consideration should be given to microscopic colitis, and the potential offending agent should be discontinued. A further consideration for patients with celiac disease is the potential presence of gluten or gluten-containing excipients and binders in prescription medications (Cruz et al. 2015; King and University of Kansas Drug Information Center Experiential Rotation Students, August 2012, 2013). Patients may need to consult with their local pharmacist or the prescription delivery company they utilize in order to determine whether their medications are gluten-free.

Inflammatory Bowel Disease

The inflammatory bowel diseases (IBDs) include Crohn's disease and ulcerative colitis. Crohn's disease can affect both the large and small intestine and is characterized by transmural inflammation and a tendency to form fistulae and

Table 4–1. Medication absorption after Roux-en-Y gastric bypass surgery

Greater after surgery	Unchanged after surgery	Reduced after surgery
Bupropion	Buspirone	Amitriptyline
Lithium	Citalopram	Clonazepam
	Diazepam	Clozapine
	Haloperidol	Fluoxetine
	Lorazepam	Olanzapine
	Methylphenidate	Paroxetine
	Oxcarbazepine	Quetiapine
	Trazodone	Risperidone
	Venlafaxine	Sertraline
	Zolpidem	Ziprasidone

Source. Roerig et al. 2013; Seaman et al. 2005.

strictures. Ulcerative colitis typically begins in the rectum and extends caudally, affecting only the mucosal layer of the bowel. Patients with IBD have rates of depression up to three times that of the general population (Fuller-Thomson and Sulman 2006), and depression may be a risk factor for nonresponse to treatment with infliximab, an antibody against tumor necrosis factor alpha (Persoons et al. 2005).

Antidepressants have been used in IBD both to treat depression that is comorbid with the disease and to treat symptoms of IBD itself. For example, paroxetine has been reported to improve quality of life by treating the underlying psychiatric disorder (Mikocka-Walus et al. 2006). On the other hand, there have been case reports of disease remission with bupropion and phenelzine (Kast 1998; Kast and Altschuler 2001). Possible mechanisms include phenelzine reducing gut permeability, thereby limiting the passage of antigens that activate inflammation (Mikocka-Walus et al. 2006), and bupropion decreasing levels of tumor necrosis factor alpha (Kast and Altschuler 2001). TCAs have been found to improve residual symptoms in 60% of IBD patients with controlled inflammation (Iskandar et al. 2014). The response was unrelated to the presence of depression prior to initiating the medication. Conversely, anti-inflammatory therapy has been found to improve depressive symptoms in patients with IBD and to significantly decrease the percentage of patients with moderate to severe depression after a month of treatment (Horst et al. 2014).

Irritable Bowel Syndrome

IBS is the most common of the functional GI disorders, with prevalence estimates ranging from 4% to 22% (Drossman et al. 2002). Symptoms include abdominal pain or discomfort that is relieved by defecation and is associated with altered stool frequency or form. Psychiatric disorders have been found in 40%–94% of IBS patients seen in specialty clinics (Palsson and Drossman 2005). Depression, anxiety, and somatic symptom disorders are commonly reported as being more prevalent in patients with IBS, but attention-deficit/hyperactivity disorder, adjustment disorders, and substance abuse are also found more frequently in patients with IBS than in the general population (Whitehead et al. 2007).

A considerable body of evidence supports the efficacy of antidepressants among IBS patients (Chao and Zhang 2013; Enck et al. 2010; Ford and Vandvik 2012; Ford et al. 2009, 2014b; Rahimi et al. 2009; Ruepert et al. 2011; Saha 2014; Trinkley and Nahata 2014; Vanuytsel et al. 2014). Both SSRIs and TCAs have demonstrated the ability to reduce global symptoms of IBS as well as abdominal pain independent of their effects on anxiety and depression (Chao and Zhang 2013; Enck et al. 2010; Ford and Vandvik 2012; Ford et al. 2009, 2014b; Rahimi et al. 2009; Ruepert et al. 2011; Saha 2014; Trinkley and Nahata 2014; Vanuytsel et al. 2014). The underlying mechanism responsible for these benefits remains unknown, however. TCAs have often been chosen for IBS patients with predominant diarrhea and abdominal spasms because of their anticholinergic effects. At doses lower than those typically prescribed for treatment of anxiety and depression, TCAs have demonstrated benefits among patients studied in randomized placebo-controlled trials (Chao and Zhang 2013; Ford et al. 2014b; Rahimi et al. 2009; Saha 2014). Although the evidence is positive overall, there are studies that have failed to demonstrate significant benefits compared with placebo. In a head-to-head comparison of imipramine and citalopram, imipramine produced greater improvement in both GI symptoms and mood than citalopram, but neither agent had a positive effect compared with placebo on the global impact of IBS (Talley et al. 2008). Because of the risk of worsening GI symptoms, TCAs should not be prescribed to patients with constipation-predominant IBS.

Alosetron, a 5-HT$_3$ antagonist, was approved for the treatment of IBS but was later withdrawn because of rare cases of ischemic colitis and severe constipation (Palsson and Drossman 2005). It is now available under a risk-management plan that requires close supervision by the prescriber. Mirtazapine, which is also a 5-HT$_3$ antagonist, may have similar features and a better safety profile; there are case reports supporting its use in IBS (Spiegel and Kolb 2011; Thomas 2000). Compared with the evidence regarding the use of TCAs, there is a smaller body of evidence supporting use of SSRIs in IBS, although fluoxetine, citalopram, and paroxetine have proven helpful in randomized controlled trials (Ford et al. 2009, 2014b). Minimal data exist regarding the role of SNRIs for IBS, with a pilot study showing improvement but poor tolerability and significant dropout (Brennan et al. 2009). Practically speaking, available data suggest that patients with constipation-predominant IBS may benefit from SSRIs, whereas patients with diarrhea-predominant IBS should be prescribed TCAs.

Incontinence

Fecal incontinence occurs in 0.3%–2.2% of community-dwelling adults and is much more common in nursing homes, where rates may approach 50% (Whitehead et al. 2001). Incontinence adversely affects quality of life as well as occupational and social functioning. A workshop paper found that loperamide and diphenoxylate (which are both opioid agonists), fiber supplements for bulking, and amitriptyline were all recommended for incontinence (Whitehead et al. 2015). Amitriptyline at low dosages (20 mg/day) decreased incontinence in 80% of patients and decreased the strength and frequency of rectal motor discharges (Santoro et al. 2000).

Diarrhea

Functional diarrhea can be part of IBS or a stand-alone, painless syndrome. In addition to loperamide and centrally acting opioids, desipramine has also been recommended at dosages of 25–200 mg/day (Dellon and Ringel 2006).

Constipation

Constipation can result from diet; metabolic diseases such as diabetes or hypothyroidism; neurological disease; and medications, including many psychotropics (Wald 2007) (see discussion in the section "Gastrointestinal Side Effects of Psychiatric Drugs"). Behavioral interventions include increased fiber and fluid intake, physical activity, and use of bulking agents. Stool softeners and osmotic laxatives (e.g., polyethylene glycol, nonabsorbable sugars) may also be considered. Evidence for the use of antidepressants is not as strong for functional constipation as in IBS (Ford et al. 2014a).

Liver Disorders

General Pharmacokinetics in Liver Disease

Impaired hepatic function will have an impact on many critical aspects of pharmacokinetics, from absorption through first-pass metabolism and hepatic biotransformation to the production of drug-binding plasma proteins as well as overall fluid status, which will determine the volume of drug distribution. *Bioavailability* describes the rate and extent (proportion of the dose) of drug delivered to the systemic circulation. For oral dosing, bioavailability is influenced mainly by gut function and first-pass metabolism (See Chapter 1, "Pharmacokinetics, Pharmacodynamics, and Principles of Drug-Drug Interactions" for a discussion of pharmacokinetics).

The small intestine is the major site of absorption for most orally administered psychotropic drugs. Some patients with liver disease may have gastroparesis or impaired GI motility, delaying drug delivery to the intestine. Absorption may also be slowed because of vascular congestion, which may exist in cirrhotic patients with portal hypertension and/or portal hypertensive gastropathy. In hepatic insufficiency, both first-pass metabolism before the drug reaches the systemic circulation and subsequent hepatic biotransformation may be slowed, resulting in higher plasma concentrations. Cirrhotic patients may have portosystemic shunting that will circumvent first-pass metabolism and result in higher systemic drug levels. Although liver disease reduces the amounts of plasma proteins produced and alters protein binding, compensatory changes in metabolism and excretion result in only transient and generally clinically insignificant changes in free drug levels (Adedoyin and

Branch 1996; Blaschke 1977). However, disease-related changes in metabolism, excretion, and volume of distribution do alter plasma drug levels, often in complex ways. Ascites and peripheral edema increase the volume of distribution of water-soluble drugs and reduce their plasma concentration. In contrast, hepatic disease may impair P450-mediated drug metabolism, reducing drug clearance and increasing drug levels. Because most psychotropic drugs are highly protein bound (often 80%–90% or more), less albumin and α_1-acid glycoprotein results in a larger proportion being free and pharmacologically active. Although more free drug in circulation increases the risks of side effects and intoxication (e.g., increased sedation with benzodiazepines) (Greenblatt and Koch-Weser 1974), it also makes more drug available for enzymatic metabolism.

Drug-Specific Issues and Dosing

The clinician prescribing psychotropic medications for a patient with liver disease should consider the severity of the liver disease, the medication being considered, the margin between therapeutic and toxic plasma levels, and whether hepatic encephalopathy is present or at high risk. Clinical response and signs of toxicity should guide dosage. Therapeutic drug monitoring may be of value, but results must be interpreted with caution because changes in protein binding may lead to falsely low estimates of active drug levels. Ideally, therapeutic drug monitoring methods selective for unbound drug should be used. In general, drugs with a small therapeutic window (e.g., lithium) should be used with caution or avoided.

Patients with hepatic encephalopathy may have additional psychiatric disorders that require treatment. An initial assessment is necessary to establish whether affective symptoms represent an underlying mood disorder versus affective dysregulation associated with encephalopathy. In some cases, treatment of encephalopathy will resolve mood symptoms. If additional psychotropic medication is needed, drugs that can worsen encephalopathy (e.g., sedatives, tranquilizers, and anticholinergic medications) should be avoided.

Unlike the creatinine clearance rate that can be used to adjust the dosages of drugs that are primarily excreted by the kidneys, there is no biochemical marker or measure to estimate hepatic clearance of drugs or specifically the decrement in drug metabolism in liver disease. However, one measure of hepatic functioning, the Child-Pugh score (CPS; Table 4–2), has often been used

Table 4–2.   Grading the severity of liver disease using the Child-Pugh score

	1 point	2 points	3 points
Albumin (g/dL)	>3.5	2.8–3.5	<2.8
Ascites	None	Mild	Moderate
Bilirubin (mg/dL)	<2.0	2–3	>3.0
Encephalopathy	None	Mild to moderate (grade 1–2)	Severe (grade 3–4)
International normalized ratio	<1.7	1.7–2.3	>2.3

Note.   Grades: A = 5–6 points; B = 7–9 points; C = 10–15 points.
Source.   Adapted from Albers et al. 1989.

to estimate the degree of cirrhosis, thereby providing some guidance regarding hepatic clearance. The CPS reflects the severity of cirrhosis (rated as mild, moderate, or severe), not hepatic clearance or drug kinetics (Albers et al. 1989). Nevertheless, the degree of cirrhosis as measured by the CPS has been used as a proxy for the potential decrease in drug metabolism, and some of the clinical variables used to calculate the CPS reflect aspects of liver disease important to drug dosing considerations (e.g., albumin, ascites, encephalopathy).

The safest strategy is to begin with lower initial doses and perhaps longer dosing intervals and then gradually titrate the dose because it may take longer for medications to reach steady state (see Table 4–3). From our clinical experience, we have found patients rated with CPS-A (mild) liver failure can usually tolerate 75%–100% of a standard initial dose. Those with CPS-B (moderate) disease should be dosed more cautiously. A 50%–75% reduction in the normal starting dose is prudent. Prolongation of the elimination half-life will delay drug levels from reaching steady state; thus, smaller incremental dosing increases are recommended. Patients with CPS-B cirrhosis can often be successfully treated with 50% of a typical psychotropic dose. Patients with CPS-C (severe) cirrhosis will commonly have some degree of hepatic encephalopathy, and medications must be cautiously monitored to avoid toxicity or worsening of the encephalopathy. Patients will require dose reductions as their liver function deteriorates over time. Certain drugs require more consideration than others. Dosing of drugs that require multistep biotransformation

Table 4–3. Psychotropic drug dosing in hepatic insufficiency (HI)

Medication	Dosing information
Antidepressants	
MAOIs	Potentially hepatotoxic. No dosing guidelines.
SSRIs	Extensively metabolized; decreased clearance and prolonged half-life. Initial dose should be reduced by 50%, with potentially longer dosing intervals between subsequent doses. Target doses are typically substantially lower than usual.
TCAs	Extensively metabolized. Potentially serious hepatic effects. No dosing guidelines.
Bupropion	Extensively metabolized; decreased clearance. In even mild cirrhosis, use at reduced dose and/or frequency. In severe cirrhosis, do not exceed 75 mg/day for conventional tablets or 100 mg/day for sustained-release formulations.
Desvenlafaxine	Primarily metabolized by conjugation. No adjustment in starting dose needed in HI. Do not exceed 100 mg/day in severe HI.
Duloxetine	Extensively metabolized; reduced metabolism and elimination. Do not use in patients with any HI.
Mirtazapine	Extensively metabolized; decreased clearance. No dosing guidelines.
Nefazodone	May cause hepatic failure. Avoid use in patients with active liver disease.
Selegiline	Extensively metabolized; use caution in HI. No dosing guidelines.
Trazodone	Extensively metabolized. No dosing guidelines.
Venlafaxine	Decreased clearance of venlafaxine and its active metabolite O-desmethylvenlafaxine. Reduce dosage by 50% in mild to moderate HI, per manufacturer.

Table 4–3. Psychotropic drug dosing in hepatic insufficiency (HI) *(continued)*

Medication	Dosing information
Atypical antipsychotics	
Aripiprazole	Extensively metabolized. No dosage adjustment needed in mild to severe HI, per manufacturer.
Clozapine	Extensively metabolized. Discontinue in patients with marked transaminase elevations or jaundice. No dosing guidelines.
Iloperidone	Extensively metabolized. Unknown pharmacokinetics in mild or moderate HI. Not recommended in patients with HI, per manufacturer.
Olanzapine	Extensively metabolized. Periodic assessment of transaminases recommended. No dosage adjustment needed, per manufacturer.
Paliperidone	Primarily renally excreted. No dosage adjustment needed in mild to moderate HI. No dosing guidelines in severe HI.
Quetiapine	Extensively metabolized; clearance decreased 30%. Start at 25 mg/day; increase by 25–50 mg/day.
Risperidone	Extensively metabolized; free fraction increased 35%. Starting dosage and dose increments not to exceed 0.5 mg twice daily. Increases > 1.5 mg twice daily should be made at intervals of ≥ 1 week.
Ziprasidone	Extensively metabolized; increased half-life and serum level in mild to moderate HI. In spite of this, manufacturer recommends no dosage adjustment.
Conventional antipsychotics	
Haloperidol, etc.	All metabolized in the liver. No specific dosing recommendations. Avoid phenothiazines (e.g., thioridazine, trifluoperazine). If nonphenothiazines are used, reduce dosage and titrate more slowly than usual.

Table 4–3. Psychotropic drug dosing in hepatic insufficiency (HI) *(continued)*

Medication	Dosing information
Anxiolytic and sedative-hypnotic drugs	
Alprazolam	Decreased metabolism and increased half-life. Reduce dosage by 50%. Avoid use in patients with cirrhosis.
Buspirone	Extensively metabolized; half-life may be prolonged. Reduce dosage and frequency in mild to moderate cirrhosis. Do not use in patients with severe impairment.
Chlordiazepoxide, clonazepam, diazepam, flurazepam, and triazolam	Extensively metabolized; reduced clearance and prolonged half-life. Avoid use if possible.
Lorazepam, oxazepam, and temazepam	Metabolized by conjugation; clearance not affected. No dosage adjustment needed. Lorazepam preferred choice.
Ramelteon	Extensively metabolized. Exposure to ramelteon increased fourfold in mild HI and tenfold in moderate HI. Use with caution in patients with moderate HI. Not recommended in severe HI.
Zaleplon and zolpidem	Metabolized in liver. Reduced clearance. Usual ceiling dose 5 mg. Not recommended in severe HI.
Eszopiclone and zopiclone	Metabolized in liver. No dosage adjustment needed for mild to moderate HI. Reduce dose by 50% in severe HI.
Mood stabilizers	
Carbamazepine	Extensively metabolized. Perform baseline liver function tests and periodic evaluations during therapy. Discontinue for active liver disease or aggravation of liver dysfunction. No dosing guidelines.
Oxcarbazepine	No dosage adjustment needed in mild to moderate HI, per manufacturer.

Table 4–3.   Psychotropic drug dosing in hepatic insufficiency (HI) *(continued)*

Medication	Dosing information
Mood stabilizers *(continued)*	
Gabapentin	Renally excreted; not appreciably metabolized. No dosage adjustment needed.
Lamotrigine	Initial, escalation, and maintenance dosages should be reduced by 50% in moderate HI (Child-Pugh B) and by 75% in severe HI (Child-Pugh C).
Lithium	Renally excreted; not metabolized. Adjust dosage on basis of fluid status.
Topiramate	Reduced clearance. No dosing guidelines.
Valproate	Extensively metabolized; reduced clearance and increased half-life. Reduce dosage; monitor liver function tests frequently, especially in first 6 months of therapy. Avoid in patients with substantial hepatic dysfunction. Caution in patients with prior history of hepatic disease.
Cholinesterase inhibitors and memantine	
Donepezil	Mildly reduced clearance in cirrhosis. No specific recommendations for dosage adjustment.
Galantamine	Use with caution in mild to moderate HI. Dose should not exceed 16 mg/day in moderate HI (Child-Pugh 7–9). Use not recommended in severe HI (Child-Pugh 10–15).
Rivastigmine	Clearance reduced 60%–65% in mild to moderate HI, but dose adjustment may not be necessary.
Memantine	Primarily renally eliminated. No dosage adjustment expected, per manufacturer.
Psychostimulants	
Atomoxetine	Extensively metabolized. Reduce initial and target dose by 50% in moderate HI and 75% in severe HI, per manufacturer.

Table 4–3. Psychotropic drug dosing in hepatic insufficiency (HI) *(continued)*

Medication	Dosing information
Psychostimulants *(continued)*	
Methylphenidate	Unclear association with hepatotoxicity, particularly when coadministered with other adrenergic drugs. No dosing guidelines.
Armodafinil, modafinil	Decreased clearance. Reduce dose by 50% in severe HI.

Note. MAOIs=monoamine oxidase inhibitors; SSRIs=selective serotonin reuptake inhibitors; TCAs=tricyclic antidepressants.
Source. Compiled from manufacturers' product information and Crone et al. 2006; Jacobson 2002; Monti and Pandi-Perumal 2007.

or those that are metabolized into active metabolites (e.g., amitriptyline, imipramine, venlafaxine, bupropion) may be more complicated to adjust than dosing of those that undergo only one-step biotransformation or are converted to inactive drug with the first biotransformation step (e.g., most SSRIs). Drugs with long half-lives, such as fluoxetine, usually should be avoided. Extended- or slow-release drug formulations usually should be avoided because the pharmacokinetics is less predictable in liver insufficiency. Benzodiazepines should be avoided in patients at risk for hepatic encephalopathy, but when they are needed (e.g., for delirium tremens), a benzodiazepine requiring only Phase II glucuronidation and not oxidative metabolism should be prescribed, specifically, lorazepam, temazepam, or oxazepam. Glucuronidation is generally preserved in cirrhosis (Pacifici et al. 1990).

Caution is warranted even for drugs not requiring hepatic metabolism. Drugs distributed in total body water (e.g., lithium) or drugs that require renal clearance of the parent drug (e.g., gabapentin) or active metabolites can be difficult to manage in cirrhotic patients with fluid overload. In addition, even patients with mild cirrhosis can have impaired renal function (due to hepatorenal syndrome or secondary hyperaldosteronism), including a reduced glomerular filtration rate. Possible abnormal renal hemodynamics, an increase in volume of distribution, and dramatic changes in fluid status may make maintaining stable therapeutic levels of renally excreted drugs difficult, if not impossible. For example, rapid changes in fluid status may occur in the routine medical management of cirrhotic patients (e.g., paracentesis, adjustment of diuretics or aggressive diuresis, fluid loss from diarrhea caused by medications used for the treatment of hepatic encephalopathy). In these situations, as the volume of total body fluid contracts, a previously therapeutic drug level could rise dramatically to a toxic level. This may be due to the slow equilibration of the drug between intracellular and extracellular fluid compartments (Anderson et al. 1976).

Hepatitis C

Chronic infection with hepatitis C virus (HCV) is one of the leading causes of progressive liver disease in the United States and remains the most common indication for liver transplantation. HCV liver disease is also the primary cause of hepatocellular carcinoma. The most common route of infection in the United States is intravenous drug usage, which accounts for well over half of all cases of HCV. Psychiatric comorbidity is common among HCV patients.

Prior to 2011, when direct-acting antiviral agents began to play a role, treatment of HCV was based on a combination of interferon (IFN) and ribavirin. Treatment with this regimen was challenging because of often intolerable side effects, including anemia, fatigue, flu-like symptoms, anorexia, insomnia, cognitive impairment, irritability, and depression, as well as the length of treatment (24–48 weeks) required. IFN-induced depression arose in approximately 25%–30% of patients and tended to develop early and persist throughout the length of therapy (Sockalingam et al. 2013, 2015). Most often rated moderate in severity, it was nonetheless a significant cause of impaired quality of life and premature treatment discontinuation. Concerns about IFN-induced depression contributed to reluctance about treating HCV-infected patients with comorbid psychiatric or substance use disorders. Collaborative treatment involving medical staff and mental health providers was able to demonstrate that successful treatment was possible. Although the presence of subthreshold depressive symptoms before IFN treatment was shown to increase the risk of developing IFN-induced depression, clinical trials demonstrated that prophylactic treatment with SSRIs could reduce the incidence and severity of depression in patients with or without a preexisting history of mood disorder (Al-Omari et al. 2013; de Knegt et al. 2011; Hou et al. 2013; Mahajan et al. 2014; Morasco et al. 2010; Schaefer et al. 2012; Udina et al. 2012, 2014). Rarely, there have also been reports of IFN-induced mania, delirium, and psychosis (Cheng et al. 2009; Goh et al. 2011; Patten 2006). In most cases, IFN-induced psychiatric symptoms abate soon after treatment discontinuation, although there are infrequent reports of persistent symptomatology (Cheng et al. 2009).

Currently, IFN-based treatment is falling out of favor with the advancement of direct-acting antiviral regimens that offer marked improvement in treatment tolerability, length of therapy, and sustained virological response (American Association for the Study of Liver Diseases 2015; Chopra and Muir 2015; Gogela et al. 2015; Stahmeyer et al. 2015). IFN-free regimens continue to evolve, but at present there are three that are commonly used: ledipasvir with sofosbuvir; paritaprevir/ritonavir/ombitasvir and dasabuvir with or without ribavirin (referred to as 3D regimen); and sofosbuvir with simeprevir (American Association for the Study of Liver Diseases 2015; Chopra and Muir 2015; Gogela et al. 2015; Stahmeyer et al. 2015). In addition, elbasvir/grazoprevir was approved by the U.S. Food and Drug Administration in 2016. Side effects are usually mild, consisting of fatigue, headache, insomnia, and nausea.

Compared with IFN-based regimens, direct-acting antiviral regimens pose a greater need for caution because of the risk of drug-drug interactions. This is primarily an issue with the 3D regimen because of the presence of ritonavir and, to a lesser extent, dasabuvir, as well as simeprevir (Dick et al. 2015; Menon et al. 2015; Soriano et al. 2015; UCSF HIV InSite 2015). Simeprevir is a mild inhibitor of intestinal CYP3A4 and can increase levels of CYP3A4 substrates such as midazolam and triazolam, increasing the risk of oversedation. With dasabuvir, there is a reported risk of increased buprenorphine and alprazolam levels when these drugs are combined with dasabuvir, but the mechanism behind the interactions is unclear (Dick et al. 2015; Menon et al. 2015; Soriano et al. 2015; UCSF HIV InSite 2015). For ritonavir, there are a large number of potential drug-drug interactions, primarily due to its ability to strongly inhibit CYP3A4 and also inhibit CYP2D6. This can result in increased exposure to a number of psychotropic medications, including but not limited to alprazolam, aripiprazole, midazolam, diazepam, vilazodone, TCAs, lurasidone, quetiapine, trazodone, eszopiclone, zolpidem, and clomipramine (Dick et al. 2015; Menon et al. 2015; Soriano et al. 2015; UCSF HIV InSite 2015). Not all of these increased exposures will necessarily be clinically significant and require dose adjustment, but they will need closer monitoring (American Association for the Study of Liver Diseases 2015; Chopra and

Muir 2015). Carbamazepine and St. John's wort are contraindicated because they can reduce antiviral levels and clinical effects because of CYP3A4 induction (Menon et al. 2015; UCSF HIV InSite 2015).

Gastrointestinal Side Effects of Psychiatric Drugs

Psychopharmacological agents cause a range of GI side effects, from mild to moderate and from transient to severe. Persistent and more severe effects are covered here and in Chapter 2, "Severe Drug Reactions," and are summarized in Table 4–4.

Nausea and Vomiting

Many psychiatric medications, including SSRIs, SNRIs, mood stabilizers, psychostimulants, and cognitive enhancers, have nausea as an early side effect. In fact, GI distress is arguably the leading cause of acute discontinuation of drugs by patients starting treatment with SSRIs and SNRIs. Lithium may cause nausea and/or vomiting, but changing the formulation to lithium citrate often helps. Providing divided doses of carbamazepine throughout the day may be helpful, as can changing sodium valproate to valproic acid. Notably, the presence of nausea, vomiting, and diarrhea may herald psychiatric medication toxicity, such as early signs of lithium toxicity or serotonin syndrome. For patients in whom nausea and vomiting prevent adequate intake of psychiatric medication, alternative routes of administration must be considered (see Chapter 3).

Diarrhea

Diarrhea occurs as a side effect of lithium at therapeutic levels and is an early sign of lithium toxicity. A cross-sectional population-based study found that 33% of patients treated with lithium reported diarrhea (Fosnes et al. 2011). Slow-release formulations of lithium can decrease the likelihood of diarrhea as a side effect. Paradoxically, lithium has also been reported to effectively treat chronic unexplained diarrhea, perhaps by modulating cyclic adenosine monophosphate activity in the gut (Owyang 1984). Diarrhea occurred in 25% of patients treated with carbamazepine in the same population-based study (Fosnes et al. 2011). Clinically, valproate, cholinesterase inhibitors, and SSRIs can also cause diarrhea (Chial et al. 2003; McCain et al. 2007).

Table 4–4. Gastrointestinal adverse effects of psychiatric drugs

Medication	Gastrointestinal adverse effects
Anxiolytics/sedative-hypnotics	
Buspirone	Nausea
Eszopiclone and zopiclone	Bitter taste, dry mouth, nausea
Zolpidem	Nausea, dyspepsia
Antidepressants	
SSRIs	
General	Nausea, diarrhea
Paroxetine	Nausea, diarrhea, constipation
Vilazodone	Nausea, abdominal pain, diarrhea, flatulence
Vortioxetine	Nausea, vomiting, constipation
SNRIs and novel action agents	
Bupropion, desvenlafaxine, duloxetine, and venlafaxine	Nausea, constipation, dry mouth
Levomilnacipran	Nausea, vomiting, constipation
Mirtazapine	Dry mouth, constipation, increased appetite
Nefazodone	Dry mouth, nausea, constipation, hepatotoxicity
TCAs	Dry mouth, constipation; more severe GI adverse effects with tertiary-amine TCAs (e.g., amitriptyline, imipramine, doxepin, clomipramine) than with secondary amine agents (e.g., desipramine, nortriptyline)
MAOI	
Selegiline (transdermal)	Diarrhea, dyspepsia, dry mouth
Substance use agents	
Buprenorphine	Abdominal pain, nausea

Table 4–4.   Gastrointestinal adverse effects of psychiatric drugs *(continued)*

Medication	Gastrointestinal adverse effects
Substance use agents *(continued)*	
Naltrexone	Abdominal pain, nausea, vomiting, diarrhea, anorexia
Varenicline	Nausea, vomiting, flatulence, constipation
Antipsychotics	
Atypical agents	
General	Dry mouth, constipation
Clozapine	Hypersalivation, constipation
Low-potency typical agents	Dry mouth, constipation, reversible cholestatic hepatotoxicity (especially with chlorpromazine)
Anticholinergics for EPS	
Benztropine, biperiden, diphenhydramine, and trihexyphenidyl	Dry mouth, constipation
Mood stabilizers	
Carbamazepine	Nausea, vomiting, dyspepsia, diarrhea, hepatotoxicity
Lamotrigine	Nausea, vomiting, dyspepsia, diarrhea
Lithium	Nausea, vomiting, diarrhea, decreased appetite
Oxcarbazepine	Nausea, vomiting, dyspepsia, diarrhea (less than carbamazepine)
Valproate	Nausea, vomiting, dyspepsia, diarrhea, hyperammonemia, hepatotoxicity
Cholinesterase inhibitors and memantine	
Cholinesterase inhibitors	Nausea, vomiting, diarrhea, anorexia; most common with rivastigmine
Memantine	Constipation

Table 4–4.   Gastrointestinal adverse effects of psychiatric drugs *(continued)*

Medication	Gastrointestinal adverse effects
Psychostimulants	
Amphetamines and methylphenidate	Stomachache, appetite suppression
Armodafinil and modafinil	Nausea, dry mouth, anorexia
Atomoxetine	Nausea, constipation, dry mouth, decreased appetite

Note.   EPS = extrapyramidal symptoms; GI = gastrointestinal; MAOI = monoamine oxidase inhibitor; SNRIs = serotonin-norepinephrine reuptake inhibitor; SSRIs = selective serotonin reuptake inhibitors; TCAs = tricyclic antidepressants.

Constipation

Constipation is often caused by psychotropic medications, particularly those with significant anticholinergic activity (e.g., TCAs, paroxetine, low-potency antipsychotics, olanzapine, benztropine). Even among relatively newer antidepressants, such as venlafaxine, bupropion, and mirtazapine, constipation can be a problematic side effect. If dietary and medication remedies described earlier in the section "Intestinal Disorders," subsection "Constipation," are ineffective, switching to a drug with less risk of constipation should be considered. Constipation can be problematic with second-generation antipsychotics, particularly clozapine, which has led to serious complications at times. Because of this, co-prescription of laxatives for patients on clozapine has been recommended as prophylaxis (Cohen et al. 2012).

Psychotropic Drug–Induced Gastrointestinal Complications

SSRIs and Upper Gastrointestinal Bleeding

In recent years, concerns have been raised about SSRIs posing an increased risk of upper GI bleeding. However, results gathered from a number of case-control and cohort studies suggest that the overall risk is more modest than originally feared (Andrade et al. 2010; Anglin et al. 2014; Dall et al. 2009; de Abajo 2011; de Abajo and García-Rodríguez 2008; Targownik et al. 2009; Vidal et al. 2008). The underlying mechanism behind this increased risk of bleeding is thought to be reduced platelet serotonin levels interfering with platelet aggregation and hemostasis (Anglin et al. 2014). Alternatively, SSRIs increase gastric acidity, which may increase the risk of peptic ulcer disease and GI bleeding (Andrade et al. 2010; Anglin et al. 2014). Whichever the mechanism, concurrent use with NSAIDs significantly increases the risk of upper GI bleeding, particularly among those considered to be at high risk (e.g., the elderly; individuals with a history of GI bleed, peptic ulcer disease, or cirrhosis) (Andrade et al. 2010; Anglin et al. 2014; Dall et al. 2009; de Abajo and García-Rodríguez 2008). The addition of proton pump inhibitors appears to help counteract this risk. Data regarding combined use of SSRIs with antiplatelet (e.g., aspirin) and anticoagulant (e.g., warfarin) drugs have yielded conflicting results as to whether there is an increased risk of GI bleeding, although some researchers feel there is probable elevated risk (Andrade et al. 2010). Overall, current information suggests that the risk of upper GI bleeding with SSRIs is low among healthy adults, but risks and benefits should be weighed for patients at higher risk for upper GI bleeding.

Psychotropic Drug–Induced Hepatitis, Hepatic Dysfunction, and Hepatic Failure

Most psychotropic medication–induced liver injury is of the idiosyncratic type and as such cannot be predicted from specific risk factors or drug dose (DeSanty and Amabile 2007). Drug-induced liver injury occurs in fewer than 1 per 1,000 to 1 per 100,000 treated patients and is usually not caused by overdose (DeSanty and Amabile 2007; Russo and Watkins 2004). Although almost all antidepressants have been implicated in cases of drug-induced hepatotoxicity, only nefazodone and duloxetine have received additional scrutiny. With duloxetine, 1% of patients developed a threefold increase in alanine transaminase compared with 0.2% receiving placebo. The findings suggest a higher risk of duloxetine-mediated hepatotoxicity in patients with preexisting chronic liver disease and in those who consume large amounts of alcohol (DeSanty and Amabile 2007). In an independent study funded by Eli Lilly that included matched comparator groups of venlafaxine, other antidepressants, and no antidepressant use, duloxetine use was associated with a four- to fivefold greater incidence of less severe hepatic outcomes (e.g., liver enzyme elevations) but not hepatic-related death or potential acute hepatic failure (Xue et al. 2011). In addition, duloxetine patients who developed severe hepatic injuries were found to have greater prevalence of baseline hepatic risk factors (e.g., hepatic insufficiency or cirrhosis), and cases with baseline hepatic risk factors had earlier onset of hepatic events (Xue et al. 2011). Because of a significant number of nefazodone-induced liver injury cases (1 case of death or transplant per 250,000–300,000 patient-years of treatment), Bristol-Myers Squibb stopped manufacturing it in 2004, although generic nefazodone is still available (DeSanty and Amabile 2007).

Valproate is associated with an overall 1:20,000 incidence of liver toxicity, although the frequency can be as high as 1:600 in certain groups (i.e., infants younger than 2 years, patients undergoing anticonvulsant polytherapy) (Zaccara et al. 2007). The risk of carbamazepine-induced hepatotoxicity is estimated at 16 cases per 100,000 treatment years, and 20 cases of severe lamotrigine-induced liver toxicity have been reported (Zaccara et al. 2007). Chlorpromazine and, less commonly, other phenothiazines may cause reversible cholestatic hepatotoxicity in up to 2% of patients, typically within the first 4 weeks of therapy. Because this reaction is believed to be due to impaired sulfoxidation, patients with primary biliary cirrhosis, who often have impaired sulfoxidation, should not be given these drugs (Leipzig 1990). Most other antipsychotics, including the atypical antipsychotics, have been implicated in cases of drug-induced elevations in liver transaminases (Marwick et al. 2012). In most cases, transaminase elevations were asymptomatic and arose within the first 6 weeks of treatment (Marwick et al. 2012). In the United States over the past 12 years, fewer than 500 patients with acute drug-induced liver toxicity developed acute hepatic failure requiring liver transplantation. The majority of these cases of acute toxicity were due to acetaminophen (mostly in overdose); only 3% were due to phenytoin, 3% were due to valproate, and < 1% were due to nefazodone (Russo et al. 2004). Thus, even severe drug-induced liver injury is usually reversible and rarely results in fatality if the drug is discontinued.

Despite the potential risk of liver injury, there is no justification to routinely monitor liver enzymes for most psychotropics (with the exception of valproate) because hepatic adverse effects are unpredictable and occur abruptly at varying times following drug initiation (Russo and Watkins 2004). Routine laboratory monitoring of hepatic enzymes and liver functions may be indicated 1) before starting treatment to establish baseline liver enzymes, 2) in high-risk groups, 3) in patients with impaired ability to communicate, or 4) in the presence of early symptoms or prodromal signs of a possible adverse reaction (Zaccara et al. 2007). Although most episodes are asymptomatic, patients can be instructed on the signs and symptoms of liver injury (e.g., right upper quadrant pain, dark urine, itching, jaundice, nausea, anorexia) when prescribed a medication that may cause such an adverse effect.

Because there are no specific biomarkers and the clinical presentation of drug-induced liver injury can mimic many other hepatological disorders, the diagnosis is essentially one of clinical suspicion after exclusion of common causes of liver disease (e.g., alcohol, viruses) (Hussaini and Farrington 2014). Instances of idiosyncratic hepatocellular jaundice are almost always associated with minor and asymptomatic aminotransferase elevations, exceeding three times the upper limit of normal in up to 15% of patients treated with drugs capable of causing these reactions (Russo and Watkins 2004). Inexplicably, the aminotransferase elevations, which reflect liver injury, often reverse even if drug therapy is continued, although a minority will develop progressive liver injury (Hussaini and Farrington 2014; Russo and Watkins 2004). Nevertheless, because it is impossible to predict the smaller subset of individuals who are actually susceptible to progressive injury from the drug, patients who develop aminotransferase elevations two to three times the upper limit of normal should be removed from therapy. In most cases, the liver injury spontaneously resolves on drug discontinuation, but in some cases the enzymes continue to rise for several days. Therefore, clinical symptoms and liver enzymes should be followed closely after the drug is discontinued. However, the combination of high aminotransferase (representing hepatocellular injury) and jaundice has been associated with a high mortality rate of 10%–15%, and any patient with drug-induced injury and jaundice should be carefully monitored for signs of acute hepatic failure, particularly coagulopathy or encephalopathy (Hussaini and Farrington 2014).

It is unclear if patients with preexisting liver disease are more susceptible to idiosyncratic drug-induced liver injury, although the manufacturer of duloxetine has recommended avoidance of its use for patients with hepatic dysfunction, and a recent database analysis supports the theory that those with preexisting liver disease are at higher risk (Xue et al. 2011). Conventional wisdom has usually held that these idiosyncratic drug reactions are based on other factors (e.g., genetics) and are not dose- or clearance-dependent (Russo and Watkins 2004). Nevertheless, caution is recommended because these patients may be less able to handle the additional loss of hepatic function caused by drug-induced injury. Another consideration is the challenge of interpreting elevations in hepatic enzyme levels in patients with preexisting liver dysfunction. If a drug-induced injury occurs in a patient with significant cirrhosis, the resulting elevation in aminotransferases may underestimate the true severity of the insult (Russo and Watkins 2004).

Drug-Induced Pancreatitis

Drug-induced pancreatitis is an infrequent cause of acute pancreatitis, representing only 0.1%–2% of cases (Dhir et al. 2007). Although most cases are mild, prompt recognition is necessary to reduce the risk of serious complications, including systemic inflammation, chronic pancreatitis, multiple organ failure, and death (Kaurich 2008). Accurate diagnosis is challenging because the clinical presentation is not readily distinguishable from other causes of acute pancreatitis (Dhir et al. 2007; Nitsche et al. 2010). Time of onset is variable, often occurring within a few weeks to months after starting a particular drug. There is no dose-response relationship for drug-induced pancreatitis because it can develop over a wide range of drug doses. Certain patient populations are at greater risk for drug-induced pancreatitis, including women, children, the elderly, and those with advanced HIV infection or IBD (Balani and Grendell 2008; Nitsche et al. 2010).

Valproic acid is the psychotropic agent with the greatest number of reported cases of drug-induced pancreatitis, the majority involving children (Gerstner et al. 2007). The true incidence is considered to be 1 in 40,000, and patients present with symptoms that typically include abdominal pain, nausea, vomiting, diarrhea, and anorexia. Transient asymptomatic hyperamylasemia occurs in 20% of adults taking valproic acid, but this does not correlate with a greater risk for pancreatitis (Zaccara et al. 2007). Infrequent case reports have linked other anticonvulsants to pancreatitis, including carbamazepine, lamotrigine, topiramate, levetiracetam, gabapentin, and vigabatrin (Zaccara et al. 2007).

Numerous cases of antipsychotic-induced pancreatitis have been reported, most involving clozapine and olanzapine, with fewer related to risperidone, haloperidol, and quetiapine (Alastal et al. 2014; Kawabe and Ueno 2014; Kerr et al. 2007; Liou et al. 2014; Potolidis et al. 2012; Rashid et al. 2009). Rarely, ziprasidone and aripiprazole have also been implicated. Despite these reports, population-based studies have yielded conflicting results as to whether antipsychotic medications are a cause of drug-induced pancreatitis (Bodén et al. 2012; Gasse et al. 2008). A Danish case-control study found an increased risk of hospitalization for acute pancreatitis with conventional antipsychotics, particularly low-potency ones (Gasse et al. 2008). However, a large Swedish study failed to find an association between antipsychotic agents and acute pancreatitis when confounding factors (e.g., gallstone disease, history of excessive alcohol use) were taken into account (Bodén et al. 2012).

Among antidepressants, mirtazapine has been implicated in several cases of drug-induced pancreatitis, whereas bupropion, venlafaxine, and SSRIs have been infrequently implicated (Hussain and Burke 2008; Sevastru et al. 2012; Spigset et al. 2003). Rechallenge with the offending drug after an episode of pancreatitis is not advised, even using lower doses or a different route of administration, because of the risk of recurrence. However, substitution with another drug of the same class is considered an acceptable option (Dhir et al. 2007).

Intestinal or Colonic Toxicity

Psychotropic medications often produce constipation as a troublesome side effect, but in some cases more serious complications may arise. In particular, antipsychotic-induced GI hypomotility can develop and infrequently progress to paralytic ileus, intestinal obstruction, bowel ischemia, megacolon, or perforation (De Hert et al. 2011; Fayad and Bruijnzeel 2012; Flanagan and Ball 2011; Hibbard et al. 2009; Palmer et al. 2008; Peyrière et al. 2009; Ramamourthy et al. 2013). The initial presentation with intermittent abdominal pain, vomiting, and bloody or malodorous diarrhea may not reflect the underlying seriousness of the condition, which can subsequently progress to peritonitis or septic shock (Peyrière et al. 2009). The mortality rate is high, with a French pharmacovigilance database reporting a mortality rate of 37% among 38 cases identified as antipsychotic-induced ischemia or necrosis (Peyrière et al. 2009). Both typical and atypical antipsychotics can cause impaired bowel motility from a combination of anticholinergic and $5-HT_3$ antagonistic effects. A considerable number of serious cases of GI hypomotility have been reported with clozapine. In a review of 102 cases of GI hypomotility (Palmer et al. 2008), more than one-third occurred within the first 4 months of treatment, and more than half occurred within 1 year; the mortality rate was 27.5%. The authors identified other potential risk factors, including high doses or serum drug levels, concomitant anticholinergic use, and concurrent physical illness (Palmer et al. 2008). Serious GI complications from clozapine appear to be more common than agranulocytosis or neutropenia. A separate study by Nielsen and Meyer identified risk factors for development of paralytic ileus among schizophrenic patients, including increasing age, female sex, use of clozapine, high-potency first-generation antipsychotics (e.g., haloperidol), TCAs, anticholinergics (e.g., benztropine), and opioids (Nielsen and Meyer 2012). Careful attention to bowel habits, keeping the dose of medication as low as possible, and trying to limit use of other anticholinergic agents are recommended approaches to reducing the risk of intestinal complications. Patients who have developed intestinal ischemia or necrosis with clozapine can potentially be rechallenged with clozapine, but risks versus benefits must be carefully considered (Ikai et al. 2013). Less frequently, colonic ischemia has been associated with barbiturates, TCAs, or cocaine, and pseudo-obstruction has also been reported with TCA treatment (Cappell 2004; Gollock and Thomson 1984; Olson et al. 1984).

Psychiatric Side Effects of Gastrointestinal Medications

In addition to psychiatric medications causing GI disorders, GI medications can have psychiatric side effects. Although much has been written about IFN, psychiatrists need to be alert to the potential effects of other GI medications because they may alter a patient's clinical presentation and require medication adjustments. Potential adverse effects of GI medications are listed in Table 4–5.

Drug-Drug Interactions

Potential interactions between GI and psychotropic medications are summarized in Tables 4–6 and 4–7. Drug interactions for antibiotics used for *H. pylori* regimens (e.g., metronidazole, tetracycline, clarithromycin, amoxicillin) are reviewed in Chapter 12, "Infectious Diseases." Additional information on

Table 4–5.   Psychiatric adverse effects of gastrointestinal drugs

Medication	Psychiatric adverse effects
Antidiarrheal agents	
Diphenoxylate	Sedation, lethargy, insomnia, depression, euphoria, confusion
Loperamide	Dizziness
Antiemetics	
Aprepitant	Dizziness
Corticosteroids (e.g., dexamethasone)	Mania, anxiety, irritability, psychosis (acute), depression (chronic)
Dimenhydrinate	Drowsiness, ataxia, disorientation, convulsions, stupor
Diphenhydramine	Drowsiness, dizziness, confusion, cognitive impairment
Dolasetron	Headache, fatigue, dizziness
Domperidone	Acute dystonic reactions (rare)
Dronabinol and nabilone	Dizziness, euphoria, paranoid reaction, abnormal thinking, somnolence, confusion
Droperidol	EPS
Granisetron	Headache, asthenia, somnolence
Metoclopramide	Restlessness, drowsiness, fatigue, dystonic reactions, dyskinesia
Palonosetron	Anxiety
Prochlorperazine	Drowsiness, dizziness, headache (common); EPS, seizures, confusion, insomnia, neuroleptic malignant syndrome
Promethazine	Drowsiness, confusion, hyperexcitability, EPS, seizures, confusion, neuroleptic malignant syndrome
Trimethobenzamide	Drowsiness, dizziness, disorientation, depression, seizure, EPS

Table 4–5.   Psychiatric adverse effects of gastrointestinal drugs *(continued)*

Medication	Psychiatric adverse effects
Histamine H$_2$-receptor antagonists	
Cimetidine	Headache, dizziness
Nizatidine	Dizziness, somnolence, anxiety, nervousness
Ranitidine	Headache, malaise, dizziness
Irritable bowel drugs	
Alosetron	Headache
Antispasmodics (dicyclomine, glycopyrrolate, and methscopolamine)	Dizziness, blurred vision, drowsiness, weakness, confusion, excitement (especially in the elderly)
Lubiprostone	Headache
Renzapride	Headache, dizziness
Sulfasalazine	Headache, anorexia
Tegaserod	Headache, dizziness
Inflammatory bowel drugs	
Adalimumab	Headache, CNS demyelinating disease
Balsalazide	Depression (uncommon), headache
Certolizumab pegol	Anxiety, CNS demyelinating disease, mood instability (rare)
Cyclosporine	Delirium, tremor, depression, mania, seizure, PML (rare)
Golimumab	CNS demyelinating disease
Infliximab	Fatigue, headache, CNS demyelinating disease, seizure (rare)
Mesalamine	Dizziness, headache
Natalizumab	Depression, headache, PML, herpes encephalitis (rare)

Table 4–5.   Psychiatric adverse effects of gastrointestinal drugs *(continued)*

Medication	Psychiatric adverse effects
Inflammatory bowel drugs *(continued)*	
Olsalazine	Insomnia, irritability, mood swings, tremor (rare)
Vedolizumab	Headache, PML
Proton pump inhibitors	
Esomeprazole, lansoprazole, omeprazole, and pantoprazole	Dizziness

Note.   CNS = central nervous system; EPS = extrapyramidal symptoms; PML = progressive multifocal leukoencephalopathy.

corticosteroids is presented in Chapter 10, "Endocrine and Metabolic Disorders." See Chapter 1 for a discussion of pharmacokinetics, pharmacodynamics, and principles of drug-drug interactions.

Conclusion

GI disorders include a wide range of physiological and functional disturbances that span multiple organ systems, from the mouth to the colorectal region. Often, psychological stress or comorbid psychopathology appears to influence the level of GI symptomatology that a patient experiences. Psychopharmacological treatment can be beneficial in improving quality of life, reducing physical discomfort, and/or controlling anxiety and depression. The selection of pharmacological agent, however, requires consideration of potential undesirable side effects (e.g., dysphagia, xerostomia, nausea, vomiting), tolerability, and safety.

Table 4–6. Gastrointestinal drug–psychotropic drug interactions

Medication	Interaction mechanism	Effects on psychotropic drugs and management
Medications for gastric acidity, peptic ulcers, and GERD		
Antacids	Increased gastric pH and delayed gastric emptying Increased sodium excretion	May reduce drug absorption; take antacids 2–3 hours apart from other drugs. Sodium bicarbonate may increase renal excretion of lithium.
Cimetidine	Inhibits CYP1A2, CYP2C9/19, CYP2D6, and CYP3A4	Inhibits oxidative metabolism of most drugs. Reduce psychotropic dose. Avoid cimetidine or use psychotropics eliminated by conjugation.
Esomeprazole	Induces CYP1A2	Increased elimination and reduced levels of clozapine and olanzapine.
Lansoprazole	Induces CYP1A2	Increased elimination and reduced levels of clozapine and olanzapine.
Omeprazole	Inhibits CYP2C19	Increased levels and toxicity of diazepam, flunitrazepam, phenytoin, and mephenytoin.
Sucralfate	Drug binding	May reduce drug absorption; take at least 2 hours prior to other drugs.
Antidiarrheal agents		
Kaolin/attapulgite	Drug binding	May bind drugs and reduce absorption; avoid within 2–3 hours of taking other medications.

Table 4–6.   Gastrointestinal drug–psychotropic drug interactions *(continued)*

Medication	Interaction mechanism	Effects on psychotropic drugs and management
Medications for irritable bowel syndrome		
Tegaserod	Inhibits CYPA2 and CYP2D6	May reduce metabolism and increase levels of atomoxetine, clozapine, chlorpromazine, olanzapine, risperidone, TCAs, maprotiline, mirtazapine, trazodone, and venlafaxine.
Antispasmodics (clidinium-chlordiazepoxide, dicyclomine, glycopyrrolate, hyoscyamine, and methscopolamine)	Additive anticholinergic effects	Increased risk of cognitive impairment and delirium in combination with anticholinergic psychotropics (TCAs, antipsychotics, benztropine, tranylcypromine). Reduced therapeutic effect of cholinesterase inhibitors and memantine.
Medications for inflammatory bowel disease		
Adalimumab, golimumab, infliximab	Increased CYP enzymes by suppression of inflammation	May reduce levels of pimozide and iloperidone.
Cyclosporine	CYP3A4 inhibition	Increased risk of oversedation with alprazolam, midazolam, or triazolam.

Table 4–6. Gastrointestinal drug–psychotropic drug interactions *(continued)*

Medication	Interaction mechanism	Effects on psychotropic drugs and management
Antinauseants/antiemetic agents		
5-HT$_3$ antagonists (dolasetron, granisetron, ondansetron, palonosetron, and ramosetron)	QT prolongation	Increased risk of cardiac arrhythmias with other QT-prolonging agents, including TCAs, typical antipsychotics, pimozide, risperidone, paliperidone, iloperidone, quetiapine, ziprasidone, and lithium.
Aprepitant	Inhibition of CYP3A4, CYP2D6, CYP1A2	Increased risk of side effects with alprazolam, midazolam, triazolam, clozapine, vilazodone, donepezil, carbamazepine, aripiprazole, quetiapine, lurasidone, and pimozide (contraindicated).
Dimenhydrinate and diphenhydramine	Additive anticholinergic effects	Increased risk of cognitive impairment and delirium in combination with anticholinergic psychotropics (TCAs, antipsychotics, benztropine, tranylcypromine). Reduced therapeutic effect of cholinesterase inhibitors and memantine.
Prochlorperazine, promethazine, trimethobenzamide	Additive anticholinergic effects	Increased risk of cognitive impairment and delirium in combination with anticholinergic psychotropics (TCAs, antipsychotics, benztropine, tranylcypromine). Reduced therapeutic effect of cholinesterase inhibitors and memantine.

Table 4–6. Gastrointestinal drug–psychotropic drug interactions (*continued*)

Medication	Interaction mechanism	Effects on psychotropic drugs and management
Antinauseants/antiemetic agents (continued)		
Domperidone and droperidol	Dopamine antagonist QT prolongation	Increased risk of EPS when combined with antipsychotics. Increased risk of cardiac arrhythmias with other QT-prolonging agents, including TCAs, typical antipsychotics, pimozide, risperidone, paliperidone, iloperidone, quetiapine, ziprasidone, and lithium.
Metoclopramide	Dopamine antagonist	Increased risk of EPS when combined with antipsychotics.
Glucocorticoids	Induce CYP3A4	Increased metabolism and reduced levels of oxidatively metabolized benzodiazepines, buspirone, carbamazepine, quetiapine, ziprasidone, and pimozide. Adjust benzodiazepine dose or consider oxazepam, lorazepam, or temazepam. Monitor carbamazepine levels. Adjust antipsychotic dose or switch to another agent.
Dronabinol and nabilone	Additive sympathomimetic effects	Additive hypertension, tachycardia, and possible cardiotoxicity with amphetamines, methylphenidate, and other sympathomimetics. Additive hypertension, tachycardia, and drowsiness with TCAs. Additive drowsiness and CNS depression with benzodiazepines, lithium, opioids, buspirone, and other CNS depressants.

Table 4–6. Gastrointestinal drug–psychotropic drug interactions (*continued*)

Medication	Interaction mechanism	Effects on psychotropic drugs and management
Direct-acting antiviral agents		
Simeprevir	Inhibition of CYP3A4	Increased risk of oversedation with alprazolam, midazolam, or triazolam.
Dasabuvir	Unknown mechanism	Increased levels of buprenorphine and alprazolam.
Ritonavir	Inhibition of CYP3A4, CYP2D6	Increased risk of side effects with alprazolam, aripiprazole, quetiapine, midazolam, diazepam, TCAs, lurasidone, trazodone, eszopiclone, zolpidem, clomipramine, and nefazodone.

Note.   CNS=central nervous system;   CYP=cytochrome P450;   EPS=extrapyramidal symptoms;   GERD=gastroesophageal reflux disease; TCAs=tricyclic antidepressants.
Source.   Compiled from Cozza et al. 2003; Wynn et al. 2007; and product monographs.

Table 4–7. Psychotropic drug–gastrointestinal drug interactions

Medication	Interaction mechanism	Effect on gastrointestinal drugs and management
Antidepressants		
Fluoxetine	Inhibits CYP1A2, CYP2C19, CYP2D6, CYP3A4	Increased levels of aprepitant, granisetron, ondansetron, palonosetron, tropisetron, and corticosteroids, including budesonide.
Fluvoxamine	Inhibits CYP1A2, CYP2C9/19, CYP3A4	Increased levels and toxicity of alosetron. Coadministration is not advised. May increase levels and toxicity of aprepitant, alosetron, granisetron, ondansetron, palonosetron, and corticosteroids, including budesonide. Increased cyclosporine levels and toxicity.
Nefazodone	Inhibits CYP3A4	Increased levels and toxicity of aprepitant, granisetron, and corticosteroids, including budesonide.
Bupropion, duloxetine, moclobemide, and paroxetine	Inhibits CYP2D6	Increased levels and toxicity of tropisetron.
TCAs	QT prolongation	Increased risk of cardiac arrhythmias with other QT-prolonging agents, including domperidone, droperidol, dolasetron, granisetron, ondansetron, palonosetron, and ramosetron.

Table 4–7. Psychotropic drug–gastrointestinal drug interactions *(continued)*

Medication	Interaction mechanism	Effect on gastrointestinal drugs and management
Antipsychotics		
Typical antipsychotics (iloperidone, paliperidone, pimozide, quetiapine, risperidone, and ziprasidone)	QT prolongation	Increased risk of cardiac arrhythmias with other QT-prolonging agents, including domperidone, droperidol, dolasetron, granisetron, ondansetron, palonosetron, and ramosetron.
Mood stabilizers		
Carbamazepine, phenytoin, and oxcarbazepine	Induces CYP1A2, CYP2C9/19, CYP3A4	Increased metabolism and reduced therapeutic effects of aprepitant, alosetron, ondansetron, palonosetron, granisetron, cyclosporine, direct-acting antiviral agents for hepatitis C, and corticosteroids, including budesonide.
Lithium	QT prolongation	Increased risk of cardiac arrhythmias with other QT-prolonging agents, including domperidone, droperidol, dolasetron, granisetron, ondansetron, palonosetron, and ramosetron.
Psychostimulants		
Armodafinil and modafinil	Induces CYP3A4	Increased metabolism and reduced therapeutic effects of aprepitant, granisetron, and corticosteroids, including budesonide.
Atomoxetine	Inhibits CYP2D6	Increased levels and toxicity of tropisetron.

Note. CYP=cytochrome P450; TCAs=tricyclic antidepressants.
Source. Compiled from Cozza et al. 2003; Wynn et al. 2007; and product monographs.

Key Clinical Points

- Dysphagia secondary to antipsychotic-induced extrapyramidal side effects can lead to life-threatening aspiration and pneumonia, particularly in the elderly.

- Non-GERD noncardiac chest pain may respond to agents that modulate pain sensitivity and pain perception. Trazodone, TCAs, SSRIs, and SNRIs have demonstrated effectiveness.

- Non-ulcer dyspepsia may respond to antidepressants and anxiolytics for pain reduction. Data are strongest for TCAs, but buspirone might also have a role.

- Nausea and vomiting due to pregnancy, cancer, or cancer treatment may respond to antipsychotics or mirtazapine. Patients should be monitored for extrapyramidal symptoms with antipsychotic agents.

- Gastric bypass and celiac disease may alter drug absorption, reducing therapeutic effect. Liquid or orally disintegrating tablets should be used instead of extended-release preparations.

- Patients with celiac disease should consult with their local pharmacist or prescription delivery service to determine whether their medications are gluten-free.

- Paroxetine, bupropion, phenelzine, and low-dose TCAs may improve quality of life in inflammatory bowel disease. Bupropion and phenelzine may induce disease remission.

- Although the effectiveness of antidepressants for irritable bowel syndrome (IBS) without comorbid psychopathology is debatable, these agents are frequently prescribed. If used, SSRIs are preferable for constipation-predominant IBS, and TCAs are preferred for diarrhea-predominant IBS.

- Direct-acting antiviral regimens have replaced interferon-based regimens and their associated psychiatric side effects. However, greater care is needed with psychotropic drug dosing because of risk of drug-drug interactions.

- Psychotropic drug dosing may need to be reduced in hepatic impairment. The Child-Pugh score, a clinical measure that estimates the severity of cirrhosis, can help guide dosing.
- The risk of upper gastrointestinal bleeding due to SSRIs appears to be much lower than first thought, although caution should be used in patient groups considered to be at high risk for upper gastrointestinal bleeding (e.g., history of upper gastrointestinal bleeds, use of NSAIDs, elderly age).
- Drug-induced pancreatitis, although rare, has been linked to some antidepressants and anticonvulsants and possibly to antipsychotic agents as well. If a patient develops drug-induced pancreatitis, rechallenge with the same agent is not recommended.
- Patients taking clozapine are at risk for serious gastrointestinal complications arising from constipation. Attention to bowel habits, drug dosage, the use of other anticholinergic agents, and coadministration of laxatives is advisable.

References

Abdulkader A, Voronovich Z, Carley J: A review of therapeutic uses of mirtazapine in psychiatric and medical conditions. Prim Care Companion CNS Disord 15(5) doi: 10.4088/PCCC.13r101525, 2013 24511451

Adedoyin A, Branch RA: Pharmacokinetics, in Hepatology: A Textbook of Liver Disease, 3rd Edition. Edited by Zakim D, Boyer TD. Philadelphia, PA, WB Saunders, 1996, pp 307–322

Aksoy H, Aksoy Ü, Karadağ OI, et al: Depression levels in patients with hyperemesis gravidarum: a prospective case-control study. Springerplus 4:34, 2015 25646155

Alastal Y, Hasan S, Chowdhury MA, et al: Hypertriglyceridemia-induced pancreatitis in psychiatric patients: case report and review of literature. Am J Ther July 1, 2014 [Epub ahead of print] 24987947

Albers I, Hartmann H, Bircher J, Creutzfeldt W: Superiority of the Child-Pugh classification to quantitative liver function tests for assessing prognosis of liver cirrhosis. Scand J Gastroenterol 24(3):269–276, 1989 2734585

Al-Omari A, Cowan J, Turner L, Cooper C: Antidepressant prophylaxis reduces depression risk but does not improve sustained virological response in hepatitis C interferon recipients without depression at baseline: a systematic review and meta-analysis. Can J Gastroenterol 27:575–581, 2013 24106729

American Association for the Study of Liver Diseases: Initial treatment of HCV infection, 2015. Available at: http://www.hcvguidelines.org/full-report/initial-treatment-hcv-infection. Accessed April 8, 2016.

Amos K, Yeoh SC, Farah CS: Combined topical and systemic clonazepam therapy for the management of burning mouth syndrome: a retrospective pilot study. J Orofac Pain 25(2):125–130, 2011 21528119

Anderson RJ, Gambertoglio JG, Schrier RW: Clinical Use of Drugs in Renal Failure. Springfield, IL, Charles C Thomas, 1976

Andrade C, Sandarsh S, Chethan KB, Nagesh KS: Serotonin reuptake inhibitor antidepressants and abnormal bleeding: a review for clinicians and a reconsideration of mechanisms. J Clin Psychiatry 71(12):1565–1575, 2010 21190637

Anglin R, Yuan Y, Moayyedi P, et al: Risk of upper gastrointestinal bleeding with selective serotonin reuptake inhibitors with or without concurrent nonsteroidal anti-inflammatory use: a systematic review and meta-analysis. Am J Gastroenterol 109(6):811–819, 2014 24777151

Badar T, Cortes J, Borthakur G, et al: Phase II open label, randomized comparative trial of ondansetron alone versus the combination of ondansetron and aprepitant for the prevention of nausea and vomiting in patients with hematologic malignancies receiving regiment containing high-dose cytarabine. Biomed Res Int doi: 10.1155/2015/497597, 2015 25654108

Balani AR, Grendell JH: Drug-induced pancreatitis: incidence, management and prevention. Drug Saf 31(10):823–837, 2008 18759507

Bashashati M, Hejazi RA, Andrews CN, Storr MA: Gastroesophageal reflux symptoms not responding to proton pump inhibitor: GERD, NERD, NARD, esophageal hypersensitivity or dyspepsia? Can J Gastroenterol Hepatol 28(6):335–341, 2014 24719900

Bielefeldt K: Gastroparesis: concepts, controversies, and challenges. Scientifica doi: 10.6064/2012/424802, 2012 24278691

Blaschke TF: Protein binding and kinetics of drugs in liver diseases. Clin Pharmacokinet 2(1):32–44, 1977 322909

Bodén R, Bexelius TS, Mattsson F, et al: Antidopaminergic drugs and acute pancreatitis: a population-based study. BMJ Open 2(3):e000914, 2012 22581796

Braak B, Klooker TK, Wouters MM, et al: Randomised clinical trial: the effects of amitriptyline on drinking capacity and symptoms in patients with functional dyspepsia, a double-blind placebo-controlled study. Aliment Pharmacol Ther 34(6):638–648, 2011 21767283

Brahm NC, Kelly-Rehm MC: Antidepressant-mediated gastroesophageal reflux disease. Consult Pharm 26(4):274–278, 2011 21486738

Brennan BP, Fogarty KV, Roberts JL, et al: Duloxetine in the treatment of irritable bowel syndrome: an open-label pilot study. Hum Psychopharmacol 24(5):423–428, 2009 19548294

Brietzke E, Lafer B: Long-acting injectable risperidone in a bipolar patient submitted to bariatric surgery and intolerant to conventional mood stabilizers (letter). Psychiatry Clin Neurosci 65(2):205, 2011 21414098

Burgstaller JM, Jenni BF, Steurer J, et al: Treatment efficacy for non-cardiovascular chest pain: a systematic review and meta-analysis. PLoS One 9(8):e104722, 2014 25111147

Camilleri M: Pharmacological agents currently in clinical trials for disorders in neuro-gastroenterology. J Clin Invest 123(10):4111–4120, 2013 24084743

Camilleri M, Stanghellini V: Current management strategies and emerging treatments for functional dyspepsia. Nat Rev Gastroenterol Hepatol 10(3):187–194, 2013 23381190

Canaparo R, Finnström N, Serpe L, et al: Expression of CYP3A isoforms and P-glycoprotein in human stomach, jejunum and ileum. Clin Exp Pharmacol Physiol 34(11):1138–1144, 2007 17880367

Cappell MS: Colonic toxicity of administered drugs and chemicals. Am J Gastroenterol 99(6):1175–1190, 2004 15180742

Celinski K, Konturek SJ, Konturek PC, et al: Melatonin or L-tryptophan accelerates healing of gastroduodenal ulcers in patients treated with omeprazole. J Pineal Res 50(4):389–394, 2011 21362032

Cha JM, Kozarek RA, Lin OS: Case of cannabinoid hyperemesis syndrome with long-term follow-up. World J Clin Cases 2(12):930–933, 2014 25516874

Chao GQ, Zhang S: A meta-analysis of the therapeutic effects of amitriptyline for treating irritable bowel syndrome. Intern Med 52(4):419–424, 2013 23411695

Charleston L IV: Burning mouth syndrome: a review of recent literature. Curr Pain Headache Rep 17(6):336, 2013 23645183

Cheng YC, Chen CC, Ho AS, Chiu NY: Prolonged psychosis associated with interferon therapy in a patient with hepatitis C: case study and literature review. Psychosomatics 50(5):538–542, 2009 19855041

Chepyala P, Svoboda RP, Olden KW: Treatment of cyclic vomiting syndrome. Curr Treat Options Gastroenterol 10(4):273–282, 2007 17761120

Chial HJ, Camilleri M, Burton D, et al: Selective effects of serotonergic psychoactive agents on gastrointestinal functions in health. Am J Physiol Gastrointest Liver Physiol 284(1):G130–G137, 2003 12488239

Chopra S, Muir AJ: Treatment regimens for chronic hepatitis C virus genotype 1. UpToDate, 2015. Available at: http://www.uptodate.com/contents/treatment-regimens-for-chronic-hepatitis-c-virus-genotype-1?source=search_result&search=Treatment+regimens+for+chronic+hepatitis+C+virus+genotype+1&selectedTitle=1%7E150. Accessed June 10, 2015.

Ciovica R, Riedl O, Neumayer C, et al: The use of medication after laparoscopic antireflux surgery. Surg Endosc 23(9):1938–1946, 2009 19169748

Clavé P, Shaker R: Dysphagia: current reality and scope of the problem. Nat Rev Gastroenterol Hepatol 12(5):259–270, 2015 25850008

Clouse RE, Sayuk GS, Lustman PJ, Prakash C: Zonisamide or levetiracetam for adults with cyclic vomiting syndrome: a case series. Clin Gastroenterol Hepatol 5(1):44–48, 2007 17157078

Cohen D, Bogers JPAM, van Dijk D, et al: Beyond white blood cell monitoring: screening in the initial phase of clozapine therapy. J Clin Psychiatry 73(10):1307–1312, 2012 23140648

Coss-Adame E, Erdogan A, Rao SSC: Treatment of esophageal (noncardiac) chest pain: an expert review. Clin Gastroenterol Hepatol 12(8):1224–1245, 2014 23994670

Cozza KL, Armstrong S, Oesterheld J: Concise Guide to the Cytochrome P450 System: Drug Interaction Principles for Medical Practice. Washington, DC, American Psychiatric Publishing, 2003

Crone CC, Gabriel GM, DiMartini A: An overview of psychiatric issues in liver disease for the consultation-liaison psychiatrist. Psychosomatics 47(3):188–205, 2006 16684936

Cruz JE, Cocchio C, Lai PT, Hermes-DeSantis E: Gluten content of medications. Am J Health Syst Pharm 72(1):54–60, 2015 25511839

Dall M, Schaffalitzky de Muckadell OB, Lassen AT, et al: An association between selective serotonin reuptake inhibitor use and serious upper gastrointestinal bleeding. Clin Gastroenterol Hepatol 7(12):1314–1321, 2009 19716436

Dall M, Schaffalitzky de Muckadell OB, Lassen AT, Hallas J: There is an association between selective serotonin reuptake inhibitor use and uncomplicated peptic ulcers: a population-based case-control study. Aliment Pharmacol Ther 32(11–12):1383–1391, 2010 21050241

Dantas RO, Nobre Souza MA: Dysphagia induced by chronic ingestion of benzodiazepine. Am J Gastroenterol 92(7):1194–1196, 1997 9219798

de Abajo FJ: Effects of selective serotonin reuptake inhibitors on platelet function: mechanisms, clinical outcomes and implications for use in elderly patients. Drugs Aging 28(5):345–367, 2011 21542658 de Abajo FJ, García-Rodríguez LA: Risk of upper gastrointestinal tract bleeding associated with selective serotonin reuptake inhibitors and venlafaxine therapy: interaction with nonsteroidal anti-inflammatory drugs and effect of acid-suppressing agents. Arch Gen Psychiatry 65(7):795–803, 2008 18606952

De Hert M, Hudyana H, Dockx L, et al: Second-generation antipsychotics and constipation: a review of the literature. Eur Psychiatry 26(1):34–44, 2011 20542667

de Knegt RJ, Bezemer G, Van Gool AR, et al: Randomised clinical trial: escitalopram for the prevention of psychiatric adverse events during treatment with peginterferon-alfa-2a and ribavirin for chronic hepatitis C. Aliment Pharmacol Ther 34(11–12):1306–1317, 2011 21999489

Dellon ES, Ringel Y: Treatment of functional diarrhea. Curr Treat Options Gastroenterol 9(4):331–342, 2006 16836952

den Hollander WJ, Kuipers EJ: Current pharmacotherapy options for gastritis. Expert Opin Pharmacother 13(18):2625–2636, 2012 23167300

DeSanty KP, Amabile CM: Antidepressant-induced liver injury. Ann Pharmacother 41(7):1201–1211, 2007 17609231

de Souza FTA, Teixeira AL, Amaral TMP, et al: Psychiatric disorders in burning mouth syndrome. J Psychosom Res 72(2):142–146, 2012 22281456

Dhir R, Brown DK, Olden KW: Drug-induced pancreatitis: a practical review. Drugs Today (Barc) 43(7):499–507, 2007 17728850

Dick TB, Lindberg LS, Ramirez DD, et al: A clinician's guide to drug-drug interactions with direct acting antiviral agents for the treatment of hepatitis C virus. Hepatology 63(2):634–643, 2015 26033675

Drossman DA: The functional gastrointestinal disorders and the Rome III process. Gastroenterology 130(5):1377–1390, 2006 16678553

Drossman DA, Camilleri M, Mayer EA, Whitehead WE: AGA technical review on irritable bowel syndrome. Gastroenterology 123(6):2108–2131, 2002 12454866

Ducasse D, Courtet P, Olie E: Burning mouth syndrome: current clinical, physiopathologic, and therapeutic data. Reg Anesth Pain Med 38(5):380–390, 2013 23970045

Duggal HS, Mendhekar DN: Risperidone-induced tardive pharyngeal dystonia presenting with persistent dysphagia: a case report. Prim Care Companion J Clin Psychiatry 10(2):161–162, 2008 18458730

Dziewas R, Warnecke T, Schnabel M, et al: Neuroleptic-induced dysphagia: case report and literature review. Dysphagia 22(1):63–67, 2007 17024549

Einarson A, Maltepe C, Boskovic R, Koren G: Treatment of nausea and vomiting in pregnancy: an updated algorithm. Can Fam Physician 53(12):2109–2111, 2007 18077743

Enck P, Junne F, Klosterhalfen S, et al: Therapy options in irritable bowel syndrome. Eur J Gastroenterol Hepatol 22(12):1402–1411, 2010 21389791

Enweluzo C, Aziz F: Gastroparesis: a review of current and emerging treatment options. Clin Exp Gastroenterol 6:161–165, 2013 24039443

Faramarzi M, Kheirkhah F, Shokri-Shirvani J, et al: Psychological factors in patients with peptic ulcer and functional dyspepsia. Caspian J Intern Med 5(2):71–76, 2014 24778780

Fayad SM, Bruijnzeel DM: A fatal case of adynamic ileus following initiation of clozapine. Am J Psychiatry 169(5):538–539, 2012 22549212

Fernández-Bañares F, de Sousa MR, Salas A, et al; RECOMINA Project, GETECCU Grupo Español de Enfermedades de Crohn y Colitis Ulcerosa: Epidemiological risk factors in microscopic colitis: a prospective case-control study. Inflamm Bowel Dis 19(2):411–417, 2013 23344243

Flanagan RJ, Ball RY: Gastrointestinal hypomotility: an under-recognised life-threatening adverse effect of clozapine. Forensic Sci Int 206(1–3):e31–e36, 2011 20719440

Ford AC, Moayyedi P: Dyspepsia. Curr Opin Gastroenterol 29(6):662–668, 2013 24100727

Ford AC, Vandvik PO: Irritable bowel syndrome. BMJ Clin Evid pii: 0410, 2012 22296841

Ford AC, Talley NJ, Schoenfeld PS, et al: Efficacy of antidepressants and psychological therapies in irritable bowel syndrome: systematic review and meta-analysis. Gut 58(3):367–378, 2009 19001059

Ford AC, Moayyedi P, Lacy BE, et al; Task Force on the Management of Functional Bowel Disorders: American College of Gastroenterology monograph on the management of irritable bowel syndrome and chronic idiopathic constipation. Am J Gastroenterol 109 (suppl 1):S2–S26, quiz S27, 2014a 25091148

Ford AC, Quigley EMM, Lacy BE, et al: Effect of antidepressants and psychological therapies, including hypnotherapy, in irritable bowel syndrome: systematic review and meta-analysis. Am J Gastroenterol 109(9):1350–1365, quiz 1366, 2014b 24935275

Fosnes GS, Lydersen S, Farup PG: Constipation and diarrhoea—common adverse drug reactions? A cross sectional study in the general population. BMC Clin Pharmacol 11:2, 2011 21332973

Fratto G, Manzon L: Use of psychotropic drugs and associated dental diseases. Int J Psychiatry Med 48(3):185–197, 2014 25492713

Fuller-Thomson E, Sulman J: Depression and inflammatory bowel disease: findings from two nationally representative Canadian surveys. Inflamm Bowel Dis 12(8):697–707, 2006 16917224

Galli JA, Sawaya RA, Friedenberg FK: Cannabinoid hyperemesis syndrome. Curr Drug Abuse Rev 4(4):241–249, 2011 22150623

Gasse C, Jacobsen J, Pedersen L, et al: Risk of hospitalization for acute pancreatitis associated with conventional and atypical antipsychotics: a population-based case-control study. Pharmacotherapy 28(1):27–34, 2008 18154471

Gerstner T, Büsing D, Bell N, et al: Valproic acid–induced pancreatitis: 16 new cases and a review of the literature. J Gastroenterol 42(1):39–48, 2007 17322992

Gogela NA, Lin MV, Wisocky JL, Chung RT: Enhancing our understanding of current therapies for hepatitis C virus (HCV). Curr HIV/AIDS Rep 12(1):68–78, 2015 25761432

Goh T, Dhillon R, Bastiampillai T: Manic induction with interferon alpha therapy (letter). Aust N Z J Psychiatry 45(11):1004, 2011 21981775

Gollock JM, Thomson JP: Ischaemic colitis associated with psychotropic drugs. Postgrad Med J 60(706):564–565, 1984 6473240

Greenblatt DJ, Koch-Weser J: Clinical toxicity of chlordiazepoxide and diazepam in relation to serum albumin concentration: a report from the Boston Collaborative Drug Surveillance Program. Eur J Clin Pharmacol 7(4):259–262, 1974 4851053

Gremeau-Richard C, Woda A, Navez ML, et al: Topical clonazepam in stomatodynia: a randomised placebo-controlled study. Pain 108(1–2):51–57, 2004 15109507

Gwillim EC, Bowyer BA: Duloxetine-induced lymphocytic colitis. J Clin Gastroenterol 46(8):717–718, 2012 22874808

Hallbäck I, Hägg S, Eriksson AC, Whiss PA: In vitro effects of serotonin and noradrenaline reuptake inhibitors on human platelet adhesion and coagulation. Pharmacol Rep 64(4):979–983, 2012 23087151

Hamad GG, Helsel JC, Perel JM, et al: The effect of gastric bypass on the pharmacokinetics of serotonin reuptake inhibitors. Am J Psychiatry 169(3):256–263, 2012 22407114

Han P, Suarez-Durall P, Mulligan R: Dry mouth: a critical topic for older adult patients. J Prosthodont Res 59(1):6–19, 2015 25498205

Heckmann SM, Kirchner E, Gruschka M, et al: A double-blind study on clonazepam in patients with burning mouth syndrome. Laryngoscope 122(4): 813–816, 2012 22344742

Hejazi RA, McCallum RW: Cyclic vomiting syndrome: treatment options. Exp Brain Res 232(8):2549–2552, 2014 24862509

Hejazi RA, Reddymasu SC, Namin F, et al: Efficacy of tricyclic antidepressant therapy in adults with cyclic vomiting syndrome: a two-year follow-up study. J Clin Gastroenterol 44(1):18–21, 2010 20027010

Hershcovici T, Achem SR, Jha LK, Fass R: Systematic review: the treatment of noncardiac chest pain. Aliment Pharmacol Ther 35(1):5–14, 2012 22077344

Hibbard KR, Propst A, Frank DE, Wyse J: Fatalities associated with clozapine-related constipation and bowel obstruction: a literature review and two case reports. Psychosomatics 50(4):416–419, 2009 19687183

Horst S, Chao A, Rosen M, et al: Treatment with immunosuppressive therapy may improve depressive symptoms in patients with inflammatory bowel disease. Dig Dis Sci 60(2):465–470, 2014 25274158

Hou XJ, Xu JH, Yu YY: Can antidepressants prevent pegylated interferon-alpha/ribavirin-associated depression in patients with chronic hepatitis C: meta-analysis of randomized, double-blind, placebo-controlled trials? PLoS One 8(10):e76799, 2013 24204676

Hussain A, Burke J: Mirtazapine associated with recurrent pancreatitis—a case report. J Psychopharmacol 22(3):336–337, 2008 18208920

Hussaini SH, Farrington EA: Idiosyncratic drug-induced liver injury: an update on the 2007 overview. Expert Opin Drug Saf 13(1):67–81, 2014 24073714

Iacopetti CL, Packer CD: Cannabinoid hyperemesis syndrome: a case report and review of pathophysiology. Clin Med Res 12(1–2):65–67, 2014 24667219

Ikai S, Suzuki T, Uchida H, et al: Reintroduction of clozapine after perforation of the large intestine—a case report and review of the literature. Ann Pharmacother 47(7–8):e31, 2013 23757383

Iskandar HN, Cassell B, Kanuri N, et al: Tricyclic antidepressants for management of residual symptoms in inflammatory bowel disease. J Clin Gastroenterol 48(5):423–429, 2014 24406434

Jacobson S: Psychopharmacology: prescribing for patients with hepatic or renal dysfunction. Psych Times 12:65–70, 2002

Jones MP: The role of psychosocial factors in peptic ulcer disease: beyond Helicobacter pylori and NSAIDs. J Psychosom Res 60(4):407–412, 2006 16581366

Jones MP, Crowell MD, Olden KW, Creed F: Functional gastrointestinal disorders: an update for the psychiatrist. Psychosomatics 48(2):93–102, 2007 17329601

Jordan K, Schaffrath J, Jahn F, et al: Neuropharmacology and management of chemotherapy-induced nausea and vomiting in patients with breast cancer. Breast Care (Basel) 9(4):246–253, 2014 25404883

Kashyap P, Farrugia G: Diabetic gastroparesis: what we have learned and had to unlearn in the past 5 years. Gut 59(12):1716–1726, 2010 20871131

Kast RE: Crohn's disease remission with phenelzine treatment. Gastroenterology 115(4):1034–1035, 1998 9786733

Kast RE, Altschuler EL: Remission of Crohn's disease on bupropion. Gastroenterology 121(5):1260–1261, 2001 11706830

Kaurich T: Drug-induced acute pancreatitis. Proc (Bayl Univ Med Cent) 21(1):77–81, 2008 18209761

Kawabe K, Ueno S: A case of acute pancreatitis associated with risperidone treatment. Clin Psychopharmacol Neurosci 12(1):67–68, 2014 24851124

Kerr TA, Jonnalagadda S, Prakash C, Azar R: Pancreatitis following olanzapine therapy: a report of three cases. Case Rep Gastroenterol 1(1):15–20, 2007 21487466

Kim SW, Shin IS, Kim JM, et al: Mirtazapine for severe gastroparesis unresponsive to conventional prokinetic treatment. Psychosomatics 47(5):440–442, 2006 16959934

Kim S-W, Shin I-S, Kim J-M, et al: Effectiveness of mirtazapine for nausea and insomnia in cancer patients with depression. Psychiatry Clin Neurosci 62(1):75–83, 2008 18289144

King AR; University of Kansas Drug Information Center Experiential Rotation Students, August 2012: Gluten content of the top 200 medications: follow-up to the influence of gluten on a patient's medication choices. Hosp Pharm 48(9):736–743, 2013 24421547

Kirkcaldy RD, Kim TJ, Carney CP: A somatoform variant of obsessive-compulsive disorder: a case report of OCD presenting with persistent vomiting. Prim Care Companion J Clin Psychiatry 6(5):195–198, 2004 15514688

Kohen I, Lester P: Quetiapine-associated dysphagia. World J Biol Psychiatry 10(4 Pt 2):623–625, 2009 18615368

Kumar N, Bashar Q, Reddy N, et al: Cyclic vomiting syndrome (CVS): is there a difference based on onset of symptoms—pediatric versus adult? BMC Gastroenterol 12:52, 2012 22639867

Lee LY, Abbott L, Mahlangu B, et al: The management of cyclic vomiting syndrome: a systematic review. Eur J Gastroenterol Hepatol 24(9):1001–1006, 2012 22634989

Leipzig RM: Psychopharmacology in patients with hepatic and gastrointestinal disease. Int J Psychiatry Med 20(2):109–139, 1990 2203695

Levenstein S, Rosenstock S, Jacobsen RK, Jorgensen T: Psychological stress increases risk for peptic ulcer, regardless of Helicobacter pylori infection or use of nonsteroidal anti-inflammatory drugs. Clin Gastroenterol Hepatol 13(3):498–506.e1, 2015 25111233

Levy RL, Olden KW, Naliboff BD, et al: Psychosocial aspects of the functional gastrointestinal disorders. Gastroenterology 130(5):1447–1458, 2006 16678558

Lichtwark IT, Newnham ED, Robinson SR, et al: Cognitive impairment in coeliac disease improves on a gluten-free diet and correlates with histological and serological indices of disease severity. Aliment Pharmacol Ther 40(2):160–170, 2014 24889390

Lin TW, Lee BS, Liao YC, et al: High dosage of aripiprazole-induced dysphagia. Int J Eat Disord 45(2):305–306, 2012 21541978

Liou LS, Hung YJ, Hsieh CH, Hsiao FC: Aggravation of hypertriglyceridemia and acute pancreatitis in a bipolar patient treated with quetiapine. Yonsei Med J 55(3):831–833, 2014 24719155

Logemann JA: Dysphagia in movement disorders. Adv Neurol 49:307–316, 1988 2964174

Lohr L: Chemotherapy-induced nausea and vomiting. Cancer J 14(2):85–93, 2008 18391612

López-D'alessandro E, Escovich L: Combination of alpha lipoic acid and gabapentin, its efficacy in the treatment of burning mouth syndrome: a randomized, double-blind, placebo controlled trial. Med Oral Patol Oral Cir Bucal 16(5):e635–e640, 2011 20711135

Mackay HP, Mitchell KG, Pickard WR, et al: The effect of trimipramine (Surmontil) on the gastric secretion of acid and pepsin in patients with duodenal ulceration. J Int Med Res 12(5):303–306, 1984 6437892

Mahajan L, Wyllie R, Goldblum J: Lymphocytic colitis in a pediatric patient: a possible adverse reaction to carbamazepine. Am J Gastroenterol 92(11):2126–2127, 1997 9362214

Mahajan S, Avasthi A, Grover S, Chawla YK: Role of baseline depressive symptoms in the development of depressive episode in patients receiving antiviral therapy for hepatitis C infection. J Psychosom Res 77(2):109–115, 2014 25077851

Maina G, Vitalucci A, Gandolfo S, Bogetto F: Comparative efficacy of SSRIs and amisulpride in burning mouth syndrome: a single-blind study. J Clin Psychiatry 63(1):38–43, 2002 11838624

Martín-Merino E, Ruigómez A, García Rodríguez LA, et al: Depression and treatment with antidepressants are associated with the development of gastro-oesophageal reflux disease. Aliment Pharmacol Ther 31(10):1132–1140, 2010 20199498

Martucci S, Biagi F, Di Sabatino A, Corazza GR: Coeliac disease. Dig Liver Dis 34 (suppl 2):S150–S153, 2002 12408460

Marwick KFM, Taylor M, Walker SW: Antipsychotics and abnormal liver function tests: systematic review. Clin Neuropharmacol 35(5):244–253, 2012 22986798

Masters KJ: Pilocarpine treatment of xerostomia induced by psychoactive medications (letter). Am J Psychiatry 162(5):1023, 2005 15863819

McCain KR, Sawyer TS, Spiller HA: Evaluation of centrally acting cholinesterase inhibitor exposures in adults. Ann Pharmacother 41(10):1632–1637, 2007 17848422

McCarthy FP, Lutomski JE, Greene RA: Hyperemesis gravidarum: current perspectives. Int J Womens Health 6:719–725, 2014 25125986

Menon RM, Badri PS, Wang T, et al: Drug-drug interaction profile of the all-oral anti-hepatitis C virus regimen of paritaprevir/ritonavir, ombitasvir, and dasabuvir. J Hepatol 63(1):20–29, 2015 25646891

Mikocka-Walus AA, Turnbull DA, Moulding NT, et al: Antidepressants and inflammatory bowel disease: a systematic review. Clin Pract Epidemiol Ment Health 2:24, 2006 16984660

Monti JM, Pandi-Perumal SR: Eszopiclone: its use in the treatment of insomnia. Neuropsychiatr Dis Treat 3(4):441–453, 2007 19300573

Morasco BJ, Loftis JM, Indest DW, et al: Prophylactic antidepressant treatment in patients with hepatitis C on antiviral therapy: a double-blind, placebo-controlled trial. Psychosomatics 51(5):401–408, 2010 20833939

Nagashima W, Kimura H, Ito M, et al: Effectiveness of duloxetine for the treatment of chronic nonorganic orofacial pain. Clin Neuropharmacol 35(6):273–277, 2012 23123692

Nguyen TMT, Eslick GD: Systematic review: the treatment of noncardiac chest pain with antidepressants. Aliment Pharmacol Ther 35(5):493–500, 2012 22239853

Nielsen J, Meyer JM: Risk factors for ileus in patients with schizophrenia. Schizophr Bull 38(3):592–598, 2012 21112965

Nieves JE, Stack KM, Harrison ME, Gorman JM: Dysphagia: a rare form of dyskinesia? J Psychiatr Pract 13(3):199–201, 2007 17522565

Nitsche CJ, Jamieson N, Lerch MM, Mayerle JV: Drug induced pancreatitis. Best Pract Res Clin Gastroenterol 24(2):143–155, 2010 20227028

North CS, Hong BA, Alpers DH: Relationship of functional gastrointestinal disorders and psychiatric disorders: implications for treatment. World J Gastroenterol 13(14):2020–2027, 2007 17465442

Nwokediuko SC: Current trends in the management of gastroesophageal reflux disease: a review. ISRN Gastroenterol doi:10.5402/2012/391631, 2012 22844607

Oh JH, Pasricha PJ: Recent advances in the pathophysiology and treatment of gastroparesis. J Neurogastroenterol Motil 19(1):18–24, 2013 23350043

Oka Y, Okamoto K, Kawashita N, et al: Meta-analysis of the risk of upper gastrointestinal hemorrhage with combination therapy of selective serotonin reuptake inhibitors and non-steroidal anti-inflammatory drugs. Biol Pharm Bull 37(6):947–953, 2014 24681541

Olden KW, Crowell MD: Chronic nausea and vomiting: new insights and approach to treatment. Curr Treat Options Gastroenterol 8(4):305–310, 2005 16009031

Olson KR, Pond SM, Verrier ED, Federle M: Intestinal infarction complicating phenobarbital overdose. Arch Intern Med 144(2):407–408, 1984 6696580

O'Neill JL, Remington TL: Drug-induced esophageal injuries and dysphagia. Ann Pharmacother 37(11):1675–1684, 2003 14565800

Oustamanolakis P, Tack J: Dyspepsia: organic versus functional. J Clin Gastroenterol 46(3):175–190, 2012 22327302

Overland MK: Dyspepsia. Med Clin North Am 98(3):549–564, 2014 24758960

Owyang C: Treatment of chronic secretory diarrhea of unknown origin by lithium carbonate. Gastroenterology 87(3):714–718, 1984 6430744

Ozdemir HH, Bulut S, Berilgen MS, et al: Resistant cyclic vomiting syndrome successfully responding to chlorpromazine. Acta Medica (Hradec Kralove) 57(1):28–29, 2014 25006660

Pacifici GM, Viani A, Franchi M, et al: Conjugation pathways in liver disease. Br J Clin Pharmacol 30(3):427–435, 1990 2223421

Padwal R, Brocks D, Sharma AM: A systematic review of drug absorption following bariatric surgery and its theoretical implications. Obes Rev 11(1):41–50, 2010 19493300

Palmer SE, McLean RM, Ellis PM, Harrison-Woolrych M: Life-threatening clozapine-induced gastrointestinal hypomotility: an analysis of 102 cases. J Clin Psychiatry 69(5):759–768, 2008 18452342

Palsson OS, Drossman DA: Psychiatric and psychological dysfunction in irritable bowel syndrome and the role of psychological treatments. Gastroenterol Clin North Am 34(2):281–303, 2005 15862936

Pardi DS: Microscopic colitis. Clin Geriatr Med 30(1):55–65, 2014 24267602

Pardi DS, Ramnath VR, Loftus EV Jr, et al: Lymphocytic colitis: clinical features, treatment, and outcomes. Am J Gastroenterol 97(11):2829–2833, 2002 12425555

Park MI, Camilleri M: Gastroparesis: clinical update. Am J Gastroenterol 101(5):1129–1139, 2006 16696789

Parker LA, Rock EM, Limebeer CL: Regulation of nausea and vomiting by cannabinoids. Br J Pharmacol 163(7):1411–1422, 2011 21175589

Passmore MJ, Devarajan S, Ghatavi K, et al: Serotonin syndrome with prolonged dysphagia. Can J Psychiatry 49(1):79–80, 2004 14763689

Patrick A, Epstein O, Ghatavi K, et al: Review article: gastroparesis. Aliment Pharmacol Ther 27(9):724–740, 2008 18248660

Patten SB: Psychiatric side effects of interferon treatment. Curr Drug Saf 1(2):143–150, 2006 18690925

Peery AF, Dellon ES, Lund J, et al: Burden of gastrointestinal disease in the United States: 2012 update. Gastroenterology 143(5):1179–1187.e1–3, 2012 22885331

Persoons P, Vermeire S, Demyttenaere K, et al: The impact of major depressive disorder on the short- and long-term outcome of Crohn's disease treatment with infliximab. Aliment Pharmacol Ther 22(2):101–110, 2005 16011668

Peyrière H, Roux C, Ferard C, et al; French Network of the Pharmacovigilance Centers: Antipsychotics-induced ischaemic colitis and gastrointestinal necrosis: a review of the French pharmacovigilance database. Pharmacoepidemiol Drug Saf 18(10):948–955, 2009 19572384

Piacentino D, Cantarini R, Alfonsi M, et al: Psychopathological features of irritable bowel syndrome patients with and without functional dyspepsia: a cross sectional study. BMC Gastroenterol 11:94, 2011 21871075

Potolidis E, Mandros C, Karakitsos D, et al: Quetiapine-associated pancreatitis in a geriatric critical care patient with delirium. Case Rep Psychiatry 625954, 2012 22934221

Prakash C, Staiano A, Rothbaum RJ, Clouse RE: Similarities in cyclic vomiting syndrome across age groups. Am J Gastroenterol 96(3):684–688, 2001 11280534

Quigley EMM, Lacy BE: Overlap of functional dyspepsia and GERD—diagnostic and treatment implications. Nat Rev Gastroenterol Hepatol 10(3):175–186, 2013 23296247

Rahimi R, Nikfar S, Rezaie A, Abdollahi M: Efficacy of tricyclic antidepressants in irritable bowel syndrome: a meta-analysis. World J Gastroenterol 15(13):1548–1553, 2009 19340896

Ramamourthy P, Kumaran A, Kattimani S: Risperidone associated paralytic ileus in schizophrenia. Indian J Psychol Med 35(1):87–88, 2013 23833349

Rashid J, Starer PJ, Javaid S: Pancreatitis and diabetic ketoacidosis with quetiapine use. Psychiatry (Edgmont) 6(5):34–37, 2009 19724733

Remes-Troche JM: The hypersensitive esophagus: pathophysiology, evaluation, and treatment options. Curr Gastroenterol Rep 12(5):417–426, 2010 20669058

Rodriguez-Cerdeira C, Sanchez-Blanco E: Treatment of burning mouth syndrome with amisulpride. J Clin Med Res 4(3):167–171, 2012 22719802

Roerig JL, Steffen K, Zimmerman C, et al: Preliminary comparison of sertraline levels in postbariatric surgery patients versus matched nonsurgical cohort. Surg Obes Relat Dis 8(1):62–66, 2012 21256091

Roerig JL, Steffen KJ, Zimmerman C, et al: A comparison of duloxetine plasma levels in postbariatric surgery patients versus matched nonsurgical control subjects. J Clin Psychopharmacol 33(4):479–484, 2013 23771193

Ruepert L, Quartero AO, de Wit NJ, et al: Bulking agents, antispasmodics, and antidepressants for the treatment of irritable bowel syndrome. Cochrane Database of Systematic Reviews 2011, Issue 8. Art. No.: CD003460. DOI: 10.1002/14651858.CD003460.pub3 21833945

Russo MW, Watkins PB: Are patients with elevated liver tests at increased risk of drug-induced liver injury? Gastroenterology 126(5):1477–1480, 2004 15131809

Russo MW, Galanko JA, Shrestha R, et al: Liver transplantation for acute liver failure from drug induced liver injury in the United States. Liver Transpl 10(8):1018–1023, 2004 15390328

Saha L: Irritable bowel syndrome: pathogenesis, diagnosis, treatment, and evidence-based medicine. World J Gastroenterol 20(22):6759–6773, 2014 24944467

Santoro GA, Eitan BZ, Pryde A, Bartolo DC: Open study of low-dose amitriptyline in the treatment of patients with idiopathic fecal incontinence. Dis Colon Rectum 43(12):1676–1681, discussion 1681–1682, 2000 11156450

Schaefer M, Sarkar R, Knop V, et al: Escitalopram for the prevention of peginterferon-alpha2a-associated depression in hepatitis C virus-infected patients without previous psychiatric disease: a randomized trial. Ann Intern Med 157(2):94–103, 2012 22801672

Schwarzer V, Heep A, Gembruch U, Rohde A: Treatment resistant hyperemesis gravidarum in a patient with type 1 diabetes mellitus: neonatal withdrawal symptoms after successful antiemetic therapy with mirtazapine. Arch Gynecol Obstet 277(1):67–69, 2008 17628816

Seaman JS, Bowers SP, Dixon P, Schindler L: Dissolution of common psychiatric medications in a Roux-en-Y gastric bypass model. Psychosomatics 46(3):250–253, 2005 15883146

Sevastru S, Wakatsuki M, Fennell J, et al: Plasma exchange in the management of a case of hypertriglyceridemic pancreatitis triggered by venlafaxine. BMJ Case Rep doi: 101136/bcr.11.2011.5208, 2012 22892234

Shamash J, Miall L, Williams F, et al: Dysphagia in the neuroleptic malignant syndrome. Br J Psychiatry 164(6):849–850, 1994 7953002

Shrivastava RK, Siegal H, Lawlor R, et al: Doxepin therapy for duodenal ulcer: a controlled trial in patients who failed to respond to cimetidine. Clin Ther 7(3):319–326, 1985 3888393

Sico JJ, Patwa H: Risperidone-induced bulbar palsy–like syndrome. Dysphagia 26(3):340–343, 2011 20922432

Simonetto DA, Oxentenko AS, Herman ML, Szostek JH: Cannabinoid hyperemesis: a case series of 98 patients. Mayo Clin Proc 87(2):114–119, 2012 22305024

Sockalingam S, Tseng A, Giguere P, Wong D: Psychiatric treatment considerations with direct acting antivirals in hepatitis C. BMC Gastroenterol 13:86, 2013 23672254

Sockalingam S, Sheehan K, Feld JJ, Shah H: Psychiatric care during hepatitis C treatment: the changing role of psychiatrists in the era of direct-acting antivirals. Am J Psychiatry 172(6):512–516, 2015 26029803

Soriano V, Labarga P, Barreiro P, et al: Drug interactions with new hepatitis C oral drugs. Expert Opin Drug Metab Toxicol 11(3):333–341, 2015 25553890

Spiegel DR, Kolb R: Treatment of irritable bowel syndrome with comorbid anxiety symptoms with mirtazapine. Clin Neuropharmacol 34(1):36–38, 2011 21242743

Spiegel DR, Webb K: A case of treatment refractory hyperemesis gravidarum in a patient with comorbid anxiety, treated successfully with adjunctive gabapentin: a review and the potential role of neurogastroenterology in understanding its pathogenesis and treatment. Innov Clin Neurosci 9(11–12):31–38, 2012 23346516

Spieker MR: Evaluating dysphagia. Am Fam Physician 61(12):3639–3648, 2000 10892635

Spigset O, Hägg S, Bate A: Hepatic injury and pancreatitis during treatment with serotonin reuptake inhibitors: data from the World Health Organization (WHO) database of adverse drug reactions. Int Clin Psychopharmacol 18(3):157–161, 2003 12702895

Srivastava M, Brito-Dellan N, Davis MP, et al: Olanzapine as an antiemetic in refractory nausea and vomiting in advanced cancer. J Pain Symptom Manage 25(6):578–582, 2003 12782438

Stahmeyer JT, Rossol S, Krauth C: Outcomes, costs and cost-effectiveness of treating hepatitis C with direct acting antivirals. J Comp Eff Res 4:1–11, 2015 25960028

Stein B, Everhart KK, Lacy BE: Treatment of functional dyspepsia and gastroparesis. Curr Treat Options Gastroenterol 12(4):385–397, 2014 25169218

Sun S, Zimmermann AE: Cannabinoid hyperemesis syndrome. Hosp Pharm 48(8):650–655, 2013 24421535

Tack J, Janssen P, Masaoka T, et al: Efficacy of buspirone, a fundus-relaxing drug, in patients with functional dyspepsia. Clin Gastroenterol Hepatol 10(11):1239–1245, 2012 22813445

Talley NJ, Kellow JE, Boyce P, et al: Antidepressant therapy (imipramine and citalopram) for irritable bowel syndrome: a double-blind, randomized, placebo-controlled trial. Dig Dis Sci 53(1):108–115, 2008 17503182

Tandra S, Chalasani N, Jones DR, et al: Pharmacokinetic and pharmacodynamic alterations in the Roux-en-Y gastric bypass recipients. Ann Surg 258(2):262–269, 2013 23222033

Targownik LE, Bolton JM, Metge CJ, et al: Selective serotonin reuptake inhibitors are associated with a modest increase in the risk of upper gastrointestinal bleeding. Am J Gastroenterol 104(6):1475–1482, 2009 19491861

Thomas SG: Irritable bowel syndrome and mirtazapine. Am J Psychiatry 157(8):1341–1342, 2000 10910804

Thoppay JR, De Rossi SS, Ciarrocca KN: Burning mouth syndrome. Dent Clin North Am 57(3):497–512, 2013 23809306

Titus R, Kastenmeier A, Otterson MF: Consequences of gastrointestinal surgery on drug absorption. Nutr Clin Pract 28(4):429–436, 2013 23835364

Trinkley KE, Nahata MC: Medication management of irritable bowel syndrome. Digestion 89(4):253–267, 2014 24992947

Tripp AC: Lithium toxicity after Roux-en-Y gastric bypass surgery. J Clin Psychopharmacol 31(2):261–262, 2011 21364348

UCSF HIV InSite: Database of antiretroviral drug interactions. Available at: http://hivinsite.ucsf.edu/insite?page=ar-00-02&post=4&param=8. Accessed June 10, 2015.

Udina M, Castellví P, Moreno-España J, et al: Interferon-induced depression in chronic hepatitis C: a systematic review and meta-analysis. J Clin Psychiatry 73(8):1128–1138, 2012 22967776

Udina M, Hidalgo D, Navinés R, et al: Prophylactic antidepressant treatment of interferon-induced depression in chronic hepatitis C: a systematic review and meta-analysis. J Clin Psychiatry 75(10):e1113–e1121, 2014 25373120

van Soest EM, Dieleman JP, Siersema PD, et al: Tricyclic antidepressants and the risk of reflux esophagitis. Am J Gastroenterol 102(9):1870–1877, 2007 17511756

Vanuytsel T, Tack JF, Boeckxstaens GE: Treatment of abdominal pain in irritable bowel syndrome. J Gastroenterol 49(8):1193–1205, 2014 24845149

van Veggel M, Olofinjana O, Davies G, Taylor D: Clozapine and gastro-oesophageal reflux disease (GORD)—an investigation of temporal association. Acta Psychiatr Scand 127(1):69–77, 2013 22901096

Viazis N, Keyoglou A, Kanellopoulos AK, et al: Selective serotonin reuptake inhibitors for the treatment of hypersensitive esophagus: a randomized, double-blind, placebo-controlled study. Am J Gastroenterol 107(11):1662–1667, 2012 21625270

Vidal X, Ibáñez L, Vendrell L, et al; Spanish-Italian Collaborative Group for the Epidemiology of Gastrointestinal Bleeding: Risk of upper gastrointestinal bleeding and the degree of serotonin reuptake inhibition by antidepressants: a case-control study. Drug Saf 31(2):159–168, 2008 18217791

Villa A, Connell CL, Abati S: Diagnosis and management of xerostomia and hyposalivation. Ther Clin Risk Manag 11:45–51, 2014 25653532

Wald A: Chronic constipation: advances in management. Neurogastroenterol Motil 19(1):4–10, 2007 17187583

Wang SY, Yang ZJ, Zhang L: Olanzapine for preventing nausea and vomiting induced by moderately and highly emetogenic chemotherapy. Asian Pac J Cancer Prev 15(22):9587–9592, 2014 25520071

Warr DG: Chemotherapy- and cancer-related nausea and vomiting. Curr Oncol 15 (suppl 1):S4–S9, 2008 18231647

Weijenborg PW, de Schepper HS, Smout AJ, Bredenoord AJ: Effects of antidepressants in patients with functional esophageal disorders or gastroesophageal reflux disease: a systematic review. Clin Gastroenterol Hepatol 13(2):251–259.e1, 2015 24997325

Whitehead WE, Wald A, Norton NJ: Treatment options for fecal incontinence. Dis Colon Rectum 44(1):131–142, discussion 142–144, 2001 11805574

Whitehead WE, Palsson OS, Levy RR, et al: Comorbidity in irritable bowel syndrome. Am J Gastroenterol 102(12):2767–2776, 2007 17900326

Whitehead WE, Rao SSC, Lowry A, et al: Treatment of fecal incontinence: state of the science summary for the National Institute of Diabetes and Digestive and Kidney Diseases workshop. Am J Gastroenterol 110(1):138–146, 2015 25331348

Wright MT: Antiemetics, akathisia, and pregnancy. Psychosomatics 48(6):461–466, 2007 18071091

Wynn GH, Sandson NB, Cozza KL: Gastrointestinal medications. Psychosomatics 48(1):79–85, 2007 17209156

Xue F, Strombom I, Turnbull B, et al: Duloxetine for depression and the incidence of hepatic events in adults. J Clin Psychopharmacol 31(4):517–522, 2011 21694615

Yamazaki Y, Hata H, Kitamori S, et al: An open-label, noncomparative, dose escalation pilot study of the effect of paroxetine in treatment of burning mouth syndrome. Oral Surg Oral Med Oral Pathol Oral Radiol Endod 107(1):e6–e11, 2009 18996028

Yin J, Song J, Lei Y, et al: Prokinetic effects of mirtazapine on gastrointestinal transit. Am J Physiol Gastrointest Liver Physiol 306(9):G796–G801, 2014 24627566

Zaccara G, Franciotta D, Perucca E: Idiosyncratic adverse reactions to antiepileptic drugs. Epilepsia 48(7):1223–1244, 2007 17386054

5

Renal and Urological Disorders

James L. Levenson, M.D.

James A. Owen, Ph.D.

Renal disease and the procedures and medications used to manage renal and urological disorders frequently cause psychiatric symptoms, including depression, anxiety, sleep disorders, and cognitive impairment. Surprisingly, the literature provides little specific guidance on the management of psychiatric symptoms in patients with renal disease, even though pharmacotherapy is confounded by disease-related alterations in pharmacokinetics (metabolism, excretion) for both hepatically and renally eliminated drugs, medication adverse effects, and drug interactions. Similar issues surround the safe and effective use of psychotropics in patients with urological disorders. The purpose of this chapter is to review psychiatric symptoms related to renal and urological disorders, psychopharmacotherapy in renal disease, and interactions between psychiatric drugs and renal and urological drugs.

Differential Diagnosis

Psychiatric Symptoms in Patients With Renal Disease

The diagnosis of psychiatric disorders in patients with end-stage renal disease (ESRD) is complicated because many somatic symptoms are extremely common as a result of renal insufficiency itself or comorbid medical disorders (especially diabetes). A systematic review of symptoms in ESRD found the following weighted mean prevalence rates: fatigue, 71%; pruritus, 55%; constipation, 53%; anorexia, 49%; pain, 47%; sleep disturbance, 44%; dyspnea, 35%; and nausea, 33% (Murtagh et al. 2007). It is not easy to determine the etiology of a particular symptom, which is often multifactorial in any case.

Depression is the most common psychiatric disorder in patients with ESRD (Kimmel et al. 2007). Prevalence estimates vary depending on definitions and methods, but the prevalence of major depression may be as high as 20%–30% (Palmer et al. 2013), with minor depression in another 25% of patients. Metabolic, psychological, and social factors all contribute to increased risk for depression in ESRD. The diagnosis of depression in uremic patients is complicated because anorexia, anergia, insomnia, constipation, poor concentration, and diminished libido may all be caused by renal insufficiency. Depression in dialysis patients may be intermittent or chronic (Cukor et al. 2008b). Depression in patients with chronic kidney disease has been shown to be associated with multiple poor outcomes, including increased mortality and hospitalization rates, as well as poorer treatment compliance and quality of life (Bautovich et al. 2014).

Significant anxiety is also frequent in almost half of patients with ESRD, intermittent in one-third, and persistent in 15% (Cukor et al. 2008a, 2008b). As with depression, metabolic, psychological, and social factors contribute to etiology. Fluid and electrolyte shifts that are too rapid may physiologically cause anxiety. Specific phobic anxiety may arise from a fear of needles or the sight of blood, as well as a reaction to removal of blood into a machine and its return to the patient's body. In one study, the prevalence of posttraumatic stress disorder symptoms was 17%, with most related to the experience of hemodialysis (Tagay et al. 2007).

Acute renal failure with uremia often causes delirium with cognitive dysfunction and, at times, psychotic symptoms. Acute onset of renal failure accompanied by hallucinations should lead to consideration of a toxic exposure (e.g., poisonous mushrooms, herbal "remedies," insecticides). Psychotic symptoms in patients with ESRD may be due to a primary psychotic disorder (10% of patients at one urban dialysis center; Cukor et al. 2007), electrolyte disturbance, comorbid medical disorder (e.g., stroke, dementia), or toxicity of a renally excreted drug (e.g., acyclovir; Yang et al. 2007).

Subtle cognitive dysfunction is often present in patients with partial renal insufficiency (Elias et al. 2009). Cognitive disorders are common in patients with ESRD as a consequence of uremia, electrolyte disturbances, toxicity of renally excreted drugs, and comorbid medical disorders (e.g., cerebrovascular disease). The signs and symptoms of uremia vary in severity, depending on both the extent to and the rapidity with which renal function is lost. Mild or chronic uremia may cause mild cognitive dysfunction, fatigue, and headache. Untreated uremia progresses to lethargy, hypoactive delirium, and coma. Up to 70% of hemodialysis patients older than age 55 have moderate to severe chronic cognitive impairment (Murray 2008). Vascular dementia is especially common because of the high prevalence of diabetes, hypertension, and atherosclerosis in patients with ESRD.

Sleep disorders, most commonly insomnia, affect 50%–80% of dialysis patients (Novak et al. 2006; Losso et al. 2015). Metabolic changes, lifestyle factors, depression, anxiety, and other underlying sleep disorders may all contribute to the development of chronic insomnia. Restless legs syndrome (RLS) is especially common, affecting 10%–30% of patients on maintenance hemodialysis and up to 50% of those on ambulatory peritoneal dialysis (Losso et al. 2015; Molnar et al. 2006; Murtagh et al. 2007) (see the subsection "Dopamine Agonists and Restless Legs Syndrome" later in this chapter). Antidepressants and antipsychotics are associated with increased risk for RLS in ESRD (Bliwise et al. 2014).

Renal Symptoms of Psychiatric Disorders: Psychogenic Polydipsia

Psychogenic polydipsia (PPD), also called primary polydipsia, occurs in 6%–20% of psychiatric patients, most commonly in patients with schizophrenia (Verghese et al. 1996). Excessive thirst, likely due to abnormal hypothalamic thirst control, causes chronic and excessive fluid intake, often beyond the renal ability to excrete dilute urine. Hyponatremia, present in 10%–20% of compulsive drinkers, is often mild and asymptomatic unless accompanied by the syndrome of inappropriate antidiuretic hormone secretion (SIADH) or other impairment of water excretion. PPD can be distinguished from diabetes insipidus by water restriction. Although both PPD and diabetes insipidus have low urine osmolality before water restriction (<100 mOsm/L), after water restriction urine becomes very concentrated with PPD (>600 mOsm/L) but remains dilute with diabetes insipidus (<600 mOsm/L) (Dundas et al. 2007). PPD can be managed by water restriction, although compliance is problematic, or by pharmacotherapy. Case reports suggest efficacy for atypical antipsychotics (clozapine, risperidone, olanzapine) and β-blockers. Acetazolamide was effective in a small case series (Takagi et al. 2011). In a small randomized controlled trial of clonidine or enalapril in chronically psychotic patients with PPD, both agents demonstrated improvement of measures reflecting fluid consumption in 60% of patients (Greendyke et al. 1998). Demeclocycline was reported to be effective in case reports but was ineffective in randomized controlled trials. Vasopressin V_2 antagonists (vaptans), including tolvaptan and conivaptan, have been shown to be effective for the treatment of hyponatremia resulting from PPD (Bhardwaj et al. 2013).

Pharmacotherapy in Renal Disease

Pharmacokinetics in Renal Disease

Although most psychotropic drugs, as the parent compounds, do not depend on the kidney for excretion, renal failure may alter the pharmacokinetics of practically all drugs through changes in distribution, protein binding, and metabolism (see Chapter 1, "Pharmacokinetics, Pharmacodynamics, and Principles of Drug-Drug Interactions"). Edema present in ESRD will increase the volume of distribution for hydrophilic drugs. Uremic products circulating in ESRD may displace highly bound drugs from plasma proteins, increasing the proportion of drug circulating free in plasma. This shift in ratio of free to bound drugs may cause therapeutic drug monitoring methods that measure total drug to suggest lower, possibly subtherapeutic levels. For those highly bound drugs for which therapeutic drug monitoring guides dosing (e.g., phenytoin, valproate), clinicians should use drug monitoring methods that are selective for free drug (see Chapter 1); otherwise, seemingly lower levels might prompt a dosage increase, with possibly toxic results.

Renal disease can also significantly modify Phase I hepatic drug metabolism, although the effects vary markedly. In general, hepatic metabolism mediated by cytochrome P450 2C9 (CYP2C9), CYP2C19, CYP2D6, and CYP3A4 is reduced in chronic renal disease, possibly through reduced CYP gene expression. Phase II metabolic reactions, including acetylation, glucuronidation, sulfation, and methylation, are also impaired in chronic renal disease (Pichette and Leblond 2003). The metabolic impact of renal disease on renal metabolism is often overlooked. Renal metabolism, which ordinarily represents about 15% of hepatic metabolic capacity, is reduced in renal insufficiency (Anders 1980).

Despite the complexity of pharmacokinetic changes in renal failure, most psychotropics do not require drastic dosage adjustment. The exceptions include drugs for which the parent compound or active metabolites undergo significant renal elimination (lithium, gabapentin, pregabalin, topiramate, paliperidone, risperidone, paroxetine, desvenlafaxine, venlafaxine, and memantine) (see Table 5–1). However, many problems associated with use of psychotropics in patients with ESRD are related to comorbid illnesses rather than to the renal failure per se. Specific dosing guidelines based on creatinine clearance are not available for most psychotropics, but many clinicians use the rule of "two-thirds" (Levy 1990)—that is, for patients with renal insufficiency, use two-thirds of the dosage (except for drugs listed in Table 5–1) used for patients with normal renal function. Table 5–1 provides recommendations for dosing psychotropics in patients with renal disease.

Drug clearance also may be influenced by hemodialysis or peritoneal dialysis. Most psychotropics are not dialyzable because of their lipophilicity and large volumes of distribution. Dialyzable psychotropics are listed in Table 5–2. Significant fluid shifts occur during and several hours after each hemodialysis treatment, making dialysis patients more prone to orthostasis. Hence, drugs that frequently cause orthostatic hypotension ideally should be avoided.

Pharmacodynamics in Renal Disease

Electrolyte disturbances associated with renal failure or diuretic therapy may increase the risk of cardiac arrhythmias. Significant QT prolongation is observed with tricyclic antidepressants (TCAs), lithium (van Noord et al. 2009), and typical and atypical antipsychotics (for a listing of QT-prolonging drugs, see CredibleMeds 2016).

Table 5–1. Psychotropic drugs in renal insufficiency (RI)

Medication	Effect and management
Antidepressants	
SSRIs	
Most	Mild to moderate RI: no dosage adjustment needed. Severe RI: may need to reduce dosage or lengthen dosing interval.
Paroxetine	Mild RI: no dosage adjustment needed. Moderate RI: 50%–75% of usual dosage. Severe RI: initial dosage of 10 mg/day; increase as needed by 10 mg at weekly intervals to a maximum of 40 mg/day. Controlled-release formulation: initial dosage of 12.5 mg/day; increase as needed by 12.5 mg at weekly intervals to a maximum of 50 mg/day.
SNRIs and novel agents	
Bupropion	Water-soluble active metabolites may accumulate. Reduce initial dosage.
Desvenlafaxine	Approximately 45% of desvenlafaxine is excreted unchanged in urine. No dosage adjustment is required in mild RI. The dosage should not exceed 50 mg/day in moderate RI or 50 mg every other day in severe RI, per manufacturer.
Duloxetine	Mild RI: population CPK analyses suggest no significant effect on apparent clearance. No data regarding use in moderate to severe RI. Not recommended for patients with end-stage renal disease.
Levomilnacipran	Moderate RI: maximum dose 80 mg. Severe RI: clearance maximum dose 40 mg.
Mirtazapine	Moderate RI: clearance decreased by 30%. Severe RI: clearance decreased by 50%.
Nefazodone	No dosage adjustment needed.

Table 5–1. Psychotropic drugs in renal insufficiency
(RI) *(continued)*

Medication	Effect and management
SNRIs and novel agents (continued)	
Trazodone	Mild RI: use with caution. No data regarding use in moderate to severe RI.
Venlafaxine	Mild to moderate RI: 75% of usual dosage. Severe RI: 50% of usual dosage. Hemodialysis patients should have dosage reduced by 50% and be dosed after dialysis session.
Vilazodone	No dosage adjustment needed.
Vortioxetine	No dosage adjustment needed.
MAOIs	May accumulate in RI.
Selegiline	Active metabolite (methamphetamine) renally eliminated. Use with caution in renal impairment. No dosing guidelines.
TCAs	Water-soluble active metabolites may accumulate. No recommended dosage adjustments.
Antipsychotics	
Atypical agents	
Aripiprazole, asenapine, clozapine, olanzapine, and quetiapine	No dosage adjustment needed.
Iloperidone	Dosage adjustment not needed in mild to moderate RI, per manufacturer. No recommendations for dosing in severe RI.
Lurasidone	Moderate to severe impairment: reduce by 50%.
Paliperidone	Clearance decreased in RI. Mild impairment: start at 3 mg/day, increasing to a maximum of 6 mg/day. Moderate to severe impairment: start at 1.5 mg/day, increasing to 3 mg/day, as tolerated.

Table 5–1. Psychotropic drugs in renal insufficiency (RI) *(continued)*

Medication	Effect and management
Atypical agents (continued)	
Risperidone	Clearance decreased in RI. Initiate therapy at 0.25–0.5 mg bid.
	Increases beyond 1.5 mg should be made at intervals of at least 7 days.
Ziprasidone	No recommendations made regarding dosage adjustment.
Typical agents	
Haloperidol, etc.	No dosage adjustment needed.
Anxiolytics and sedative-hypnotics	
Benzodiazepines	
Most	No dosage adjustment needed.
Chlordiazepoxide	Severe RI: 50% of usual dosage.
Nonbenzodiazepines	
Buspirone	Use in severe RI not recommended.
Ramelteon	No dosage adjustment needed.
Suvorexant	No dosage adjustment needed.
Zaleplon	Mild to moderate RI: no dosage adjustment needed. Severe RI: not adequately studied.
Zolpidem	Dosage adjustment may not be needed in RI.
Zopiclone and eszopiclone	No dosage adjustment needed.

Table 5–1.   Psychotropic drugs in renal insufficiency
(RI) *(continued)*

Medication	Effect and management
Anticonvulsant and antimanic agents	
Carbamazepine	Severe RI: 75% of usual dosage.
Gabapentin	$Cl_{cr} > 60$ mL/min: 1,200 mg/day (400 mg tid). Cl_{cr} 30–60 mL/min: 600 mg/day (300 mg bid). Cl_{cr} 15–30 mL/min: 300 mg/day. $Cl_{cr} < 15$ mL/min: 150 mg/day (300 mg every other day). Hemodialysis: 300–400 mg loading dose to patients who have never received gabapentin, then 200–300 mg after each dialysis session.
Lamotrigine	Reduced dosage may be effective in significant RI.
Lithium	Moderate RI: 50%–75% of usual dosage. Hemodialysis: supplemental dose of 300 mg once after each dialysis session.
Oxcarbazepine	Initiate therapy at 300 mg/day (50% of usual starting dosage).
Pregabalin	Cl_{cr} 30–60 mL/min: 50% of usual dosage. Cl_{cr} 15–30 mL/min: 25% of usual dosage. $Cl_{cr} < 15$ mL/min: 12.5% of usual dosage. Hemodialysis: supplemental dose may be needed after each 4-hour dialysis session. See manufacturer's recommendations.
Topiramate	Mild RI: 100% of usual dosage. Moderate RI: 50% of usual dosage. Severe RI: 25% of usual dosage. Supplemental dose may be needed after hemodialysis.
Valproate	No dosage adjustment needed in RI, but valproate level measurements are misleading.

Table 5–1. Psychotropic drugs in renal insufficiency (RI) *(continued)*

Medication	Effect and management
Cholinesterase inhibitors and memantine	
Donepezil	Limited data suggest no dosage adjustment needed.
Galantamine	Moderate RI: maximum dosage 16 mg/day. Severe RI: use not recommended.
Memantine	Extensive renal elimination. Mild to moderate RI: no dosage reduction needed. Severe RI: reduce dosage to 5 mg bid.
Rivastigmine	Dosage adjustment not recommended.
Psychostimulants	
Dextroamphetamine	No dosage adjustment needed.
Atomoxetine	No dosage adjustment needed.
Lisdexamfetamine	Mild RI: no dosage adjustment needed. Moderate RI: maximum dose 50 mg. Severe RI: maximum dose 30 mg.
Methylphenidate	No dosage adjustment needed.
Modafinil and armodafinil	No dosage adjustment needed.
Dopamine agonists	
Amantadine	Cl_{cr} 80 mL/min: 100 mg bid. Cl_{cr} 60 mL/min: 100 mg qd alternated with 100 mg bid every other day. Cl_{cr} 40 mL/min: 100 mg/day. Cl_{cr} 30 mL/min: 200 mg twice weekly. Cl_{cr} 20 mL/min: 100 mg three times weekly. Cl_{cr} 10 mL/min: 200 mg alternated with 100 mg every 7 days.

Table 5–1. Psychotropic drugs in renal insufficiency (RI) *(continued)*

Medication	Effect and management
Dopamine agonists *(continued)*	
Pramipexole	90% renal elimination: Clearance of pramipexole is 75% lower in severe renal impairment (Cl_{cr} 20 mL/min) and 60% lower in patients with moderate impairment (Cl_{cr} 40 mL/min) compared with healthy volunteers. The interval between titration steps should be increased to 14 days in RLS patients with severe and moderate renal impairment (Cl_{cr} 20–60 mL/min).

Note. Mild RI is >50 mL/min; moderate RI is 10–50 mL/min; severe RI is <10 mL/min. bid=twice a day; Cl_{cr}=creatinine clearance; CPK=creatine phosphokinase; MAOIs=monoamine oxidase inhibitors; qd=once a day; RLS=restless legs syndrome; SNRIs=serotonin-norepinephrine reuptake inhibitors; SSRIs=selective serotonin reuptake inhibitors; TCAs=tricyclic antidepressants; tid=three times a day.
Source. Cohen et al. 2004; Crone et al. 2006; Jacobson 2002; Periclou et al. 2006; and manufacturers' product information.

Psychotropic Drugs in Renal Disease

Antidepressants

Despite the high prevalence of depression, few studies have been done of the effectiveness of antidepressants in dialysis patients. One small randomized controlled trial of low-dose paroxetine (10 mg/day) combined with psychotherapy showed a small benefit in reducing depressive symptoms (Koo et al. 2005). Another tiny randomized controlled trial of fluoxetine (Blumenfield et al. 1997) and a tiny open trial of TCAs (Kennedy et al. 1989) were encouraging but were too small and too brief, as was a trial of citalopram (Hosseini et al. 2012). Two large randomized controlled trials of sertraline in dialysis patients are currently under way (Friedli et al. 2015; Jain et al. 2013).

Virtually all antidepressants may be used in patients with renal failure. Patients with ESRD tend to be more sensitive to the side effects of TCAs, including sedation, anticholinergic toxicity (urinary retention, dry mouth that encourages excessive drinking), orthostatic hypotension, and QT prolongation. Hydroxylated metabolites have been shown to be markedly elevated in patients with ESRD and may be responsible for some TCA side effects. Nor-

Table 5–2.   Dialyzable psychotropic drugs

Medication	Conventional hemodialysis	High-permeability hemodialysis	Peritoneal dialysis
Carbamazepine		Yes	
Gabapentin	Yes	Likely	
Lamotrigine		Clearance increased 20%	
Lithium	Yes	Yes	Yes
Pregabalin	Yes	Likely	
Topiramate	Yes	Likely	
Valproate	Yes	Likely	

Note. Likely=no data, but increased clearance likely on the basis of conventional hemodialysis observations; Yes=studies indicate clearance increased by ≥30%.

Source. Bassilios et al. 2001; Israni et al. 2006; Lacerda et al. 2006; MedlinePlus 2015; Ward et al. 1994.

triptyline and desipramine are considered preferred TCAs for patients with renal failure because these drugs are less likely than other TCAs to cause anticholinergic effects or orthostatic hypotension (Gillman 2007). Limited data are available on the use of newer antidepressants in patients with renal failure. The half-life of venlafaxine is prolonged in renal insufficiency; its clearance is reduced by more than 50% in patients undergoing dialysis. Desvenlafaxine undergoes significant renal elimination, requiring dosage reduction in patients with moderate and severe renal impairment. Paroxetine levels are two to four times higher in renal insufficiency. Because most antidepressants are metabolized by the liver and excreted by the kidney, the prudent action is to initially reduce the dosage for all antidepressants to minimize the potential accumulation of active metabolites. However, a large retrospective study found no increased adverse effects of higher versus lower doses of paroxetine, mirtazapine, and venlafaxine (Dev et al. 2014).

Antipsychotics

All antipsychotics may be used in patients with renal failure. Paliperidone clearance, however, is significantly decreased in all degrees of renal impairment, requiring a reduction in initial and target dosage. Difficulties with other antipsychotics can arise from the complications of renal failure and dialysis or from the chronic disease causing renal failure (e.g., diabetes). For example, patients with ESRD who also have diabetic autonomic neuropathy will be at higher risk for drug side effects, including postural hypotension and bladder, gastrointestinal, and sexual dysfunction. Antipsychotics associated with hyperglycemia (e.g., clozapine, olanzapine) should be avoided in patients with comorbid diabetes. In patients with electrolyte disturbances, risk of cardiac arrhythmias can be minimized by using antipsychotics with the least QT-prolonging effect.

Anxiolytics and Sedative-Hypnotics

We found no clinical trials of pharmacotherapy for anxiety in patients with ESRD. Benzodiazepine and zolpidem use in dialysis patients has been associated with a 15% increase in mortality, but this appeared to be partially explained by increased use of these medications by patients with comorbid chronic obstructive pulmonary disease (Winkelmayer et al. 2007). In Japan, benzodiazepines were associated with higher mortality (relative risk 1.27, 95% confidence interval 1.01–1.59) in hemodialysis patients with symptoms of depression, most of whom had not received antidepressants, even after controlling for confounders (Fukuhara et al. 2006). Fukuhara et al. (2006) suggested that these benzodiazepine-related deaths may have been caused by inappropriate use of benzodiazepines instead of antidepressants to treat depression and the drugs' adverse cognitive and psychomotor effects.

Virtually all sedative-hypnotics except barbiturates can be used in patients with renal failure. Barbiturates should be avoided because they may increase osteomalacia and because of excessive sedation. Preferred benzodiazepines include those with inactive metabolites, such as lorazepam and oxazepam; however, there is a risk of propylene glycol toxicity with continuous infusion of lorazepam (Horinek et al. 2009). Other benzodiazepines with inactive metabolites include clonazepam and temazepam, but less is known about changes in their half-lives in ESRD.

Mood Stabilizers

Lithium is almost entirely excreted by the kidneys. It is contraindicated in patients with acute renal failure but not in those with chronic renal failure. For patients with stable partial renal insufficiency, clinicians should dose conservatively and monitor renal function frequently. For patients on dialysis, lithium is completely dialyzed and may be given as a single oral dose (300–600 mg) following hemodialysis treatment. Lithium levels should not be checked until at least 2–3 hours after dialysis because reequilibration from tissue stores occurs in the immediate postdialysis period. For patients on peritoneal dialysis, lithium can be given in the dialysate. Lithium prolongs the QT interval and may increase the risk of cardiac arrhythmias in patients with electrolyte disturbances. Dosage adjustment recommendations based on creatinine clearance are available for gabapentin, lithium, topiramate, and carbamazepine (Jacobson 2002).

Cholinesterase Inhibitors and Memantine

It appears, from the limited data available, that dosage adjustment of donepezil and rivastigmine is not required. Galantamine should be used cautiously in patients with moderate renal insufficiency; according to the manufacturer, its use in patients with severe renal insufficiency is not recommended. Memantine undergoes extensive renal elimination, requiring a dosage reduction in patients with severe renal insufficiency.

Psychostimulants

Methylphenidate and atomoxetine do not require dosage adjustment. The maximum recommended dose of mixed amphetamine salts in severe renal impairment is 20 mg. Recommendations for lisdexamfetamine are shown in Table 5–1.

Dopamine Agonists and Restless Legs Syndrome

Dopaminergic therapy (levodopa or the dopamine receptor agonists pramipexole, ropinirole, and rotigotine) has been recommended as first-line treatment for RLS. Although dopamine agonists and gabapentin have been found to be effective in reducing RLS symptoms in the general population, data supporting their use in patients with ESRD come from small, mostly unblinded trials (Aurora et al. 2012; Giannaki et al. 2014). Side effects of dopamine agonists can be problematic but are less frequent with other dopamine agonists than with levodopa. Alternative treatment options for RLS include benzodiazepines (especially clonazepam), opioids, and other anticonvulsants, but only very limited data are available on their effectiveness and side-effect profile in patients with ESRD (Molnar et al. 2006). If iron deficiency is present, repletion of iron will improve RLS.

Psychiatric Adverse Effects of Renal and Urological Agents

Drugs used in the treatment of renal and urological disorders sometimes have psychiatric adverse effects. The following subsections describe these effects for a variety of drug classes. Psychiatric adverse effects of other medications frequently used to treat patients with renal disease are covered elsewhere in this book: corticosteroids for autoimmune nephritis in Chapter 10, "Endocrine and Metabolic Disorders," antihypertensives in Chapter 6, "Cardiovascular Disorders," and immunosuppressants after renal transplant in Chapter 16, "Organ Transplantation."

Antispasmodics

Anticholinergic agents commonly used to treat overactive bladder are associated with psychiatric adverse effects, including cognitive impairment, confusion, fatigue, and psychosis (see Table 5–3). Cumulative use of strong anticholinergics, including bladder antimuscarinics, is associated with an increase in incident dementia (Gray et al. 2015). Among the available agents, penetration of the blood-brain barrier appears to be highest for oxybutynin; lower for tolterodine, solifenacin, and darifenacin; and lowest for fesoterodine and trospium chloride (Kerdraon et al. 2014). A large longitudinal cohort study identified mild cognitive impairment in 80% of patients receiving anticholinergics for overactive bladder compared with 35% of age-matched control subjects (Ancelin et al. 2006). Cognitive impairment is well documented, and cases of frank psychosis have been reported for first-generation anticholinergics, such as oxybutynin (Gulsun et al. 2006; Kay et al. 2006) and tolterodine (Salvatore et al. 2007; Tsao and Heilman 2003; Womack and Heilman 2003). Oxybutynin appears to be most likely to cause cognitive impairment (Kay and Ebinger 2008). Few central nervous system side effects have been reported in clinical trials of the newer agents. However, it should be remembered that elderly patients with dementia would have been excluded from the trials, and they would be most vulnerable to anticholinergic effects on cognition.

Diuretics

Thiazide diuretics are the most common cause of hyponatremia (Liamis et al. 2008). Psychiatric symptoms of hyponatremia include lethargy, stupor, confusion, psychosis, irritability, and seizures.

The α_1-Adrenergic Antagonists

The α_1 antagonists, including alfuzosin, doxazosin, silodosin, tamsulosin, and terazosin, are used in the treatment of benign prostatic hyperplasia and prostatitis. All α-blockers can cause hypotension. Doxazosin and tamsulosin have also been associated with insomnia and impotence. Increased anxiety may occur with doxazosin.

5-α-Reductase Inhibitors

Dutasteride and finasteride, indicated for benign prostatic hyperplasia, may cause impotence and decreased libido.

Vasopressin Antagonists

Conivaptan, a vasopressin V_2-selective receptor antagonist, is associated with confusion and insomnia in safety and efficacy trials (Cumberland Pharmaceuticals 2009). Tolvaptan appears to have a more benign psychiatric adverse-effect profile (Gheorghiade et al. 2003).

Table 5–3. Psychiatric adverse effects of renal and urological drugs

Medication	Psychiatric adverse effects
Urinary antispasmodics	
Oxybutynin > tolterodine, solifenacin, darifenacin > fesoterodine > trospium chloride	Cognitive impairment, confusion, fatigue, psychosis
Thiazide and thiazide-like diuretics	
Bendroflumethiazide, chlorothiazide, chlorthalidone, hydrochlorothiazide, hydroflumethiazide, indapamide, metolazone, and trichlormethiazide	Hyponatremia-induced lethargy, stupor, confusion, psychosis, irritability, seizures
α_1 Antagonists	
Doxazosin	Anxiety, insomnia, impotence
Tamsulosin	Insomnia, impotence
5-α-Reductase inhibitors	
Dutasteride and finasteride	Impotence, decreased libido
Vasopressin antagonists	
Conivaptan	Confusion, insomnia

Renal and Urological Adverse Effects of Psychotropics

Psychotropic drugs have a variety of renal and urological adverse effects (see Table 5–4), including hyponatremia or hypernatremia, nephropathy, urinary retention or incontinence, and sexual dysfunction.

Renal Effects of Psychotropics

Hyponatremia, which can manifest as lethargy, stupor, confusion, psychosis, irritability, and seizures, has many different precipitants, including thiazide diuretics (see Table 5–3), but two have particular psychiatric relevance: 1) SIADH, which can be caused by many psychotropic drugs, especially oxcarbazepine

Table 5–4.   Renal and urological adverse effects of psychiatric drugs

Medication	Renal/urological adverse effects
Mood stabilizers	
Lithium	Nephrogenic diabetes insipidus, hypernatremia
Carbamazepine and oxcarbazepine	SIADH, psychogenic polydipsia, hyponatremia
Antidepressants	
SSRIs or SNRIs	Sexual dysfunction, SIADH, psychogenic polydipsia, hyponatremia
Duloxetine	Urinary retention
TCAs	Urinary hesitancy, urinary retention, SIADH, psychogenic polydipsia, hyponatremia
Antipsychotics	SIADH, psychogenic polydipsia, hyponatremia
Low-potency typical antipsychotics	Urinary hesitancy, urinary retention
Anticholinergic agents for EPS	
Trihexyphenidyl, benztropine, etc.	Urinary hesitancy, urinary retention

Note.   EPS = extrapyramidal symptoms; SIADH = syndrome of inappropriate antidiuretic hormone secretion; SNRIs = serotonin-norepinephrine reuptake inhibitors; SSRIs = selective serotonin reuptake inhibitors; TCAs = tricyclic antidepressants.

and carbamazepine but also selective serotonin reuptake inhibitors (SSRIs), TCAs, and antipsychotics, and 2) PPD (discussed earlier in the subsection "Renal Symptoms of Psychiatric Disorders: Psychogenic Polydipsia"). In an acutely psychotic patient with hyponatremia, urinary concentration can help distinguish drug-induced SIADH from psychogenic polydipsia: the concentration will be high in the former and low in the latter (Atsariyasing and Goldman 2014). Hyponatremia is most common with oxcarbazepine and is more common in elderly patients. Among antidepressants, SSRIs and serotonin-norepinephrine reuptake inhibitors are much more likely than TCAs to cause hyponatremia (De Picker et al. 2014). The risk increases considerably if the patient is also taking other drugs that cause hyponatremia, such as thiazide diuretics (Letmaier et al. 2012). Acute-onset symptomatic hyponatremia may require emergent treatment with hypertonic (3%) saline. In chronic cases, correction should be gradual to minimize the risk of pontine myelinolysis, relying on fluid restriction and vasopressin receptor antagonists (Siegel 2008).

Hypernatremia can result in cognitive dysfunction, delirium, seizures, and lethargy, progressing to stupor and coma. Hypernatremia is usually caused by dehydration with significant total body water deficits. The only psychotropic drug that causes hypernatremia is lithium, via nephrogenic diabetes insipidus (NDI). Most patients receiving lithium have polydipsia and polyuria, reflecting mild benign NDI. Lithium-induced NDI sometimes has persisted long after lithium discontinuation and varies from mild polyuria to hyperosmolar coma. NDI has been treated with nonsteroidal anti-inflammatory drugs, thiazides, and amiloride, as well as sodium restriction (Grünfeld and Rossier 2009; Liamis et al. 2008). Amiloride is considered the treatment of choice for lithium-induced NDI.

The effect of lithium on renal function is controversial, with variable results from recent retrospective and cohort studies (Aiff et al. 2014; Aprahamian et al. 2014; Close et al. 2014; Rej et al. 2014a, 2014b; Roxanas et al. 2014). Some studies report that longer duration of lithium therapy is predictive of a decrease in estimated glomerular filtration ("creeping creatinine"), whereas others do not. Although chronic lithium use may result in altered kidney morphology, including interstitial fibrosis, tubular atrophy, urinary casts, and occasionally glomerular sclerosis, in 10%–20% of patients (Bendz et al. 1996), these changes are not generally associated with impaired renal function. In one meta-analysis, Paul et al. (2009) concluded that any lithium-induced effect on renal function is quantitatively small and probably clinically insignificant. Although long-term lithium treatment is the only well-established factor associated with lithium-induced nephropathy, changes in renal function are often associated with other factors, including age, episodes of lithium toxicity, other medications (analgesics, substance abuse), and the presence of comorbid disorders (hypertension, diabetes). Lithium dosage is not strongly related to nephrotoxic effects (Freeman and Freeman 2006). The progression of lithium nephrotoxicity to ESRD is rare (0.2%–0.7%) and requires lithium use for several decades (Presne et al. 2003). Lithium is so efficacious in bipolar disorder that the risk of renal dysfunction during chronic use is considered acceptable with yearly monitoring of renal function.

Urological Effects of Psychotropics

Many psychotropics cause disorders of micturition. Urinary retention is associated with drugs with significant anticholinergic activity, including TCAs and antipsychotics, especially low-potency typical agents but also atypical agents. Urinary incontinence and other lower urinary tract symptoms (frequency, urgency, incomplete emptying) occur in approximately 40% of patients taking clozapine but in only 15% of the general population (Jeong et al. 2008) and may persist for the duration of treatment. The prevalence of urinary frequency and urgency is significantly higher in women taking atypical antipsychotics in general (Hall et al. 2012). Treatment of clozapine-induced urinary incontinence with sympathomimetics, anticholinergics, and desmopressin has not proved consistently useful.

SSRIs and serotonin-norepinephrine reuptake inhibitors cause sexual side effects (delayed or absent orgasm or ejaculation or reduced libido) in 30%–70% of users. Bupropion and mirtazapine appear not to be associated with sexual dysfunction (Clayton et al. 2014; Serretti et al. 2009). Antidepressant-induced sexual dysfunction can be managed by switching to a less problematic agent or by as-needed use of the phosphodiesterase type 5 (PDE5) inhibitor sildenafil, which has been shown to be effective in controlled trials in men and women (Nurnberg et al. 2003, 2008). Antipsychotics, TCAs, and irreversible monoamine oxidase inhibitors (MAOIs) also can impair sexual function (see the subsection "Hyperprolactinemia" in Chapter 10, "Endocrine and Metabolic Disorders").

Drug-Drug Interactions

A number of pharmacodynamic and pharmacokinetic drug interactions frequently occur between drugs prescribed for renal and urological disorders and psychotropic drugs (see Tables 5–5 and 5–6). See Chapter 1 for a discussion of pharmacokinetics, pharmacodynamics, and principles of drug-drug interactions.

Pharmacodynamic Interactions

A number of urological agents have effects on cardiac conduction (see Table 5–5). Thiazides and loop diuretics may cause conduction abnormalities through electrolyte disturbances, including hypokalemia and hypomagnese-

Table 5–5. Renal and urological drug–psychotropic drug interactions

Medication	Interaction mechanism	Effects on psychotropic drugs and management
Diuretics		
All	Additive hypotensive effect	Increased risk of hypotensive effects with antipsychotics, TCAs, and MAOIs.
Thiazide diuretics	Blocked sodium/lithium reabsorption	Reduced lithium clearance leads to increased lithium levels and risk of toxicity. Monitor lithium levels.
	Additive hyponatremia	Potential for additive hyponatremic effects when combined with oxcarbazepine, carbamazepine, and, to a lesser degree, SSRIs, TCAs, and antipsychotics. Monitor electrolytes.
	Electrolyte abnormalities, hypokalemia, hypomagnesemia	Increased risk of cardiac arrhythmias with other QT-prolonging agents, including TCAs, typical antipsychotics, pimozide, risperidone, paliperidone, iloperidone, quetiapine, ziprasidone, and lithium.
Indapamide	QT prolongation	Increased risk of cardiac arrhythmias with other QT-prolonging agents, including TCAs, typical antipsychotics, pimozide, risperidone, paliperidone, iloperidone, quetiapine, ziprasidone, and lithium.
Loop diuretics	Electrolyte abnormalities, hypokalemia, hypomagnesemia	Increased risk of cardiac arrhythmias with other QT-prolonging agents, including TCAs, typical antipsychotics, pimozide, risperidone, paliperidone, iloperidone, quetiapine, ziprasidone, and lithium.
	Urine acidification	Increased excretion and reduced effect of amphetamine, amitriptyline, imipramine, meperidine, methadone, memantine, and flecainide.

Table 5–5. Renal and urological drug–psychotropic drug interactions *(continued)*

Medication	Interaction mechanism	Effects on psychotropic drugs and management
Diuretics *(continued)*		
Carbonic anhydrase inhibitors	Urine alkalinization	Reduced excretion and prolonged effect of amphetamine, amitriptyline, imipramine, meperidine, methadone, memantine, and flecainide.
Eplerenone, osmotic diuretics, and spironolactone	Increased lithium clearance	Reduced lithium levels and possible loss of therapeutic effect. Monitor lithium levels. Amiloride has little effect on lithium levels.
Phosphate binders		
Calcium acetate, calcium carbonate, and lanthanum carbonate	Urine alkalinization	Reduced excretion and prolonged effect of amphetamine, amitriptyline, imipramine, meperidine, methadone, memantine, and flecainide.
Anticholinergic urinary antispasmodics		
Darifenacin, oxybutynin, solifenacin, tolterodine, and trospium	Additive anticholinergic effects	Increased peripheral and central anticholinergic adverse effects of TCAs and antipsychotics. Reduced therapeutic effects of cognitive enhancers. Avoid combination if possible. Darifenacin has less central effect and is preferred.

Table 5–5. Renal and urological drug–psychotropic drug interactions (*continued*)

Medication	Interaction mechanism	Effects on psychotropic drugs and management
PDE5 inhibitors		
Sildenafil and tadalafil	Additive hypotensive effect	Increased risk of hypotensive effects with antipsychotics, TCAs, and MAOIs.
Vardenafil	Additive hypotensive effect QT prolongation	Increased risk of hypotensive effects with antipsychotics, TCAs, and MAOIs. Increased risk of cardiac arrhythmias with other QT-prolonging agents, including TCAs, typical antipsychotics, pimozide, risperidone, paliperidone, iloperidone, quetiapine, ziprasidone, and lithium.
α₁ Antagonists for BPH		
All	Additive hypotensive effect	Increased risk of hypotensive effects with antipsychotics, TCAs, and MAOIs.
Alfuzosin	QT prolongation	Increased risk of cardiac arrhythmias with other QT-prolonging agents, including TCAs, typical antipsychotics, pimozide, risperidone, paliperidone, iloperidone, quetiapine, ziprasidone, and lithium.

Table 5–5.   Renal and urological drug–psychotropic drug interactions *(continued)*

Medication	Interaction mechanism	Effects on psychotropic drugs and management
Vasopressin antagonists		
Conivaptan	Inhibits CYP3A4	Reduced metabolism of oxidatively metabolized benzodiazepines, buspirone, carbamazepine, quetiapine, ziprasidone, and pimozide. Midazolam AUC is increased two- to threefold. Adjust benzodiazepine dosage or consider oxazepam, lorazepam, or temazepam. Avoid combination with buspirone or pimozide. Monitor carbamazepine levels. Adjust antipsychotic dosage or switch to another agent.

Note.   AUC = area under the concentration-time curve; BPH = benign prostatic hypertrophy; CYP = cytochrome P450; MAOIs = monoamine oxidase inhibitors; PDE5 = phosphodiesterase type 5; SSRIs = selective serotonin reuptake inhibitors; TCAs = tricyclic antidepressants.

Table 5–6.   Psychotropic drug–renal and urological drug interactions

Medication	Interaction mechanism	Effects on renal/urological drugs and management
Antidepressants		
Fluoxetine	Inhibits CYP3A4	Increased levels of the following: Vasopressin antagonists—conivaptan, tolvaptan α_1 Antagonists for BPH—alfuzosin, doxazosin, tamsulosin 5-α-Reductase inhibitors—dutasteride, finasteride PDE5 inhibitors—sildenafil, tadalafil, vardenafil Anticholinergic urinary antispasmodics—darifenacin, oxybutynin, solifenacin Potassium-sparing diuretics—eplerenone Avoid concurrent use of CYP3A4 inhibitors.
	Inhibits CYP2D6	Increased levels of tamsulosin, possibly increasing hypotensive adverse effect. Caution with strong CYP3A4 or CYP2D6 inhibitors.
Nefazodone	Inhibits CYP3A4	Increased levels of the following: Vasopressin antagonists—conivaptan, tolvaptan α_1 Antagonists for BPH—alfuzosin, doxazosin, tamsulosin 5-α-Reductase inhibitors—dutasteride, finasteride PDE5 inhibitors—sildenafil, tadalafil, vardenafil Anticholinergic urinary antispasmodics—darifenacin, oxybutynin, solifenacin Potassium-sparing diuretics—eplerenone Avoid concurrent use of CYP3A4 inhibitors.

Table 5–6. Psychotropic drug–renal and urological drug interactions *(continued)*

Medication	Interaction mechanism	Effects on renal/urological drugs and management
Antidepressants *(continued)*		
Bupropion, duloxetine, moclobemide, and paroxetine	Inhibits CYP2D6	Increased levels of tamsulosin, possibly increasing hypotensive adverse effect. Paroxetine increased AUC by 1.6-fold. Caution with strong CYP3A4 or CYP2D6 inhibitors.
TCAs	Additive hypotensive effects	Increased risk of severe hypotension with the following: PDE5 inhibitors—sildenafil, tadalafil, vardenafil α_1 Antagonists for BPH—alfuzosin, doxazosin, tamsulosin, terazosin
	QT prolongation	Increased risk of cardiac arrhythmias with other QT-prolonging agents, including alfuzosin, indapamide, and vardenafil
MAOIs	Additive hypotensive effects	Increased risk of severe hypotension with the following: PDE5 inhibitors—sildenafil, tadalafil, vardenafil α_1 Antagonists for BPH—alfuzosin, doxazosin, tamsulosin, terazosin
St. John's wort	Induces CYP3A4	Decreased conivaptan and tolvaptan levels. Avoid use of CYP3A4 inducers.

Table 5–6.   Psychotropic drug–renal and urological drug interactions *(continued)*

Medication	Interaction mechanism	Effects on renal/urological drugs and management
Antipsychotics		
Typical and atypical: pimozide, risperidone, paliperidone, iloperidone, quetiapine, and ziprasidone	QT prolongation	Increased risk of cardiac arrhythmias with other QT-prolonging agents, including alfuzosin, indapamide, and vardenafil.
Typical and atypical	Additive hypotensive effects	Increased risk of severe hypotension with the following: PDE5 inhibitors—sildenafil, tadalafil, vardenafil α_1 antagonists for BPH—alfuzosin, doxazosin, tamsulosin, terazosin
Mood stabilizers		
Carbamazepine, oxcarbazepine, and phenytoin	Induces CYP3A4	Decreased conivaptan and tolvaptan levels. Avoid use of CYP3A4 inducers.
Lithium	QT prolongation	Increased risk of cardiac arrhythmias with other QT-prolonging agents, including alfuzosin, indapamide, and vardenafil.

Table 5–6. Psychotropic drug–renal and urological drug interactions *(continued)*

Medication	Interaction mechanism	Effects on renal/urological drugs and management
Psychostimulants		
Armodafinil and modafinil	Induces CYP3A4	Decreased conivaptan and tolvaptan levels. Avoid use of CYP3A4 inducers.
Atomoxetine	Inhibits CYP2D6	Increased levels of tamsulosin, possibly increasing hypotensive adverse effect. Caution with strong CYP3A4 or CYP2D6 inhibitors.

Note. AUC=area under the concentration-time curve; BPH=benign prostatic hypertrophy; CYP=cytrochome P450; MAOIs=monoamine oxidase inhibitors; PDE5=phosphodiesterase type 5; TCAs=tricyclic antidepressants.

mia. Alfuzosin, indapamide, and vardenafil prolong the QT interval (for a listing of QT-prolonging drugs, see CredibleMeds 2016). These agents should be used with caution in the presence of psychotropic drugs with QT-prolonging effects, such as TCAs, antipsychotics, and lithium (Kane et al. 2008; van Noord et al. 2009). The anticholinergic properties of urinary antispasmodics can interact in an additive manner to increase the anticholinergic adverse effects of TCAs and antipsychotics (dry mouth, dry eyes, urinary retention, constipation, decreased sweating, and cognitive impairment). Anticholinergic antispasmodics may impair cognitive function and diminish the cognitive benefits of cholinesterase inhibitors and memantine. The hypotensive adverse effects of α_1 antagonists (e.g., doxazosin) for benign prostatic hyperplasia and PDE5 inhibitors (sildenafil, vardenafil, and tadalafil) may exacerbate hypotensive effects of psychotropic agents, including TCAs, antipsychotics, and MAOIs. Hyponatremic effects of thiazide diuretics may be enhanced in combination with oxcarbazepine and carbamazepine and, to a lesser degree, with SSRIs, TCAs, and antipsychotics.

Pharmacokinetic Interactions

Diuretics alter lithium excretion but not in a consistent direction. Thiazide diuretics reduce lithium excretion, giving rise to clinically significant increases in lithium levels. Acute administration of loop diuretics (furosemide, ethacrynic acid, bumetanide) increases lithium excretion, causing a drop in lithium levels; with chronic use of loop diuretics, compensatory changes leave lithium levels somewhat unpredictable but not greatly changed. Carbonic anhydrase inhibitors (acetazolamide, dichlorphenamide, methazolamide) and osmotic diuretics (e.g., mannitol) reduce lithium levels. Potassium-sparing diuretics, including both epithelial sodium channel blockers (amiloride, triamterene) and aldosterone antagonists (spironolactone, eplerenone), may increase lithium excretion (Eyer et al. 2006; Finley et al. 1995). Furosemide and amiloride are considered to have the least effect on lithium excretion.

Metabolic drug interactions can change the levels of drugs used to treat renal and urological disorders, thereby increasing the drugs' toxicity or reducing their therapeutic effect. Many renal and urological agents are CYP3A4 substrates (see Table 5–6); coadministration of a CYP3A4 inhibitor (fluoxetine, nefazodone) may increase renal and urological drug bioavailability and blood levels and exacerbate toxicity. Inhibition of CYP3A4 (and likely P-glycoprotein) has the potential to greatly increase oxybutynin's bioavailability (normally only 6%) and exacerbate anticholinergic toxicity. CYP3A4 inhibitors increase alfuzosin and vardenafil blood levels and enhance cardiac conduction toxicity (QT prolongation). Severe hypotensive effects have been reported with sildenafil in the presence of potent CYP3A4 inhibitors; PDE5 inhibitors (sildenafil, tadalafil, vardenafil) should not be combined with potent CYP3A4 inhibitors. Tamsulosin, a substrate for CYP3A4 and CYP2D6, may exhibit increased toxicity when combined with CYP3A4 or CYP2D6 inhibitors (e.g., paroxetine). Conversely, the therapeutic effect of these CYP3A4 substrates may be diminished in patients also receiving CYP3A4 inducers (e.g. carbamazepine). Coadministration of conivaptan, a potent CYP3A4 inhibitor as well as a substrate, increases the systemic exposure (area under the curve) of midazolam up to threefold (Cumberland Pharmaceuticals 2009). Similar effects would be expected with other oxidatively metabolized benzodiazepines, buspirone, carbamazepine, quetiapine, ziprasidone, and pimozide.

Changes in urine pH can modify the elimination of those compounds whose ratio of ionized to un-ionized forms is dramatically altered across the physiological range of urine pH (4.6–8.2) (i.e., the compound has a pK_a within this pH range). Un-ionized forms of drugs undergo greater glomerular resorption, whereas ionized drug forms have less resorption and greater urinary excretion. Thiazide and loop diuretics decrease urine pH and promote the excretion of amphetamines and possibly other basic drugs such as amitriptyline, imipramine, meperidine, methadone (Nilsson et al. 1982), and memantine (Cadwallader 1983; Freudenthaler et al. 1998). Conversely, carbonic anhydrase inhibitors and phosphate binders (calcium carbonate, calcium acetate, and lanthanum carbonate) alkalinize urine, which may reduce clearance and prolong the effect of these drugs.

Key Clinical Points

- Unless specific information is available for dosing of psychotropic drugs in renal failure, clinicians should start patients with two-thirds the dosage recommended for patients with normal renal function.

- Renal failure alters not only renal elimination of drugs but also hepatic metabolism. Clinicians should employ therapeutic drug monitoring (methods selective for free drug) when possible in patients with renal disease.

- Lithium levels should be regularly monitored in patients receiving diuretic therapy. Furosemide and amiloride are considered to have the least effect on lithium excretion.

- Disease- and medication-induced electrolyte disturbances increase the risk of cardiac arrhythmias. Psychotropics should be chosen for their lack of QT-prolonging effects.

- Many renal and urological drugs are metabolized by CYP3A4. Inhibitors of CYP3A4 should be avoided. This is especially relevant for alfuzosin and vardenafil, which prolong the QT interval.

- Amiloride is considered the treatment of choice for lithium-induced diabetes insipidus.

- Lorazepam and oxazepam are preferred benzodiazepines in patients with ESRD because of absence of active metabolites. Because the half-lives of lorazepam and oxazepam may increase up to fourfold, smaller-than-usual dosages are required.

- Of the common anticholinergic urinary antispasmodics, oxybutynin has the most anticholinergic adverse effects on the central nervous system.

References

Aiff H, Attman PO, Aurell M, et al: End-stage renal disease associated with prophylactic lithium treatment. Eur Neuropsychopharmacol 24(4):540–544, 2014 24503277

Ancelin ML, Artero S, Portet F, et al: Non-degenerative mild cognitive impairment in elderly people and use of anticholinergic drugs: longitudinal cohort study. BMJ 332(7539):455–459, 2006 16452102

Anders MW: Metabolism of drugs by the kidney. Kidney Int 18(5):636–647, 1980 7463957

Aprahamian I, Santos FS, dos Santos B, et al: Long-term, low-dose lithium treatment does not impair renal function in the elderly: a 2-year randomized, placebo-controlled trial followed by single-blind extension. J Clin Psychiatry 75(7):e672–e678, 2014 25093483

Cumberland Pharmaceuticals: Vaprisol (conivaptan). Nashville, NT, Cumberland Pharmaceuticals, 2009. Available at: http://www.vaprisol.com. Accessed April 12, 2016.

Atsariyasing W, Goldman MB: A systematic review of the ability of urine concentration to distinguish antipsychotic- from psychosis-induced hyponatremia. Psychiatry Res 217(3):129–133, 2014 24726819

Aurora RN, Kristo DA, Bista SR, et al: American Academy of Sleep Medicine: The treatment of restless legs syndrome and periodic limb movement disorder in adults—an update for 2012: practice parameters with an evidence-based systematic review and meta-analyses: an American Academy of Sleep Medicine Clinical Practice Guideline. Sleep 35(8):1039–1062, 2012 22851801

Bassilios N, Launay-Vacher V, Khoury N, et al: Gabapentin neurotoxicity in a chronic haemodialysis patient. Nephrol Dial Transplant 16(10):2112–2113, 2001 11572915

Bautovich A, Katz I, Smith M, et al: Depression and chronic kidney disease: a review for clinicians. Aust N Z J Psychiatry 48(6):530–541, 2014 24658294

Bendz H, Sjödin I, Aurell M: Renal function on and off lithium in patients treated with lithium for 15 years or more: a controlled, prospective lithium-withdrawal study. Nephrol Dial Transplant 11(3):457–460, 1996 8671815

Bhardwaj SB, Motiwala FB, Morais M, Lippmann SB: Vaptans for hyponatremia induced by psychogenic polydipsia. Prim Care Companion CNS Disord 15(1) pii: PCC.12l01444, 2013 23724348

Bliwise DL, Zhang RH, Kutner NG: Medications associated with restless legs syndrome: a case-control study in the US Renal Data System (USRDS). Sleep Med 15(10):1241–1245, 2014 25156752

Blumenfield M, Levy NB, Spinowitz B, et al: Fluoxetine in depressed patients on dialysis. Int J Psychiatry Med 27(1):71–80, 1997 9565715

Cadwallader DE: Biopharmaceutics and Drug Interactions. New York, Raven, 1983

Clayton AH, El Haddad S, Iluonakhamhe JP, et al: Sexual dysfunction associated with major depressive disorder and antidepressant treatment. Expert Opin Drug Saf 13(10):1361–1374, 2014 25148932

Close H, Reilly J, Mason JM, et al: Renal failure in lithium-treated bipolar disorder: a retrospective cohort study. PLoS One 9(3):e90169, 2014 24570976

Cohen LM, Tessier EG, Germain MJ, Levy NB: Update on psychotropic medication use in renal disease. Psychosomatics 45(1):34–48, 2004 14709759

CredibleMeds: Risk categories for drugs that prolong QT and induce torsades de pointes (TdP), June 15, 2016. Available at: https://crediblemeds.org. Accessed July 7, 2016.

Crone CC, Gabriel GM, DiMartini A: An overview of psychiatric issues in liver disease for the consultation-liaison psychiatrist. Psychosomatics 47(3):188–205, 2006 16684936

Cukor D, Coplan J, Brown C, et al: Depression and anxiety in urban hemodialysis patients. Clin J Am Soc Nephrol 2(3):484–490, 2007 17699455

Cukor D, Coplan J, Brown C, et al: Anxiety disorders in adults treated by hemodialysis: a single-center study. Am J Kidney Dis 52(1):128–136, 2008a 18440682

Cukor D, Coplan J, Brown C, et al: Course of depression and anxiety diagnosis in patients treated with hemodialysis: a 16-month follow-up. Clin J Am Soc Nephrol 3(6):1752–1758, 2008b 18684897

De Picker L, Van Den Eede F, Dumont G, et al: Antidepressants and the risk of hyponatremia: a class-by-class review of literature. Psychosomatics 55(6):536–547, 2014 25262043

Dev V, Dixon SN, Fleet JL, et al: Higher anti-depressant dose and major adverse outcomes in moderate chronic kidney disease: a retrospective population-based study. BMC Nephrol 15:79, 2014 24884589

Dundas B, Harris M, Narasimhan M: Psychogenic polydipsia review: etiology, differential, and treatment. Curr Psychiatry Rep 9(3):236–241, 2007 17521521

Elias MF, Elias PK, Seliger SL, et al: Chronic kidney disease, creatinine and cognitive functioning. Nephrol Dial Transplant 24(8):2446–2452, 2009 19297357

Eyer F, Pfab R, Felgenhauer N, et al: Lithium poisoning: pharmacokinetics and clearance during different therapeutic measures. J Clin Psychopharmacol 26(3):325–330, 2006 16702900

Finley PR, Warner MD, Peabody CA: Clinical relevance of drug interactions with lithium. Clin Pharmacokinet 29(3):172–191, 1995 8521679

Freeman MP, Freeman SA: Lithium: clinical considerations in internal medicine. Am J Med 119(6):478–481, 2006 16750958

Freudenthaler S, Meineke I, Schreeb KH, et al: Influence of urine pH and urinary flow on the renal excretion of memantine. Br J Clin Pharmacol 46(6):541–546, 1998 9862242

Friedli K, Almond M, Day C, et al: A study of sertraline in dialysis (ASSertID): a protocol for a pilot randomised controlled trial of drug treatment for depression in patients undergoing haemodialysis. BMC Nephrol 16:172, 2015 26503099

Fukuhara S, Green J, Albert J, et al: Symptoms of depression, prescription of benzodiazepines, and the risk of death in hemodialysis patients in Japan. Kidney Int 70(10):1866–1872, 2006 17021611

Gheorghiade M, Niazi I, Ouyang J, et al; Tolvaptan Investigators: Vasopressin V2-receptor blockade with tolvaptan in patients with chronic heart failure: results from a double-blind, randomized trial. Circulation 107(21):2690–2696, 2003 12742979

Giannaki CD, Hadjigeorgiou GM, Karatzaferi C, et al: Epidemiology, impact, and treatment options of restless legs syndrome in end-stage renal disease patients: an evidence-based review. Kidney Int 85(6):1275–1282, 2014 24107848

Gillman PK: Tricyclic antidepressant pharmacology and therapeutic drug interactions updated. Br J Pharmacol 151(6):737–748, 2007 17471183

Gray SL, Anderson ML, Dublin S, Larson EB: Cumulative use of strong anticholinergics and incident dementia: a prospective cohort study. JAMA Intern Med 175(3):401–407, 2015 25621434

Greendyke RM, Bernhardt AJ, Tasbas HE, Lewandowski KS: Polydipsia in chronic psychiatric patients: therapeutic trials of clonidine and enalapril. Neuropsychopharmacology 18(4):272–281, 1998 9509495

Grünfeld JP, Rossier BC: Lithium nephrotoxicity revisited. Nat Rev Nephrol 5(5):270–276, 2009 19384328

Gulsun M, Pinar M, Sabanci U: Psychotic disorder induced by oxybutynin: presentation of two cases. Clin Drug Investig 26(10):603–606, 2006 17163294

Hall SA, Maserejian NN, Link CL, et al: Are commonly used psychoactive medications associated with lower urinary tract symptoms? Eur J Clin Pharmacol 68(5):783–791, 2012 22138718

Horinek EL, Kiser TH, Fish DN, et al: Propylene glycol accumulation in critically ill patients receiving continuous intravenous lorazepam infusions. Ann Pharmacother 43(12):1964–1971, 2009 19920159

Hosseini SH, Espahbodi F, Mirzadeh Goudarzi SM: Citalopram versus psychological training for depression and anxiety symptoms in hemodialysis patients. Iran J Kidney Dis 6(6):446–451, 2012 23146983

Israni RK, Kasbekar N, Haynes K, Berns JS: Use of antiepileptic drugs in patients with kidney disease. Semin Dial 19(5):408–416, 2006 16970741

Jacobson S: Psychopharmacology: prescribing for patients with hepatic or renal dysfunction. Psychiatr Times 19:65–70, 2002

Jain N, Trivedi MH, Rush AJ, et al: Rationale and design of the Chronic Kidney Disease Antidepressant Sertraline Trial (CAST). Contemp Clin Trials 34(1):136–144, 2013 23085503

Jeong SH, Kim JH, Ahn YM, et al: A 2-year prospective follow-up study of lower urinary tract symptoms in patients treated with clozapine. J Clin Psychopharmacol 28(6):618–624, 2008 19011429

Kane JM, Lauriello J, Laska E, et al: Long-term efficacy and safety of iloperidone: results from 3 clinical trials for the treatment of schizophrenia. J Clin Psychopharmacol 28(2 suppl 1):S29–S35, 2008 18334910

Kay GG, Ebinger U: Preserving cognitive function for patients with overactive bladder: evidence for a differential effect with darifenacin. Int J Clin Pract 62(11):1792–1800, 2008 18699842

Kay G, Crook T, Rekeda L, et al: Differential effects of the antimuscarinic agents darifenacin and oxybutynin ER on memory in older subjects. Eur Urol 50(2):317–326, 2006 16687205

Kennedy SH, Craven JL, Rodin GM: Major depression in renal dialysis patients: an open trial of antidepressant therapy. J Clin Psychiatry 50(2):60–63, 1989 2644243

Kerdraon J, Robain G, Jeandel C, et al: Impact on cognitive function of anticholinergic drugs used for the treatment of overactive bladder in the elderly [in French]. Prog Urol 24(11):672–681, 2014 25214448

Kimmel PL, Cukor D, Cohen SD, Peterson RA: Depression in end-stage renal disease patients: a critical review. Adv Chronic Kidney Dis 14(4):328–334, 2007 17904499

Koo JR, Yoon JY, Joo MH, et al: Treatment of depression and effect of antidepression treatment on nutritional status in chronic hemodialysis patients. Am J Med Sci 329(1):1–5, 2005 15654172

Lacerda G, Krummel T, Sabourdy C, et al: Optimizing therapy of seizures in patients with renal or hepatic dysfunction. Neurology 67(12) (suppl 4):S28–S33, 2006 17190918

Letmaier M, Painold A, Holl AK, et al: Hyponatraemia during psychopharmacological treatment: results of a drug surveillance programme. Int J Neuropsychopharmacol 15(6):739–748, 2012

Levy NB: Psychopharmacology in patients with renal failure. Int J Psychiatry Med 20(4):325–334, 1990 2086520

Liamis G, Milionis H, Elisaf M: A review of drug-induced hyponatremia. Am J Kidney Dis 52(1):144–153, 2008 18468754

Losso RL, Minhoto GR, Riella MC: Sleep disorders in patients with end-stage renal disease undergoing dialysis: comparison between hemodialysis, continuous ambulatory peritoneal dialysis and automated peritoneal dialysis. Int Urol Nephrol 47(2):369–375, 2015 25358390

MedlinePlus: Lamotrigine, 2015. Bethesda, MD, U.S. National Library of Medicine. Available at: https://www.nlm.nih.gov/medlineplus/druginfo/meds/a695007.html. Accessed July 6, 2016.

Molnar MZ, Novak M, Mucsi I: Management of restless legs syndrome in patients on dialysis. Drugs 66(5):607–624, 2006 16620140

Murray AM: Cognitive impairment in the aging dialysis and chronic kidney disease populations: an occult burden. Adv Chronic Kidney Dis 15(2):123–132, 2008 18334236

Murtagh FE, Addington-Hall J, Higginson IJ: The prevalence of symptoms in end-stage renal disease: a systematic review. Adv Chronic Kidney Dis 14(1):82–99, 2007 17200048

Nilsson MI, Widerlöv E, Meresaar U, Anggård E: Effect of urinary pH on the disposition of methadone in man. Eur J Clin Pharmacol 22(4):337–342, 1982 6286317

Novak M, Shapiro CM, Mendelssohn D, Mucsi I: Diagnosis and management of insomnia in dialysis patients. Semin Dial 19(1):25–31, 2006 16423179

Nurnberg HG, Hensley PL, Gelenberg AJ, et al: Treatment of antidepressant-associated sexual dysfunction with sildenafil: a randomized controlled trial. JAMA 289(1):56–64, 2003 12503977

Nurnberg HG, Hensley PL, Heiman JR, et al: Sildenafil treatment of women with antidepressant-associated sexual dysfunction: a randomized controlled trial. JAMA 300(4):395–404, 2008 18647982

Palmer S, Vecchio M, Craig JC, et al: Prevalence of depression in chronic kidney disease: systematic review and meta-analysis of observational studies. Kidney Int 84(1):179–191, 2013

Paul R, Minay J, Cardwell C, et al: Meta-analysis of the effects of lithium usage on serum creatinine levels. J Psychopharmacol 24(10):1425–1431, 2009 19395432

Periclou A, Ventura D, Rao N, Abramowitz W: Pharmacokinetic study of memantine in healthy and renally impaired subjects. Clin Pharmacol Ther 79(1):134–143, 2006 16413248

Pichette V, Leblond FA: Drug metabolism in chronic renal failure. Curr Drug Metab 4(2):91–103, 2003 12678690

Presne C, Fakhouri F, Noël LH, et al: Lithium-induced nephropathy: fate of progression and prognostic factors. Kidney Int 64(2):585–592, 2003 12846754

Rej S, Li BW, Looper K, Segal M: Renal function in geriatric psychiatry patients compared to non-psychiatric older adults: effects of lithium use and other factors. Aging Ment Health 18(7):847–853, 2014a 24533667

Rej S, Shulman K, Herrmann N, et al: Prevalence and correlates of renal disease in older lithium users: a population-based study. Am J Geriatr Psychiatry 22(11):1075–1082, 2014b 24566239

Roxanas M, Grace BS, George CR: Renal replacement therapy associated with lithium nephrotoxicity in Australia. Med J Aust 200(4):226–228, 2014 24580527

Salvatore S, Serati M, Cardozo L, et al: Cognitive dysfunction with tolterodine use. Am J Obstet Gynecol 197(2):e8, 2007 17689620

Serretti A, Chiesa A, Cardozo L, et al: Treatment-emergent sexual dysfunction related to antidepressants: a meta-analysis. J Clin Psychopharmacol 29(3):259–266, 2009 19440080

Siegel AJ: Hyponatremia in psychiatric patients: update on evaluation and management. Harv Rev Psychiatry 16(1):13–24, 2008 18306096

Tagay S, Kribben A, Hohenstein A, et al: Posttraumatic stress disorder in hemodialysis patients. Am J Kidney Dis 50(4):594–601, 2007 17900459

Takagi S, Watanabe Y, Imaoka T, et al: Treatment of psychogenic polydipsia with acetazolamide: a report of 5 cases. Clin Neuropharmacol 34(1):5–7, 2011 18306096

Tsao JW, Heilman KM: Transient memory impairment and hallucinations associated with tolterodine use. N Engl J Med 349(23):2274–2275, 2003 14657444

van Noord C, Straus SM, Sturkenboom MC, et al: Psychotropic drugs associated with corrected QT interval prolongation. J Clin Psychopharmacol 29(1):9–15, 2009 19142100

Verghese C, de Leon J, Josiassen RC: Problems and progress in the diagnosis and treatment of polydipsia and hyponatremia. Schizophr Bull 22(3):455–464, 1996 8873296

Ward ME, Musa MN, Bailey L: Clinical pharmacokinetics of lithium. J Clin Pharmacol 34(4):280–285, 1994 8006194

Winkelmayer WC, Mehta J, Wang PS: Benzodiazepine use and mortality of incident dialysis patients in the United States. Kidney Int 72(11):1388–1393, 2007 17851463

Womack KB, Heilman KM: Tolterodine and memory: dry but forgetful. Arch Neurol 60(5):771–773, 2003 12756144

Yang HH, Hsiao YP, Shih HC, Yang JH: Acyclovir-induced neuropsychosis successfully recovered after immediate hemodialysis in an end-stage renal disease patient. Int J Dermatol 46(8):883–884, 2007 17651180

6

Cardiovascular Disorders

Peter A. Shapiro, M.D.

Comorbidity of psychiatric disorders and heart disease is extremely common. Psychopharmacological treatment for psychiatric disorders in patients with cardiovascular disease has been an important topic of active investigation from the beginning of the modern era of psychopharmacology, in the mid-twentieth century, when psychoactive agents such as chlorpromazine, tricyclic antidepressants (TCAs), and lithium were noted to have significant cardiovascular effects. In the last 20 years, psychiatric disorders, especially depression, have been found to be associated with increased cardiovascular morbidity and mortality in patients with existing heart disease, spurring even greater interest in the effects of psychopharmacological treatment in cardiac patients.

The most common psychiatric problems in patients with heart disease are adjustment disorders, anxiety disorders, depressive disorders, and neurocognitive disorders (delirium and dementia). Posttraumatic stress disorder is increasingly recognized as both a risk factor for incident coronary disease and a complication of cardiac events that in turn increases the risk of recurrent events. Patients who undergo long-term treatment with antipsychotic medications are at risk for heart disease due to metabolic side effects. Nicotine dependence, substance use disorders, and sexual dysfunction may also be problems that require intervention.

Most clinical trials in psychopharmacology exclude patients with significant medical comorbidity, so most psychopharmacotherapy practice for patients with cardiovascular disease is based on inferences from studies of patients without heart disease or on clinical lore alone. More specific evidence about treatment in patients with heart disease is needed. Nevertheless, some general guidelines apply.

Differential Diagnostic Considerations

In general, differential diagnosis of psychiatric problems in patients with cardiac disease begins with phenomenological characterization of the psychopathology. Next, one must evaluate whether the condition is secondary to a general medical condition or substance (including medications used to treat the medical condition) or is a primary psychiatric problem. Finally, comorbidity will help to define treatment plans.

Some common errors involve misattribution of symptoms to a primary psychiatric diagnosis rather than to the cardiac problem. For example, patients with paroxysmal supraventricular tachycardia may appear to be anxious or to be having panic attacks. Patients with unrecognized congestive heart failure, pulmonary congestion, and nocturnal dyspnea may complain of insomnia and receive a diagnosis of depression or panic attacks. These patients will respond better to effective heart failure management than to psychotropics.

The workup of psychiatric symptoms in cardiac patients should include assessment of cardiac rhythm; blood pressure; fluid and electrolyte status; glycemic control; blood gases; blood count; and hepatic, renal, and thyroid function. Hypotension and arrhythmias may reduce cerebral blood flow and perfusion of other vital organs, resulting in organic mental syndromes. Severe hyponatremia and anemia may lead to a variety of psychiatric symptoms. Hepatic and renal dysfunction often cause mood or cognitive disturbances. Hypothyroidism, which may occur as a complication of amiodarone therapy, causes mood and cognitive problems. The presence of infections and the role of medications and substance use or withdrawal symptoms should be considered.

Consideration should be given to the presence of central nervous system (CNS) disease, including cerebrovascular disease and primary degenerative brain disorders (e.g., Alzheimer's disease, Parkinson's disease). The prevalence of small vessel ischemic cerebrovascular disease is high in patients with ischemic heart disease, even in patients without a known history of transient ischemic attack or stroke (Lazar et al. 2001). Electroencephalograms are often useful to distinguish encephalopathies (hypoactive delirium, dementia, recurring seizures, and interictal states) from depression with apathy, psychomotor retardation, or apparent cognitive impairment.

Neuropsychiatric Side Effects of Cardiac Medications

Neuropsychiatric effects of cardiovascular medications should be considered in the differential diagnosis (see Table 6–1). α-Adrenergic blocking agents may cause depression and sexual dysfunction. The purported association of β-adrenergic blocking agents with depression was disproven in a quantitative review of randomized trials (Ko et al. 2002). This study, reviewing 15 trials with a total of more than 35,000 subjects treated for acute myocardial infarction, hypertension, or congestive heart failure, found no effect of β-blocker treatment on reported depressive symptoms. For fatigue and sexual dysfunction, the estimated numbers needed to treat to cause one additional case of these adverse events were 57 and 199 patients per year, respectively. Withdrawal of therapy because of fatigue or sexual dysfunction occurred in fewer than 6 cases per 1,000 patient-years of treatment. Similarly, a comparison of post–myocardial infarction patients taking β-blockers with matched patients not taking β-blockers found no effect of β-blocker therapy on incident depressive symptoms or cases of depressive disorder (van Melle et al. 2006). However, a trend was noted toward higher depression symptom scores with long-term use or higher dosages.

Digoxin may produce visual hallucinations, often of colored rings around objects. Some antiarrhythmic agents (especially lidocaine) cause confusion, hallucinations, or delirium. Angiotensin-converting enzyme (ACE) inhibitors are occasionally associated with mood elevation or depression. Amiodarone treatment often leads to hypothyroidism; these thyroid disturbances may result in cognitive dulling or depression symptoms. Hypokalemia and hypona-

Table 6–1.   Selected adverse neuropsychiatric effects of cardiac medications

Cardiac medication	Neuropsychiatric effects
α-Adrenergic blockers	Depression, sexual dysfunction
Amiodarone	Mood disorders secondary to thyroid effects
Angiotensin-converting enzyme inhibitors	Mood elevation or depression (rare)
Antiarrhythmic agents	Hallucinations, confusion, delirium
β-Adrenergic blockers	Fatigue, sexual dysfunction
Digoxin	Visual hallucinations, delirium, depression
Diuretics	Anorexia, weakness, apathy secondary to electrolyte disturbances

tremia from diuretic therapy may result in anorexia, weakness, and apathy; thiazide diuretics sometimes cause erectile dysfunction. For more extensive discussion, see the reviews by Brown and Stoudemire (1998) and Keller and Frishman (2003).

Alterations in Pharmacokinetics in Heart Disease

For most patients, heart disease per se does not result in alterations in drug absorption, distribution, metabolism, and elimination, but there are some important exceptions (see Table 6–2). These are severe right-sided heart failure with secondary hepatic congestion, ascites, or marked peripheral edema; severe left-sided heart failure with low cardiac output; and use of diuretics.

Right-sided congestive heart failure may result in elevated central venous pressure and impaired venous drainage from the hepatic venous system and the gut wall. Resulting gut wall edema may reduce drug absorption. Mild to moderate hepatic congestion has a limited effect on drug metabolism, but cirrhosis secondary to hepatic congestion leads to reduced serum albumin, relatively increased α_1 acid glycoprotein level, and ascites, which may alter drug

Table 6-2. Pharmacokinetic changes in heart disease

Condition	Physiological consequences	Pharmacokinetic effects	Significance
Drug absorption			
Right-sided heart failure	Hepatic congestion, gut wall edema	Decreased absorption	Uncertain
Drug distribution			
"Cardiac cirrhosis"	Reduced albumen, ascites, increased α_1 acid glycoprotein	Increased or decreased free drug levels	Uncertain
Drug metabolism			
Left-sided heart failure	Decreased hepatic artery blood flow, decreased Phase I hepatic metabolism	Reduced elimination of parent drug	Important for drugs with low therapeutic index and high hepatic extraction
Drug elimination			
Left-sided heart failure	Decreased renal artery blood flow, decreased glomerular filtration rate	Reduced elimination of water-soluble molecules	Risk of lithium toxicity

distribution and serum levels of free drug. Because the effects of diminished absorption and variable changes in drug distribution may be additive or off-setting, it is difficult to predict net effects. In general, as serum total protein and albumin levels fall with more advanced disease, the prudent action is to use smaller than usual dosages of psychotropic agents and increase dosages cautiously. When the ratio of free to protein-bound drug changes, the total plasma drug level is reduced, even though the amount of free drug, which is the amount that determines drug activity, remains the same. Therapeutic drug monitoring that measures only the total drug level would result in a lower level and may mislead the physician to increase drug dosage.

Left-sided heart failure results in reduced cardiac output and reduced blood flow through the hepatic and renal arteries. Decreased hepatic artery blood flow results in reduced drug metabolism, particularly Phase I processes—that is, ox-idation (e.g., cytochrome P450 [CYP]) and reduction reactions. Conjugation reactions (Phase II metabolism) that make drug metabolites water-soluble and subject to excretion through the kidneys are relatively spared. Because most psy-chotropic agents undergo hepatic Phase I metabolism, they will tend to accu-mulate. Even agents that rely on Phase II metabolism (e.g., lorazepam, oxazepam) tend to accumulate, albeit less than agents metabolized by Phase I processes (e.g., diazepam, amitriptyline). Again, as cardiac output falls, reduced dosage of most psychotropic agents may be necessary. Severe left-sided heart failure results in renal dysfunction due to hypotension and reduced renal artery blood flow. Thus, management of combined left- and right-sided heart failure, with combinations of β-blockers, ACE inhibitors, or angiotensin II receptor blockers and diuretics, is often limited by progressive renal dysfunction, requir-ing inotropic support. Lithium is the most important psychotropic agent elim-inated primarily by renal excretion—gabapentin, pregabalin, paliperidone, and memantine are others—and excretion of lithium and these other drugs falls along with creatinine clearance.

Diuretic use itself affects excretion of lithium. Thiazide diuretics block so-dium reabsorption in the glomerular proximal convoluted tubule; as serum sodium is depleted, tubular reuptake of lithium from the glomerular filtrate is enhanced. Thus, thiazide diuretics increase the serum lithium level and may increase risk of lithium toxicity. Loop diuretics (furosemide, ethacrynic acid, bumetanide) have little effect on serum lithium levels (Crabtree et al. 1991; Finley et al. 1995). However, chronic use of any diuretic in patients with heart failure may reduce creatinine clearance, raising the serum lithium level and increasing risk of lithium toxicity (Finley et al. 1995). Lithium dosing should be closely monitored or withheld entirely in patients with congestive heart failure whose fluid and electrolyte status is unstable. Use of hepatically metabolized mood stabilizers (e.g., valproate) may be preferred in these patients.

Psychotropic Medication Use in Heart Disease

Mackin (2008) provides a comprehensive discussion of cardiac side effects of psychotropic drugs. Some important effects are summarized in Table 6–3.

Anxiolytics and Sedative-Hypnotics

Relevant Treatment Literature

Although anxiety symptoms are common in patients with heart disease, studies are lacking of benzodiazepine and buspirone treatment efficacy in treatment of anxiety in patients with heart disease.

Prescribing Principles

Benzodiazepines, compared with buspirone, have the advantage of rapid onset of effect. Lorazepam, oxazepam, and temazepam may be the safest benzodiazepines to prescribe in patients with heart disease because these drugs do not undergo Phase I hepatic metabolism and are therefore relatively unaffected by altered metabolism in heart failure. Longer-acting agents and agents with active metabolites that effectively extend their elimination half-life and duration of action—clonazepam, clorazepate, diazepam, chlordiazepoxide, flurazepam, halazepam, and quazepam—should be used cautiously and at low dosages because they may accumulate to a higher than expected steady-state level because of slowed elimination. Cognitive dysfunction or delirium can result when the CNS depressant effect of benzodiazepines is superimposed on a brain already compromised by microvascular disease, which may co-occur with atherosclerotic cardiovascular disease.

Desirable Secondary Effects

Benzodiazepines have no significant effects of their own on heart rate and blood pressure, but reduction in acute anxiety can lead to reduction in anxiety-associated tachycardia, myocardial irritability, and myocardial work

Table 6–3.   Cardiac adverse effects of psychotropic drugs

Medication	Cardiac effects
Antipsychotics	Hypotension, orthostatic hypotension, cardiac conduction disturbances, ventricular tachycardia/fibrillation, metabolic syndrome
Antidepressants	
Bupropion	Hypertension
Monoamine oxidase inhibitors	Orthostatic hypotension
Serotonin-norepinephrine reuptake inhibitors	Hypertension
Selective serotonin reuptake inhibitors	Reduced heart rate, occasional clinically significant sinus bradycardia or sinus arrest; QT prolongation, especially with citalopram
Tricyclic antidepressants	Hypotension, orthostatic hypotension, Type 1A antiarrhythmic effects: slowed conduction through atrioventricular node and His bundle; heart block; QT prolongation; ventricular fibrillation
Trazodone	Orthostatic hypotension
Stimulants	Hypertension, tachycardia, tachyarrhythmias
Mood stabilizers	
Lithium	Sinus node dysfunction
Carbamazepine	Type 1A antiarrhythmic effects; atrioventricular block
Phosphodiesterase type 5 inhibitors	Hypotension, myocardial ischemia

(Huffman and Stern 2003). Effects on autonomic nervous system activity and on the balance of parasympathetic to sympathetic tone are uncertain; both parasympathetic withdrawal and a shift in sympathovagal balance toward increased parasympathetic predominance have been described in response to benzodiazepines (Marty et al. 1986; Vogel et al. 1996). Buspirone has no cardiovascular effects.

Antidepressants

Relevant Treatment Literature

Many studies have examined treatment of depression in patients with heart disease. Initial investigations of TCAs demonstrated their efficacy and their significant cardiovascular side-effect profile, which was particularly pronounced in patients with heart disease: increased heart rate, orthostatic hypotension, and cardiac conduction disturbances. First-, second-, or third-degree heart block may develop, and a pacemaker may be necessary to avoid syncope, particularly in patients with a prolonged PR interval at baseline. A series of studies on depressed patients with impaired left ventricular function suggested that nortriptyline, titrated to a blood level between 50 and 150 ng/mL, is relatively well tolerated in patients with impaired left ventricular function (Roose and Glassman 1989). In overdose, TCAs can cause lethal ventricular arrhythmias associated with QRS and QT interval prolongation. TCAs have Type 1A (quinidine-like) antiarrhythmic properties (Giardina et al. 1986). Type 1A antiarrhythmic agents are associated with increased mortality in patients with ischemic heart disease (Morganroth and Goin 1991). TCA users also had increased risk of incident myocardial infarction, compared with non-antidepressant users and with users of selective serotonin reuptake inhibitors (SSRIs), in a cohort of more than 50,000 workers, with a median 4.5-year follow-up (Cohen et al. 2000).

SSRIs may reduce heart rate and may prolong the QT interval to a variable extent. Generally, the chronotropic effect is small, no more than two to three beats per minute, but occasionally it may be clinically significant. Sinus bradycardia and syncope have been reported (Glassman et al. 1998). The U.S. Food and Drug Administration (FDA) requires a warning about QT interval prolongation and risk of torsades de pointes in the manufacturer's package insert for citalopram, based on case reports of sudden cardiac death and observation of dose-dependent QT interval prolongation with citalopram and (to a lesser degree) escitalopram. In a large retrospective cross-sectional study, citalopram demonstrated significant dose-related QT interval prolongation, whereas other antidepressants did not (for bupropion, dose was inversely associated with QT interval) (Castro et al. 2013). Epidemiological studies, however, demonstrate either no or very low extra risk of sudden cardiac death associated with citalopram use even at high doses (Leonard et al. 2011; Tampi et al. 2015; Weeke et al. 2012; Zivin et al. 2013).

Three large-scale randomized placebo-controlled, double-blind trials of SSRIs in heart disease have been reported. The first, the Sertraline Antidepressant Heart Attack Randomized Trial (SADHEART), enrolled 369 patients within 30 days of an acute coronary syndrome (Glassman et al. 2002, 2006). Patients were randomly assigned to 24 weeks of treatment with sertraline or to placebo. Sertraline was dosed in a range from 50 to 200 mg/day (mean 71 mg/day). Sertraline was more effective than placebo overall, as measured by the Clinical Global Impressions Improvement scale; planned subgroup analyses demonstrated that sertraline efficacy was limited to patients with recurrent depression, depression onset before the index cardiac event, or severe depression with Hamilton Rating Scale for Depression (Ham-D) scores greater than 20. Patients with first-episode onset of depression after the index cardiac event had a high placebo response rate, and sertraline showed no advantage over placebo. Sertraline treatment did not have significant effects on heart rate, blood pressure, cardiac conduction intervals, left ventricular ejection fraction, or arrhythmias. Results were similar for patients with left ventricular ejection fraction above and below 35%. The study was not designed to have sufficient sample size to test for a difference in rates of major adverse cardiac events, but a trend toward a reduction in events in patients treated with sertraline was noted. In another study, the Enhancing Recovery in Coronary Heart Disease (ENRICHD) trial for treatment of depression and low social support after myocardial infarction, open treatment with sertraline, which was prescribed in a nonrandomized fashion, was also associated with reduced major adverse cardiac events and reduced mortality (Taylor et al. 2005).

The second study, the Canadian Cardiac Randomized Evaluation of Antidepressant and Psychotherapy Efficacy (CREATE) trial, enrolled 281 patients with stable coronary disease. Patients were randomly assigned simultaneously to citalopram versus placebo and to clinical management alone versus clinical management supplemented by interpersonal psychotherapy (Lespérance et al. 2007). Citalopram dosing ranged from 20 to 40 mg/day (mean 33.1 mg/day). Patients were followed for 12 weeks. Clinical management plus interpersonal psychotherapy had no advantage over clinical management alone, but citalopram demonstrated antidepressant efficacy superior to that of placebo. There were no differences between treatment groups in cardiovascular effects and adverse event rates.

In a recently reported Korean trial, EsDEPACS (Kim et al. 2015), 300 patients who were 2–14 weeks (mean 29 days) status post hospitalization for an acute coronary syndrome, met criteria for diagnosis of major or minor depressive disorder by structured interview, and had a Beck Depression Inventory score of 10 or more were enrolled into a randomized double-blind, placebo-controlled trial of escitalopram 5–20 mg daily for depression. The duration of treatment was 24 weeks. Subjects with at least one follow-up visit after randomization ($n=217$) were included in the data analysis. The effect of escitalopram on Ham-D ratings was significant, and no adverse cardiovascular effects were more common in escitalopram-treated subjects except for dizziness. Escitalopram treatment was also superior to placebo with respect to other measures of depression severity and functional status.

Bleeding risk is a theoretical concern when using SSRIs in patients taking warfarin or antiplatelet therapy because SSRIs themselves increase gastrointestinal bleeding and inhibit platelet activation by reducing platelet serotonin. Empirical findings in heart disease populations are mixed. A retrospective case-control comparison study in patients hospitalized for acute coronary syndromes found a reduction in in-hospital recurrent ischemic events, heart failure, and asymptomatic cardiac enzyme elevation in patients taking SSRI antidepressants during the hospital stay. SSRIs were associated with an increase in minor bleeding complications but no effect on either major cardiac event rates or major bleeding complications (Ziegelstein et al. 2007). Almost all of the patients in this study were also taking aspirin and were receiving full-dose antiplatelet therapy. There was no increase in bleeding associated with sertraline in the SADHART study, even though a majority of subjects received concomitant aspirin and/or antiplatelet therapy (Glassman et al. 2002; Serebruany et al. 2003a, 2003b), and bleeding complications were no more likely in patients who had undergone cardiac artery bypass surgery and were exposed to SSRIs than in those exposed to other antidepressants (Kim et al. 2009). Other studies, however, have found increased incidence of bleeding events in longer-term follow-up of patients treated concurrently with SSRIs and warfarin (e.g., for atrial fibrillation), antiplatelet therapy, or antiplatelet therapy plus aspirin, with hazard ratios in the range of 1.5–3 (Cochran et al. 2011; Labos et al. 2011; Schelleman et al. 2011; Wallerstedt et al. 2009).

In patients with heart failure, depression is common and is associated with lower quality of life, more rapid decline in functional status, and increased mortality. Antidepressants were linked to increased mortality and major cardiovascular events over 3-year follow-up in a prospective naturalistic follow-up study of 204 outpatients with heart failure. In a cohort of patients hospitalized for congestive heart failure, however, antidepressant use was not associated with increased mortality after adjustment for other relevant variables, including depression (O'Connor et al. 2008).

Several controlled trials have tested SSRIs for depression in patients with heart failure. In SADHART, randomization was stratified by ejection fraction. Sertraline effects were similar in subjects with left ventricular ejection fraction lower and higher than 35% (Glassman et al. 2002). A larger trial of sertraline limited to patients with heart failure did not find a beneficial effect of sertraline with respect to depression or cardiovascular outcomes (O'Connor et al. 2010). In a very small ($n=28$) randomized placebo-controlled trial, depression response to treatment was 69% at 12 weeks for subjects treated with paroxetine controlled release 12.5–25 mg/day versus only 23% for subjects treated with placebo (Gottlieb et al. 2007). A placebo-controlled trial of citalopram in elderly depressed patients with congestive heart failure was terminated prematurely after an interim analysis showed a very high placebo response rate and no separation of citalopram from placebo (Fraguas et al. 2009).

Orthostatic hypotension is a known side effect of mirtazapine in patients who do not have heart disease. Mirtazapine was tested in a randomized placebo-controlled trial involving 94 patients (Honig et al. 2007), nested within the larger Myocardial Infarction and Depression–Intervention Trial (MIND-IT; van Melle et al. 2007). Mirtazapine dosing ranged from 30 to 45 mg/day. At week 8, the effect of mirtazapine on Ham-D scores was not significantly different from that of placebo, but mirtazapine was more efficacious as measured by the Depression scale of the Symptom Checklist–90 and by the Beck Depression Inventory. Patients with inadequate response at 8 weeks were offered alternative treatment, whereas the subset of patients with adequate response at 8 weeks continued with maintenance treatment to 24-week follow-up ($n=40$). In this small subset of patients, the efficacy of mirtazapine treatment was demonstrated on all measures at 24-week follow-up. Mirtazapine was well tolerated.

Limited data are available about other antidepressants for treatment of patients with heart disease. Hypertension sufficient to cause treatment discontinuation occurred in 2 of 40 patients in an open-label study of bupropion in patients with heart disease (Roose et al. 1991). Hypertension is also a known adverse effect of venlafaxine; no studies have been reported of venlafaxine in patients with cardiac disease, but an open-label study in patients older than 60 years found significant rates of increased blood pressure and orthostatic hypotension and several instances of palpitations, dizziness, or QT prolongation (Johnson et al. 2006). Venlafaxine (but not paroxetine) treatment reduced laboratory measures of heart rate variability (an undesirable effect) in a cohort of depressed subjects who were free of heart disease (Davidson et al. 2005). Monoamine oxidase inhibitors have not been studied in patients with heart disease; their use is not appealing in view of their strong risk of orthostatic hypotension, the risk of interaction with pressors, and the risk of hypertensive reactions to dietary indiscretions.

Duloxetine did not appear to be associated with significant cardiovascular risks in the subjects in 42 placebo-controlled trials, 3 of which involved patients with diabetic neuropathy (Wernicke et al. 2007). The medication has not been studied, however, in patients with significant heart disease.

In a small open-label study in patients with congestive heart failure and depression, nefazodone produced a significant reduction in heart rate but no changes in heart rate variability (Lespérance et al. 2003).

In a small placebo-controlled trial in patients with cardiac disease, trazodone was without significant adverse cardiac effects except postural hypotension (Bucknall et al. 1988). Numerous case reports (e.g., Service and Waring 2008) have described QT prolongation and ventricular arrhythmias after trazodone overdose.

Hierarchy of Drug Choice

On the basis of the available evidence, escitalopram, citalopram, and sertraline appear to be the first-line pharmacotherapy treatment options for depression in patients with coronary artery disease, with very limited data to suggest a preferential role of paroxetine in congestive heart failure. The relative absence of CYP interactions associated with escitalopram and citalopram (and, to a lesser degree, with lower-dose sertraline) is an advantage in patients taking other medications. Citalopram requires vigilance with respect to the QT interval and arrhythmia risk. Patients who cannot tolerate or have failed to respond to these agents might logically be offered second-line treatment with mirtazapine, bupropion, venlafaxine, or duloxetine, with special attention to blood pressure response during treatment. TCAs remain the gold standard of antidepressant efficacy; however, especially in patients with ischemic heart disease, they have a substantial side-effect burden and carry increased mortality risk. Nortriptyline might be a reasonable third-line option in patients who have failed to respond to adequate trials of other first- and second-line treatments and who are sufficiently impaired by depression that the additional adverse-effect risks are worth incurring.

Prescribing Principles

The agent of choice depends on the factors described previously, the patient's comorbid conditions, and the patient's other medications. Medication should be started at a low dose—possibly below the lowest therapeutic dose—and subjective tolerability and relevant electrocardiographic effects, vital signs, physical examination, and laboratory parameters should be reassessed before the dose is increased. Dosage increases should be followed by reassessment for adverse effects. For patients in heart failure who also have hepatic or renal dysfunction, target dosages may need to be reduced to lower than normal levels because of prolonged metabolism. However, if a patient is tolerating medication well but not responding adequately, it is worthwhile to consider a dosage increase.

Desirable Secondary Effects

Antihistaminic agents (TCAs, trazodone, mirtazapine) may increase appetite and promote weight gain in patients with cardiac cachexia, and sedating effects may help patients with insomnia. Bupropion is one of the few psychotropic agents associated with weight loss and therefore may help patients who need to lose weight as part of their cardiac treatment program. Bupropion is also indicated as pharmacotherapy for smoking cessation (although the period of acute treatment of a depressive episode is probably an unfavorable time to attempt smoking cessation). Whether the anti-platelet effect of SSRIs is clinically valuable in patients with ischemic heart disease is unknown (Pollock et al. 2000; Serebruany et al. 2003b).

Antipsychotics

Relevant Treatment Literature

Delirium is frequently treated with antipsychotic medication, although such treatment is off-label. Heart disease patients with other psychiatric disorders may also require antipsychotic drug therapy. No controlled studies have been reported of the benefits of antipsychotic medications specifically in cardiac patients.

All antipsychotic agents may cause hypotension, especially orthostatic hypotension (Mackin 2008). The effect is particularly marked for low-potency agents such as chlorpromazine. Olanzapine, clozapine, and quetiapine may be associated with higher rates of orthostatic hypotension than other second-generation agents. Complaints of dizziness may occur even in the absence of hypotension or orthostatic hypotension. Increased heart rate is common in patients treated with clozapine, but bradycardia can also occur with clozapine and other second-generation antipsychotics. In a review of FDA data, syncope due to orthostatic hypotension occurred in up to 1% of patients treated with quetiapine and up to 6% of patients treated with clozapine. Most of the patients in these samples did *not* have heart disease. Tolerance to the blood pressure–lowering effects of antipsychotics may develop over time; initiating treatment at low dosages reduces the risk. Salt supplements, α-adrenergic agonists such as midodrine, and mineralocorticoids such as fludrocortisone can reduce the risk, but these agents may not be suitable for some cardiac patients; support stockings may be an acceptable alternative.

Metabolic syndrome—comprising dyslipidemia, glucose intolerance, hypertension, and abdominal obesity—is an important side effect of second-generation antipsychotics, especially olanzapine and clozapine, and a risk factor for coronary artery disease (Bobes et al. 2007; Correll et al. 2006; Newcomer and Hennekens 2007). Aripiprazole and ziprasidone are less likely to lead to these effects than other second-generation antipsychotic medications. Current recommendations for prevention of metabolic side effects associated with second-generation antipsychotics emphasize exercise and dietary modification (Newcomer and Sernyak 2007) (see also Chapter 2, "Severe Drug Reactions").

All antipsychotic medications may prolong the QT interval, with the possible exception of aripiprazole. Haloperidol, droperidol, thioridazine, sertindole, and ziprasidone tend to produce greater-magnitude QT prolongation than other agents (Glassman and Bigger 2001; Harrigan et al. 2004; Stöllberger et al. 2005). QT interval prolongation (QTc above 440 ms and especially above 500 ms) is associated with increased risk of polymorphic sustained ventricular tachycardia (torsades de pointes), which can degenerate into ventricular fibrillation. First-generation phenothiazine antipsychotics may also cause QT interval prolongation and torsades de pointes. Nevertheless, there are case reports of patients with delirium treated in intensive care units with intravenous haloperidol at dosages up to 1,000 mg/day without harm (Tesar et al. 1985), and low dosages of aripiprazole, quetiapine, and olanzapine are commonly used to treat psychotic symptoms in hospitalized patients, including cardiac patients. Pimozide, a rarely used drug, may also induce prolongation of QT interval. It is contraindicated in patients with QT syndrome or history of cardiac arrhythmias. Coadministration of pimozide with strong CYP3A4 inhibitors is also contraindicated. Women, patients with chronic heavy alcohol consumption, and patients with anorexia nervosa are at increased risk of torsades de pointes. Other easily noted risk factors for torsades de pointes include severe heart disease, hypokalemia, hypomagnesemia, and concurrent treatment with one of the myriad other drugs that prolong the QT interval (see Table 6–4) (Beach et al. 2013; Brojmohun et al. 2013; Justo et al. 2005; Stöllberger et al. 2005). A comprehensive review concluded that at therapeutic doses, antipsychotic drugs alone, in the absence of other risk factors, were unlikely to cause torsades de pointes (Hasnain and Vieweg 2014).

On the basis of Danish registry data, the risk of sudden death associated with antipsychotic medication is estimated to be only about 2–4 per 10,000 person-years of exposure in otherwise medically healthy subjects (Glassman and Bigger 2001). However, reviews of treatment studies addressing use of both first- and second-generation antipsychotic medications in behaviorally disturbed elderly patients have concluded that antipsychotic medications are associated with about a 1.9% absolute increase in short-term mortality in this patient population (4.5% vs. 2.6%, or about a 70% increase in adjusted relative risk), mostly due to cardiovascular events and infections. This resulted in an FDA-mandated warning about off-label treatment of agitation and psychotic symptoms in behaviorally disturbed elderly patients with dementia (Gill et al. 2007; Kuehn 2008; Liperoti et al. 2005; Rochon et al. 2008). A review of Tennessee Medicaid data found that nonusers of antipsychotic drugs had a sudden death rate of 0.0014 deaths per person-year, whereas antipsychotic drug users had a sudden death rate of 0.0028–0.0029 deaths per person-year. Thus, antipsychotic drugs were associated with an approximate doubling of risk for sudden death, but the absolute risk was only about 0.0015 deaths per person-year, yielding a number needed to treat to cause one additional sudden death in 1 year of 666 persons (Ray et al. 2009). The degree to which these findings apply in the treatment of delirium and acute psychotic symptoms in patients with cardiac disease is unknown.

Table 6–4. Risk factors for torsades de pointes

Familial long QT syndrome

QT prolongation

Female sex

Chronic heavy alcohol use

Anorexia nervosa

Low ejection fraction

Hypokalemia

Hypomagnesemia

Concurrent treatment with multiple drugs that prolong QT interval or inhibit metabolism of a QT-prolonging drug

Clozapine is associated with a risk of myocarditis, which has been variously estimated to occur in 1 in 10,000 to 1 in 500 to more than 1% of exposed patients (Merrill et al. 2005). Generally, clozapine-associated myocarditis occurs within the first few weeks of treatment. The mechanism of inflammation is uncertain, but an immune hypersensitivity reaction is suspected. Patients exposed to clozapine also have an increased incidence of cardiomyopathy, even in the absence of an acute myocarditis process; onset may occur months to a few years after starting treatment (Mackin 2008).

Hierarchy of Drug Choice

In light of its relative freedom from metabolic problems and QRS prolongation, aripiprazole deserves consideration as first-line treatment for psychotic symptoms in patients with heart disease or with significant coronary artery disease risk factors. However, few data are available to definitively support this impression. Olanzapine and aripiprazole are available as orally disintegrating tablets, which may be a convenient route of administration for patients who cannot swallow tablets, and many medications are available for intramuscular administration. Asenapine is absorbed through the buccal mucosa, which may obviate the need for intramuscular medication in patients unable to take oral medication. Intravenous haloperidol, in widely variable dosages, has been in use (off-label) for decades.

Prescribing Principles

Before antipsychotic drugs are prescribed, heart patients should be evaluated for risk factors for sudden cardiac death. Risk factors include history of syncope or cardiac arrest, family history of sudden death, familial long QT syndrome (Roden 2008), long QT interval, low ejection fraction, treatment with other drugs that may prolong the QT interval either directly or through drug interactions, hypokalemia, and hypomagnesemia. Vital signs and electrocardiograms should be reviewed. For patients with congestive heart failure, lower than normal dosages may be adequate.

Mood Stabilizers

No studies have been reported of mood stabilizers as treatment for depression or bipolar disorder in heart patients. Lithium can cause sinus node dysfunction, manifesting in sinus bradycardia or sinus arrest. Lithium excretion is almost entirely through the kidney and is sensitive to the effects of diuretics (see the section "Alterations in Pharmacokinetics in Heart Disease" earlier in this chapter), ACE inhibitors, and angiotensin II receptor blockers. Long-term lithium use may cause impaired renal function, which may complicate heart failure management. Valproic acid has no cardiovascular effects; however, it may cause thrombocytopenia, which may be important for patients taking anticoagulants or those receiving antiplatelet therapy. It may increase plasma warfarin levels, but this has not been shown to be of clinical significance. An interaction with aspirin has been described that results in decreased protein binding, inhibited metabolism, and elevated free valproic acid level in blood. Lamotrigine does not have significant cardiac effects. It undergoes only Phase II hepatic metabolism, which may make it easier to dose in heart failure. Carbamazepine appears to be relatively free of cardiac effects in healthy patients (Kennebäck et al. 1995), but some electrocardiographic abnormalities have occurred in patients with heart disease (Kennebäck et al. 1991). Both carbamazepine and oxcarbazepine are associated with hyponatremia, especially in elderly women (see the section "Drug-Drug Interactions" later in this chapter). Gabapentin and pregabalin have no known cardiac effects.

Psychostimulants

Relevant Treatment Literature

Despite clinical lore supporting the value of stimulants to improve mood, increase energy, and improve subjective well-being in patients who are medically ill (Emptage and Semla 1996), including patients with heart disease (e.g., Kaufmann et al. 1984), no clinical trials have been reported of the risks and benefits of stimulants for depressed cardiac patients. A Cochrane review of a number of small trials of psychostimulant treatment of depression, including several trials in subjects who were medically ill, found no association between stimulant use and adverse cardiac effects but noted significant limitations in the quantity and quality of evidence available (Candy et al. 2008). Low dosages of stimulants (e.g., methylphenidate 5–30 mg/day, dextroamphetamine 5–20 mg/day) used as treatment for depression in medical patients have minimal effects on heart rate and blood pressure (Masand and Tesar 1996). A review of data from five clinical trials of stimulant and nonstimulant drugs for treatment of attention-deficit/hyperactivity disorder in adults concluded that amphetamine and methylphenidate both raise systolic and diastolic blood pressure by about 5 mmHg; the dosages of stimulants were not described in this report (Wilens et al. 2005). Reviews of adverse events in young adults taking stimulants for attention-deficit/hyperactivity disorder reported very low rates of cardiac events (Cooper et al. 2011; Peyre et al. 2014).

Prescribing Principles

Contraindications to stimulant use in manufacturers' package inserts generally include broadly construed serious heart problems, structural cardiac abnormalities, serious cardiac rhythm abnormalities, cardiomyopathy, and coronary artery disease. Interpreting this language may require clinical judgment and consultation with a cardiologist. Stimulant treatment should not be started without a medical consultation in a patient with history of heart disease or hypertension; symptoms of chest pain, palpitations, or shortness of breath; or physical exam findings of tachycardia, elevated blood pressure, or irregular heart rhythm. Stimulant treatment should be avoided in patients with acute ischemia, unstable angina, frequent ventricular premature contractions, or tachyarrhythmias. However, with concurrent medical supervision, in inpatient settings with cardiac monitoring, I have employed stimulants in the treatment of numerous patients within days after coronary artery bypass graft surgery, myocardial infarction, heart transplantation, and admission for decompensated heart failure and acute coronary events. Even ill patients can start with methylphenidate at dosages of 5 mg/day, with the dosage increased over a few days up to 20–30 mg/day. Vital signs and heart rhythm should be assessed with dosage changes. Benefit from stimulant medications for depressed cardiac patients should be observable within several days.

With respect to newer agents, such as modafinil and atomoxetine, almost no data are available. Potential hemodynamic effects, especially increased systolic blood pressure, could be problematic for patients with heart failure or coronary artery disease (Heitmann et al. 1999; Shibao et al. 2007; Taneja et al. 2005).

Cognitive Enhancers

Cognitive enhancers have not been studied in trials for patients with heart disease. The cholinesterase inhibitors donepezil, rivastigmine, and galantamine have modest benefit for treatment of mild to moderate dementia. Their procholinergic effects reduce heart rate and may rarely result in sinus bradycardia, heart block, and syncope. Clinical trials of cholinesterase inhibitors have largely excluded patients with cardiovascular disease, although there is some evidence of increased mortality and treatment discontinuation due to cardiovascular side effects in elderly patients with heart disease treated with cholinesterase inhibitors (Malone and Lindesay 2007). For the N-methyl-D-aspartate receptor antagonist memantine, which is indicated for treatment of moderate dementia, the manufacturer reported hypertension as a rare event in premarketing trials.

Other Agents

Varenicline, a nicotinic receptor partial agonist, was introduced in 2006 as a medication to aid smoking cessation, with data from two studies showing short-term cessation rates significantly better than those achieved with bupropion or placebo (Gonzales et al. 2006; Jorenby et al. 2006). A third study demonstrated that for patients who achieved abstinence during 12 weeks of acute treatment, adding an additional 12 weeks of maintenance treatment improved abstinence at 24 and 52 weeks (Tonstad et al. 2006). Important side effects of varenicline are nausea and worsening of depression. Varenicline does not have significant cardiac effects. Varenicline should be titrated over 7 days from a starting dosage of 0.5 mg once daily to 1 mg twice daily.

Naltrexone hydrochloride, an opioid antagonist, is sometimes used to reduce craving and help prevent relapse in patients with a history of alcohol dependence. This may be useful for patients with alcoholic cardiomyopathy, in concert with other measures to promote and maintain abstinence. Naltrexone has no cardiovascular effects in this situation. Intravenous naloxone, given as a competitive opioid receptor inhibitor in patients with opioid intoxication or overdose, may cause hypertension, hypotension, pulmonary edema, and cardiac arrest.

Acamprosate is indicated for maintenance of abstinence in patients with alcohol dependence. Acamprosate has no cardiovascular effects.

Topiramate was recently reported to improve maintenance of abstinence from alcohol (Johnson et al. 2007). Topiramate has no cardiovascular side effects. Hydrochlorothiazide increases topiramate blood levels. Topiramate reduces digoxin blood levels slightly.

The phosphodiesterase type 5 (PDE5) inhibitors sildenafil, vardenafil, and tadalafil, used for the treatment of erectile dysfunction, cause vasodilatation and increased blood flow into the penile corpus cavernosum. PDE5 inhibitors are also systemic and pulmonary arterial vasodilators and interact with numerous other agents that lower blood pressure. PDE5 inhibitors are also useful for treatment of pulmonary hypertension (Wilkins et al. 2008). Concurrent use of nitrates is contraindicated because of severe hypotension, and extreme caution must be used when combining α-blocking agents with PDE5 inhibitors. PDE5 inhibitor use in patients with cardiovascular disease has resulted in syncope, chest pain, myocardial infarction, tachycardia, and death, usually in conjunction with sexual activity.

Drug-Drug Interactions

The discussion of drug interactions in this section is based on several comprehensive reviews (Robinson and Owen 2005; Strain et al. 1999, 2002; Williams et al. 2007). Interactions between psychotropic and cardiac medications are due to pharmacodynamic properties of the drugs (i.e., they have overlapping and additive or offsetting effects) or pharmacokinetic effects (i.e., one drug affects metabolism, distribution, or elimination of the other), including but not limited to effects on hepatic metabolism by the CYP system (see Tables 6–5 and 6–6). For a complete review of drug-drug interactions, including cardiac medications, see Chapter 1, "Pharmacokinetics, Pharmacodynamics, and Principles of Drug-Drug Interactions."

Common pharmacodynamic interactions are additive effects on heart rate, blood pressure, and cardiac conduction. Many psychotropic drugs reduce blood pressure, and combining them with antihypertensive medications will increase the hypotensive effect. SSRI antidepressants tend to reduce heart rate; combining them with β-blockers may exacerbate the bradycardic effect. TCAs and mirtazapine suppress the centrally mediated antihypertensive effects of clonidine; the combination of TCA or mirtazapine with clonidine may result in severe hypertension. Drugs that prolong cardiac conduction—TCAs, phenothiazines, and atypical antipsychotics—may interact with amiodarone, Type 1A antiarrhythmic drugs, and ibutilide, resulting in atrioventricular block or prolonged QT interval. Several antibiotics, antifungal agents, methadone, tacrolimus, and cocaine also prolong the QT interval. Trazodone combined with amiodarone has resulted in QT prolongation and ventricular tachycardia.

Lithium clearance is an important example of a pharmacokinetic interaction that does not involve the hepatic CYP system. Thiazide diuretics, nifedipine, verapamil, lisinopril, ACE inhibitors, and angiotensin II receptor blockers all reduce lithium clearance and raise serum lithium levels. Acetazolamide and osmotic diuretics such as mannitol increase lithium clearance. Lithium toxicity may occur even when serum levels are not elevated in patients also taking diltiazem or verapamil.

Hyponatremia, a common side effect of SSRIs, oxcarbazepine, and carbamazepine, can be significantly exacerbated by interaction with the added hyponatremic effect of diuretics (Dong et al. 2005; Jacob and Spinler 2006; Ranta and Wooten 2004; Rosner 2004).

Many benzodiazepines, fluoxetine, paroxetine, and nefazodone can increase blood levels of digoxin, by an unknown mechanism.

Donepezil, rivastigmine, and galantamine have systemic and CNS procholinergic effects; these may be antagonized by medicines with anticholinergic activity, including disopyramide, procainamide, quinidine, isosorbide dinitrate, digoxin, and furosemide, resulting in cognitive worsening. Cholinesterase inhibitors plus β-blockers have additive bradycardic effects and could cause syncope.

Numerous pharmacokinetic interactions involve inhibition or induction of CYP isozymes involved in the metabolism of psychotropic and cardiac medications (see Chapter 1). The following discussion is limited to a few specific interactions of clinical importance.

Most β-blockers, including carvedilol, propranolol, and metoprolol, are metabolized mainly by CYP2D6, which is strongly inhibited by fluoxetine, paroxetine, and bupropion. Significant bradycardia could result. Most antiarrhythmic drugs are also metabolized by CYP2D6.

Table 6–5. Clinically relevant cardiac drug–psychotropic drug interactions

Cardiac drug	Mechanism of interaction	Clinical effects and management
ACE inhibitors	Reduced lithium clearance	Elevated lithium levels. Monitor serum lithium levels.
Angiotensin II receptor blockers	Reduced lithium clearance	Elevated lithium levels. Monitor serum lithium levels.
Antianginals		
Isosorbide dinitrate	Anticholinergic activity	Impaired cognition. Reduced therapeutic effect of cholinesterase inhibitors and memantine.
Antiarrhythmics		
Amiodarone	Inhibition of CYP2C9, CYP2D6, and CYP3A4	Increased levels of phenytoin, TCAs, opiates, risperidone, aripiprazole, atomoxetine, benzodiazepines, buspirone, alfentanil, zopiclone, eszopiclone, modafinil. Impaired activation of codeine to morphine.
Disopyramide	Anticholinergic activity	Impaired cognition. Reduced therapeutic effect of cholinesterase inhibitors and memantine.
Mexiletine	CYP1A2 inhibition	Increased levels of olanzapine and clozapine.
Procainamide	Anticholinergic activity	Impaired cognition. Reduced therapeutic effect of cholinesterase inhibitors and memantine.
Propafenone	CYP1A2 inhibition	Increased levels of olanzapine and clozapine.

Table 6–5.   Clinically relevant cardiac drug–psychotropic drug interactions *(continued)*

Cardiac drug	Mechanism of interaction	Clinical effects and management
Antiarrhythmics *(continued)*		
Quinidine	CYP2D6 inhibition	Increased levels of TCAs, opiates, risperidone, aripiprazole, atomoxetine. Impaired activation of codeine to morphine.
	Anticholinergic activity	Impaired cognition. Reduced therapeutic effect of cholinesterase inhibitors and memantine.
Antihyperlipidemics		
Fluvastatin, gemfibrozil, lovastatin, and simvastatin	CYP2C9 inhibition	Increased levels of phenytoin. Monitor phenytoin levels.
Calcium channel blockers		
Diltiazem	CYP3A4 inhibition	Increased levels of benzodiazepines, buspirone, alfentanil, zopiclone, eszopiclone, modafinil.
Nifedipine and verapamil	Reduced lithium clearance	Elevated lithium levels. Monitor serum lithium levels.
Cardiac glycosides		
Digoxin	Anticholinergic activity	Impaired cognition. Reduced therapeutic effect of cholinesterase inhibitors and memantine.

Table 6–5. Clinically relevant cardiac drug–psychotropic drug interactions (*continued*)

Cardiac drug	Mechanism of interaction	Clinical effects and management
Diuretics		
Acetazolamide and osmotic diuretics	Increased lithium clearance	Reduced lithium levels. Monitor serum lithium levels. Carbonic anhydrase inhibitors may decrease excretion of amphetamines.
Furosemide	Anticholinergic activity	Impaired cognition. Reduced therapeutic effect of cholinesterase inhibitors and memantine.
Thiazides	Reduced lithium clearance	Elevated lithium levels. Monitor serum lithium levels.

Note. ACE=angiotensin-converting enzyme; CYP=cytochrome P450; TCAs=tricyclic antidepressants.

Table 6–6. Clinically relevant psychotropic drug–cardiac drug interactions

Psychotropic drug	Mechanism of interaction	Clinical effects and management
Antidepressants		
Bupropion	CYP2D6 inhibition	Increased β-blocker levels→decreased heart rate. Increased levels of many antiarrhythmics with possible conduction abnormalities.
Duloxetine	CYP2D6 inhibition	Increased β-blocker levels→decreased heart rate. Increased levels of many antiarrhythmics with possible conduction abnormalities.
Fluoxetine	CYP3A4 inhibition	Increased statin levels→myopathy, hepatic injury. Increased calcium channel blocker levels→hypotension.
Fluvoxamine	CYP2C9 inhibition	Increased warfarin levels, increased INR→possible increased bleeding risk. Fluvoxamine contraindicated in patients receiving warfarin.
Mirtazapine	Unknown	Possible severe hypertension with clonidine; avoid this combination.
Moclobemide	CYP2D6 inhibition	Increased β-blocker levels→decreased heart rate. Increased levels of many antiarrhythmics with possible conduction abnormalities.
Nefazodone	CYP3A4 inhibition	Increased statin levels→myopathy, hepatic injury. Increased calcium channel blocker levels→hypotension.

Table 6–6. Clinically relevant psychotropic drug–cardiac drug interactions (*continued*)

Psychotropic drug	Mechanism of interaction	Clinical effects and management
Antidepressants (*continued*)		
Paroxetine	CYP2D6 inhibition	Increased β-blocker levels →decreased heart rate. Increased levels of many antiarrhythmics with possible conduction abnormalities.
Trazodone	Type 1A antiarrhythmic effects	QT prolongation, AV block with amiodarone, ibutilide, and Type 1A antiarrhythmic agents. Monitor QT interval. Avoid trazodone in conjunction with antiarrhythmic therapy.
MAOIs	MAO inhibition increases monoamine effect	Increased pressor effects of epinephrine and dopamine→hypertension.
SSRIs and SNRIs	Pharmacodynamic synergism: SIADH plus sodium wasting	SSRI/SNRI-induced SIADH and hyponatremia. Exacerbated with thiazide diuretic–induced sodium wasting. Monitor sodium levels. Consider nonthiazide diuretics.
TCAs	Type 1A antiarrhythmic effects	QT prolongation, AV block with amiodarone, ibutilide, and Type 1A antiarrhythmic agents. Monitor QT interval. Avoid TCAs in conjunction with antiarrhythmic therapy.
	Unknown	Possible severe hypertension with clonidine; avoid this combination.

Table 6–6. Clinically relevant psychotropic drug–cardiac drug interactions *(continued)*

Psychotropic drug	Mechanism of interaction	Clinical effects and management
Antipsychotics		
Atypical and typical antipsychotics	Type 1A antiarrhythmic effects	QT prolongation; AV block with amiodarone, ibutilide, and Type 1A antiarrhythmic agents. Monitor QT interval. Use antipsychotics with minimal QT-prolonging effect (olanzapine, aripiprazole).
Mood stabilizers		
Carbamazepine	Pan-inducer of CYP metabolic enzymes	Increased metabolism and lower levels of most cardiac medications, including warfarin, β-blockers, antiarrhythmics, statins, calcium channel blockers. Avoid carbamazepine if possible. Monitor cardiovascular function. Increase cardiac agent dosage as necessary.
	Pharmacodynamic synergism: SIADH plus sodium wasting	SSRI/SNRI-induced SIADH and hyponatremia. Exacerbated with thiazide diuretic–induced sodium wasting. Monitor sodium levels. Consider nonthiazide diuretics.
Oxcarbazepine	Pharmacodynamic synergism: SIADH plus sodium wasting	SSRI/SNRI-induced SIADH and hyponatremia. Exacerbated with thiazide diuretic–induced sodium wasting. Monitor sodium levels. Consider nonthiazide diuretics.
Phenytoin	Pan-inducer of CYP metabolic enzymes	Increased metabolism and lower levels of most cardiac medications, including warfarin, β-blockers, antiarrhythmics, statins, calcium channel blockers. Avoid phenytoin if possible. Monitor cardiovascular function.

Table 6–6. Clinically relevant psychotropic drug–cardiac drug interactions *(continued)*

Psychotropic drug	Mechanism of interaction	Clinical effects and management
Cholinesterase inhibitors	Pharmacodynamic synergism: increased vagal tone	Increased β-blocker effect on heart rate. Monitor heart rate. Reduce β-blocker dosage as necessary.

Note. AV=atrioventricular; CYP=cytochrome P450; INR=international normalized ratio; MAOIs=monoamine oxidase inhibitors; SIADH=syndrome of inappropriate antidiuretic hormone secretion; SNRIs=serotonin-norepinephrine reuptake inhibitors; SSRIs=selective serotonin reuptake inhibitors; TCAs=tricyclic antidepressants.

Warfarin is metabolized mainly by CYP2C9 and to a lesser extent through several other CYP isenozymes. Fluvoxamine inhibition and carbamazepine induction of CYP2C9 may cause clinically significant increase or decrease, respectively, in the international normalized ratio. Clopidogrel, argatroban, and heparin have not been reported to have interactions with psychotropic medications.

Most statins are metabolized by CYP3A4. Myopathy and hepatic injury as a result of statin toxicity may theoretically result from interaction with fluvoxamine, nefazodone, or other strong CYP3A4 inhibitors.

Although added QT prolongation could occur if metabolism of an antipsychotic drug were inhibited by a second agent, the clinical significance of this effect is uncertain. Cautious electrocardiographic monitoring would be especially appropriate in patients who begin with a QT interval near the upper limits of normal (Harrigan et al. 2004).

The combination of β-blockers and phenothiazines results in increased blood levels of both due to mutual metabolic inhibition. Heart rate and blood pressure effects, as well as CNS effects, may be increased.

Key Clinical Points

- Hypotension and QT interval prolongation should be monitored, particularly with TCAs, citalopram, and antipsychotic medications.
- Serum lithium levels need to be closely monitored.
- Many relevant cardiac medications are metabolized through CYP2D6; bupropion, fluoxetine, duloxetine, moclobemide, and paroxetine are CYP2D6 inhibitors.
- Many relevant cardiac medications are metabolized through CYP3A4; nefazodone, fluoxetine, fluvoxamine, and diltiazem are strong CYP3A4 inhibitors.
- Carbamazepine, phenytoin, and barbiturates are strong inducers of multiple CYP enzymes and increase metabolism of many cardiac drugs.
- Sertraline, escitalopram, and citalopram are the agents that have demonstrated effectiveness for treatment of depression in patients with coronary artery disease.

References

Beach SR, Celano CM, Noseworthy PA, et al: QTc prolongation, torsades de pointes, and psychotropic medications. Psychosomatics 54(1):1–13, 2013 23295003

Bobes J, Arango C, Aranda P, et al; CLAMORS Study Collaborative Group: Cardiovascular and metabolic risk in outpatients with schizophrenia treated with antipsychotics: results of the CLAMORS Study. Schizophr Res 90(1–3):162–173, 2007 17123783

Brojmohun A, Lou JY, Zardkoohi O, Funk MC: Protected from torsades de pointes? What psychiatrists need to know about pacemakers and defibrillators. Psychosomatics 54(5):407–417, 2013 23756118

Brown TM, Stoudemire A: Cardiovascular agents, in Psychiatric Side Effects of Prescription and Over-the-Counter Medications. Washington, DC, American Psychiatric Press, 1998, pp 209–238

Bucknall C, Brooks D, Curry PV, et al: Mianserin and trazodone for cardiac patients with depression. Eur J Clin Pharmacol 33(6):565–569, 1988 3284752

Candy M, Jones L, Williams R, et al: Psychostimulants for depression. Cochrane Database of Systematic Reviews 2008, Issue 2. Art. No.: CD006722. DOI: 10.1002/14651858.CD006722.pub2 18425966

Castro VM, Clements CC, Murphy SN, et al: QT interval and antidepressant use: a cross sectional study of electronic health records. BMJ 346:f288, 2013 23360890

Cochran KA, Cavallari LH, Shapiro NL, Bishop JR: Bleeding incidence with concomitant use of antidepressants and warfarin. Therap Drug Monit 33:433–438, 2011

Cohen HW, Gibson G, Alderman MH: Excess risk of myocardial infarction in patients treated with antidepressant medications: association with use of tricyclic agents. Am J Med 108(1):2–8, 2000 11059434

Cooper WO, Habel LA, Sox CM, et al: ADHD drugs and serious cardiovascular events in children and young adults. N Engl J Med 365(20):1896–1904, 2011 22043968

Correll CU, Frederickson AM, Kane JM: Metabolic syndrome and the risk of coronary heart disease in 367 patients treated with second-generation antipsychotic drugs. J Clin Psychiatry 67:575–583, 2006

Crabtree BL, Mack JE, Johnson CD, Amyx BC: Comparison of the effects of hydrochlorothiazide and furosemide on lithium disposition. Am J Psychiatry 148:1060–1063, 1991 1853956

Davidson J, Watkins L, Owens M, et al: Effects of paroxetine and venlafaxine XR on heart rate variability in depression. J Clin Psychopharmacol 25(5):480–484, 2005 16160626

Dong X, Leppik IE, White J, Rarick J: Hyponatremia from oxcarbazepine and carbamazepine. Neurology 65(12):1976–1978, 2005 16380624

Emptage RE, Semla TP: Depression in the medically ill elderly: a focus on methylphenidate. Ann Pharmacother 30(2):151–157, 1996 8835049

Finley PR, Warner MD, Peabody CA: Clinical relevance of drug interactions with lithium. Clin Pharmacokinet 29(3):172–191, 1995 8521679

Fraguas R, da Silva Telles RM, Alves TC, et al: A double-blind, placebo-controlled
treatment trial of citalopram for major depressive disorder in older patients with
heart failure: the relevance of the placebo effect and psychological symptoms.
Contemp Clin Trials 30(3):205–211, 2009 19470312

Giardina EG, Barnard T, Johnson L, et al: The antiarrhythmic effect of nortriptyline
in cardiac patients with premature ventricular depolarizations. J Am Coll Cardiol
7:1363–1369, 1986 3711494

Gill SS, Bronskill SE, Normand SL, et al: Antipsychotic drug use and mortality in
older adults with dementia. Ann Intern Med 146(11):775–786, 2007
17548409

Glassman AH, Bigger JT Jr: Antipsychotic drugs: prolonged QTc interval, torsade de
pointes, and sudden death. Am J Psychiatry 158(11):1774–1782, 2001 11691681

Glassman AH, Rodriguez AI, Shapiro PA: The use of antidepressant drugs in patients
with heart disease. J Clin Psychiatry 59 (suppl 10):16–21, 1998 9720478

Glassman AH, O'Connor CM, Califf RM, et al; Sertraline Antidepressant Heart Attack Randomized Trial (SADHEART) Group: Sertraline treatment of major depression in patients with acute MI or unstable angina. JAMA 288(6):701–709,
2002 12169073

Glassman AH, Bigger JTJ, Gaffney M, et al: Onset of major depression associated with
acute coronary syndromes: relationship of onset, major depressive disorder history, and episode severity to sertraline benefit. Arch Gen Psychiatry 63(3):283–
288, 2006 16520433

Gonzales D, Rennard SI, Nides M, et al; Varenicline Phase 3 Study Group: Varenicline, an alpha4beta2 nicotinic acetylcholine receptor partial agonist, vs sustained-release bupropion and placebo for smoking cessation: a randomized
controlled trial. JAMA 296(1):47–55, 2006 16820546

Gottlieb SS, Kop WJ, Thomas SA, et al: A double-blind placebo-controlled pilot study
of controlled-release paroxetine on depression and quality of life in chronic heart
failure. Am Heart J 153(5):868–873, 2007 17452166

Harrigan EP, Miceli JJ, Anziano R, et al: A randomized evaluation of the effects of six
antipsychotic agents on QTc, in the absence and presence of metabolic inhibition. J Clin Psychopharmacol 24(1):62–69, 2004 14709949

Hasnain M, Vieweg WV: QTc interval prolongation and torsade de pointes associated
with second-generation antipsychotics and antidepressants: a comprehensive review. CNS Drugs 28(10):887–920, 2014 25168784

Heitmann J, Cassel W, Grote L, et al: Does short-term treatment with modafinil affect blood pressure in patients with obstructive sleep apnea? Clin Pharmacol Ther 65(3):328–335, 1999 10096265

Honig A, Kuyper AMG, Schene AH, et al; MIND-IT investigators: Treatment of post-myocardial infarction depressive disorder: a randomized, placebo-controlled trial with mirtazapine. Psychosom Med 69(7):606–613, 2007 17846258

Huffman JC, Stern TA: The use of benzodiazepines in the treatment of chest pain: a review of the literature. J Emerg Med 25(4):427–437, 2003 14654185

Jacob S, Spinler SA: Hyponatremia associated with selective serotonin-reuptake inhibitors in older adults. Ann Pharmacother 40(9):1618–1622, 2006 16896026

Johnson BA, Rosenthal N, Capece JA, et al; Topiramate for Alcoholism Advisory Board; Topiramate for Alcoholism Study Group: Topiramate for treating alcohol dependence: a randomized controlled trial. JAMA 298(14):1641–1651, 2007 17925516

Johnson EM, Whyte E, Mulsant BH, et al: Cardiovascular changes associated with venlafaxine in the treatment of late-life depression. Am J Geriatr Psychiatry 14(9):796–802, 2006 16943176

Jorenby DE, Hays JT, Rigotti NA, et al; Varenicline Phase 3 Study Group: Efficacy of varenicline, an alpha4beta2 nicotinic acetylcholine receptor partial agonist, vs placebo or sustained-release bupropion for smoking cessation: a randomized controlled trial. JAMA 296(1):56–63, 2006 16820547

Justo D, Prokhorov V, Heller K, Zeltser D: Torsade de pointes induced by psychotropic drugs and the prevalence of its risk factors. Acta Psychiatr Scand 111(3):171–176, 2005 15701100

Kaufmann MW, Cassem N, Murray G, MacDonald D: The use of methylphenidate in depressed patients after cardiac surgery. J Clin Psychiatry 45(2):82–84, 1984 6693366

Keller S, Frishman WH: Neuropsychiatric effects of cardiovascular drug therapy. Cardiol Rev 11(2):73–93, 2003 12620132

Kennebäck G, Bergfeldt L, Vallin H, et al: Electrophysiologic effects and clinical hazards of carbamazepine treatment for neurologic disorders in patients with abnormalities of the cardiac conduction system. Am Heart J 121(5):1421–1429, 1991 2017974

Kennebäck G, Bergfeldt L, Tomson T: Electrophysiological evaluation of the sodium-channel blocker carbamazepine in healthy human subjects. Cardiovasc Drugs Ther 9(5):709–714, 1995 8573554

Kim DH, Daskalakis C, Whellan DJ, et al: Safety of selective serotonin reuptake inhibitor in adults undergoing coronary artery bypass grafting. Am J Cardiol 103(10):1391–1395, 2009 19427434

Kim JM, Bae KY, Stewart R, et al: Escitalopram treatment for depressive disorder following acute coronary syndrome: a 24-week double-blind, placebo-controlled trial. J Clin Psychiatry 76(1):62–68, 2015 25375836

Ko DT, Hebert PR, Coffey CS, et al: Beta-blocker therapy and symptoms of depression, fatigue, and sexual dysfunction. JAMA 288(3):351–357, 2002 12117400

Kuehn BM: FDA: Antipsychotics risky for elderly. JAMA 300(4):379–380, 2008 18647971

Labos C, Dasgupta K, Nedjar H, et al: Risk of bleeding associated with combined use of selective serotonin reuptake inhibitors and antiplatelet therapy following acute myocardial infarction. CMAJ 183(16):1835–1843, 2011 21948719

Lazar RM, Shapiro PA, Moskowitz A, et al: Randomized trial of on- vs off-pump CABG reveals baseline memory dysfunction. Paper presented at the annual meeting of the American Heart Association, Anaheim, CA, November 2001

Leonard CE, Bilker WB, Newcomb C, et al: Antidepressants and the risk of sudden cardiac death and ventricular arrhythmia. Pharmacoepidemiol Drug Saf 20(9):903–913, 2011 21796718

Lespérance F, Frasure-Smith N, Laliberté MA, et al: An open-label study of nefazodone treatment of major depression in patients with congestive heart failure. Can J Psychiatry 48(10):695–701, 2003 14674053

Lespérance F, Frasure-Smith N, Koszycki D, et al; CREATE Investigators: Effects of citalopram and interpersonal psychotherapy on depression in patients with coronary artery disease: the Canadian Cardiac Randomized Evaluation of Antidepressant and Psychotherapy Efficacy (CREATE) trial. JAMA 297(4):367–379, 2007 17244833

Liperoti R, Gambassi G, Lapane KL, et al: Conventional and atypical antipsychotics and the risk of hospitalization for ventricular arrhythmias or cardiac arrest. Arch Intern Med 165(6):696–701, 2005 15795349

Mackin P: Cardiac side effects of psychiatric drugs. Hum Psychopharmacol 23 (suppl 1):3–14, 2008 18098218

Malone DM, Lindesay J: Cholinesterase inhibitors and cardiovascular disease: a survey of old age psychiatrists' practice. Age Ageing 36(3):331–333, 2007 17350975

Marty J, Gauzit R, Lefevre P, et al: Effects of diazepam and midazolam on baroreflex control of heart rate and on sympathetic activity in humans. Anesth Analg 65(2):113–119, 1986 2935050

Masand PS, Tesar GE: Use of stimulants in the medically ill. Psychiatr Clin North Am 19(3):515–547, 1996 8856815

Merrill DB, Dec GW, Goff DC: Adverse cardiac effects associated with clozapine. J Clin Psychopharmacol 25(1):32–41, 2005 15643098

Morganroth J, Goin JE: Quinidine-related mortality in the short-to-medium-term treatment of ventricular arrhythmias. A meta-analysis. Circulation 84(5):1977–1983, 1991 1834365

Newcomer JW, Hennekens CH: Severe mental illness and risk of cardiovascular disease. JAMA 298(15):1794–1796, 2007 17940236

Newcomer JW, Sernyak MJ: Identifying metabolic risks with antipsychotics and monitoring and management strategies. J Clin Psychiatry 68(7):e17, 2007 17685728

O'Connor CM, Jiang W, Kuchibhatla M, et al: Antidepressant use, depression, and survival in patients with heart failure. Arch Intern Med 168(20):2232–2237, 2008 19001200

O'Connor CM, Jiang W, Kuchibhatla M, et al; SADHART-CHF Investigators: Safety and efficacy of sertraline for depression in patients with heart failure: results of the SADHART-CHF (Sertraline Against Depression and Heart Disease in Chronic Heart Failure) trial. J Am Coll Cardiol 56(9):692–699, 2010 20723799

Peyre H, Hoertel N, Hatteea H, et al: Adulthood self-reported cardiovascular risk and ADHD medications: results from the 2004-2005 National Epidemiologic Survey on Alcohol and Related Conditions. J Clin Psychiatry 75(2):181–182, 2014 24602253

Pollock BG, Laghrissi-Thode F, Wagner WR: Evaluation of platelet activation in depressed patients with ischemic heart disease after paroxetine or nortriptyline treatment. J Clin Psychopharmacol 20(2):137–140, 2000 10770450

Ranta A, Wooten GF: Hyponatremia due to an additive effect of carbamazepine and thiazide diuretics. Epilepsia 45(7):879, 2004 15230718

Ray WA, Chung CP, Murray KT, et al: Atypical antipsychotic drugs and the risk of sudden cardiac death. N Engl J Med 360(3):225–235, 2009 19144938

Robinson MJ, Owen JA: Psychopharmacology, in The American Psychiatric Publishing Textbook of Psychosomatic Medicine. Edited by Levenson JL. Washington, DC, American Psychiatric Publishing, 2005, pp 871–922

Rochon PA, Normand S-L, Gomes T, et al: Antipsychotic therapy and short-term serious events in older adults with dementia. Arch Intern Med 168(10):1090–1096, 2008 18504337

Roden DM: Clinical practice: long-QT syndrome. N Engl J Med 358(2):169–176, 2008 18184962

Roose SP, Glassman AH: Cardiovascular effects of tricyclic antidepressants in depressed patients with and without heart disease. J Clin Psychiatry 50:S1–S18, 1989

Roose SP, Dalack GW, Glassman AH, et al: Cardiovascular effects of bupropion in depressed patients with heart disease. Am J Psychiatry 148(4):512–516, 1991 1900980

Roose SP, Glassman AH, Attia E, Woodring S: Comparative efficacy of selective serotonin reuptake inhibitors and tricyclics in the treatment of melancholia. Am J Psychiatry 151(12):1735–1739, 1994 7977878

Roose SP, Glassman AH, Attia E, et al: Cardiovascular effects of fluoxetine in depressed patients with heart disease. Am J Psychiatry 155(5):660–665, 1998a 9585718

Roose SP, Laghrissi-Thode F, Kennedy JS, et al: Comparison of paroxetine and nortriptyline in depressed patients with ischemic heart disease. JAMA 279(4):287–291, 1998b 9450712

Rosner MH: Severe hyponatremia associated with the combined use of thiazide diuretics and selective serotonin reuptake inhibitors. Am J Med Sci 327(2):109–111, 2004 14770031

Schelleman H, Brensinger CM, Bilker WB, Hennessy S: Antidepressant-warfarin interaction and associated gastrointestinal bleeding risk in a case-control study. PLoS One 6(6):e21447, 2011 DOI: 10.1371/journal.pone.0021447 21731754

Serebruany VL, Glassman AH, Malinin AI, et al; Sertraline AntiDepressant Heart Attack Randomized Trial Study Group: Platelet/endothelial biomarkers in depressed patients treated with the selective serotonin reuptake inhibitor sertraline after acute coronary events: the Sertraline AntiDepressant Heart Attack Randomized Trial (SADHART) Platelet Substudy. Circulation 108(8):939–944, 2003a 12912814

Serebruany VL, Glassman AH, Malinin AI, et al: Selective serotonin reuptake inhibitors yield additional antiplatelet protection in patients with congestive heart failure treated with antecedent aspirin. Eur J Heart Fail 5(4):517–521, 2003b 12921813

Service JA, Waring WS: QT prolongation and delayed atrioventricular conduction caused by acute ingestion of trazodone. Clin Toxicol (Phila) 46(1):71–73, 2008 18167038

Sherwood A, Blumenthal JA, Trivedi R, et al: Relationship of depression to death or hospitalization in patients with heart failure. Arch Intern Med 167(4):367–373, 2007 17325298

Shibao C, Raj SR, Gamboa A, et al: Norepinephrine transporter blockade with atomoxetine induces hypertension in patients with impaired autonomic function. Hypertension 50(1):47–53, 2007 17515448

Stöllberger C, Huber JO, Finsterer J: Antipsychotic drugs and QT prolongation. Int Clin Psychopharmacol 20(5):243–251, 2005 16096514

Strain JJ, Caliendo G, Alexis JD, et al: Cardiac drug and psychotropic drug interactions: significance and recommendations. Gen Hosp Psychiatry 21(6):408–429, 1999 10664901

Strain JJ, Karim A, Caliendo G, et al: Cardiac drug-psychotropic drug update. Gen Hosp Psychiatry 24(5):283–289, 2002 12220794

Strik JJ, Honig A, Lousberg R, et al: Efficacy and safety of fluoxetine in the treatment of patients with major depression after first myocardial infarction: findings from a double-blind, placebo-controlled trial. Psychosom Med 62(6):783–789, 2000 11138997

Tampi RR, Balderas M, Carter KV, et al: Citalopram, QTc prolongation, and torsades de pointes. Psychosomatics 56(1):36–43, 2015 25619672

Taneja I, Diedrich A, Black BK, et al: Modafinil elicits sympathomedullary activation. Hypertension 45(4):612–618, 2005 15753235

Taylor CB, Youngblood ME, Catellier D, et al; ENRICHD Investigators: Effects of antidepressant medication on morbidity and mortality in depressed patients after myocardial infarction. Arch Gen Psychiatry 62(7):792–798, 2005 15997021

Tesar GE, Murray GB, Cassem NH: Use of high-dose intravenous haloperidol in the treatment of agitated cardiac patients. J Clin Psychopharmacol 5(6):344–347, 1985 4067002

Tonstad S, Tønnesen P, Hajek P, et al; Varenicline Phase 3 Study Group: Effect of maintenance therapy with varenicline on smoking cessation: a randomized controlled trial. JAMA 296(1):64–71, 2006 16820548

van Melle JP, Verbeek DEP, van den Berg MP, et al: Beta-blockers and depression after myocardial infarction: a multicenter prospective study. J Am Coll Cardiol 48(11):2209–2214, 2006 17161247

van Melle JP, de Jonge P, Honig A, et al; MIND-IT investigators: Effects of antidepressant treatment following myocardial infarction. Br J Psychiatry 190:460–466, 2007 17541103

Vogel LR, Muskin PR, Collins ED, Sloan RP: Lorazepam reduces cardiac vagal modulation in normal subjects. J Clin Psychopharmacol 16(6):449–453, 1996 8959471

Wallerstedt SM, Gleerup H, Sundström A, et al: Risk of clinically relevant bleeding in warfarin-treated patients—influence of SSRI treatment. Pharmacoepidemiol Drug Saf 18(5):412–416, 2009 19301238

Weeke P, Jensen A, Folke F, et al: Antidepressant use and risk of out-of-hospital cardiac arrest: a nationwide case-time-control study. Clin Pharmacol Ther 92(1):72–79, 2012 22588605

Wernicke J, Lledó A, Raskin J, et al: An evaluation of the cardiovascular safety profile of duloxetine: findings from 42 placebo-controlled studies. Drug Saf 30(5):437–455, 2007 17472422

Wilens TE, Hammerness PG, Biederman J, et al: Blood pressure changes associated with medication treatment of adults with attention-deficit/hyperactivity disorder. J Clin Psychiatry 66(2):253–259, 2005 15705013

Wilkins MR, Wharton J, Grimminger F, Ghofrani HA: Phosphodiesterase inhibitors for the treatment of pulmonary hypertension. Eur Respir J 32(1):198–209, 2008 18591337

Williams S, Wynn G, Cozza K, Sandson NB: Cardiovascular medications. Psychosomatics 48(6):537–547, 2007 18071104

Yeragani VK, Pesce V, Jayaraman A, Roose S: Major depression with ischemic heart disease: effects of paroxetine and nortriptyline on long-term heart rate variability measures. Biol Psychiatry 52(5):418–429, 2002 12242058

Ziegelstein RC, Meuchel J, Kim TJ, et al: Selective serotonin reuptake inhibitor use by patients with acute coronary syndromes. Am J Med 120(6):525–530, 2007 17524755

Zivin K, Pfeiffer PN, Bohnert ASB, et al: Evaluation of the FDA warning against prescribing citalopram at doses exceeding 40 mg. Am J Psychiatry 170(6):642–650, 2013 23640689

7

Respiratory Disorders

Yvette L. Smolin, M.D.

Catherine Daniels-Brady, M.D.

Wendy L. Thompson, M.D.

James L. Levenson, M.D.

The modern era of treatment for depression was ushered in by the serendipitous discovery in 1952 that iproniazid, a potential anti-tubercular agent, caused an elevation of mood in patients with tuberculosis (TB; Lieberman 2003). Iproniazid was a poor anti-tubercular drug, but its secondary activity as a monoamine oxidase inhibitor opened the door to the use of drugs to treat depression.

In this chapter we focus on asthma, chronic obstructive pulmonary disease (COPD), cystic fibrosis, TB, obstructive sleep apnea (OSA), and vocal cord dysfunction (VCD). For both psychological and physiological reasons, patients with these disorders may present with symptoms that are a focus of psychopharmacological treatment (see Table 7–1). Most conditions discussed (except cystic fibrosis, or if the patient smokes) do not alter the metabolism of pulmonary or other drugs. The main concern is to avoid medications that decrease respiratory drive or otherwise adversely affect ventilation. Psychiatric side effects of the medications used to treat pulmonary disease and drug-drug interactions are also reviewed.

Differential Diagnostic Considerations

All respiratory disorders discussed in this chapter are frequently associated with psychiatric symptoms that may require psychotropic medication. There is a complex interplay between psychiatric conditions and pulmonary diseases, with comorbidities often found to have a bidirectional association (Atlantis et al. 2013; Jain and Lolak 2009). These comorbidities may occur because of the following factors: reaction to an illness and treatment, direct physiological consequence of an illness, complication of treatment, or psychiatric illness that may coincide with the respiratory illness without being etiologically related. Which diagnosis came first may be difficult to determine.

Anxiety

Dyspnea, chest tightness, and the sensation of choking are common both in anxiety disorders and in respiratory diseases (Shanmugam et al. 2007). Thus, anxiety symptoms may be due to a comorbid anxiety disorder, an anxious response to a respiratory disease, an anxious response to the treatment of the disease, or the respiratory disease itself. Differentiation is important whenever possible; if the symptoms have a physiological basis (e.g., hypoxia), then this condition must be treated, either independently or in conjunction with treatment of the associated anxiety. For example, a patient with pulmonary embolus may present with dyspnea and hyperventilation in the absence of chest pain, which could be mistaken for a panic attack (Mehta et al. 2000). Anxiety disorders, especially panic disorder, are included in the differential diagnosis for VCD (Hicks et al. 2008). Anxiety disorders occur in almost one-third of asthmatics in primary care, and anxiety may precipitate asthma attacks (Cooper et al. 2007 Liu et al. 2014; Roy-Byrne et al. 2008; Scott et al. 2007). Theophylline and many β-agonists may induce or exacerbate anxiety (Thompson and

Table 7–1.   Psychiatric symptoms often associated with respiratory diseases

Illness	Symptoms
Asthma	Anxiety, depression, substance abuse (marijuana, crack cocaine), sleep disturbance
Chronic obstructive pulmonary disease	Anxiety, depression, nicotine dependence, cognitive impairment, sleep disturbance, sexual dysfunction, fatigue
Cystic fibrosis	Depression, anxiety, eating disorder
Functional respiratory disorders	
Vocal cord dysfunction	Stress, anxiety, depression, conversion disorder
Hyperventilation syndrome	Anxiety, depression, pseudoseizure
Sleep apnea	Somnolence, sleep disturbance, irritability, depression, cognitive impairment
Tuberculosis	Psychosis, sleep disturbance, substance abuse, cognitive impairment, fatigue, lethargy, mania, delirium

Sullivan 2006). In addition, theophylline and psychosocial risk factors may contribute to an increase in suicidal ideation, independent of depressive disorders (Favreau et al. 2012). There is a higher risk of anxiety with patients with COPD, and the anxiety may exert a negative impact on health outcomes (Eisner et al. 2010).

Depression

The evaluation of depression in a patient with respiratory illness poses challenges in that it is sometimes difficult to determine if the vegetative symptoms of depression (weight loss, fatigue, poor sleep, loss of interest in activities) are evidence of the psychiatric disorder or symptoms of the somatic disorder or both (Pachi et al. 2013). In patients with the pulmonary diseases discussed in this chapter, the prevalence of depression is higher than in the general population. The prevalence rate of depression has been reported as 23% in patients with COPD (Schneider et al. 2010), 22% in patients with cystic fibrosis

(Quon et al. 2015), 30% in asthmatics (Kumar et al. 2013), and 45% in patients with TB (Ige and Lasebikan 2011).

Sleep Disturbance

Sleep disturbance may be caused by sleep apnea, nocturnal cough, nocturnal asthma attacks, medication side effect, or restless legs syndrome, as well as by comorbid anxiety or depression (Lo Coco et al. 2009). More than 50% of patients with COPD have pronounced sleep complaints (George and Bayliff 2003). Many patients with COPD are found to have OSA, referred to as *overlap syndrome* (McNicholas et al. 2013). These patients have more severe sleep-related hypoxia and hypercapnea than if they had just one of the disorders. This syndrome also produces excessive daytime sleepiness, insomnia, and, very frequently, irritability and depressive symptoms (Baran and Richert 2003). Such patients may have significant difficulty with attention, psychomotor speed, and executive skills (Andreou et al. 2014).

Cognitive Deficits

Decreased pulmonary function contributes to decreased cognitive function (Emery et al. 2012). COPD is associated with an increased risk of cognitive impairment, cognitive decline, and dementia (Dodd 2015). Cognitive dysfunction occurs frequently in COPD patients, even those without chronic hypoxia or hypercapnea (Zheng et al. 2008). In a longitudinal cohort study, the cognitive performance of patients with severe COPD declined over a 6-year period (Hung et al. 2009). Oxygen therapy may help to minimize cognitive deficits in patients with mild hypoxia (Kozora et al. 1999). Other patients may have potentially reversible causes of cognitive deficits such as hypercapnea or exacerbation of coexisting cardiac disease. OSA is associated with cessation or reduction of airflow during sleep and thus can contribute to neurocognitive deficits (Lal et al. 2012).

Neuropsychiatric Side Effects of Drugs Used to Treat Respiratory Diseases

Medications used to treat respiratory illnesses often cause neuropsychiatric side effects. These drugs and side effects are discussed in detail in this section and are summarized in Table 7–2.

Table 7–2. Neuropsychiatric side effects of drugs used to treat respiratory diseases

Drug	Symptoms
Antibiotics	Minimal side effects: rare cases of psychosis, mania, delirium, or mental status changes
Anticholinergics	
Atropine	Paranoia; tactile, visual, and auditory hallucinations; memory loss; delirium; agitation
Antituburculars	
Cycloserine and isoniazid	Depression, hallucinations, psychosis
Ethambutol	Confusion; auditory and visual hallucinations (rare)
Rifampin	May reduce effectiveness of other medications
Bronchodilators	
β-Agonists	
Albuterol and levalbuterol	Anxiety, insomnia, paranoia, hallucinations, tremor, palpitations
Formoterol and arformoterol	Insomnia, anxiety, tremor, palpitations
Isoproterenol	Anxiety, insomnia, tremor
Metaproterenol	Anxiety, insomnia
Pirbuterol	Anxiety, tremor
Salmeterol	Anxiety, tremor, palpitations
Other Bronchodilators	
Theophylline and aminophylline	Anxiety, insomnia, tremor, restlessness, withdrawal, hyperactivity, psychosis, delirium, mutism
Corticosteroids	
Inhaled	Uncommon
Oral (e.g., prednisone, prednisolone, dexamethasone)	Depression, mania, lability, anxiety, insomnia, psychosis, hallucinations, paranoia, personality changes

Table 7–2.   Neuropsychiatric side effects of drugs used to treat respiratory diseases *(continued)*

Drug	Symptoms
Leukotriene inhibitors	
Montelukast, zafirlukast, and zileuton	Fatigue, asthenia, suicidal ideation
Mixed α- and β-agonists	
Epinephrine	Anxiety, tremor, psychosis
Phenylephrine	Depression, hallucinations, paranoia
Phenylpropanolamine	Restlessness, anxiety, insomnia, psychosis, hallucinations, aggressiveness

Source.   American Thoracic Society et al. 2003; Breen et al. 2006; Flume et al. 2007; Pachi et al. 2013; Polosa 2008; Thompson and Sullivan 2006.

Antibiotics

Antibiotics are used to treat infections associated with asthma, COPD, and cystic fibrosis. Although they usually have minimal side effects, there are case studies reporting psychosis, mania, delirium, or changes in behavior related to antibiotic treatment (Lally and Mannion 2013; Tomé and Filipe 2011). Psychiatric side effects of antibiotics are discussed in detail in Chapter 12, "Infectious Diseases."

Anticholinergics

Atropine, an anticholinergic that is used rarely for the treatment of asthma, can cause paranoia; visual, tactile, and auditory hallucinations; memory loss; delirium; and agitation. Inhaled tiotropium, also an anticholinergic, has a duration of action that is much longer than that of ipratropium bromide, which has not been reported to cause psychiatric side effects.

Antitubercular Drugs

Drugs such as isoniazid and cycloserine produce side effects such as depression, hallucinations, and psychosis (Carroll et al. 2012; Sharma et al. 2014).

There is a single case report of a drug-induced violent suicide (Behara et al. 2014). Rifampin, another antitubercular drug, may reduce the effectiveness of other medications by enhancing enzyme induction actions. Ethambutol can cause confusion, and there have been case reports of this drug causing auditory or visual hallucinations (Doherty et al. 2013; Testa et al. 2013).

Bronchodilators

The most common side effects of the β-adrenergic bronchodilators are nervousness and tremor. Albuterol can also cause insomnia. Mixed α- and β-agonists are often used in over-the-counter asthma medications. Epinephrine, ephedrine, phenylephrine, and phenylpropanolamine can cause anxiety, insomnia, tremor, and, in high doses, psychosis.

Aminophylline and Theophylline

Aminophylline is a less potent and shorter acting xanthine than theophylline. These drugs can produce dose-related side effects such as anxiety, insomnia, tremor, psychosis, delirium, and mutism. Theophylline has a narrow therapeutic window. Adverse effects can occur even at therapeutic serum levels. This is one of the reasons that the use of theophylline has decreased significantly. Toxicity is characterized by marked anxiety, severe nausea, and insomnia and may progress to psychosis and delirium. When there are signs of toxicity, theophylline should be stopped until the symptoms abate and the blood level returns to the therapeutic range. Theophylline may induce tremor or exacerbate essential tremor. There is an association with an increased risk of suicide attempts with adult asthmatics taking theophylline, which should be considered when this medication is being prescribed (Favreau et al. 2012).

Corticosteroids

It is uncommon to have side effects from inhaled steroids. Steroids such as prednisone, prednisolone, and dexamethasone can produce neuropsychiatric symptoms that are most likely linked to the dose of steroids: the higher the dose, the greater the likelihood of psychiatric symptoms. The side effects can include euphoria, irritability, anxiety, mania, psychosis, delirium, and mixed states. Cognitive deficits can also be noted (Dubovsky et al. 2012). Discontinuation of long-term glucocorticoid therapy is associated with increased risk of depression, delirium, and confusion (Fardet et al. 2013). Corticosteroid-induced psychiatric symptoms are reviewed in more detail in Chapter 10, "Endocrine and Metabolic Disorders."

Leukotriene Inhibitors

Montelukast, zafirlukast, and zileuton are leukotriene inhibitors, which can cause fatigue, dizziness, and suicidal ideation, as well as sleep disorders, behavioral disorders, and depression. The greatest adverse effects have been related to montelukast. However, there is no evidence of an increase in suicide (Schumock et al. 2011, 2012).

Alteration of Pharmacokinetics

For the most part, respiratory illnesses do not have an impact on pharmacokinetics, with two major exceptions: cystic fibrosis and smoking. Cystic fibrosis–related abnormalities in cellular ion transport may alter drug pharmacokinetics because of abnormalities in the ion transport function of the cell membrane. The rate of drug absorption is slowed, but the extent of absorption is generally unchanged, and bioavailability and volume of distribution are unaffected. Cystic fibrosis increases oxidative hepatic metabolism, but only for drug substrates of cytochrome P450 1A2 (CYP1A2) and CYP2C8; metabolism by other cytochromes is unchanged (Rey et al. 1998). There is little in the literature about the use of lithium in patients with cystic fibrosis, and what is there is contradictory. Brager et al. (1996) reported that renal clearance is reduced, resulting in higher lithium levels. However, in a case report by Turkel and Cafaro (1992), there was no alteration in the lithium level with standard dosages. It appears prudent for patients with cystic fibrosis to be started on a low dosage of lithium, with careful monitoring to avoid toxicity.

Smoking affects both the pharmacodynamics and the pharmacokinetics of many drugs. Smoking-induced bronchoconstriction is countertherapeutic, resulting in a poorer response to bronchodilators. In addition, the therapeutic response to corticosteroids is impaired in smokers with asthma compared with nonsmokers with asthma and in patients with COPD (Braganza et al. 2008). Smoking induces CYP1A2, which enhances the metabolism of drug substrates of this hepatic enzyme, including clozapine, olanzapine, duloxetine, and theophylline. Unless drug dosage is increased accordingly, lower, possibly subtherapeutic, drug levels will result. If the patient stops smoking, a week or more is required before CYP1A2 activity declines to normal (Kroon 2007). In this case, substrate drugs may require a dosage reduction to prevent toxicities.

Effects of Psychotropic Drugs on Pulmonary Function

Antidepressants

Because very few studies have examined the safety and efficacy of antidepressants in patients with pulmonary disease, their safety can only be inferred by the lack of published reports of drug-disease interactions. There have been individual case reports of eosinophilic pneumonia associated with various antidepressants, but this appears to be a very rare adverse event (Ben-Noun 2000; Salerno et al. 1995). The major concerns with monoamine oxidase inhibitors are drug-drug interactions, which are addressed later in the chapter in the section "Drug-Drug Interactions."

Anxiolytics and Sedative-Hypnotics

Respiratory depression resulting from sedative-hypnotics and opioids is the most common adverse respiratory effect associated with psychotropic medications. The respiratory depressant effects of benzodiazepines can significantly reduce the ventilatory response to hypoxia. This may precipitate respiratory failure in a patient with marginal respiratory reserve and contraindicates their use in patients with carbon dioxide retention. Reports are mixed regarding the safety of benzodiazepines in COPD, with studies raising significant concerns about the potential of benzodiazepines to decrease tidal volume, oxygen saturation, and minute ventilation and their potential to depress respiratory functions that participate in maintaining homeostasis of blood gases during sleep (Roth 2009). A prospective cohort study showed that in patients with COPD on long-term oxygen therapy, benzodiazepine use was associated with a 20% increase in mortality over patients who did not use benzodiazepines (Ekström et al. 2014). Benzodiazepines may also precipitate cough. Zolpidem did not impair respiratory drive or pulmonary function tests in patients with mild to moderate COPD (Girault et al. 1996). One small randomized controlled trial (RCT) showed ramelteon to be free of respiratory effects in patients with moderate to severe COPD (Kryger et al. 2009). Suvorexant had no adverse respiratory effects in patients with mild to moderate COPD (Sun et al. 2015).

Barbiturates for alcohol withdrawal, especially phenobarbital, should be avoided in patients with impaired respiratory drive, severe COPD, or OSA. Chronic treatment of epilepsy with phenobarbital may be an exception. Attention is required when combining sedating antidepressants and other sedating drugs such as anxiolytics and sedative-hypnotics in patients with severe COPD or OSA; the additive sedating effects may reduce respiratory drive.

In a small RCT in patients with mild COPD, buspirone was shown to improve exercise tolerance and the sensation of dyspnea (Argyropoulou et al. 1993). Buspirone was also reported to be well tolerated in combination with bronchodilators (Kiev and Domantay 1988). Despite these early encouraging studies, there have been no reports of the use of buspirone in respiratory diseases since then.

Antipsychotics

In a Canadian study, patients using atypical antipsychotics were found to have a significantly greater risk of death or near death from asthma (Joseph et al. 1996). Patients who had recently discontinued antipsychotic use were at a particularly high risk. Patients with asthma and COPD are particularly susceptible to cardiac arrhythmias (De Bruin et al. 2003). If antipsychotic medications are used, those most likely to cause QTc prolongation (ziprasidone, thioridazine) should be avoided, or the patients should be monitored. Abrupt discontinuation of antipsychotics with significant anticholinergic activity, such as clozapine, may cause cholinergic rebound, impairing the effectiveness of anticholinergic asthma medication (Szafrański and Gmurkowski 1999).

Acute pulmonary edema has been reported with phenothiazine overdose (Li and Gefter 1992). Several reports suggest that antipsychotics may be associated with increased risk for pulmonary embolism (Borras et al. 2008; Waage and Gedde-Dahl 2003). A recent meta-analysis revealed that exposure to both first- and second-generation antipsychotics was associated with a 50% increase in the risk of development of venous thromboembolism; antipsychotic exposure was not associated with a significantly increased rate of pulmonary embolus, but there was a wide confidence interval that included the possibility of substantial harm (Barbui et al. 2014). A subsequent large case-control study by the same authors found that current use of either typical or atypical anti-psychotics was associated with a twofold increased risk of pulmonary embolus compared with past use of antipsychotics and that patients who concurrently received prescriptions for both typical and atypical antipsychotics had a four-fold increased risk of pulmonary embolus (Conti et al. 2015).

Laryngeal dystonia, presenting as acute dyspnea, is a rare form of acute dys-tonic reaction. It is usually associated with high-potency typical antipsychotics but has also been reported with atypical antipsychotics (Ganesh et al. 2015; Goga et al. 2012). It generally occurs, like other dystonic reactions, within 24–48 hours after antipsychotic therapy is initiated or, in a small number of cases, when dosage is increased. The reaction can be life threatening but usu-ally responds dramatically to intramuscular injection of anticholinergic agents. Tardive laryngeal dystonia has also been very rarely reported (Matsuda et al. 2012). Tardive dyskinesia affecting the respiratory musculature is rare, generally occurs with long-term typical antipsychotic use, and can severely im-pede breathing in patients with reduced respiratory capacity (Jann and Bitar 1982; Kruk et al. 1995). Several cases of respiratory muscle dyskinesia were re-ported to occur when the antipsychotic was discontinued (e.g., Mendhekar and Inamdar 2010).

Weight gain caused by antipsychotics may further impair respiratory capac-ity in patients with decreased respiratory function, especially in restrictive lung disease. A U.S. Food and Drug Administration black box warning on antipsy-chotic medications cautions against their use in elderly patients with dementia because of increased risk for death secondary to cardiovascular complications and infection, particularly pneumonia. The latter may be due to aspiration of secretions secondary to sedation and dysphagia.

Mood Stabilizers

Carbamazepine may cause cough, dyspnea, pulmonary infiltrates, and idio-pathic pulmonary fibrosis.

Psychostimulants

Methylphenidate has been reported to cause dyspnea, asthma, pulmonary in-filtrates, respiratory failure from idiopathic pulmonary fibrosis, and pulmo-nary vascular disease (Ben-Noun 2000).

Cognitive Enhancers

There is scant literature on the use of cognitive enhancers in patients with respiratory illnesses. A number of pulmonary side effects have been reported with these drugs, frequently dyspnea and bronchitis and infrequently pneumonia, hyperventilation, pulmonary congestion, wheezing, hypoxia, pleurisy, pulmonary collapse, sleep apnea, and snoring.

Prescribing Psychotropic Medications in Respiratory Disease

Asthma

Antidepressants

The selective serotonin reuptake inhibitors (SSRIs) citalopram and escitalopram have been studied for the treatment of depression in patients with asthma in randomized, double-blind trials (Brown et al. 2005, 2012). Remission rates for depression were numerically higher, but not statistically significantly higher, in the active medication groups. Both SSRIs were well tolerated. Patients treated with citalopram had a significant decrease in corticosteroid use. Depressed asthmatic patients receiving open-label bupropion experienced improvement in depressive and asthmatic symptoms (Brown et al. 2007), as did depressed and nondepressed patients treated with sertraline (Smoller et al. 1998).

Sedative-Hypnotics

A recent study found that benzodiazepine or zopiclone use by asthmatic patients was significantly associated with the occurrence of asthma exacerbations and an increase in 2-year all-cause mortality (Nakafero et al. 2015). There are no studies of trazodone or mirtazapine for insomnia in patients with respiratory disorders. Two small studies report inconsistent effects of melatonin on pulmonary function in patients with asthma; in one study melatonin increased inflammation and decreased lung function (Sutherland et al. 2003), and in the other it produced no change in asthma symptoms while improving sleep (Campos et al. 2004).

Antipsychotics

Inhaled loxapine is contraindicated in patients with asthma (Teva 2013). In a study of inhaled loxapine in patients with asthma, 53% of subjects experienced symptomatic bronchospasm of mild or moderate severity. Eleven out of 15 of these respiratory events responded to rescue bronchodilator (albuterol) (Gross et al. 2014). There are no other published clinical trials of antipsychotics in patients with asthma.

Chronic Obstructive Pulmonary Disease

Antidepressants

The tricyclic antidepressant (TCA) nortriptyline was found to be safe and effective for depression and improved functional outcomes in COPD (Borson et al. 1992). There have been multiple other studies of SSRIs and TCAs in COPD patients with depression and anxiety, but these studies have been limited in utility because of methodological issues, and there is little clarity about the effectiveness of antidepressants in patients with COPD (Usmani et al. 2011; Yohannes and Alexopoulos 2014). The studies have not consistently shown improvements in respiratory symptoms or physiological measures of respiratory function in patients treated with antidepressants. No major safety issues have emerged from the existing studies.

Sedative-Hypnotics

Benzodiazepine use in patients with COPD requires caution. Although benzodiazepines are very often prescribed to patients with COPD (Vozoris et al. 2013), reports of their safety are mixed (Roth 2009). Adverse respiratory effects of benzodiazepines in COPD are more likely to occur in the elderly and in patients with more severe disease (Ekström et al. 2014; Vozoris et al. 2014). A population-based retrospective cohort study found that patients with COPD were at increased risk for outpatient COPD exacerbations or emergency department visits for COPD or pneumonia within the first 30 days after receiving a benzodiazepine prescription (Vozoris et al. 2014). This study and another study (Ekström et al. 2014) showed that rates of hospital admission were not increased in patients with COPD who were prescribed benzodiazepines. Benzodiazepine prescription has been associated with a modest increase in mortality in patients with severe COPD (Ekström et al. 2014).

In spite of these findings, benzodiazepines should not be rejected automatically for use in all patients with COPD. A few small studies found short-term use of low-dose benzodiazepines safe in patients with stable normocapnic COPD and no comorbid sleep apnea (Stege et al. 2010). Anxiety can reduce respiratory efficiency, and benzodiazepines may actually improve respiratory status in some patients, especially those with asthma or emphysema ("pink puffers") (Mitchell-Heggs et al. 1980).

In patients with stable COPD, zopiclone moderately increased the carbon dioxide pressure without reducing minimum oxygen saturation and improved sleep quality. In patients with combined features of COPD and OSA, zopiclone reduced apnea and hypopnea (Holmedahl et al. 2014). In patients with COPD, ramelteon and melatonin have been found to improve length of sleep and sleep quality with no worsening of pulmonary function (Halvani et al. 2013; Kryger et al. 2007; Nunes et al. 2008).

Mood Stabilizers

There is a theoretical concern that the inhibition of histone deacetylase by valproic acid could worsen pulmonary function in COPD patients. However, a recent study did not show an increase in hospital admissions or emergency department visits for COPD exacerbation or a change in the initiation of oral corticosteroids in patients commencing treatment with valproic acid versus phenytoin (Antoniou et al. 2015).

Antipsychotics

Inhaled loxapine is contraindicated in patients with COPD (Teva 2013). In a study of inhaled loxapine in patients with COPD, symptomatic bronchospasm of mild to moderate severity occurred in 19% of patients with COPD (Gross et al. 2014). There are no other published clinical trials of antipsychotics in patients with COPD.

Cognitive Enhancers

Because of their cholinomimetic effects, cholinesterase inhibitors increase acetylcholine levels and would be expected to cause bronchoconstriction. Also, they are likely to block the therapeutic effects of bronchodilators, especially anticholinergic agents such as ipratropium and tiotropium. However, a population-based cohort study did not show an increase in COPD-related emergency department visits or hospitalizations in new users of cholinesterase inhibitors versus dementia patients who were not prescribed these drugs (Stephenson et al. 2012). Caution is still advised in using cholinesterase inhibitors in patients with COPD; however, memantine does not have respiratory side effects.

Sleep Apnea

Antidepressants

Mirtazapine may be an effective treatment for OSA in stroke patients but may worsen central and mixed sleep apnea (Brunner 2008). One randomized crossover double-blind study of mirtazapine in patients with OSA found it to reduce the apnea-hypopnea index and reduce sleep fragmentation (Carley et al. 2007). However, in this study and two follow-up studies with negative OSA outcomes, there were high dropout rates due to increased daytime lethargy and weight gain (Marshall et al. 2008). Mirtazapine should therefore be avoided in patients with OSA. In small RCTs, paroxetine and protriptyline (one of two studies) improved apnea-hypopnea index scores relative to placebo, with multiple other antidepressants yielding negative results (Smith et al. 2006). Trazodone was studied as a hypnotic agent at a dose of 100 mg in patients with OSA. It was found that trazodone increased the respiratory arousal threshold (a favorable outcome in OSA patients) but did not alter the apnea-hypopnea index (Eckert et al. 2014).

Sedative-Hypnotics

In patients with sleep apnea, the melatonin agonist ramelteon improved length of sleep with no worsening of their pulmonary function (Kryger et al. 2007). Zolpidem, on an acute basis, has been shown in patients with severe OSA to promote sleep without disturbing the efficiency of continuous positive airway pressure (CPAP) therapy (Berry and Patel 2006). A double-blind, placebo-controlled study of zaleplon use during CPAP titration in patients with OSA found an improvement in sleep latency without adverse effects on apnea-hypopnea index or oxygenation (Park et al. 2013). An open-label study of zolpidem in patients with idiopathic central sleep apnea showed an overall improvement in apnea or hypopnea and sleep efficiency. In this study there were large individual differences in the response to zolpidem, with some patients having an overall increase in apnea or hypopnea events with fewer central events and more obstructive apnea or hypopneas (Quadri et al. 2009). In patients with mild to moderate sleep apnea, zopiclone has been found to improve sleep while not worsening breathing (Rosenberg et al. 2007).

In contrast, benzodiazepine-induced respiratory suppression occurs when patients with OSA are awake as well as asleep, potentially prolonging sleep apneic episodes with dangerous consequences. Benzodiazepines have muscle relaxant properties, which can cause worsening of upper airway collapsibility in patients with OSA. Buspirone may improve the respiratory status of patients with sleep apnea (Mendelson et al. 1991).

Antipsychotics

Weight gain with olanzapine, quetiapine, and other atypical antipsychotics is particularly problematic in patients with OSA; the additional weight will worsen the sleep apnea. A recent pilot study was designed to identify confounding factors that may explain the association between atypical antipsychotic usage and OSA. It was found that atypical antipsychotic use was associated with increased rates of OSA diagnosis in depressed patients but not in those who had other psychiatric diagnoses. The severity of OSA was not found to be associated with antipsychotic use (Shirani et al. 2011).

Stimulants

Chronic respiratory illnesses often lead to insomnia and daytime sleepiness. The few studies of stimulants have been in sleep apnea. Modafinil (and also armodafinil, the R-enantiomer of modafinil) was found to increase daytime wakefulness when used as an adjunctive treatment for patients with OSA who were benefiting from CPAP but who still experienced daytime sleepiness. Behavioral alertness and functional impairment also improved, and sleep architecture remained intact (Hirshkowitz et al. 2007). Armodafinil was found to improve driving performance and subjective sleepiness in patients with OSA who were not receiving CPAP treatment (Chapman et al. 2014; Kay and Feldman 2013). Atomoxetine improved wakefulness in patients with mild to moderate OSA without worsening the respiratory distress index (Bart Sangal et al. 2008). In spite of these encouraging findings, psychostimulants should be used with caution in this population given the limited breadth of this literature and the increased risk for cardiac arrhythmia in chronic respiratory disease.

Cognitive Enhancers

Two small randomized, double-blind, placebo-controlled studies found that donepezil improved sleep apnea, increased rapid eye movement sleep, and improved cognition in patients with Alzheimer's disease (Moraes et al. 2006, 2008).

Cystic Fibrosis

Scant literature exists regarding the use of psychotropic medications in patients with cystic fibrosis. In theory, the anticholinergic effects of TCAs could exacerbate the difficulty that patients with cystic fibrosis have with clearing their secretions. However, there is interest in use of amitriptyline as a therapeutic agent for cystic fibrosis, and several studies demonstrate that amitriptyline is safe and well tolerated (Nährlich et al. 2013; Riethmüller et al. 2009). In a single case study of lithium treatment for bipolar mania in a patient with cystic fibrosis, mood improved with no apparent impact on pulmonary function (Turkel and Cafaro 1992).

Vocal Cord Dysfunction

Benzodiazepines can be used to terminate a severe episode of VCD (Hicks et al. 2008). If a benzodiazepine is prescribed, reduced doses of a shorter-acting benzodiazepine (e.g., lorazepam) should be used so that adverse effects are mild and rapidly reversible with drug discontinuation.

Dyspnea in Advanced and Terminal Disease

A number of pharmacological agents, including opioids, have been tried in patients with advanced pulmonary disease whose dyspnea could not be managed by treating the underlying disease. A meta-analysis of 18 small studies in COPD showed a statistically significant positive effect of opioids on the sensation of dyspnea, especially when the agents were administered orally or parenterally rather than nebulized (Jennings et al. 2002). There was no evidence to suggest a deleterious effect on arterial blood gases or oxygen saturation. The use of low-dose oral or parenteral opioids to treat dyspnea associated with end-stage pulmonary disease has been confirmed in other studies (Abernethy et al. 2003; Lorenz et al. 2008). A retrospective chart survey found that sedatives, hypnotics, and morphine were frequently used in patients with terminal malignant and nonmalignant pulmonary disease (Kanemoto et al. 2007). Although these drugs were useful and effective, the authors emphasized the need to weigh comfort against the potential shortening of life due to respiratory depression. Opioids (usually morphine) are also used in terminal weaning from ventilatory support (Campbell 2007). Benzodiazepines are considered second- or third-line interventions for relief of dyspnea in terminal weaning of ventilator support (Simon et al. 2010).

Drug-Drug Interactions

A number of pharmacokinetic and pharmacodynamic drug interactions may occur between drugs prescribed for chronic respiratory disease and psychotropic drugs (Table 7–3).

It is important to note that smoking, a cause or contributor to multiple respiratory illnesses, can enhance the metabolism of multiple psychotropic drugs via induction of CYP1A2, CYP2B6, and CYP2D6 (Kroon 2007). This includes benzodiazepines; zolpidem; antipsychotics (notable exceptions are aripiprazole, quetiapine, risperidone, and ziprasidone); and antidepressants, including fluvoxamine, duloxetine, TCAs, and mirtazapine. Reduction or cessation of smoking may necessitate reduction in dosage of psychotropic medications whose metabolism has been induced.

Many anti-infective agents, including macrolide and fluoroquinolone antibacterials and conazole antifungals, are potent inhibitors of one or more CYP isozymes, whereas several rifamycins such as rifampin induce multiple CYP enzymes. Anti-infective drugs can cause significant psychotropic drug toxicities or loss of therapeutic effect unless the psychotropic drug dose is suitably adjusted.

Although there is no evidence that isoniazid causes serotonin syndrome when combined with serotonergic antidepressants, dietary tyramine restriction should be used when isoniazid is combined with an antidepressant (DiMartini 1995). In patients taking isoniazid, sympathomimetics such as epinephrine, ephedrine, and pseudoephedrine, especially common in many over-the-counter cold, cough, and sinus preparations, should be avoided (Dawson et al. 1995). Inhaled β-agonists appear to be safe to use because little is absorbed systemically. SSRI and serotonin-norepinephrine reuptake inhibitor antidepressants are safe to use with the selective β_2-agonists (e.g., terbutaline, metaproterenol, albuterol, isoetharine).

Theophylline can lower alprazolam and possibly other benzodiazepine levels (Tuncok et al. 1994) and may counteract the therapeutic effects of benzodiazepines by exacerbating anxiety and insomnia. Theophylline may also increase lithium clearance (Cook et al. 1985; Holstad et al. 1988; Perry et al. 1984); lithium levels should be monitored when these drugs are coadministered.

Several psychotropic medications, including TCAs, low-potency typical antipsychotics, and anticholinergic agents for extrapyramidal symptoms, have

Table 7–3. Respiratory drug–psychotropic drug interactions

Drug	Mechanism of interaction	Clinical effect
Anticholinergics		
Atropine (systemic)	Additive anticholinergic effect	Additive anticholinergic effects with TCAs, antipsychotics, and other anticholinergic agents. Countertherapeutic effects with cholinesterase inhibitor cognitive enhancers.
β-Agonists		
Albuterol	QT prolongation	Increased QT interval: avoid QT-prolonging drugs (TCAs, antipsychotics [pimozide, quetiapine, risperidone, ziprasidone]).
Bronchodilators		
Theophylline	Increased renal clearance	Increased clearance and lower levels of renally eliminated drugs (lithium, gabapentin, pregabalin, paliperidone, memantine, desvenlafaxine).
Leukotriene inhibitors		
Zafirlukast	Moderate inhibitor of CYP2C9, CYP2C8, CYP3A4	Possible increased levels of carbamazepine, phenytoin, benzodiazepines, pimozide, quetiapine, ziprasidone.

Source. Wynn et al. 2009.

anticholinergic effects that may enhance the bronchodilator effects of atropine and inhaled anticholinergic bronchodilators such as ipratropium and tiotropium.

Respiratory disease drugs are also susceptible to pharmacokinetic interactions from psychotropic drugs. Fluvoxamine inhibits CYP1A2 and can significantly increase theophylline levels (Dawson et al. 1995). Carbamazepine and phenobarbital, both general metabolic inducers, significantly reduce blood levels of many drugs, including theophylline and doxycycline. St. John's wort is also a CYP1A2 inducer and can lower theophylline levels to subtherapeutic values (Hu et al. 2005).

Key Clinical Points

- Most antidepressants have little or no effect on respiratory status; however, anticholinergic antidepressants may have functional and bronchodilating benefits.
- Generally, avoid sedating agents in CO_2 retainers. If necessary, short-acting benzodiazepines with no active metabolites, prescribed at low dose, are best tolerated.
- Polypharmacy contributes to unwanted drug-drug interactions and increases risk for respiratory side effects.
- Drugs known to cause QTc prolongation should be avoided in patients with asthma and COPD. If these drugs are used, cardiac status should be carefully monitored.
- Smoking induces CYP1A2, CYP2B6, and CYP2D6, thereby lowering the levels of many psychotropic medications. When smoking is reduced or stopped, psychotropic side effects and blood levels should be monitored and doses adjusted as necessary.
- Rifampin induces metabolism of some psychiatric drugs. Higher dosages of these psychiatric medications may be required for adequate response in patients treated for tuberculosis.
- Isoniazid is a weak irreversible monoamine oxidase inhibitor that may cause serotonin syndrome or hypertensive crisis when combined with SSRIs and sympathomimetic psychotropics and agents used to treat pulmonary diseases.

- Theophylline has multiple activating psychiatric side effects. Its levels can be reduced by CYP1A2 inducers such as carbamazepine and increased by CYP1A2 inhibitors such as fluvoxamine.
- The side effects of steroids can include euphoria, irritability, depression, mania, psychosis, and mixed states. It is important to remember that discontinuation after long-term therapy can be associated with increased risk of depression, delirium, and confusion.

References

Abernethy AP, Currow DC, Frith P, et al: Randomised, double blind, placebo controlled crossover trial of sustained release morphine for the management of refractory dyspnoea. BMJ 327(7414):523–528, 2003 12958109

American Thoracic Society; CDC; Infectious Diseases Society of America: Treatment of tuberculosis. MMWR Recomm Rep 52:1–77, 2003 12836625

Andreou G, Vlachos F, Makanikas K: Effects of chronic obstructive pulmonary disease and obstructive sleep apnea on cognitive functions: evidence for a common nature. Sleep Disord 2014:768210, 2014 24649370

Antoniou T, Yao Z, Camacho X, et al: Safety of valproic acid in patients with chronic obstructive pulmonary disease: a population-based cohort study. Pharmacoepidemiol Drug Saf 24(3):256–261, 2015 25656984

Argyropoulou P, Patakas D, Koukou A, et al: Buspirone effect on breathlessness and exercise performance in patients with chronic obstructive pulmonary disease. Respiration 60(4):216–220, 1993 8265878

Atlantis E, Fahey P, Cochrane B, Smith S: Bidirectional associations between clinically relevant depression or anxiety and COPD: a systematic review and meta-analysis. Chest 144(3):766–777, 2013 23429910

Baran AS, Richert AC: Obstructive sleep apnea and depression. CNS Spectr 8(2):128–134, 2003 12612498

Barbui C, Conti V, Cipriani A: Antipsychotic drug exposure and risk of venous thromboembolism: a systematic review and meta-analysis of observational studies. Drug Saf 37(2):79–90, 2014 24403009

Bart Sangal R, Sangal JM, Thorp K: Atomoxetine improves sleepiness and global severity of illness but not the respiratory disturbance index in mild to moderate obstructive sleep apnea with sleepiness. Sleep Med 9(5):506–510, 2008 17900980

Behara C, Krishna K, Singh H: Antitubercular drug-induced violent suicide of a hospitalized patient. BMJ Case Rep Jan 6 doi: 10.1136/bcr-2013-201469, 2014 24395874

Ben-Noun L: Drug-induced respiratory disorders: incidence, prevention and management. Drug Saf 23(2):143–164, 2000 10945376

Berry RB, Patel PB: Effect of zolpidem on the efficacy of continuous positive airway pressure as treatment for obstructive sleep apnea. Sleep 29(8):1052–1056, 2006 16944674

Borras L, Eytan A, de Timary P, et al: Pulmonary thromboembolism associated with olanzapine and risperidone. J Emerg Med 35(2):159–161, 2008 18281175

Borson S, McDonald GJ, Gayle T, et al: Improvement in mood, physical symptoms, and function with nortriptyline for depression in patients with chronic obstructive pulmonary disease. Psychosomatics 33(2):190–201, 1992 1557484

Braganza G, Chaudhuri R, Thomson NC: Treating patients with respiratory disease who smoke. Ther Adv Respir Dis 2(2):95–107, 2008 19124362

Brager NP, Campbell NR, Reisch H, et al: Reduced renal fractional excretion of lithium in cystic fibrosis. Br J Clin Pharmacol 41(2):157–159, 1996 8838443

Breen RA, Miller RF, Gorsuch T, et al: Adverse events and treatment interruption in tuberculosis patients with and without HIV co-infection. Thorax 61(9):791–794, 2006 16844730

Brown ES, Vigil L, Khan DA, et al: A randomized trial of citalopram versus placebo in outpatients with asthma and major depressive disorder: a proof of concept study. Biol Psychiatry 58(11):865–870, 2005 15993860

Brown ES, Vornik LA, Khan DA, Rush AJ: Bupropion in the treatment of outpatients with asthma and major depressive disorder. Int J Psychiatry Med 37(1):23–28, 2007 17645195

Brown ES, Howard C, Khan DA, Carmody TJ: Escitalopram for severe asthma and major depressive disorder: a randomized, double-blind, placebo-controlled proof-of-concept study. Psychosomatics 53(1):75–80, 2012 22221724

Brunner H: Success and failure of mirtazapine as alternative treatment in elderly stroke patients with sleep apnea—a preliminary open trial. Sleep Breath 12(3):281–285, 2008 18369672

Campbell ML: How to withdraw mechanical ventilation: a systematic review of the literature. AACN Adv Crit Care 18(4):397–403, quiz 344–345, 2007 17978613

Campos FL, da Silva-Júnior FP, de Bruin VM, de Bruin PF: Melatonin improves sleep in asthma: a randomized, double-blind, placebo-controlled study. Am J Respir Crit Care Med 170(9):947–951, 2004 15306531

Carley DW, Olopade C, Ruigt GS, Radulovacki M: Efficacy of mirtazapine in obstructive sleep apnea syndrome. Sleep 30(1):35–41, 2007 17310863

Carroll MW, Lee M, Cai Y, et al: Frequency of adverse reactions to first- and second-line anti-tuberculosis chemotherapy in a Korean cohort. Int J Tuberc Lung Dis 16(7):961–966, 2012 22584241

Chapman JL, Kempler L, Chang CL, et al: Modafinil improves daytime sleepiness in patients with mild to moderate obstructive sleep apnoea not using standard treatments: a randomised placebo-controlled crossover trial. Thorax 69(3):274–279, 2014 24287166

Conti V, Venegoni M, Cocci A, et al: Antipsychotic drug exposure and risk of pulmonary embolism: a population-based, nested case-control study. BMC Psychiatry 15:92, 2015 25924683

Cook BL, Smith RE, Perry PJ, Calloway RA: Theophylline-lithium interaction. J Clin Psychiatry 46(7):278–279, 1985 4008452

Cooper CL, Parry GD, Saul C, et al: Anxiety and panic fear in adults with asthma: prevalence in primary care. BMC Fam Pract 8:62–68, 2007 17963505

Dawson JK, Earnshaw SM, Graham CS: Dangerous monoamine oxidase inhibitor interactions are still occurring in the 1990s. J Accid Emerg Med 12(1):49–51, 1995 7640830

De Bruin ML, Hoes AW, Leufkens HG: QTc-prolonging drugs and hospitalizations for cardiac arrhythmias. Am J Cardiol 91(1):59–62, 2003 12505572

DiMartini A: Isoniazid, tricyclics and the "cheese reaction". Int Clin Psychopharmacol 10(3):197–198, 1995 8675973

Dodd JW: Lung disease as a determinant of cognitive decline and dementia. Alzheimers Res Ther 7(1):32, 2015 25798202

Doherty AM, Kelly J, McDonald C, et al: A review of the interplay between tuberculosis and mental health. Gen Hosp Psychiatry 35(4):398–406, 2013 23660587

Dubovsky AN, Arvikar S, Stern TA, Axelrod L: The neuropsychiatric complications of glucocorticoid use: steroid psychosis revisited. Psychosomatics 53(2):103–115, 2012 22424158

Eckert DJ, Malhotra A, Wellman A, White DP: Trazodone increases the respiratory arousal threshold in patients with obstructive sleep apnea and a low arousal threshold. Sleep 37(4):811–819, 2014 24899767

Eisner MD, Blanc PD, Yelin EH, et al: Influence of anxiety on health outcomes in COPD. Thorax 65(3):229–234, 2010 20335292

Ekström MP, Bornefalk-Hermansson A, Abernethy AP, Currow DC: Safety of benzodiazepines and opioids in very severe respiratory disease: national prospective study. BMJ 348:g445, 2014 24482539

Emery CF, Finkel D, Pedersen NL: Pulmonary function as a cause of cognitive aging. Psychol Sci 23(9):1024–1032, 2012 22864997

Fardet L, Nazareth I, Whitaker HJ, Petersen I: Severe neuropsychiatric outcomes following discontinuation of long-term glucocorticoid therapy: a cohort study. J Clin Psychiatry 74(4):e281–e286, 2013 23656853

Favreau H, Bacon SL, Joseph M, et al: Association between asthma medications and suicidal ideation in adult asthmatics. Respir Med 106(7):933–941, 2012 22495109

Flume PA, O'Sullivan BP, Robinson KA, et al; Cystic Fibrosis Foundation, Pulmonary Therapies Committee: Cystic fibrosis pulmonary guidelines: chronic medications for maintenance of lung health. Am J Respir Crit Care Med 176(10):957–969, 2007 17761616

Ganesh M, Jabbar U, Iskander FH: Acute laryngeal dystonia with novel antipsychotics: a case report and review of literature. J Clin Psychopharmacol 35(5):613–615, 2015 26252439

George CF, Bayliff CD: Management of insomnia in patients with chronic obstructive pulmonary disease. Drugs 63(4):379–387, 2003 12558460

Girault C, Muir JF, Mihaltan F, et al: Effects of repeated administration of zolpidem on sleep, diurnal and nocturnal respiratory function, vigilance, and physical performance in patients with COPD. Chest 110(5):1203–1211, 1996 8915222

Goga JK, Seidel L, Walters JK, et al: Acute laryngeal dystonia associated with aripiprazole. J Clin Psychopharmacol 32(6):837–839, 2012 23131892

Gross N, Greos LS, Meltzer EO, et al: Safety and tolerability of inhaled loxapine in subjects with asthma and chronic obstructive pulmonary disease—two randomized controlled trials. J Aerosol Med Pulm Drug Deliv 27(6):478–487, 2014 24745666

Halvani A, Mohsenpour F, Nasiriani K: Evaluation of exogenous melatonin administration in improvement of sleep quality in patients with chronic obstructive pulmonary disease. Tanaffos 12(2):9–15, 2013 25191456

Hicks M, Brugman SM, Katial R: Vocal cord dysfunction/paradoxical vocal fold motion. Prim Care 35(1):81–103, vii, 2008 18206719

Hirshkowitz M, Black JE, Wesnes K, et al: Adjunct armodafinil improves wakefulness and memory in obstructive sleep apnea/hypopnea syndrome. Respir Med 101(3):616–627, 2007 16908126

Holmedahl NH, Øverland B, Fondenes O, et al: Zopiclone effects on breathing at sleep in stable chronic obstructive pulmonary disease. Sleep Breath 19(3):921–230, 2014 25501294

Holstad SG, Perry PJ, Kathol RG, et al: The effects of intravenous theophylline infusion versus intravenous sodium bicarbonate infusion on lithium clearance in normal subjects. Psychiatry Res 25(2):203–211, 1988 2845461

Hu Z, Yang X, Ho PC, et al: Herb-drug interactions: a literature review. Drugs 65(9):1239–1282, 2005 15916450

Hung WW, Wisnivesky JP, Siu AL, Ross JS: Cognitive decline among patients with chronic obstructive pulmonary disease. Am J Respir Crit Care Med 180(2):134–137, 2009 19423714

Ige OM, Lasebikan VO: Prevalence of depression in tuberculosis patients in comparison with non-tuberculosis family contacts visiting the DOTS clinic in a Nigerian tertiary care hospital and its correlation with disease pattern. Ment Health Fam Med 8(4):235–241, 2011 23205064

Jain A, Lolak S: Psychiatric aspects of chronic lung disease. Curr Psychiatry Rep 11(3):219–225, 2009 19470284

Jann MW, Bitar AH: Respiratory dyskinesia. Psychosomatics 23(7):764–765, 1982 6126912

Jennings AL, Davies AN, Higgins JP, et al: A systematic review of the use of opioids in the management of dyspnoea. Thorax 57(11):939–944, 2002 12403875

Joseph KS, Blais L, Ernst P, Suissa S: Increased morbidity and mortality related to asthma among asthmatic patients who use major tranquillisers. BMJ 312(7023):79–82, 1996 8555932

Kanemoto K, Satoh H, Kagohashi K, et al: Psychotropic drugs for terminally ill patients with respiratory disease. Tuberk Toraks 55(1):5–10, 2007 17401788

Kay GG, Feldman N: Effects of armodafinil on simulated driving and self-report measures in obstructive sleep apnea patients prior to treatment with continuous positive airway pressure. J Clin Sleep Med 9(5):445–454, 2013 23674935

Kiev A, Domantay AG: A study of buspirone coprescribed with bronchodilators in 82 anxious ambulatory patients. J Asthma 25(5):281–284, 1988 3053607

Kozora E, Filley CM, Julian LJ, Cullum CM: Cognitive functioning in patients with chronic obstructive pulmonary disease and mild hypoxemia compared with patients with mild Alzheimer disease and normal controls. Neuropsychiatry Neuropsychol Behav Neurol 12(3):178–183, 1999 10456802

Kroon LA: Drug interactions with smoking. Am J Health Syst Pharm 64(18):1917–1921, 2007 17823102

Kruk J, Sachdev P, Singh S: Neuroleptic-induced respiratory dyskinesia. J Neuropsychiatry Clin Neurosci 7(2):223–229, 1995 7626967

Kryger M, Wang-Weigand S, Roth T: Safety of ramelteon in individuals with mild to moderate obstructive sleep apnea. Sleep Breath 11(3):159–164, 2007 17294232

Kryger M, Roth T, Wang-Weigand S, Zhang J: The effects of ramelteon on respiration during sleep in subjects with moderate to severe chronic obstructive pulmonary disease. Sleep Breath 13(1):79–84, 2009 18584227

Kumar P, Misra S, Kundu S, et al: Prevalence of depression among asthma patients and effects of asthma control on severity of depression. World Allergy Organ J 6 (suppl 1):23, 2013

Lal C, Strange C, Bachman D: Neurocognitive impairment in obstructive sleep apnea. Chest 141(6):1601–1610, 2012 22670023

Lally L, Mannion L: The potential for antimicrobials to adversely affect mental state. BMJ Case Rep 2013(July):5, 2013 23833088

Li C, Gefter WB: Acute pulmonary edema induced by overdosage of phenothiazines. Chest 101(1):102–104, 1992 1729053

Lieberman JA III: History of the use of antidepressants in primary care. Prim Care Companion J Clin Psychiatry 5 (suppl 7):6–10, 2003

Lima OM, Oliveira-Souza Rd, Santos Oda R, et al: Subclinical encephalopathy in chronic obstructive pulmonary disease. Arq Neuropsiquiatr 65(4B):1154–1157, 2007 18345421

Liu S, Wu R, Li L, et al: The prevalence of anxiety and depression in Chinese asthma patients. PLoS One 9(7):e103014, 2014 25054657

Lo Coco D, Mattaliano A, Lo Coco A, Randisi B: Increased frequency of restless legs syndrome in chronic obstructive pulmonary disease patients. Sleep Med 10(5):572–576, 2009 18996743

Lorenz KA, Lynn J, Dy SM, et al: Evidence for improving palliative care at the end of life: a systematic review. Ann Intern Med 148(2):147–159, 2008 18195339

Marshall NS, Yee BJ, Desai AV, et al: Two randomized placebo-controlled trials to evaluate the efficacy and tolerability of mirtazapine for the treatment of obstructive sleep apnea. Sleep 31(6):824–831, 2008 18548827

Matsuda N, Hashimoto N, Kusumi I, et al: Tardive laryngeal dystonia associated with aripiprazole monotherapy. J Clin Psychopharmacol 32(2):297–298, 2012 22388164

McNicholas WT, Verbraecken J, Marin JM: Sleep disorders in COPD: the forgotten dimension. Eur Respir Rev 22(129):365–375, 2013 23997063

Mehta TA, Sutherland JG, Hodgkinson DW: Hyperventilation: cause or effect? J Accid Emerg Med 17(5):376–377, 2000 11005417

Mendelson WB, Maczaj M, Holt J: Buspirone administration to sleep apnea patients. J Clin Psychopharmacol 11(1):71–72, 1991 2040719

Mendhekar DN, Inamdar A: Withdrawal-emergent respiratory dyskinesia with risperidone treated with clozapine. J Neuropsychiatry Clin Neurosci 22(2):E24, 2010 20463136

Mitchell-Heggs P, Murphy K, Minty K, et al: Diazepam in the treatment of dyspnoea in the 'Pink Puffer' syndrome. Q J Med 49(193):9–20, 1980 6776586

Moraes W dos S, Poyares DR, Guilleminault C, et al: The effect of donepezil on sleep and REM sleep EEG in patients with Alzheimer disease: a double-blind placebo-controlled study. Sleep 29(2):199–205, 2006 16494088

Moraes W dos, Poyares D, Sukys-Claudino L, et al: Donepezil improves obstructive sleep apnea in Alzheimer disease: a double-blind, placebo-controlled study. Chest 133(3):677–683, 2008 18198262

Nährlich L, Mainz JG, Adams C, et al: Therapy of CF-patients with amitriptyline and placebo—a randomised, double-blind, placebo-controlled Phase IIb multicenter, cohort-study. Cell Physiol Biochem 31(4–5):505–512, 2013 23572075

Nakafero G, Sanders RD, Nguyen-Van-Tam JS, Myles PR: Association between benzodiazepine use and exacerbations and mortality in patients with asthma: a matched case-control and survival analysis using the United Kingdom Clinical Practice Research Datalink. Pharmacoepidemiol Drug Saf 24(8):793–802, 2015 26013409

Nunes DM, Mota RM, Machado MO, et al: Effect of melatonin administration on subjective sleep quality in chronic obstructive pulmonary disease. Braz J Med Biol Res 41(10):926–931, 2008 19030713

Pachi A, Bratis D, Moussas G, Tselebis A: Psychiatric morbidity and other factors affecting treatment adherence in pulmonary tuberculosis patients. Tuberc Res Treat 2013:489865, 2013 23691305

Park JG, Olson EJ, Morgenthaler TI: Impact of zaleplon on continuous positive airway pressure therapy compliance. J Clin Sleep Med 9(5):439–444, 2013 23674934

Perry PJ, Calloway RA, Cook BL, Smith RE: Theophylline precipitated alterations of lithium clearance. Acta Psychiatr Scand 69(6):528–537, 1984 6741601

Polosa R: An overview of chronic severe asthma. Intern Med J 38(3):190–198, 2008 18028366

Quadri S, Drake C, Hudgel DW: Improvement of idiopathic central sleep apnea with zolpidem. J Clin Sleep Med 5(2):122–129, 2009 19968044

Quon BS, Bentham WD, Unutzer J, et al: Prevalence of symptoms of depression and anxiety in adults with cystic fibrosis based on the PHQ-9 and GAD-7 screening questionnaires. Psychosomatics 56(4):345–353, 2015 25556569

Rey E, Tréluyer JM, Pons G: Drug disposition in cystic fibrosis. Clin Pharmacokinet 35(4):313–329, 1998 9812180

Riethmüller J, Anthonysamy J, Serra E, et al: Therapeutic efficacy and safety of amitriptyline in patients with cystic fibrosis. Cell Physiol Biochem 24(1-2):65–72, 2009 19590194

Rosenberg R, Roach JM, Scharf M, Amato DA: A pilot study evaluating acute use of eszopiclone in patients with mild to moderate obstructive sleep apnea syndrome. Sleep Med 8(5):464–470, 2007 17512799

Roth T: Hypnotic use for insomnia management in chronic obstructive pulmonary disease. Sleep Med 10(1):19–25, 2009 18693067

Roy-Byrne PP, Davidson KW, Kessler RC, et al: Anxiety disorders and comorbid medical illness. Gen Hosp Psychiatry 30(3):208–225, 2008 18433653

Salerno SM, Strong JS, Roth BJ, Sakata V: Eosinophilic pneumonia and respiratory failure associated with a trazodone overdose. Am J Respir Crit Care Med 152(6 Pt 1):2170–2172, 1995 8520792

Schneider C, Jick SS, Bothner U, Meier CR: COPD and the risk of depression. Chest 137(2):341–347, 2010 19801582

Schumock GT, Lee TA, Joo MJ, et al: Association between leukotriene-modifying agents and suicide: what is the evidence? Drug Saf 34(7):533–544, 2011 21663330

Schumock GT, Stayner LT, Valuck RJ, et al: Risk of suicide attempt in asthmatic children and young adults prescribed leukotriene-modifying agents: a nested case-control study. J Allergy Clin Immunol 130(2):368–375, 2012 22698520

Scott KM, Von Korff M, Ormel J, et al: Mental disorders among adults with asthma: results from the World Mental Health Survey. Gen Hosp Psychiatry 29(2):123–133, 2007 17336661

Sharma B, Handa R, Nagpal K, et al: Cycloserine-induced psychosis in a young female with drug-resistant tuberculosis. Gen Hosp Psychiatry 36(4):451.e3–451.e4, 2014 24766906

Shirani A, Paradiso S, Dyken ME: The impact of atypical antipsychotic use on obstructive sleep apnea: a pilot study and literature review. Sleep Med 12(6):591–597, 2011 21645873

Simon ST, Higginson IJ, Booth S, et al: Benzodiazepines for the relief of breathlessness in advanced malignant and non-malignant diseases in adults. Cochrane Database of Systematic Reviews 2010, Issue 1. Art. No.: CD007354. DOI: 10.1002/14651858.CD007354.pub2 20091630

Smith I, Lasserson TJ, Wright J: Drug therapy for obstructive sleep apnoea in adults. Cochrane Database of Systematic Reviews 2006, Issue 2. Art. No.: CD003002. DOI: 10.1002/14651858.CD003002.pub3 21645873

Smoller JW, Pollack MH, Systrom D, Kradin RL: Sertraline effects on dyspnea in patients with obstructive airways disease. Psychosomatics 39(1):24–29, 1998 9538672

Stege G, Heijdra YF, van den Elshout FJ, et al: Temazepam 10mg does not affect breathing and gas exchange in patients with severe normocapnic COPD. Respir Med 104(4):518–524, 2010 19910177

Stephenson A, Seitz DP, Fischer HD, et al: Cholinesterase inhibitors and adverse pulmonary events in older people with chronic obstructive pulmonary disease and concomitant dementia: a population-based, cohort study. Drugs Aging 29(3):213–223, 2012 22332932

Sun H, Palcza J, Rosenberg R, et al: Effects of suvorexant, an orexin receptor antagonist, on breathing during sleep in patients with chronic obstructive pulmonary disease. Respir Med 109(3):416–426, 2015 25661282

Sutherland ER, Ellison MC, Kraft M, Martin RJ: Elevated serum melatonin is associated with the nocturnal worsening of asthma. J Allergy Clin Immunol 112(3):513–517, 2003 13679809

Szafrański T, Gmurkowski K: Clozapine withdrawal. A review [in Polish]. Psychiatr Pol 33(1):51–67, 1999 10786215

Testa A, Giannuzzi R, Sollazzo F, et al: Psychiatric emergencies (part II): psychiatric disorders coexisting with organic diseases. Eur Rev Med Pharmacol Sci 17 (suppl 1):65–85, 2013 23436669

Teva: Adasuve [package insert]. Horsham, PA, Teva Pharmaceuticals USA, December 2013

Thompson WL, Sullivan SP: Pulmonary disease, in Psychosomatic Medicine. Edited by Blumenfield M, Strain JJ. Philadelphia, PA, Lippincott, Williams & Wilkins, 2006, pp 193–212

Tomé AM, Filipe A: Quinolones: review of psychiatric and neurological adverse reactions. Drug Saf 34(6):465–488, 2011 21585220

Tuncok Y, Akpinar O, Guven H, Akkoclu A: The effects of theophylline on serum alprazolam levels. Int J Clin Pharmacol Ther 32(12):642–645, 1994 7881701

Turkel SB, Cafaro DR: Lithium treatment of a bipolar patient with cystic fibrosis. Am J Psychiatry 149(4):574, 1992 1554052

Usmani ZA, Carson KV, Cheng JN, et al: Pharmacological interventions for the treatment of anxiety disorders in chronic obstructive pulmonary disease. Cochrane Database of Systematic Reviews 2011, Issue 11. Art. No.: CD008483. DOI: 10.1002/14651858.CD008483.pub2 22071851

Vozoris NT, Fischer HD, Wang X, et al: Benzodiazepine use among older adults with chronic obstructive pulmonary disease: a population-based cohort study. Drugs Aging 30(3):183–192, 2013 23371396

Vozoris NT, Fischer HD, Wang X, et al: Benzodiazepine drug use and adverse respiratory outcomes among older adults with COPD. Eur Respir J 44(2):332–340, 2014 24743966

Waage IM, Gedde-Dahl A: Pulmonary embolism possibly associated with olanzapine treatment. BMJ 327(7428):1384, 2003 14670884

Wynn G, Oesterheld JR, Cozza KL, Armstrong SC: Clinical Manual of Drug Interaction: Principles for Medical Practice. Washington, DC, American Psychiatric Publishing, 2009

Yohannes AM, Alexopoulos GS: Pharmacological treatment of depression in older patients with chronic obstructive pulmonary disease: impact on the course of the disease and health outcomes. Drugs Aging 31(7):483–492, 2014 24902934

Zheng GQ, Wang Y, Wang XT: Chronic hypoxia-hypercapnia influences cognitive function: a possible new model of cognitive dysfunction in chronic obstructive pulmonary disease. Med Hypotheses 71(1):111–113, 2008 18331781

8

Oncology

Philip A. Bialer, M.D.

Stephen J. Ferrando, M.D.

Shirley Qiong Yan, Pharm.D., BCOP

Psychiatric symptoms are common in many cancer patients, especially in those with advanced cancer. Several factors, including the emotional stress of the cancer diagnosis, the effects of central nervous system (CNS) tumors, neurotoxicity from immune reactions to non-CNS tumors, and the adverse effects of cancer chemotherapy or radiotherapy, may contribute to psychiatric comorbidity. In most situations, psychiatric symptoms can be safely managed with psychotropics; however psychotropic agents must be carefully selected to avoid adverse interactions with chemotherapeutic agents, including interactions that potentially limit the therapeutic efficacy of chemotherapy. In this chapter we review psychiatric symptoms related to cancer and cancer treatment, psychopharmacological treatment of psychiatric comorbidity, and interactions between psychiatric and oncological drugs.

Differential Diagnosis of Psychiatric Manifestations of Cancers

Cancer-Related Depression and Fatigue

Emotional distress accompanies the diagnosis of cancer and adversely affects the patient's quality of life. Surveys suggest that about 50% of patients with advanced cancer have symptoms that meet criteria for a psychiatric disorder, most commonly adjustment disorder (11%–35%), major depression (5%–26%), and anxiety disorders (6%–10%) (Traeger et al. 2012). Pancreatic, oropharnyngeal, and breast cancers are often associated with symptoms of depression (Carvalho et al. 2014; Chen et al. 2013). The diagnosis of cancer may also exacerbate preexisting psychiatric disorders. Depression and fatigue are frequent adverse effects of cancer chemotherapy and radiation therapy (discussed in the section "Neuropsychiatric Adverse Effects of Oncology Treatments").

Differentiating transient adjustment-related depression and anxiety warranting at most short-term pharmacotherapy (e.g., benzodiazepines) from major depression or generalized anxiety disorder requiring ongoing pharmacotherapy can be challenging. Further, differentiating neurovegetative symptoms of depression and anxiety such as anorexia or fatigue from those produced by cancer or its treatment is often difficult. Addressing potential underlying causes of fatigue such as anemia and close monitoring of these symptoms during pharmacotherapy is warranted. On the one hand, these symptoms may be ameliorated with pharmacotherapy; however, if residual neurovegetative symptoms persist, adjunctive treatment should be initiated.

Psychiatric Symptoms of Brain Tumors

Brain tumors typically cause generalized or focal neurological symptoms and signs. However, some tumors, especially in neurologically silent areas, may give rise only to psychiatric symptoms such as depression, anxiety disorders, mania, psychosis, personality changes, anorexia, or cognitive dysfunction. Although there have been attempts in the past to categorize psychiatric symptoms according to tumor location or histological type, a review indicated a lack of specific association (Madhusoodanan et al. 2007). Brain imaging should be considered for patients presenting with atypical psychiatric symptoms, onset of psychiatric symptoms after age 40, or a change in the clinical presentation of existing psychiatric symptoms (Gupta and Kumar 2004; Hollister and Boutros 1991; Moise and Madhusoodanan 2006). (See also Chapter 9, "Central Nervous System Disorders").

Paraneoplastic Limbic Encephalitis

Paraneoplastic limbic encephalitis (PLE) is a consequence of CNS damage from antineuronal antibodies expressed as an immune response to a non–nervous system cancer. Symptoms include rapidly progressive confusion and short-term memory deficits, depression, visual and auditory hallucinations, delusions, paranoia, and seizures (Voltz 2007). PLE occurs most often in small-cell lung cancer (40%) and seminoma (20%) but also in lymphoma and tumors of the breast and thymus (Gultekin et al. 2000). In most cases of PLE, neuropsychiatric symptoms precede cancer diagnosis, often by several years. PLE is identified by characteristic findings on magnetic resonance imaging, with supporting evidence from electroencephalogram and cerebrospinal fluid antibody studies. Symptoms have limited response to psychopharmacotherapy (Foster and Caplan 2009). Although antipsychotics and anticonvulsants have been tried, treatment is focused on eradication of the tumor and on immunosuppressant therapy.

Psychopharmacological Treatment of Psychiatric Disorders in Cancer Patients

The research literature on psychopharmacological treatment of psychiatric disorders in cancer is relatively sparse and is focused primarily on depression and somatic symptoms, including pain, nausea, and fatigue (for general clinical reviews of major psychotropic drug classes in cancer, see Berney et al. 2000; Buclin et al. 2001; Caruso et al. 2013; Mazzocato et al. 2000; and Stiefel et al. 1999). Psychopharmacological treatment of pain and nausea is covered in Chapter 17, "Pain Management," and Chapter 4, "Gastrointestinal Disorders," respectively. Psychopharmacological treatment of depression, anxiety, cancer-related fatigue (CRF), and cognitive impairment is covered in the following subsections.

Depression

Depression has a prevalence ranging from 10.8% to 24% in cancer patients (Ng et al. 2011) and a prevalence of 13.7% among cancer survivors (Zhao et al. 2014). Multiple case series and case reports suggest effectiveness of tricyclic antidepressants (TCAs) and selective serotonin reuptake inhibitors (SSRIs) in a range of cancers; however, a relatively small number of randomized controlled trials (RCTs) have been conducted. Generally, RCTs have included predominantly women with breast and gynecological malignancies, many have been relatively brief in duration (5–6 weeks), and several studies have been underpowered to detect drug-drug or drug-placebo differences. Of note, a large multicenter study that randomly assigned cancer patients with depression either to a manualized program of collaborative depression care or to usual care by their oncologists found a significantly (and substantially) higher response rate in the depression care group (Sharpe et al. 2014; Walker et al. 2014).

Cyclic Antidepressants

Mianserin (a tetracyclic antideprssant) up to 60 mg/day in depressed women with breast cancer has been reported by two groups to be superior to placebo in improving both depression and quality of life (Costa et al. 1985; van Heeringen and Zivkov 1996). Mianserin was well tolerated, and dropouts were greater in placebo-treated patients because of lack of response. In a clinical sample, patients with gynecological malignancies and depression who were adherent to imipramine treatment (minimum 150 mg/day for 4 weeks) had significantly decreased depressive symptoms when compared with patients who did not adhere to the treatment (Evans et al. 1988).

Selective Serotonin Reuptake Inhibitors

A 5-week RCT of fluoxetine ($n=45$) versus placebo ($n=46$) for depression in cancer patients did not find a difference in the primary depression endpoint on the Montgomery-Åsberg Depression Rating Scale (MADRS); however, fluoxetine yielded greater reduction in general distress as measured by the Symptom Checklist–90 (SCL-90; Razavi et al. 1996). In a 6-week multisite RCT comparing fluoxetine (20–40 mg/day, $n=21$) and desipramine (25–100 mg/day, $n=17$) in depressed women with breast, colorectal, and gynecological malignancies, both treatments yielded significant improvements in depression, anxiety, and quality of life endpoints (Holland et al. 1998). However, 29% of patients treated with fluoxetine and 41% of patients treated with desipramine withdrew because of adverse events. The results of both of these studies were hampered by their brief duration. In two large RCTs of treatment for depressive and/or fatigue symptoms in women with breast cancer who were actively undergoing chemotherapy, paroxetine 20 mg/day initiated just after starting chemotherapy and discontinued a week after ending chemotherapy was more effective than placebo in reducing depressive symptoms but not fatigue (Morrow et al. 2003; Roscoe et al. 2005). A small multicenter RCT comparing paroxetine (n=13) with desipramine (n=11) and placebo (n=11) showed no group differences, likely a result of high placebo response and lack of statistical power (Musselman et al. 2006).

Fluoxetine was superior to placebo in an oncologist-driven RCT for the treatment of nonmajor depression and diminished quality of life in advanced cancer patients (3–24 months estimated survival) (Fisch et al. 2003); however, this effect was accounted for by improvement in the patients with the most severe depression at baseline. Nausea and vomiting were also more common in the fluoxetine group. In another oncologist-driven RCT comparing sertraline 50 mg/day with placebo for the amelioration of mild depression, anxiety, and other quality-of-life symptoms, sertraline showed no benefit over placebo and was associated with higher dropout (Stockler et al. 2007). This study was stopped because of higher mortality in the sertraline group at the first interim analysis on a subset of the patients; however, survival did not differ between the treatment groups when all enrolled patients were analyzed with a longer duration of follow-up.

Other Antidepressants

In a 6-week unblinded randomized trial in advanced cancer patients with multiple somatic and psychiatric symptoms, mirtazapine (7.5–30 mg/day), but not imipramine (5–100 mg/day) or a no-medication control, was found to reduce depression and anxiety as measured by the Hospital Anxiety and Depression Scale (HADS) as well as insomnia (Cankurtaran et al. 2008). Similarly, in a group of depressed patients with lung, breast, and gastrointestinal cancers suffering from nausea or vomiting and sleep disturbance, open-label treatment with mirtazapine (orally dissolving, 15–45 mg/day) was associated with improvement in depressive and somatic symptoms and quality of life within 7 days (Kim et al. 2008). Excessive sleepiness occurred in 36% of patients early in treatment but generally abated within 2 weeks. Mirtazapine has also been found to be useful for the treatment of cancer-related cachexia and anorexia (Riechelmann et al. 2010). Bupropion sustained release (100–300 mg/day) was effective in an open-label trial for depressive symptoms in cancer patients in which fatigue was the primary endpoint (Moss et al. 2006).

Psychostimulants

Methylphenidate and dextroamphetamine have also been found to be effective in case series and small open-label trials of depression in patients with advanced cancer, with onset of action generally within 2–5 days (Homsi et al. 2001; Olin and Masand 1996; Sood et al. 2006). Methylphenidate and modafinil have been found to improve depression in RCTs in which CRF was the primary endpoint (Kaleita et al. 2006; Kerr et al. 2012; Meyers et al. 1998).

Cholinesterase Inhibitors

In a small clinical trial with irradiated brain tumor patients, donepezil demonstrated limited improvements in acute fatigue, depression, and cognitive impairment (Shaw et al. 2006).

Melatonin

One RCT showed that melatonin may reduce the risk of breast cancer patients developing depression (Hansen et al. 2014).

Conclusion

The limited clinical trial literature generally supports the use of standard antidepressants for the treatment of moderate to severe depression in cancer patients. However, it should be kept in mind that those currently receiving chemotherapy and/or who have widespread disease are likely to be sensitive to adverse effects such as nausea. In patients with advanced malignancies and limited life expectancies, a psychostimulant should be considered because of rapid onset of response and benefit for accompanying symptoms such as fatigue and cognitive impairment.

Anxiety

Anxiety is also prevalent in cancer patients and is often comorbid with depression, in which case antidepressant treatment is effective in alleviating anxiety symptoms (see previous subsection, "Depression"). SSRI and serotonin-norepinephrine reuptake inhibitor (SNRI) antidepressants are the long-term treatment of choice for anxiety disorders such as generalized anxiety disorder or panic disorder. There are no studies of antidepressants among cancer patients in which anxiety is the primary endpoint. Atypical antipsychotics such as olanzapine and quetiapine have also been used to treat anxiety symptoms in the clinical setting but have not been systematically studied.

Benzodiazepines are often used clinically to treat acute anxiety-related symptoms and nausea. Alprazolam (0.5–3.4 mg/day) *and* placebo were found to decrease anxiety symptoms within 1 week in 36 patients with mixed cancers enrolled in an RCT (Wald et al. 1993). Similarly, in a 10-day multicenter RCT that included 147 inpatients and outpatients with mixed cancers, alprazolam 0.5 mg three times daily and progressive muscle relaxation were found to reduce anxiety symptoms (Holland et al. 1998). Alprazolam produced greater and more rapid symptom relief on some but not all outcome measures. In both studies the structure and attention received by the patients was thought to be instrumental in alleviating symptoms.

In clinical practice, clinicians often use lorazepam in cancer patients because of its favorable pharmacokinetics, multiple routes of administration, and putative efficacy for treating nausea and other distressing symptoms (Buzdar et al. 1994). Clonazepam is also employed because of its longer half-life. In utilizing benzodiazepines in cancer patients, excessive sedation, cognitive impairment, rebound/withdrawal, and other adverse effects should be monitored closely (Costantini et al. 2011; Stiefel et al. 1999).

When benzodiazepines are used to treat anxiety, patients with a history of previous substance or alcohol misuse must be monitored carefully. Caution is also advised for patients who may be receiving multiple sedating medications, in particular patients who may be receiving narcotics to treat pain. An alternative approach may be the use of gabapentin, which was shown to be effective in addressing anxiety in a cohort of breast cancer survivors (Lavigne et al. 2012).

Cancer-Related Fatigue

CRF affects a majority of cancer patients at some point during the course of illness. The most common disease-related correlates are active chemotherapy and anemia. Fatigue is often comorbid with anxiety and depression; however, it also occurs alone and can be a residual symptom even if the anxiety and depression are treated effectively. Anemia-related fatigue is ameliorated by treatment with erythropoietin or darbepoetin (see Mücke et al. 2015 for a review).

Psychostimulants and modafinil are the most commonly prescribed psychotropic agents for CRF. Methylphenidate 10–50 mg daily in divided doses has been studied in RCTs in patients with advanced cancer (Escalante et al. 2014; Moraska et al. 2010), palliative care patients (Bruera et al. 2013), and patients with prostate cancer (Roth et al. 2010). In palliative care patients, fatigue improved after 1 week in both methylphenidate and placebo groups, the latter attributed to the powerful effects of research nurse support. Effects were sustained up to 36 weeks during open-label methylphenidate treatment. There was a significant decrease in the prostate study. The benefits of methylphenidate in the other studies were mixed, although improvement in cognition and more severe fatigue was noted. Modafinil has been studied in four open-label trials of CRF, including breast cancer, cerebral tumor, and lung cancer patients, and in one RCT involving patients with mixed cancers receiving chemotherapy (Cooper et al. 2009; Spathis et al. 2014). In the controlled trial with 642 patients receiving concurrent chemotherapy, modafinil 200 mg/day was more efficacious than placebo in treating fatigue and excessive daytime sleepiness but not depressive symptoms (Spathis et al. 2014). Patients with the highest levels of fatigue at the beginning of their second cycle of chemotherapy benefited most. Adverse effects reported in these trials included headache, nausea, and activation symptoms such as insomnia and anxiety.

Armodafinil has been studied in two recent RCTs and did not demonstrate any significant improvement in fatigue compared with placebo (Berenson et al. 2015; Page et al. 2015). Although the patients with more baseline fatigue in the study by Page et al. did experience improved quality of life and reduced fatigue, the results of the study by Berenson et al. suggested a strong placebo effect.

Two RCTs of paroxetine (Morrow et al. 2003; Roscoe et al. 2005) (see earlier subsection "Depression") and one of donepezil (Bruera et al. 2007) failed to show superiority of these agents over placebo in the treatment of CRF. Paroxetine improved depression but not fatigue.

Although potential etiological factors for CRF (e.g., anemia, depression) should be addressed whenever possible, methylphenidate and modafinil appear to be effective treatments for CRF. Because many patients have residual symptoms of fatigue, which diminishes their quality of life, adjunctive treatment should not be unduly delayed. Excessive activation and anorexia are not a major clinical concern at usual therapeutic doses, but these potential adverse effects should be monitored.

Cognitive Impairment

Although cognitive dysfunction is documented in brain tumor and postadjuvant chemotherapy breast cancer patients, pharmacological treatment data are relatively lacking. For patients with brain tumors who are undergoing radiation therapy, donepezil 5–10 mg daily was modestly beneficial for cognitive dysfunction (Shaw et al. 2006). Although one open-label study indicated benefit of methylphenidate for brain tumor patients undergoing radiation (Meyers et al. 1998), two small RCTs, one in a similar population (Butler et al. 2007) and one in breast cancer patients undergoing chemotherapy (Mar Fan et al. 2008), yielded negative results.

Adverse Oncological Effects of Psychotropics

Antipsychotics

Evaluation of cancer risk with antipsychotic medications is confounded by the association in patients with schizophrenia of several risk factors for cancer, including alcohol abuse, obesity, smoking, and inactive lifestyle. Antipsychotic-induced hyperprolactinemia is also considered a risk factor for pituitary, breast, and endometrial cancers (see also Chapter 10, "Endocrine and Metabolic Disorders").

There have been a number of epidemiological studies reporting both increased and decreased rates of cancer in patients taking (mostly typical) antipsychotics (Dalton et al. 2006; Hippisley-Cox et al. 2007; Mortensen 1987, 1992; Wang et al. 2002). No findings have been clearly replicated.

Because of the relatively recent introduction of atypical antipsychotics, there are few studies exploring the cancer risk. Risperidone, and possibly its major metabolite paliperidone, may be associated with pituitary tumors. A retrospective pharmacovigilance study employed the FDA Adverse Event Reporting System database through March 2005 to assess the association of pituitary tumors with atypical antipsychotics. Risperidone was associated with pituitary tumors at 18.7 times the expected rate (Szarfman et al. 2006). A survey of the World Health Organization's Adverse Drug Reaction database supports this relationship between risperidone and pituitary neoplasms (Doraiswamy et al. 2007). However, a more recent retrospective review of more than 400,000 records found no increased risk for pituitary tumors with mass effect among patients taking risperidone compared with other atypical antipsychotics (McCarren et al. 2012).

One review and meta-analysis indicated that there may be a relationship between antipsychotic-induced hyperprolactinemia and breast cancer risk, but the risk is much lower than for other factors such as nulliparity, obesity, diabetes mellitus, and unhealthy lifestyle factors (De Hert et al. 2016).

Reluctance to prescribe antipsychotics because of fear of increasing cancer risk is not supported by available studies, with the possible exception of increased risk for pituitary tumors with risperidone. Animal studies suggest a relationship between pituitary tumor growth and hyperprolactinemia secondary to dopamine D_2 receptor antagonism (Szarfman et al. 2006). It would seem prudent to avoid antipsychotics with a high incidence of hyperprolactinemia (risperidone, paliperidone, ziprasidone, haloperidol, and aripiprazole) in patients with present or past history of pituitary endocrine tumors. Evidence that antipsychotics may reduce cancer risk is inconclusive.

Anxiolytics

Studies support the lack of cancer risk with benzodiazepine use for several cancers, including non-Hodgkin's lymphoma; Hodgkin's disease; malignant melanoma; and breast, large bowel, lung, endometrial, ovarian, testicular, thyroid, and liver cancer (Halapy et al. 2006; Rosenberg et al. 1995). Although a more recent population-based retrospective cohort study suggested an overall increased risk of developing cancer among individuals using benzodiazepines (Kao et al. 2012), the results may be misleading because of a lack of theoretical rationale and the presence of many confounding factors (Kao et al. 2012; Selaman et al. 2012).

Mood Stabilizers

Lithium salts frequently cause leukocytosis, which raised a concern that lithium may act as an inducer or reinducer of acute and chronic monocytic leukemia (Swierenga et al. 1987). However, no association of lithium and leukemia was observed in two retrospective studies of leukemia patients (Lyskowski and Nasrallah 1981; Resek and Olivieri 1983). A third retrospective study observed a significant inverse trend for nonepithelial cancers with lithium dose (Cohen et al. 1998). This report suggested that psychiatric patients have lower cancer prevalence than the general population and that lithium may have a protective effect. More recent retrospective studies of the risk of long-term lithium use on the development of renal cell and other upper urinary tract tumors have produced mixed findings, with one study showing an increased risk and the other showing no significant association (Pottegård et al. 2016; Zaidan et al. 2014). Other RCTs have shown that lithium may be protective and/or may actually enhance the chemotherapeutic treatment of non–small cell lung cancer, hormone-independent prostate cancer, and pancreatic ductal adenocarcinoma (Hossein et al. 2012; Lan et al. 2013; Peng et al. 2013). Valproate, similar to other short-chain fatty acids, has been known to have anticancer effects on a variety of malignant cells in vitro. Several clinical trials have confirmed the efficacy of valproate in acute myeloid leukemia and myelodysplastic syndromes (Kuendgen and Gattermann 2007). There are no human studies of carbamazepine carcinogenicity.

Antidepressants

The relationship between antidepressant use and cancer risk has been suggested, but early epidemiological studies yielded inconsistent results. Serotonin-enhancing antidepressants elevate prolactin levels, and hyperprolactinemia has been associated with increased risk of postmenopausal breast cancer. Large population-based case-control surveys and a meta-analysis reported no association between the risk of breast cancer and the use of antidepressants overall, by antidepressant class, or by individual agent (Cosgrove et al. 2011; Wernli et al. 2009). Similar methodologies have been used to examine the risk of ovarian, prostate, lung, and colorectal cancer with SSRIs and TCAs. No evidence of increased risk of ovarian cancer was observed with antidepressants in general or with SSRIs (Moorman et al. 2005). SSRI use did not increase the risk of prostate cancer (Tamim et al. 2008) and was associated with a decreased risk of lung cancer (Toh et al. 2007). Although one study found a decreased risk of colorectal cancer among SSRI users, more recent case-control studies disputed this finding (Coogan et al. 2009; Cronin-Fenton et al. 2011; Xu et al. 2006). A marginally elevated risk of lung and prostate cancer, possibly due to experimental bias, was observed among TCA users.

Conclusion

Studies to date do not support withholding any psychiatric medications on the basis of fear of increasing cancer risk, nor can any conclusions be drawn regarding their potential for reducing cancer risk.

Neuropsychiatric Adverse Effects of Oncology Treatments

Radiotherapy

Fatigue is the most common neuropsychological acute reaction to brain radiation, often occurring within several weeks of initiating therapy and generally lasting 1–3 months. Delayed reactions, including decreased energy, depression, and cognitive dysfunction, occur months or years postradiotherapy and are generally irreversible.

Methylphenidate use in brain tumor patients receiving radiation therapy did not demonstrate any improvement in fatigue or cognition (Butler et al. 2007). However, modafinil (Kaleita et al. 2006), donepezil (Shaw et al. 2006), and memantine (Day et al. 2014) have demonstrated limited improvements in acute fatigue, depression, and cognitive impairment in small clinical trials with irradiated brain tumor patients.

Chemotherapy

Delirium

Delirium is common in cancer, with many possible causes, including adverse effects of chemotherapy, infection, brain metastases, and terminal delirium. Delirium occurs frequently with chemotherapeutic agents associated with CNS toxicity and those able to cross the blood-brain barrier, including 5-fluorouracil, ifosfamide, asparaginase, chlorambucil, cytarabine, methotrexate, interferons, interleukins, vincristine, and vinblastine (Fann and Sullivan 2003). Corticosteroids (see also Chapter 10 for full discussion), antihistamines, and opioids are a few supportive medications also potentially contributing to an acute confusional state (Agar and Lawlor 2008). Medication-related delirium often responds to dosage reduction or a change of drug. The incidence of delirium and other psychiatric symptoms may be exacerbated by the interaction of tumor-related factors and treatment-induced neurotoxicity. There are no RCTs of psychotropic drugs for cancer-related delirium (Breitbart 2011) (see Breitbart 2014 for a summary of RCTs in medically ill patients). Treatment of delirium is discussed more fully in Chapter 15, "Surgery and Critical Care."

Cognitive Impairment

Chemotherapy-induced cognitive dysfunction, sometimes referred to as "chemo brain," has been identified in patients with breast, colorectal, and testicular cancers (Joly et al. 2015). Inflammatory cytokines have been implicated in the pathogenesis of the cognitive dysfunction, and the demarcation between the cancer and the therapies is not always clear.

Chemotherapeutic Agents

Psychiatric adverse effects of oncology drugs are summarized in Table 8–1 and discussed below.

Ifosfamide.   Ifosfamide encephalopathy, characterized by seizures, drowsiness, confusion, and hallucinations, occurs in 15%–30% of patients and is often dose limiting. Predisposing factors for ifosfamide-induced encephalopathy include previous cisplatin exposure, and concomitant use of opioids and cytochrome P450 2B6 (CYP2B6) inhibitors, as well as low serum albumin, increased serum creatinine, and increased hemoglobin (Szabatura et al. 2015). Case reports suggest a lack of efficacy of psychoactive agents for ifosfamide-induced neurotoxicity and delirium. Symptoms usually resolve after drug withdrawal and treatment with oral or intravenous methylene blue (Dufour et al. 2006). Although methylene blue is widely used to treat ifosfamide delirium, its efficacy has not been confirmed in controlled clinical trials, and many patients experience positive outcomes without methylene blue (Alici-Evcimen and Breitbart 2007; Brunello et al. 2007).

Nonclassic alkylating agents.   Neuropsychiatric adverse events have been reported with procarbazine and altretamine. Several case reports identify psychosis as a side effect of procarbazine chemotherapy (Carney et al. 1982; van Eys et al. 1987). Other psychiatric adverse effects, including hallucinations, anxiety, depression, confusion, and nightmares, are also associated with procarbazine use (Sigma-Tau Pharmaceuticals 2014). Altretamine was associated with fatigue (63%) and anxiety or depression (29%) of mild to moderate severity during a 6-month Phase 2 trial (Rothenberg et al. 2001).

Biological response modifiers.   The immunomodulatory agents interferon-alpha (IFN-α) and interleukin-2 (IL-2) are often associated with psychiatric adverse effects, including apathy, fatigue, cognitive impairment, depression

Table 8–1. Psychiatric adverse effects of oncology drugs

Medication	Psychiatric adverse effects
Alkylating agents	
Nitrogen mustards	
Ifosfamide	Seizures, drowsiness, confusion, hallucinations
Nonclassic alkylators	
Altretamine	Fatigue, anxiety, depression
Procarbazine	Psychosis, hallucinations, anxiety, depression, confusion, nightmares (Sigma-Tau Pharmaceuticals 2014)
Antimetabolites	
Pyrimidine analogs	
Cytarabine (cytosine arabinoside)	Confusion, somnolence, personality changes (high dose) (Baker et al. 1991; Pfizer Canada 2011)
Interferon/Interleukins	
Interferon-α-2a	Apathy, fatigue, depression, suicidal behaviors, agitation, mania, psychoses
Interferon-α-2b	Apathy, fatigue, depression, suicidal behaviors, confusion, mania
Interleukin-2 (aldesleukin)	Apathy, fatigue, confusion, sedation, anxiety, psychosis
Retinoic acid compounds	
Tretinoin (ATRA)	Anxiety, insomnia, depression, confusion, agitation, hallucinations
Enzymes	
Pegasparaginase	Somnolence, fatigue, coma, seizures, confusion, agitation, hallucinations (Baxalta 2016)

Table 8–1.   Psychiatric adverse effects of oncology
drugs *(continued)*

Medication	Psychiatric adverse effects
Monoclonal antibodies	
Bortezomib	35% incidence of psychiatric disorders: agitation, confusion, mental status change, psychotic disorder, suicidal ideation (Millennium Pharmaceuticals 2009)

Note.   ATRA = all-trans retinoic acid.

with suicidal ideation, and psychosis. Preexisting psychiatric illness increases vulnerability to psychiatric adverse effects. (See Chapter 4 for a more thorough discussion of psychiatric symptoms associated with IFN-α.)

IL-2 been found to be elevated in patients with major depressive disorder (Liu et al. 2012; Udina et al. 2014b), and therapy with this agent has been reported to cause severe depressive symptoms in >20% of cancer patients (Capuron et al. 2000). Neuropsychiatric symptoms may lead to treatment discontinuation.

IFN-α-induced depression in cancer patients is responsive to antidepressant treatment in controlled trials with paroxetine (Capuron et al. 2002; Musselman et al. 2001), but symptoms of fatigue and anorexia are less responsive to SSRI treatment (Capuron et al. 2002). Use of an adjunctive antidepressant was associated with better adherence to IFN-α therapy (Musselman et al. 2001). Other neurobehavioral side effects of IFN-α, such as anxiety and cognitive dysfunction, have also been found to respond to treatment with paroxetine (McNutt et al. 2012; Udina et al. 2014a).

Retinoic acid compounds.   Retinoic acid compounds, commonly used to treat acne (isotretinoin), are also employed systemically for acute promyelocytic leukemia (tretinoin, all-trans retinoic acid) and brain and pancreatic cancer (isotretinoin). Tretinoin frequently causes psychiatric symptoms, including anxiety (17%), insomnia (14%), depression (14%), confusion (11%), agitation (9%), and hallucinations (6%). Several studies also suggest an association between isotretinoin use and depression, suicide, and psychosis. See Chapter 13, "Dermatological Disorders," for additional discussion of isotretinoin and depression and suicide.

Hormone therapy.   Tamoxifen has been reported to impair verbal memory in several clinical trials (Jenkins et al. 2004; Schilder et al. 2009). Despite early concerns, a large placebo-controlled retrospective cohort study of women with breast cancer concluded that tamoxifen administration does not increase the risk for developing depression (Lee et al. 2007). These results support the conclusion of an earlier multicenter placebo-controlled chemoprevention trial that tamoxifen does not increase risk for or exacerbate existing depression in women (Day et al. 2001). The effect of the aromatase inhibitor anastrozole on memory is unclear, with studies showing either greater impairment than with tamoxifen (Bender et al. 2007) or little or no impairment (Jenkins et al. 2008).

Vinca alkaloids.   Posterior reversible encephalopathy syndrome has been reported in patients receiving vinflunine (Helissey et al. 2012) and vinorelbine (Chen and Huang 2012).

Drug-Drug Interactions

Drug-drug interactions are common in cancer therapy because of multiple medications, including cytotoxic chemotherapeutic agents, hormonal agents, and adjunctive medications for supportive care, as well as patients' preexisting medical problems. Because most cancer patients are elderly (Yancik 2005), the drug burden from other medical conditions can be considerable.

A number of complex pharmacokinetic and pharmacodynamic interactions can occur between chemotherapy and psychotropic medications. Pharmacokinetic interactions due to chemotherapy occur at several levels: inhibition of metabolic enzymes (CYP enzymes, monoamine oxidase), reduction of metabolism and excretion due to cytotoxic effects on hepatic and renal function, and altered distribution (hypoalbuminemia) and absorption (increased P-glycoprotein [P-gp] activity) (see Tables 8–2 and 8–3). Many cancer agents are prodrugs (i.e., compounds that require metabolic activation for clinical effect), and many of these utilize CYP enzymes for their activation (see Table 8–4). Drug-drug interactions from adjunctive medications, including psychotropic medications, can enhance or impair the metabolic activation of these prodrugs and affect their therapeutic benefit and adverse effects. Although clinicians should be vigilant about screening for any potential drug interactions, many of these interactions are theoretical in nature, and because oncological drug

Table 8–2. Oncology drug–psychotropic drug interactions

Medication	Interaction mechanism	Effects on psychotropic drugs and management
Alemtuzumab, arsenic trioxide, cetuximab, daunorubicin, denileukin, etoposide, homoharringtonine, idarubicin, mitoxantrone, nilotinib, rituximab, tamoxifen, and tretinoin (systemic)	QT prolongation	Increased QT prolongation in combination with other QT-prolonging drugs such as TCAs, citalopram, typical antipsychotics, pimozide, risperidone, paliperidone, iloperidone, quetiapine, ziprasidone, and lithium.
Asparaginase	Hypoalbuminemia	Therapeutic drug monitoring of total (free+bound) drug may give misleading results. Use methods selective for free drug levels (see Chapter 2).
Cisplatin	Nephrotoxicity	Reduced elimination of renally eliminated drugs (e.g., lithium, paliperidone, desvenlafaxine, gabapentin, pregabalin, memantine). Monitor lithium levels.
	Unknown	Decreased levels of carbamazepine, phenytoin, valproate.
Carboplatin, ifosfamide, and methotrexate	Nephrotoxicity—acute and chronic reduction in GFR	Reduced elimination of renally eliminated drugs (e.g., lithium, paliperidone, desvenlafaxine, gabapentin, pregabalin, memantine). Monitor lithium levels.

Table 8–2.   Oncology drug–psychotropic drug interactions *(continued)*

Medication	Interaction mechanism	Effects on psychotropic drugs and management
Dasatinib	Inhibits CYP3A4	Increased levels and toxicities for pimozide, quetiapine, ziprasidone, iloperidone, desvenlafaxine, oxidatively metabolized benzodiazepines, fentanyl, methadone, meperidine, tramadol.
5-Fluorouracil and capecitabine	Reduced synthesis of CYP2C9	Reduced phenytoin metabolism with increased toxicity.
Imatinib	Inhibits CYP2C9, CYP2D6, CYP3A4	Increased levels and toxicities for phenytoin, pimozide, quetiapine, risperidone, ziprasidone, iloperidone, TCAs, bupropion, paroxetine, venlafaxine, fentanyl, meperidine, tramadol, atomoxetine, and benzodiazepines except oxazepam, lorazepam, and temazepam (see Chapter 2 for expanded listing).
Interleukin-2 (aldesleukin)	QT prolongation	Increased QT prolongation in combination with other QT-prolonging drugs such as TCAs, citalopram, typical antipsychotics, pimozide, risperidone, paliperidone, iloperidone, quetiapine, ziprasidone, and lithium.
	Nephrotoxicity and reduced renal function	Reduced elimination of renally eliminated drugs (e.g., lithium, paliperidone, desvenlafaxine, gabapentin, pregabalin, memantine). Monitor lithium levels.
	Reduced hepatic and renal function	Reduced hepatic metabolism and renal elimination of most drugs.

Table 8–2. Oncology drug–psychotropic drug interactions *(continued)*

Medication	Interaction mechanism	Effects on psychotropic drugs and management
Interferon-α	General inhibition of CYP450	Increased levels and adverse effects for oxidatively metabolized drugs, especially those metabolized by CYP1A2, CYP2C19, and CYP2D6.
	QT prolongation	Increased QT prolongation in combination with other QT-prolonging drugs such as TCAs, citalopram, typical antipsychotics, pimozide, risperidone, paliperidone, iloperidone, quetiapine, ziprasidone, and lithium.
	P-gp inhibition	Possible increased oral bioavailability of P-gp substrates (e.g., carbamazepine, phenytoin, lamotrigine, olanzapine, risperidone, quetiapine).
Procarbazine	MAO inhibition	Serotonin syndrome with SSRI/SNRIs, TCAs, MAOIs, lithium, opiates (fentanyl, meperidine, methadone, tramadol, dextromethorphan, and propoxyphene), etc. Hypertensive reaction with TCAs, sympathomimetics, psychostimulants, etc.
Tamoxifen	Inhibits CYP2C9	Reduced phenytoin metabolism with increased toxicity.

Note. CYP=cytochrome P450; GFR=glomerular filtration rate; MAO=monoamine oxidase; P-gp=P-glycoprotein; SNRIs=serotonin–norepinephrine reuptake inhibitors; SSRIs=selective serotonin reuptake inhibitors; TCAs=tricyclic antidepressants.

Table 8–3.   Psychotropic drug–oncology drug interactions

Medication	Pharmacokinetic effect	Effects on oncological drug and management
Carbamazepine, phenytoin, and oxcarbazepine; armodafinil and modafinil; St. John's wort	Induction of CYP3A4 and other CYP enzymes	Increased metabolism and reduced exposure and therapeutic effect of CYP3A4 substrates, including bexarotene, dasatinib, docetaxel, doxorubicin, gefitinib, etoposide, imatinib, lapatinib, methotrexate, paclitaxel, sorafenib, sunitinib, teniposide, topotecan, toremifene, vinblastine, vincristine, and vinorelbine.
		Increased metabolism of cyclophosphamide and ThioTEPA and increased exposure to the toxic active metabolites. Reduce dosage to avoid excessive toxicity.
		Increased metabolic activation of prodrugs ifosfamide and procarbazine increases toxicity and shortens duration of effect.
		Increased metabolic inactivation of prodrug irinotecan reduces therapeutic effect.
Fluoxetine	Inhibition of CYP3A4	Reduced metabolism and increased exposure and toxicities of CYP3A4 substrates, including bexarotene, dasatinib, docetaxel, doxorubicin, gefitinib, etoposide, imatinib, lapatinib, methotrexate, paclitaxel, sorafenib, sunitinib, teniposide, topotecan, toremifene, vinblastine, vincristine, and vinorelbine.
		Reduced metabolism of cyclophosphamide and ThioTEPA and reduced exposure to toxic active metabolites.
		Reduced metabolic activation of prodrugs ifosfamide, irinotecan, and procarbazine.

Table 8–3. Psychotropic drug–oncology drug interactions *(continued)*

Medication	Pharmacokinetic effect	Effects on oncological drug and management
Fluvoxamine	Inhibition of CYP1A2	Reduced metabolism and increased exposure and toxicities of CYP1A2 substrates, including bendamustine, erlotinib, and pomalidomide.
	Anticoagulant or antiplatelet	Increased anticoagulant or antiplatelet effects in combination with other antiplatelet drugs such as dasatinib and ibrutinib.
Atomoxetine, bupropion, duloxetine, fluoxetine, moclobemide, and paroxetine	Inhibition of CYP2D6	Reduced bioactivation of prodrug tamoxifen. Decreased therapeutic effect.
Carbamazepine	Downregulation of folate carrier	Reduced methotrexate cancer treatment efficacy.
Valproate	Inhibition of UGT1A1	Reduced metabolism of irinotecan active metabolite (SN-38) and increased toxicity. Possible reduced metabolism of sorafenib.

Note. CYP = cytochrome P450; UGT = uridine 5′-diphosphate glucuronosyltransferase.

Table 8–4. Oncology prodrugs activated by cytochrome P450 (CYP) metabolism

Prodrug	Activating enzymes
Cyclophosphamide	CYP2B6
Dacarbazine	CYP1A2
Ifosfamide	CYP3A4
Procarbazine	Unidentified CYPs
Tamoxifen	CYP2D6, CYP3A4

Note. Refer to Chapter 1, "Pharmacokinetics, Pharmacodynamics, and Drug-Drug Interactions," for a listing of relevant CYP metabolic inhibitors and inducers.

interactions are rarely reported, their clinical impact is uncertain (see Chapter 1, "Pharmacokinetics, Pharmacodynamics, and Principles of Drug-Drug Interactions").

Interactions Affecting Drug Distribution

Asparaginase reduces serum albumin by approximately 25% (Petros et al. 1992; Yang et al. 2008). Reductions in serum albumin can have variable clinical effects on serum levels and clearance of highly protein bound drugs, including carbamazepine, phenytoin, and valproate (see Chapter 1). When psychotropic drugs are coadministered with asparaginase, levels of the psychotropics should be monitored using methods selective for free drug; otherwise, lower total (free+bound) drug levels may prompt an inappropriate dosage increase.

Inhibition of Drug Metabolism by Chemotherapy Agents

The protein kinase inhibitors imatinib, nilotinib, and dasatinib and the antiandrogen nilutamide inhibit several CYP isozymes. Imatinib inhibits CYP2D6 and CYP3A4, and CYP2C9 (Miguel and Albuquerque 2011; Novartis 2009), and the second-generation compound nilotinib has greater scope, inhibiting CYP2C8, CYP2C9, CYP2D6, and CYP3A4 and P-gp (Deremer et al. 2008). Nilutamide may inhibit several isoenzymes, including CYP1A2 and CYP3A4, but this has not been firmly established (Sanofi 2015). In the presence of one of these anticancer agents, many drugs, including many psychotropics, may experience increased bioavailability and reduced metabolism due to their metabolism pathways through CYP isozymes. Similarly, dasatinib is also a CYP3A4 inhibitor (Bristol-Myers Squibb 2016; Miguel and Albuquerque 2011), which may increase the bioavailability and plasma levels of several psychotropics, including pimozide, quetiapine, ziprasidone, iloperidone, desvenlafaxine, oxidatively metabolized benzodiazepines, fentanyl, and methadone, leading to unwanted toxicities and side effects.

Interferons and interleukins can give rise to drug interactions through inhibition of one or more CYP isozymes or the P-gp efflux transporter. Some small studies have shown that interferons significantly inhibit CYP1A2 and CYP2D6 immediately after the first interferon dose (Islam et al. 2002; Williams et al. 1987), followed by inhibition of CYP1A2, CYP2C19, and CYP2D6 over the course of treatment. However, other investigators have not found any consistent changes in CYP1A2 and CYP3A4 (Pageaux et al. 1998) or CYP2D6 and CYP3A4 (Becquemont et al. 2002). The reason for this variable effect is unclear. Given the wide scope of interferon's potential effects on CYP metabolism, the introduction of INF-α may require dose reduction of narrow therapeutic range drugs metabolized by CYP isozymes.

Reduction in CYP isozyme activity has also been observed with IL-2 administration. Research suggests that high-dose ($\geq 9 \times 10^6$ units/m^2) IL-2 therapy may reduce metabolism of drugs metabolized by CYP1A2 (olanzapine and clozapine) and CYP3A4 (e.g., benzodiazepines, pimozide, quetiapine, ziprasidone, iloperidone, modafinil) (Elkhawaji et al. 1999; Vanda 2016).

Procarbazine inhibits monoamine oxidase and could trigger serotonin syndrome in combination with TCAs, SSRIs, SNRIs, monoamine oxidase inhibitors (MAOIs), or opiates with serotonin reuptake–inhibiting activity (meperidine, fentanyl, tramadol, methadone, dextromethorphan, and propoxyphene). Therefore, psychostimulants and other sympathomimetics should be avoided, and patients should be instructed to follow a tyramine-restricted diet.

Inhibition of Renal Elimination by Chemotherapy Agents

Several cancer agents are nephrotoxic, including the platinating agents cisplatin, carboplatin, and oxaliplatin; methotrexate; ifosfamide; and aldesleukin (Kintzel 2001) (Table 8–2). A 20%–40% reduction in glomerular filtration rate (GFR) following cisplatin therapy is common. Surprisingly, there is little evidence to suggest these drugs (with the exception of aldeskeukin) alter renal

drug elimination. In three case reports of patients receiving lithium, the introduction of cisplatin led to a transient decrease—not the expected increase—in
lithium levels in two cases (Beijnen et al. 1992, 1994) and no change in a third
(Pietruszka et al. 1985). In a survey of 123 children and adolescents, ifosfamide was shown to cause an average reduction in GFR of about 30%
(Skinner et al. 2000). Caution is advised when administering a nephrotoxic
agent with a drug that is primarily renally eliminated, including lithium,
paliperidone, venlafaxine, desvenlafaxine, gabapentin, pregabalin, and memantine (Nagler et al. 2012).

Intentional Pharmacokinetic Interactions

Although drug-drug interactions are generally avoided in clinical practice because of unwanted side effects, some interactions or combinations of drugs are
purposely used to increase therapeutic efficacy. For example, the oral bioavailability of the anticancer agent paclitaxel can be increased tenfold by coadministering cyclosporine, a CYP3A4 and P-gp inhibitor (Helgason et al. 2006).
For other medications, including psychotropics, the pharmacokinetic effect of
coadministering drugs for their interacting properties must be considered.

Interactions of Psychotropic Drugs With Chemotherapy Agents

Drug interactions that influence oncology drug levels may increase toxicity or
reduce therapeutic effect, compromising overall survival rate. Many chemotherapy agents are CYP3A4 substrates. Coadministration of a CYP3A4 inhibitor
(e.g., fluoxetine, fluvoxamine) may increase chemotherapy drug bioavailability
and blood levels, exacerbating toxicity (Table 8–3), which can decrease patients'
medication adherence to these life-saving chemotherapy agents.

Psychotropic Induction of Chemotherapeutic Metabolism

Concurrent use of the general CYP enzyme–inducing anticonvulsants carbamazepine, phenytoin, and phenobarbital with antileukemic chemotherapy
has been shown to compromise the efficacy of the chemotherapy (Relling et
al. 2000). Patients receiving long-term anticonvulsant therapy had significantly worse event-free survival (odds ratio 2.67) than the anticonvulsant-free
group. Systemic clearance of teniposide and methotrexate was shown to be
faster in the anticonvulsant group. Other studies confirm increased clearance
of imatinib (Pursche et al. 2008), irinotecan (Mathijssen et al. 2002a, 2002b),
gefitinib (Swaisland et al. 2005), dasatinib (Johnson et al. 2010), nilotinib

(Tanaka et al. 2011), and erlotinib (Hamilton et al. 2014; Pillai et al. 2013) in the presence of CYP enzyme inducers.

Psychotropic Inhibition of Chemotherapy Prodrug Bioactivation

Many chemotherapy agents are administered as prodrugs. Cyclophosphamide, dacarbazine, ifosfamide, procarbazine, tamoxifen, and trofosfamide undergo bioactivation via the CYP pathway (Table 8–4). Drug interactions that inhibit the bioactivation of oncology prodrugs may reduce therapeutic effect and survival rate.

Tamoxifen is metabolized to the active metabolite endoxifen in a two-step process involving both CYP2D6 and CYP3A4 (Briest and Stearns 2009). In women with breast cancer taking tamoxifen, plasma levels of endoxifen were reduced following the strong CYP2D6 inhibitor paroxetine (>70%) or the mild CYP2D6 inhibitor sertraline (>40%). Conversion of tamoxifen was also reduced with even mild CYP3A4 inhibition (Jin et al. 2005). In women with breast cancer who were receiving tamoxifen therapy, concurrent use of a CYP2D6 inhibitor increased the recurrence of breast cancer 1.9-fold (Aubert et al. 2009). A large population-based cohort study of women treated with tamoxifen found that concurrent use of paroxetine was associated with increased breast cancer mortality (Kelly et al. 2010). Paroxetine, fluoxetine, sertraline (CYP2D6 inhibition at >200 mg/day), duloxetine, bupropion, moclobemide, atomoxetine, and other CYP2D6 inhibitors should be avoided during tamoxifen therapy (Goetz et al. 2007). Citalopram, escitalopram, venlafaxine, and mirtazapine are preferred because of their lack of effect on CYP metabolism (Breitbart 2011; Miguel and Albuquerque 2011). Despite this concern, paroxetine and other antidepressants that inhibit CYP2D6 continue to be prescribed frequently to women taking tamoxifen (Binkhorst et al. 2013; Dieudonné et al. 2014; Dusetzina et al. 2013).

Irinotecan, a topoisomerase I inhibitor, has complex metabolism. It is metabolized to the active cytotoxic compound SN-38 by carboxylesterases but is inactivated by CYP3A4 isozymes. Drugs that induce CYP3A4, including carbamazepine, phenytoin, phenobarbital (Kuhn 2002), and St. John's wort (Mathijssen et al. 2002b), produce significant reductions in SN-38 levels, as does valproate (de Jong et al. 2007). Dosage adjustment may be required in the presence of these and other psychotropic drugs that induce (armodafinil, modafinil) or inhibit (fluoxetine, fluvoxamine, nefazodone) CYP3A4.

Cyclophosphamide is converted by CYP2B6 metabolism to the active anticancer metabolite 4-hydroxycoumarin (4-OHC). Two case reports suggest that CYP enzyme induction by phenytoin (de Jonge et al. 2005) or carbamazepine (Ekhart et al. 2009) enhances conversion to 4-OHC and may increase toxicities. Conversely, CYP2B6 inhibitors would be expected to reduce 4-OHC levels and decrease therapeutic effect. Common psychotropic drugs, including paroxetine, fluoxetine, and fluvoxamine, are also CYP2B6 inhibitors, and concurrent administration should be avoided.

Ifosfamide and trofosfamide (an ifosfamide prodrug), in contrast to cyclophospamide, are activated by CYP3A4 and inactivated by CYP2B6 and CYP3A4. One study suggests that CYP3A4 inhibitors and inducers should be avoided when administering ifosfamide and possibly during trofosfamide therapy (Kerbusch et al. 2001).

Pharmacodynamic Interactions

A wide variety of chemotherapy agents prolong QT interval (Table 8–2) (Arbel et al. 2007; Slovacek et al. 2008; Yeh 2006; see also https://crediblemeds.org/). These agents should be used with caution in the presence of other QT-prolonging drugs such as TCAs, citalopram, typical antipsychotics, pimozide, risperidone, paliperidone, iloperidone, quetiapine, ziprasidone, and lithium (Beach et al. 2013; Kane et al. 2008; van Noord et al. 2009).

Hypotension is commonly associated with etoposide, denileukin, systemic tretinoin, alemtuzumab, cetuximab, rituximab, INF-α, and IL-2 (aldesleukin). These agents may exacerbate hypotensive effects of psychotropic agents, including TCAs, antipsychotics, and MAOIs.

Antiemetics are often used to manage chemotherapy-induced nausea and vomiting during intense chemotherapy treatment. Antiemetic drug interactions are discussed in Chapter 4.

Drug Interaction Summary

Clinically significant drug-drug interactions are rarely reported in the literature, and many are speculative in nature; however, several interactions deserve attention. The use of multiple QT-prolonging drugs should be avoided. Several chemotherapy agents inhibit metabolism of psychotropic drugs and may increase psychotropic toxicities. In this event, psychotropic clinical response and therapeutic drug level monitoring should guide dosage adjustments. SSRIs, SNRIs, TCAs, MAOIs, and other agents known to precipitate serotonin syndrome should be avoided with procarbazine. Many oncological drugs are metabolized primarily through CYP3A4 isozymes; therefore, inducers and inhibitors of CYP3A4 should be avoided. Reduced therapeutic efficacy of oncological prodrugs may occur in the presence of drugs that inhibit their metabolic activation. Prodrug interactions that reduce therapeutic efficacy are becoming increasingly recognized. Conversely, the adverse effects of oncological prodrugs may be exacerbated by metabolic inducers—especially pan-inducers such as carbamazepine, phenytoin, and phenobarbital.

Key Clinical Points

- Psychiatric comorbidities of cancer or cancer therapy are often undertreated. Anxiety, depression, and fatigue can be treated effectively with psychotropics.
- Neuropsychiatric symptoms of chemotherapy—especially depression with interferon and interleukin—may lead to treatment discontinuation. Use of an adjunctive antidepressant enhances adherence to chemotherapy.
- Studies to date do not support withholding any psychiatric medications on the basis of fear of increasing cancer risk, with the possible exception of antipsychotics with a high incidence of hyperprolactinemia in patients with present or past history of pituitary endocrine tumors.
- Many chemotherapeutic agents prolong QT interval. Coadministration of other QT-prolonging drugs, including many psychotropics, should be avoided.
- Many chemotherapy agents are metabolized by CYP3A4. Coadministration of a CYP3A4 inhibitor may exacerbate chemotherapy toxicity and should be avoided.
- Use of psychotropics that do not inhibit metabolism is preferred when in combination with oncology prodrugs such as tamoxifen (see Table 8–4).

References

Agar M, Lawlor P: Delirium in cancer patients: a focus on treatment-induced psychopathology. Curr Opin Oncol 20(4):360–366, 2008 18525328

Alici-Evcimen Y, Breitbart WS: Ifosfamide neuropsychiatric toxicity in patients with cancer. Psychooncology 16(10):956–960, 2007 17278152

Arbel Y, Swartzon M, Justo D: QT prolongation and torsades de pointes in patients previously treated with anthracyclines. Anticancer Drugs 18(4):493–498, 2007 17351403

Aubert RE, Stanek EJ, Yao J, et al: Risk of breast cancer recurrence in women initiating tamoxifen with CYP2D6 inhibitors (meeting abstracts). J Clin Oncol 27(18S):CRA508, 2009

Baker WJ, Royer GL Jr, Weiss RB: Cytarabine and neurologic toxicity. J Clin Oncol 9:679–693, 1991 1648599

Baxalta: Oncaspar (pegasparaginase) product monograph, Bannockburn, IL, Baxalta, 2016. Available at: http://www.baxalta.com/assets/documents/OncasparPI.pdf. Accessed June 15, 2016.

Beach SR, Celano CM, Noseworthy PA, et al: QTc prolongation, torsades de pointes, and psychotropic medications. Psychosomatics 54(1):1–13, 2013 23295003

Becquemont L, Chazouilleres O, Serfaty L, et al: Effect of interferon alpha-ribavirin bitherapy on cytochrome P450 1A2 and 2D6 and N-acetyltransferase-2 activities in patients with chronic active hepatitis C. Clin Pharmacol Ther 71(6):488–495, 2002 12087352

Beijnen JH, Vlasveld LT, Wanders J, et al: Effect of cisplatin-containing chemotherapy on lithium serum concentrations. Ann Pharmacother 26(4):488–490, 1992 1576384

Beijnen JH, Bais EM, ten Bokkel Huinink WW: Lithium pharmacokinetics during cisplatin-based chemotherapy: a case report. Cancer Chemother Pharmacol 33(6):523–526, 1994 7511066

Bender CM, Sereika SM, Brufsky AM, et al: Memory impairments with adjuvant anastrozole versus tamoxifen in women with early-stage breast cancer. Menopause 14(6):995–998, 2007 17898668

Berenson JR, Yellin O, Shamasunder HK, et al: A phase 3 trial of armodafinil for the treatment of cancer-related fatigue for patients with multiple myeloma. Support Care Cancer 23(6):1503–1512, 2015 25370889

Berney A, Stiefel F, Mazzocato C, Buclin T: Psychopharmacology in supportive care of cancer: a review for the clinician. III. Antidepressants. Support Care Cancer 8(4):278–286, 2000 10923767

Binkhorst L, Mathijssen RH, van Herk-Sukel MP, et al: Unjustified prescribing of CYP2D6 inhibiting SSRIs in women treated with tamoxifen. Breast Cancer Res Treat 139(3):923–929, 2013 23760858

Breitbart W: Do antidepressants reduce the effectiveness of tamoxifen? Psychooncology 20(1):1–4, 2011 21182159

Breitbart WA: Treatment of delirium and confusional states in oncology and palliative care settings, in Psychopharmacology in Oncology and Palliative Care: A Practical Manual. Edited by Grassi L, Riba M. Heidelberg, Germany, Springer, 2014, pp 203–228

Briest S, Stearns V: Tamoxifen metabolism and its effect on endocrine treatment of breast cancer. Clin Adv Hematol Oncol 7(3):185–192, 2009 19398943

Bristol-Myers Squibb: Sprycel (dasatinib), New York, Bristol-Myers Squibb, 2016. Available at: www.sprycel.com. Accessed April 14, 2016.

Bruera E, El Osta B, Valero V, et al: Donepezil for cancer fatigue: a double-blind, randomized, placebo-controlled trial. J Clin Oncol 25(23):3475–3481, 2007 17687152

Bruera E, Yennurajalingam S, Palmer JL, et al: Methylphenidate and/or a nursing telephone intervention for fatigue in patients with advanced cancer: a randomized, placebo-controlled, phase II trial. J Clin Oncol 31(19):2421–2427, 2013 23690414

Brunello A, Basso U, Rossi E, et al: Ifosfamide-related encephalopathy in elderly patients: report of five cases and review of the literature. Drugs Aging 24(11):967–973, 2007 17953463

Buclin T, Mazzocato C, Berney A, Stiefel F: Psychopharmacology in supportive care of cancer: a review for the clinician IV: other psychotropic agents. Support Care Cancer 9(4):213–222, 2001 11430416

Butler JM Jr, Case LD, Atkins J, et al: A phase III, double-blind, placebo-controlled prospective randomized clinical trial of d-threo-methylphenidate HCl in brain tumor patients receiving radiation therapy. Int J Radiat Oncol Biol Phys 69(5):1496–1501, 2007 17869448

Buzdar AU, Esparza L, Natale R, et al: Lorazepam-enhancement of the antiemetic efficacy of dexamethasone and promethazine: a placebo-controlled study. Am J Clin Oncol 17(5):417–421, 1994 8092114

Cankurtaran ES, Ozalp E, Soygur H, et al: Mirtazapine improves sleep and lowers anxiety and depression in cancer patients: superiority over imipramine. Support Care Cancer 16(11):1291–1298, 2008 18299900

Capuron L, Ravaud A, Dantzer R: Early depressive symptoms in cancer patients receiving interleukin 2 and/or interferon alfa-2b therapy. J Clin Oncol 18(10):2143–2151, 2000 10811680

Capuron L, Gumnick JF, Musselman DL, et al: Neurobehavioral effects of interferon-alpha in cancer patients: phenomenology and paroxetine responsiveness of symptom dimensions. Neuropsychopharmacology 26(5):643–652, 2002 11927189

Carney MW, Ravindran A, Lewis DS: Manic psychosis associated with procarbazine. Br Med J (Clin Res Ed) 284(6309):82–83, 1982 6797665

Caruso R, Grassi L, Nanni MG, Riba M: Psychopharmacology in psycho-oncology. Curr Psychiatry Rep 15(9):393, 2013 23949568

Carvalho AF, Hyphantis T, Sales PM, et al: Major depressive disorder in breast cancer: a critical systematic review of pharmacological and psychotherapeutic clinical trials. Cancer Treat Rev 40(3):349–355, 2014 24084477

Chen AM, Daly ME, Vazquez E, et al: Depression among long-term survivors of head and neck cancer treated with radiation therapy. JAMA Otolaryngol Head Neck Surg 139(9):885–889, 2013 23949013

Chen YH, Huang CH: Reversible posterior leukoencephalopathy syndrome induced by vinorelbine. Clin Breast Cancer 12(3):222–225, 2012 22424944

Cohen Y, Chetrit A, Cohen Y, et al: Cancer morbidity in psychiatric patients: influence of lithium carbonate treatment. Med Oncol 15(1):32–36, 1998 9643528

Coogan PF, Strom BL, Rosenberg L: Antidepressant use and colorectal cancer risk. Pharmacoepidemiol Drug Saf 18(11):1111–1114, 2009 19623565

Cooper MR, Bird HM, Steinberg M: Efficacy and safety of modafinil in the treatment of cancer-related fatigue. Ann Pharmacother 43(4):721–725, 2009 19318599

Cosgrove L, Shi L, Creasey DE, et al: Antidepressants and breast and ovarian cancer risk: a review of the literature and researchers' financial associations with industry. PLoS One 6(4):e18210, 2011 21494667

Costa D, Mogos I, Toma T: Efficacy and safety of mianserin in the treatment of depression of women with cancer. Acta Psychiatr Scand Suppl 320:85–92, 1985 3901675

Costantini C, Ale-Ali A, Helsten T: Sleep aid prescribing practices during neoadjuvant or adjuvant chemotherapy for breast cancer. J Palliat Med 14(5):563–566, 2011 21388255

Cronin-Fenton DP, Riis AH, Lash TL, et al: Antidepressant use and colorectal cancer risk: a Danish population-based case-control study. Br J Cancer 104(1):188–192, 2011 20877356

Dalton SO, Johansen C, Poulsen AH, et al: Cancer risk among users of neuroleptic medication: a population-based cohort study. Br J Cancer 95(7):934–939, 2006 16926836

Day J, Zienius K, Gehring K, et al: Interventions for preventing and ameliorating cognitive deficits in adults treated with cranial irradiation. Cochrane Database of Systematic Reviews 2014, Issue 12. Art. No.: CD011335. DOI: 10.1002/14651858.CD011335.pub2 25519950

Day R, Ganz PA, Costantino JP: Tamoxifen and depression: more evidence from the National Surgical Adjuvant Breast and Bowel Project's Breast Cancer Prevention (P-1) Randomized Study. J Natl Cancer Inst 93(21):1615–1623, 2001 11698565

De Hert M, Peuskens J, Sabbe T, et al: Relationship between prolactin, breast cancer risk, and antipsychotics in patients with schizophrenia: a critical review. Acta Psychiatr Scand 133(1):5–22, 2016 26114737

de Jong FA, van der Bol JM, Mathijssen RH, et al: Irinotecan chemotherapy during valproic acid treatment: pharmacokinetic interaction and hepatotoxicity. Cancer Biol Ther 6(9):1368–1374, 2007 17873515

de Jonge ME, Huitema AD, van Dam SM, et al: Significant induction of cyclophosphamide and thiotepa metabolism by phenytoin. Cancer Chemother Pharmacol 55(5):507–510, 2005 15685452

Deremer DL, Ustun C, Natarajan K: Nilotinib: a second-generation tyrosine kinase inhibitor for the treatment of chronic myelogenous leukemia. Clin Ther 30(11):1956–1975, 2008 19108785

Dieudonné AS, De Nys K, Casteels M, et al: How often did Belgian physicians co-prescribe tamoxifen with strong CYP2D6 inhibitors over the last 6 years? Acta Clin Belg 69(1):47–52, 2014 24635399

Doraiswamy PM, Schott G, Star K, et al: Atypical antipsychotics and pituitary neoplasms in the WHO database. Psychopharmacol Bull 40(1):74–76, 2007 17285098

Dufour C, Grill J, Sabouraud P, et al: Ifosfamide induced encephalopathy: 15 observations [in French]. Arch Pediatr 13(2):140–145, 2006 16364615

Dusetzina SB, Alexander GC, Freedman RA, et al: Trends in co-prescribing of antidepressants and tamoxifen among women with breast cancer, 2004–2010. Breast Cancer Res Treat 137(1):285–296, 2013 23149465

Ekhart C, Rodenhuis S, Beijnen JH, Huitema AD: Carbamazepine induces bioactivation of cyclophosphamide and thiotepa. Cancer Chemother Pharmacol 63(3):543–547, 2009 18437385

Elkhawaji J, Robin MA, Berson A, et al: Decrease in hepatic cytochrome P450 after interleukin-2 immunotherapy. Biochem Pharmacol 57(8):951–954, 1999 10086330

Escalante CP, Meyers C, Reuben JM, et al: A randomized, double-blind, 2-period, placebo-controlled crossover trial of a sustained-release methylphenidate in the treatment of fatigue in cancer patients. Cancer J 20(1):8–14, 2014 24445757

Evans DL, McCartney CF, Haggerty JJ Jr, et al: Treatment of depression in cancer patients is associated with better life adaptation: a pilot study. Psychosom Med 50(1):73–76, 1988 3344305

Fann JR, Sullivan AK: Delirium in the course of cancer treatment. Semin Clin Neuropsychiatry 8(4):217–228, 2003 14613049

Fisch MJ, Loehrer PJ, Kristeller J, et al; Hoosier Oncology Group: Fluoxetine versus placebo in advanced cancer outpatients: a double-blinded trial of the Hoosier Oncology Group. J Clin Oncol 21(10):1937–1943, 2003 12743146

Foster AR, Caplan JP: Paraneoplastic limbic encephalitis. Psychosomatics 50(2):108–113, 2009 19377018

Goetz MP, Knox SK, Suman VJ, et al: The impact of cytochrome P450 2D6 metabolism in women receiving adjuvant tamoxifen. Breast Cancer Res Treat 101(1):113–121, 2007 17115111

Gultekin SH, Rosenfeld MR, Voltz R, et al: Paraneoplastic limbic encephalitis: neurological symptoms, immunological findings and tumour association in 50 patients. Brain 123(Pt 7):1481–1494, 2000 10869059

Gupta RK, Kumar R: Benign brain tumours and psychiatric morbidity: a 5-years retrospective data analysis. Aust N Z J Psychiatry 38(5):316–319, 2004 15144507

Halapy E, Kreiger N, Cotterchio M, Sloan M: Benzodiazepines and risk for breast cancer. Ann Epidemiol 16(8):632–636, 2006 16406246

Hamilton M, Wolf JL, Drolet DW, et al: The effect of rifampicin, a prototypical CYP3A4 inducer, on erlotinib pharmacokinetics in healthy subjects. Cancer Chemother Pharmacol 73(3):613–621, 2014 24474302

Hansen MV, Andersen LT, Madsen MT, et al: Effect of melatonin on depressive symptoms and anxiety in patients undergoing breast cancer surgery: a randomized, double-blind, placebo-controlled trial. Breast Cancer Res Treat 145(3):683–695, 2014 24756186

Helgason HH, Kruijtzer CM, Huitema AD, et al: Phase II and pharmacological study of oral paclitaxel (Paxoral) plus ciclosporin in anthracycline-pretreated metastatic breast cancer. Br J Cancer 95(7):794–800, 2006 16969354

Helissey C, Chargari C, Lahutte M, et al: First case of posterior reversible encephalopathy syndrome associated with vinflunine. Invest New Drugs 30(5):2032–2034, 2012 21728021

Hippisley-Cox J, Vinogradova Y, Coupland C, Parker C: Risk of malignancy in patients with schizophrenia or bipolar disorder: nested case-control study. Arch Gen Psychiatry 64(12):1368–1376, 2007 18056544

Holland JC, Romano SJ, Heiligenstein JH, et al: A controlled trial of fluoxetine and desipramine in depressed women with advanced cancer. Psychooncology 7(4):291–300, 1998 9741068

Hollister LE, Boutros N: Clinical use of CT and MR scans in psychiatric patients. J Psychiatry Neurosci 16(4):194–198, 1991 1786261

Homsi J, Nelson KA, Sarhill N, et al: A phase II study of methylphenidate for depression in advanced cancer. Am J Hosp Palliat Care 18(6):403–407, 2001 11712722

Hossein G, Zavareh VA, Fard PS: Combined treatment of androgen-independent prostate cancer cell line DU145 with chemotherapeutic agents and lithium chloride: effect on growth arrest and/or apoptosis. Avicenna J Med Biotechnol 4(2):75–87, 2012 23408470

Islam M, Frye RF, Richards TJ, et al: Differential effect of IFNalpha-2b on the cytochrome P450 enzyme system: a potential basis of IFN toxicity and its modulation by other drugs. Clin Cancer Res 8(8):2480–2487, 2002 12171873

Jenkins V, Shilling V, Fallowfield L, et al: Does hormone therapy for the treatment of breast cancer have a detrimental effect on memory and cognition? A pilot study. Psychooncology 13(1):61–66, 2004 14745746

Jenkins VA, Ambroisine LM, Atkins L, et al: Effects of anastrozole on cognitive performance in postmenopausal women: a randomised, double-blind chemoprevention trial (IBIS II). Lancet Oncol 9(10):953–961, 2008 18768369

Jin Y, Desta Z, Stearns V, et al: CYP2D6 genotype, antidepressant use, and tamoxifen metabolism during adjuvant breast cancer treatment. J Natl Cancer Inst 97(1):30–39, 2005 15632378

Johnson FM, Agrawal S, Burris H, et al: Phase 1 pharmacokinetic and drug-interaction study of dasatinib in patients with advanced solid tumors. Cancer 116(6):1582–1591, 2010 20108303

Joly F, Giffard B, Rigal O, et al: Impact of cancer and its treatments on cognitive function: advances in research from the Paris International Cognition and Cancer Task Force Symposium and update since 2012. J Pain Symptom Manage 50(6):830–841, 2015 26344551

Kaleita T, Wellisch D, Graham C, et al: Pilot study of modafinil for treatment of neurobehavioral dysfunction and fatigue in adult patients with brain tumors (abstract). J Clin Oncol 24(18S)(June 20 suppl):1503, 2006

Kane JM, Lauriello J, Laska E, et al: Long-term efficacy and safety of iloperidone: results from 3 clinical trials for the treatment of schizophrenia. J Clin Psychopharmacol 28(2) (suppl 1):S29–S35, 2008 18334910

Kao CH, Sun LM, Su KP, et al: Benzodiazepine use possibly increases cancer risk: a population-based retrospective cohort study in Taiwan. J Clin Psychiatry 73(4):e555–e560, 2012 22579162

Kelly CM, Juurlink DN, Gomes T, et al: Selective serotonin reuptake inhibitors and breast cancer mortality in women receiving tamoxifen: a population based cohort study. BMJ 340:c693, 2010 20142325

Kerbusch T, Jansen RL, Mathôt RA, et al: Modulation of the cytochrome P450-mediated metabolism of ifosfamide by ketoconazole and rifampin. Clin Pharmacol Ther 70(2):132–141, 2001 11503007

Kerr CW, Drake J, Milch RA, et al: Effects of methylphenidate on fatigue and depression: a randomized, double-blind, placebo-controlled trial. J Pain Symptom Manage 43(1):68–77, 2012 22208450

Kim SW, Shin IS, Kim JM, et al: Effectiveness of mirtazapine for nausea and insomnia in cancer patients with depression. Psychiatry Clin Neurosci 62(1):75–83, 2008 18289144

Kintzel PE: Anticancer drug-induced kidney disorders. Drug Saf 24(1):19–38, 2001 11219485

Kuendgen A, Gattermann N: Valproic acid for the treatment of myeloid malignancies. Cancer 110(5):943–954, 2007 17647267

Kuhn JG: Influence of anticonvulsants on the metabolism and elimination of irinotecan: a North American Brain Tumor Consortium preliminary report. Oncology (Williston Park) 16(8, suppl 7):33–40, 2002 12199631

Lan Y, Liu X, Zhang R, et al: Lithium enhances TRAIL-induced apoptosis in human lung carcinoma A549 cells. Biometals 26(2):241–254, 2013 23378009

Lavigne JE, Heckler C, Mathews JL, et al: A randomized, controlled, double-blinded clinical trial of gabapentin 300 versus 900 mg versus placebo for anxiety symptoms in breast cancer survivors. Breast Cancer Res Treat 136(2):479–486, 2012 23053645

Lee KC, Ray GT, Hunkeler EM, Finley PR: Tamoxifen treatment and new-onset depression in breast cancer patients. Psychosomatics 48(3):205–210, 2007 17478588

Liu Y, Ho RC, Mak A: Interleukin (IL)-6, tumour necrosis factor alpha (TNF-alpha) and soluble interleukin-2 receptors (sIL-2R) are elevated in patients with major depressive disorder: a meta-analysis and meta-regression. J Affect Disord 139(3):230–239, 2012 21872339

Lyskowski J, Nasrallah HA: Lithium therapy and the risk for leukemia. Br J Psychiatry 139:256, 1981 7317712

Madhusoodanan S, Danan D, Moise D: Psychiatric manifestations of brain tumors: diagnostic implications. Expert Rev Neurother 7(4):343–349, 2007 17425489

Mar Fan HG, Clemons M, Xu W, et al: A randomised, placebo-controlled, double-blind trial of the effects of d-methylphenidate on fatigue and cognitive dysfunction in women undergoing adjuvant chemotherapy for breast cancer. Support Care Cancer 16(6):577–583, 2008 17972110

Mathijssen RH, Sparreboom A, Dumez H, et al: Altered irinotecan metabolism in a patient receiving phenytoin. Anticancer Drugs 13(2):139–140, 2002a 11901305

Mathijssen RH, Verweij J, de Bruijn P, et al: Effects of St. John's wort on irinotecan metabolism. J Natl Cancer Inst 94(16):1247–1249, 2002b 12189228

Mazzocato C, Stiefel F, Buclin T, Berney A: Psychopharmacology in supportive care of cancer: a review for the clinician: II. neuroleptics. Support Care Cancer 8(2):89–97, 2000 10739354

McCarren M, Qiu H, Ziyadeh N, et al: Follow-up study of a pharmacovigilance signal: no evidence of increased risk with risperidone of pituitary tumor with mass effect. J Clin Psychopharmacol 32(6):743–749, 2012 23131882

McNutt MD, Liu S, Manatunga A, et al: Neurobehavioral effects of interferon-alpha in patients with hepatitis-C: symptom dimensions and responsiveness to paroxetine. Neuropsychopharmacology 37(6):1444–1454, 2012 22353759

Meyers CA, Weitzner MA, Valentine AD, Levin VA: Methylphenidate therapy improves cognition, mood, and function of brain tumor patients. J Clin Oncol 16(7):2522–2527, 1998 9667273

Miguel C, Albuquerque E: Drug interaction in psycho-oncology: antidepressants and antineoplastics. Pharmacology 88(5-6):333–339, 2011 22123153

Millennium Pharmaceuticals: Velcade (bortezomib). Cambridge, MA, Millennium Pharmaceuticals, 2009. Available at: http://www.velcade.com. Accessed April 14, 2016.

Moise D, Madhusoodanan S: Psychiatric symptoms associated with brain tumors: a clinical enigma. CNS Spectr 11(1):28–31, 2006 16400253

Moorman PG, Berchuck A, Calingaert B, et al: Antidepressant medication use [corrected] and risk of ovarian cancer. Obstet Gynecol 105(4):725–730, 2005 15802397

Moraska AR, Sood A, Dakhil SR, et al: Phase III, randomized, double-blind, placebo-controlled study of long-acting methylphenidate for cancer-related fatigue: North Central Cancer Treatment Group NCCTG-N05C7 trial. J Clin Oncol 28(23):3673–3679, 2010 20625123

Morrow GR, Hickok JT, Roscoe JA, et al; University of Rochester Cancer Center Community Clinical Oncology Program: Differential effects of paroxetine on fatigue and depression: a randomized, double-blind trial from the University of Rochester Cancer Center Community Clinical Oncology Program. J Clin Oncol 21(24):4635–4641, 2003 14673053

Mortensen PB: Neuroleptic treatment and other factors modifying cancer risk in schizophrenic patients. Acta Psychiatr Scand 75(6):585–590, 1987 2887088

Mortensen PB: Neuroleptic medication and reduced risk of prostate cancer in schizophrenic patients. Acta Psychiatr Scand 85(5):390–393, 1992 1351334

Moss EL, Simpson JS, Pelletier G, Forsyth P: An open-label study of the effects of bupropion SR on fatigue, depression and quality of life of mixed-site cancer patients and their partners. Psychooncology 15(3):259–267, 2006 16041840

Mücke M, Mochamat CH, Cuhls H, et al; Mochamat: Pharmacological treatments for fatigue associated with palliative care. Cochrane Database of Systematic Reviews 2015, Issue 5. Art. No.: CD006788, DOI: 10.1002/14651858.CD006788.pub3 26026155

Musselman DL, Lawson DH, Gumnick JF, et al: Paroxetine for the prevention of depression induced by high-dose interferon alfa. N Engl J Med 344(13):961–966, 2001 11274622

Musselman DL, Somerset WI, Guo Y, et al: A double-blind, multicenter, parallel-group study of paroxetine, desipramine, or placebo in breast cancer patients (stages I, II, III, and IV) with major depression. J Clin Psychiatry 67(2):288–296, 2006 16566626

Nagler EV, Webster AC, Vanholder R, Zoccali C: Antidepressants for depression in stage 3–5 chronic kidney disease: a systematic review of pharmacokinetics, efficacy and safety with recommendations by European Renal Best Practice (ERBP). Nephrol Dial Transplant 27(10):3736–3745, 2012 22859791

Ng CG, Boks MP, Zainal NZ, de Wit NJ: The prevalence and pharmacotherapy of depression in cancer patients. J Affect Disord 131(1-3):1–7, 2011 20732716

Novartis: Gleevec (Imatinib). St Louis, MO, Novartis, 2009. Available at: www.gleevec.com. Accessed April 14, 2016.

Olin J, Masand P: Psychostimulants for depression in hospitalized cancer patients. Psychosomatics 37(1):57–62, 1996 8600496

Page BR, Shaw EG, Lu L, et al: Phase II double-blind placebo-controlled randomized study of armodafinil for brain radiation-induced fatigue. Neuro Oncol 17(10):1393–1401, 2015 25972454

Pageaux GP, le Bricquir Y, Berthou F, et al: Effects of interferon-alpha on cytochrome P-450 isoforms 1A2 and 3A activities in patients with chronic hepatitis C. Eur J Gastroenterol Hepatol 10(6):491–495, 1998 9855065

Peng Z, Ji Z, Mei F, et al: Lithium inhibits tumorigenic potential of PDA cells through targeting hedgehog-GLI signaling pathway. PLoS One 8(4):e61457, 2013 23626687

Petros WP, Rodman JH, Relling MV, et al: Variability in teniposide plasma protein binding is correlated with serum albumin concentrations. Pharmacotherapy 12(4):273–277, 1992 1518726

Pfizer Canada: Cytosar (cytarabine) product monograph. 2011. Available at: http://www.pfizer.com/files/products/uspi_cytarabine_2g.pdf. Accessed June 16, 2016.

Pietruszka LJ, Biermann WA, Vlasses PH: Evaluation of cisplatin-lithium interaction. Drug Intell Clin Pharm 19(1):31–32, 1985 4038480

Pillai VC, Venkataramanan R, Parise RA, et al: Ritonavir and efavirenz significantly alter the metabolism of erlotinib—an observation in primary cultures of human hepatocytes that is relevant to HIV patients with cancer. Drug Metab Dispos 41(10):1843–1851, 2013 23913028

Pottegård A, Hallas J, Jensen BL, et al: Long-term lithium use and risk of renal and upper urinary tract cancers. J Am Soc Nephrol 27(1):249–225, 2016 25941353

Pursche S, Schleyer E, von Bonin M, et al: Influence of enzyme-inducing antiepileptic drugs on trough level of imatinib in glioblastoma patients. Curr Clin Pharmacol 3(3):198–203, 2008 18781906

Razavi D, Allilaire JF, Smith M, et al: The effect of fluoxetine on anxiety and depression symptoms in cancer patients. Acta Psychiatr Scand 94(3):205–210, 1996 8891089

Relling MV, Pui CH, Sandlund JT, et al: Adverse effect of anticonvulsants on efficacy of chemotherapy for acute lymphoblastic leukaemia. Lancet 356(9226):285–290, 2000 11071183

Resek G, Olivieri S: No association between lithium therapy and leukemia. Lancet 1(8330):940, 1983 6132264

Riechelmann RP, Burman D, Tannock IF, et al: Phase II trial of mirtazapine for cancer-related cachexia and anorexia. Am J Hosp Palliat Care 27(2):106–110, 2010 19776373

Roscoe JA, Morrow GR, Hickok JT, et al: Effect of paroxetine hydrochloride (Paxil) on fatigue and depression in breast cancer patients receiving chemotherapy. Breast Cancer Res Treat 89(3):243–249, 2005 15754122

Rosenberg L, Palmer JR, Zauber AG, et al: Relation of benzodiazepine use to the risk of selected cancers: breast, large bowel, malignant melanoma, lung, endometrium, ovary, non-Hodgkin's lymphoma, testis, Hodgkin's disease, thyroid, and liver. Am J Epidemiol 141(12):1153–1160, 1995 7771453

Roth AJ, Nelson C, Rosenfeld B, et al: Methylphenidate for fatigue in ambulatory men with prostate cancer. Cancer 116(21):5102–5110, 2010 20665492

Rothenberg ML, Liu PY, Wilczynski S, et al: Phase II trial of oral altretamine for consolidation of clinical complete remission in women with stage III epithelial ovarian cancer: a Southwest Oncology Group trial (SWOG-9326). Gynecol Oncol 82(2):317–322, 2001 11531286

Sanofi: Anandron (nilutamide) product monograph. Laval, QC, Canada, Sanofi-Aventis, 2015. Available at: http://www.sanofi.ca/products/en/anandron.pdf. Accessed April 14, 2016.

Schilder CM, Eggens PC, Seynaeve C, et al: Neuropsychological functioning in post-menopausal breast cancer patients treated with tamoxifen or exemestane after AC-chemotherapy: cross-sectional findings from the neuropsychological TEAM-side study. Acta Oncol 48(1):76–85, 2009 18777410

Selaman Z, Bolton JM, Oswald T, Sareen J: Association of benzodiazepine use with increased cancer risk is misleading due to lack of theoretical rationale and presence of many confounding factors. J Clin Psychiatry 73(9):1264, author reply 1264–1265, 2012 23059153

Sharpe M, Walker J, Holm Hansen C, et al; SMaRT (Symptom Management Research Trials) Oncology-2 Team: Integrated collaborative care for comorbid major depression in patients with cancer (SMaRT Oncology-2): a multicentre randomised controlled effectiveness trial. Lancet 384(9948):1099–1108, 2014 25175478

Shaw EG, Rosdhal R, D'Agostino RB Jr, et al: Phase II study of donepezil in irradiated brain tumor patients: effect on cognitive function, mood, and quality of life. J Clin Oncol 24(9):1415–1420, 2006 16549835

Sigma-Tau Pharmaceuticals: Matulane (procarbazine). Gaithersburg, MD, Sigma-Tau Pharmaceuticals, 2014. Available at: http://www.matulane.com. Accessed April 14, 2016.

Skinner R, Cotterill SJ, Stevens MC; United Kingdom Children's Cancer Study Group: Risk factors for nephrotoxicity after ifosfamide treatment in children: a UKCCSG Late Effects Group study. Br J Cancer 82(10):1636–1645, 2000 10817497

Slovacek L, Ansorgova V, Macingova Z, et al: Tamoxifen-induced QT interval prolongation. J Clin Pharm Ther 33(4):453–455, 2008 18613864

Sood A, Barton DL, Loprinzi CL: Use of methylphenidate in patients with cancer. Am J Hosp Palliat Care 23(1):35–40, 2006 16450661

Spathis A, Fife K, Blackhall F, et al: Modafinil for the treatment of fatigue in lung cancer: results of a placebo-controlled, double-blind, randomized trial. J Clin Oncol 32(18):1882–1888, 2014 24778393

Stiefel F, Berney A, Mazzocato C: Psychopharmacology in supportive care in cancer: a review for the clinician. I. Benzodiazepines. Support Care Cancer 7(6):379–385, 1999 10541978

Stockler MR, O'Connell R, Nowak AK, et al; Zoloft's Effects on Symptoms and Survival Time Trial Group: Effect of sertraline on symptoms and survival in patients with advanced cancer, but without major depression: a placebo-controlled double-blind randomised trial. Lancet Oncol 8(7):603–612, 2007 17548243

Swaisland HC, Ranson M, Smith RP, et al: Pharmacokinetic drug interactions of gefitinib with rifampicin, itraconazole and metoprolol. Clin Pharmacokinet 44(10):1067–1081, 2005 16176119

Swierenga SH, Gilman JP, McLean JR: Cancer risk from inorganics. Cancer Metastasis Rev 6(2):113–154, 1987 2439222

Szabatura AH, Cirrone F, Harris C, et al: An assessment of risk factors associated with ifosfamide-induced encephalopathy in a large academic cancer center. J Oncol Pharm Pract 21(3):188–193, 2015 24664476

Szarfman A, Tonning JM, Levine JG, Doraiswamy PM: Atypical antipsychotics and pituitary tumors: a pharmacovigilance study. Pharmacotherapy 26(6):748–758, 2006 16716128

Tamim HM, Mahmud S, Hanley JA, et al: Antidepressants and risk of prostate cancer: a nested case-control study. Prostate Cancer Prostatic Dis 11(1):53–60, 2008 17684479

Tanaka C, Yin OQ, Smith T, et al: Effects of rifampin and ketoconazole on the pharmacokinetics of nilotinib in healthy participants. J Clin Pharmacol 51(1):75–83, 2011 20702754

Toh S, Rodríguez LA, Hernández-Díaz S: Use of antidepressants and risk of lung cancer. Cancer Causes Control 18(10):1055–1064, 2007 17682831

Traeger L, Greer JA, Fernandez-Robles C, et al: Evidence-based treatment of anxiety in patients with cancer. J Clin Oncol 30(11):1197–1205, 2012 22412135

Udina M, Hidalgo D, Navinés R, et al: Prophylactic antidepressant treatment of interferon-induced depression in chronic hepatitis C: a systematic review and meta-analysis. J Clin Psychiatry 75(10):e1113–e1121, 2014a 25373120

Udina M, Moreno-España J, Capuron L, et al: Cytokine-induced depression: current status and novel targets for depression therapy. CNS Neurol Disord Drug Targets 13(6):1066–1074, 2014b 24923336

van Eys J, Cangir A, Pack R, Baram T: Phase I trial of procarbazine as a 5-day continuous infusion in children with central nervous system tumors. Cancer Treat Rep 71(10):973–974, 1987 3308081

van Heeringen K, Zivkov M: Pharmacological treatment of depression in cancer patients. A placebo-controlled study of mianserin. Br J Psychiatry 169(4):440–443, 1996 8894194

van Noord C, Straus SM, Sturkenboom MC, et al: Psychotropic drugs associated with corrected QT interval prolongation. J Clin Psychopharmacol 29(1):9–15, 2009 19142100

Vanda: Fanapt (iloperidone). Washington, DC, Vanda Pharmaceuticals, 2016. Available at: http://www.fanapt.com/. Accessed April 14, 2016.

Voltz R: Neuropsychological symptoms in paraneoplastic disorders. J Neurol 254 (suppl 2):II84–II86, 2007 17503138

Wald TG, Kathol RG, Noyes R Jr, et al: Rapid relief of anxiety in cancer patients with both alprazolam and placebo. Psychosomatics 34(4):324–332, 1993 8351307

Walker J, Hansen CH, Martin P, et al; SMaRT (Symptom Management Research Trials) Oncology-3 Team: Integrated collaborative care for major depression comorbid with a poor prognosis cancer (SMaRT Oncology-3): a multicentre randomised controlled trial in patients with lung cancer. Lancet Oncol 15(10):1168–1176, 2014 25175097

Wang PS, Walker AM, Tsuang MT, et al: Dopamine antagonists and the development of breast cancer. Arch Gen Psychiatry 59(12):1147–1154, 2002 12470131

Wernli KJ, Hampton JM, Trentham-Dietz A, Newcomb PA: Antidepressant medication use and breast cancer risk. Pharmacoepidemiol Drug Saf 18(4):284–290, 2009 19226540

Williams SJ, Baird-Lambert JA, Farrell GC: Inhibition of theophylline metabolism by interferon. Lancet 2(8565):939–941, 1987 2444839

Xu W, Tamim H, Shapiro S, et al: Use of antidepressants and risk of colorectal cancer: a nested case-control study. Lancet Oncol 7(4):301–308, 2006 16574545

Yancik R: Population aging and cancer: a cross-national concern. Cancer J 11(6):437–441, 2005 16393477

Yang L, Panetta JC, Cai X, et al: Asparaginase may influence dexamethasone pharmacokinetics in acute lymphoblastic leukemia. J Clin Oncol 26(12):1932–1939, 2008 18421047

Yeh ET: Cardiotoxicity induced by chemotherapy and antibody therapy. Annu Rev Med 57:485–498, 2006 16409162

Zaidan M, Stucker F, Stengel B, et al: Increased risk of solid renal tumors in lithium-treated patients. Kidney Int 86(1):184–190, 2014 24451323

Zhao G, Okoro CA, Li J, et al: Current depression among adult cancer survivors: findings from the 2010 Behavioral Risk Factor Surveillance System. Cancer Epidemiol 38(6):757–764, 2014 25455653

9

Central Nervous System Disorders

Adam P. Pendleton, M.D., M.B.A.

Jason P. Caplan, M.D.

The delicate neuronal meshwork of the human brain mediates both neurological and psychiatric function. Diseases that affect the central nervous system (CNS) are therefore apt to cause both neurological and psychiatric symptoms, and their management requires care so as not to exacerbate symptoms in either domain. In this chapter we discuss the treatment of the common neuropsychiatric manifestations of cognitive dysfunction, depression, anxiety, psychosis, and emotional and behavioral dysregulation that are common across CNS diseases.

Dementia

Dementia is a clinical syndrome characterized by cognitive decline, emotional and behavioral dysregulation, and impairments in activities of daily living. Specific phenotypes of dementia have been identified; however, some research indicates that dementia may represent a spectrum disorder, with variance in the presentation of initial symptoms (Dodel et al. 2008). Alzheimer's disease is the most common type of dementia, accounting for almost 70% of all patients with dementia ages 65 and older. Other types of dementia include vascular dementia; Lewy body dementia; frontotemporal dementia; dementia due to Parkinson's disease (lenticulostriatal dementia); and dementias due to immune diseases, infectious diseases, or brain injury.

The American Psychiatric Association (APA) Work Group on Alzheimer's Disease and Other Dementias published a second edition of their treatment guidelines for Alzheimer's disease and other dementias in 2007 (American Psychiatric Association Work Group on Alzheimer's Disease and Other Dementias 2007). We provide an outline of the salient features of these guidelines related to pharmacotherapy.

Alzheimer's Disease

Cognitive Deficits

Currently, three cholinesterase inhibitors—donepezil, rivastigmine, and galantamine—have been approved by the U.S. Food and Drug Administration (FDA) to treat mild to moderate Alzheimer's disease, but only donepezil is approved for treatment of severe Alzheimer's disease. Acetylcholinesterase inhibitors (AchEIs) have been shown to have modest benefits in the cognitive, behavioral, and functional realms (Hansen et al. 2008; Rodda et al. 2009) and have generally mild side effects associated with cholinergic excess, such as nausea, vomiting, and diarrhea. Rivastigmine has been observed to slow the rate of cognitive decline and activities of daily living, and the transdermal patch delivery appears to have fewer side effects while retaining efficacy (Birks et al. 2015). The N-methyl-D-aspartate (NMDA) receptor antagonist memantine is FDA approved for use in moderate to severe Alzheimer's disease and has a low side-effect profile with isolated reports of delirium.

Vitamin E (α-tocopherol) is no longer recommended for the treatment of cognitive symptoms of dementia because of limited evidence for its efficacy (Farina et al. 2012) and concerns regarding its safety. Furthermore, aspirin, steroidal and nonsteroidal anti-inflammatory agents (Jaturapatporn et al. 2012), statin medications (McGuinness et al. 2014), and estrogen supplementation (Hogervorst et al. 2009) have shown a lack of efficacy and safety in placebo-controlled trials in patients with Alzheimer's disease and as a result are also not recommended.

Depression

Depression is the most common comorbid condition in dementia and can worsen cognitive deficits, resulting in a poorer quality of life, increased risk of hospitalization, and increased caregiver burnout. Selective serotonin reuptake inhibitors (SSRIs) are considered to be the first-line agents and are chosen on the basis of side-effect profile. Sertraline, citalopram, and escitalopram have the fewest drug interactions of the SSRIs and are therefore commonly prescribed. However, large multicenter randomized controlled trials (RCTs) have shown that sertraline has lack of evidence of efficacy as far as 24 weeks into treatment, with associated concern of adverse effects (Banerjee et al. 2013; Rosenberg et al. 2010; Weintraub et al. 2010). Bupropion, venlafaxine, and mirtazapine have limited evidence of efficacy; however, mirtazapine was found to lack efficacy by Banerjee et al. (2013). Despite the seemingly pessimistic evidence of SSRI use in Alzheimer's disease–associated depression, a 2012 study by Bergh et al. found that discontinuation of escitalopram, citalopram, sertraline, or paroxetine all resulted in increased depression scores, suggesting that although SSRI therapy may not improve depression, it may substantially diminish the acceleration of depressive symptoms (Bergh et al. 2012). Previously, tricyclic antidepressants (TCAs) or monoamine oxidase inhibitors (MAOIs) were considered as third-line treatment, but the 2007 APA guidelines recommend avoiding TCAs because of the danger of substantial anticholinergic effects.

Anxiety

Anxiety is a common symptom found in dementia patients, both as a comorbid condition and as a result of depression. SSRIs are generally considered to be the first-line agents. Benzodiazepines can occasionally have a role in treating patients with prominent anxiety or on an as-needed basis for patients with infrequent episodes of agitation. However, adverse effects of benzodiazepines in this population include sedation, worsening cognition, delirium, increased risk of falls, and worsening of respiratory disorders. Lorazepam and oxazepam, which have no active metabolites, are typically preferable to agents with a longer half-life such as diazepam or clonazepam. Atypical antipsychotics should be used only for the short-term management of severe anxiety until SSRIs take effect because of the black box warning of atypical antipsychotic use in the elderly, explained in the subsection "Psychosis and Agitation."

Sleep Disturbances

Sleep disturbances, including decreased nocturnal sleep, sleep fragmentation, nocturnal wandering, and daytime sleepiness, are common among Alzheimer's patients and have an impact on the quality of life for both patients and their caregivers. To date, few RCTs have been performed to guide treatment for sleep disturbances. Melatonin and ramelteon have been studied, but there is a lack of evidence supporting their use. Trazodone at low doses has some evidence to support its use, but larger studies are required (McCleery et al. 2014).

Psychosis and Agitation

Psychosis, aggression, and agitation are common in patients with moderate to severe dementia, and it is critical to consider the safety of the patient and caregivers when choosing pharmacological interventions. In 2005, the FDA added a black box warning for the use of atypical antipsychotics in elderly patients with dementia-related psychosis. In order to better understand the effectiveness of different antipsychotics for the treatment of Alzheimer's disease–related behavioral disturbance, the National Institute of Mental Health performed a landmark study, the Clinical Antipsychotic Trials of Intervention Effectiveness—Alzheimer's Disease (CATIE-AD; Schneider et al. 2006). In the multicenter CATIE-AD RCT, outpatients with Alzheimer's disease and psychosis, agitation, or aggression received olanzapine, quetiapine, risperidone, or placebo. The Clinical Global Impression of Change scale was used to measure the differences in the groups, and there was little difference between the medications and placebo. The authors thus concluded that the adverse effects of the atypical antipsychotics outweigh the benefits when used for these indications.

However, it is important to note that the effects of antipsychotics such as olanzapine and risperidone on symptoms of anger, aggression, and paranoia have been found to be effective (Ballard et al. 2006). Although management of these symptoms is helpful for patients and caregivers, these medications are not effective treatments for cognitive symptoms or improving quality of life (Sultzer et al. 2008). Very careful consideration of the use of atypical antipsychotics in this patient population must weigh the benefits of behavioral control against the significant risks already mentioned, along with the risks of weight gain and decreases in high-density lipoproteins associated with long-term use of these agents (Zheng et al. 2009). For these reasons, antipsychotics should be used sparingly, at the lowest effective dose, and should be considered a short-term adjunctive medication. These principles are underscored in a 2016 practice guideline published by the APA on the use of antipsychotics to treat agitation or psychosis in patients with dementia (American Psychiatric Association 2016).

Other classes of medications, including typical antipsychotics, benzodiazepines, and mood stabilizers, have been used for the treatment of behavioral problems in patients with Alzheimer's disease, but robust evidence of their effect is limited. There is modest evidence for the use of SSRIs in Alzheimer's disease–associated agitation. A 2011 Cochrane review reported significant reduction in agitation with the use of sertraline and citalopram (Seitz et al. 2011). A 2014 randomized controlled trial (RCT) further supported the use of citalopram for agitation in patients with Alzheimer's disease, although the authors noted that the daily dose should be limited to 30 mg to minimize adverse cardiac effects (Porsteinsson et al. 2014). Sink and colleagues (2005) evaluated the efficacy of certain medications used for the treatment of neuropsychiatric symptoms associated with dementia. They created an algorithm that suggested the use of cholinesterase inhibitors, augmented with an SSRI in depressed patients or followed by an SSRI in nondepressed but agitated patients, followed by antipsychotics, then finally mood stabilizers.

Little evidence is available regarding the use of mood stabilizers in the management of behavioral disturbances in dementia. Yeh and Ouyang (2012) reviewed the available data and found significant evidence suggesting that carbamazepine can be effective for management of agitation; however, valproate, oxcarbazepine, and lithium showed low or no evidence of efficacy. Memantine was previously suggested to be effective for agitation in patients with Alzheimer's disease, but a double-blind RCT by Herrmann and colleagues showed no superiority over placebo (Herrmann et al. 2013). A double-blind RCT examining the use of a combined formulation of dextromethorphan and quinidine (discussed in the subsection "Pseudobulbar Affect") for agitation in patients with Alzheimer's disease demonstrated clinically relevant efficacy without exacerbation of cognitive impairment or sedation (Cummings et al. 2015).

Lewy Body Dementia

Cognitive Deficits

Dementia with Lewy bodies (DLB) is a result of a disease process leading to the deposition of α-synuclein. Patients with DLB have more significant cholinergic deficits compared with patients with Alzheimer's disease (Tarawneh and Galvin 2007), and they tend to have a more rapid progression of behavioral dysregulation. Previously, DLB was considered to be a diagnostically distinct condition; however, actual Lewy body deposits have been found not only in patients with DLB but also in patients with Alzheimer's disease and patients with Parkinson's disease–related dementia. This overlap in pathology is reflected in the overlap of treatment for these diseases.

In randomized placebo-controlled trials of rivastigmine, patients with DLB showed improvement in cognitive vigilance, working memory, episodic memory, attention, and executive functions (Wesnes et al. 2002). Donepezil was found to produce a significant improvement over a 1-year span in patients with DLB, measured using the Mini-Mental State Examination (Mori et al. 2015).

Psychosis

Hallucinations occur in 60%–70% of patients with DLB and tend to occur in the first few years of the disease, compared with the end stage of Alzheimer's disease (Ballard et al. 1999). The AchEIs have been shown to improve DLB-associated hallucinations, delusions, and paranoia. Furthermore, stopping medications that worsen neuropsychiatric symptoms, including anticholinergic medications, amantadine, dopamine agonists, monoamine oxidase inhibitors, catechol-O-methyl transferase inhibitors, and levodopa is recommended (Wood et al. 2010). A slow discontinuation of dopaminergic agents is recommended to minimize the risk of neuroleptic malignant syndrome.

The use of antipsychotics in DLB is controversial because patients with DLB are exquisitely sensitive to extrapyramidal side effects in addition to having increased risk per the FDA black box warning. However, short-term use of antipsychotics can still be beneficial, specifically if there is a high risk of harm to the patient because of psychosis (Wood et al. 2010). A thorough review of the treatment of DLB published in 2015 outlines the antipsychotic options for patients with DLB, with the most evidence supporting the use of quetiapine and clozapine and clozapine being the second-line choice because of concern regarding agranulocytosis (Boot et al. 2015).

Similar to treatment options in Alzheimer's disease, the adverse effects of atypical antipsychotics should be carefully considered in the context of the overall disease burden of the individual patient, avoiding agents such as olanzapine, clozapine, and quetiapine in patients at risk for hyperlipidemia or diabetes and avoiding olanzapine and risperidone in patients with elevated cerebrovascular risk. Pimavanserin is a promising new agent for the management of psychosis in parkinsonian patients that became available in mid-2016. It functions as a selective serotonin 5-HT_{2A} inverse agonist (Cummings et al. 2014) and may prove to be a better tolerated medication for psychosis in both DLB and Parkinson's disease because of its lack of dopamine antagonism.

Frontotemporal Dementia

Cognitive Deficits

In comparison with Alzheimer's disease, the cholinergic system in patients with frontotemporal dementia (FTD) remains relatively intact, with the majority of the abnormalities occurring in the dopaminergic and serotonergic systems (Huey et al. 2006). To date, there have been no medications shown to improve or even stabilize cognitive dysfunction in patients with FTD. The sparse data on the use of cholinesterase inhibitors in FTD demonstrates possible benefit of specific areas of cognitive dysfunction. One study showed galantamine to have mild improvement of aphasia in some patients with specific FTD variants (Kertesz et al. 2008). Rivastigmine has evidence for mild improvement of executive function but not global cognition (Moretti et al. 2004). Donepezil has no evidence for treatment of FTD cognitive deficits and has evidence that its use can worsen both cognition and behavioral dysregulation in patients with FTD (Mendez et al. 2007). An RCT of memantine in this population demonstrated no improvement in symptoms, with a greater incidence of adverse cognitive effects than placebo; thus, memantine is not recommended in FTD (Boxer et al. 2013). Oxytocin has been investigated for patients with FTD, but evidence is limited, and initial reports from small samples have not shown any improvement in symptoms (Finger et al. 2015).

Behavioral Disruption

The involvement of the frontal lobe in FTD can result in behaviors such as compulsions, gambling, stealing, sexual disinhibition, apathy, and carbohydrate craving, which can place the patient at risk and create a significant level of caregiver burden. SSRIs have shown some efficacy in addressing these behaviors in case reports and small observational studies (Moretti et al. 2003). Trazodone, an atypical serotonergic antidepressant, has demonstrated improvement of neuropsychiatric symptoms of FTD in randomized double-blind studies (Lebert et al. 2004). Atypical antipsychotic use in this patient population carries the same risk-to-benefit consideration as discussed for Alzheimer's disease and DLB, as patients with FTD also have increased extrapyramidal side effect sensitivity.

AchEIs, antiepileptic medications, and MAOIs all have limited evidence for use in FTD. The available literature includes reports of both improvement and worsening of neuropsychiatric symptoms. Benzodiazepine use in this patient population is not recommended because of risks of deliriogenicity, further cognitive dulling, and paradoxical agitation.

Vascular Dementia

Given the nature of pathology in vascular dementia, the most important intervention is prevention of further vasculopathy and stroke, including smoking cessation, and control of hypertension, hyperlipidemia, and diabetes. In a meta-analysis of controlled trials in patients with vascular dementia, donepezil, galantamine, memantine, and rivastigmine have been shown to improve cognitive function as measured by the Alzheimer's Disease Assessment Scale (Kavirajan and Schneider 2007).

Stroke

Stroke patients are at significant risk for a variety of neuropsychiatric disturbances, the presentation of which is heavily dependent on the location and extent of the stroke itself. These disturbances include dementia, depression, mania, anxiety, psychosis, disinhibition, apathy, and fatigue.

Cognitive Deficits

The pathophysiology of poststroke cognitive disorders is similar to that of vascular dementia, with evidence supporting use of the AchEIs as described previously in the subsection "Vascular Dementia."

Depression

Depression can be one of the most devastating neuropsychiatric symptoms poststroke. It has a prevalence of almost 30% any time after a stroke (Ayerbe et al. 2013) and is associated with increased morbidity and mortality. It was previously thought that depression was more likely in individuals with a left hemispheric stroke than a right hemispheric stroke, but meta-analyses have not supported this association (Carson et al. 2000).

There are no current formal guidelines for the treatment of poststroke depression. TCAs, SSRIs, and mirtazapine have all demonstrated some benefit in clinical trials. A 2008 Cochrane review that examined 12 trials of antidepressant therapy for poststroke depression (Hackett et al. 2008) showed modest improvement of depression, but there was also a significantly higher incidence of adverse effects.

The prevention of poststroke depression has been studied, with evidence that mirtazapine given prophylactically and acutely after stroke may prevent depression (Niedermaier et al. 2004). An RCT showed escitalopram to be modestly effective in reducing the prevalence of poststroke depression, but the therapeutic benefit was marginal (Robinson et al. 2008). A prospective trial demonstrated that statins have a protective effect against the development of poststroke depression at 1 year (Kim et al. 2014).

Mania

Mania is a rare consequence of stroke, and no clear guidelines for treatment of poststroke mania have been published. A systematic review reported that patients most at risk for poststroke mania are males with right-sided cerebral infarct who have no personal or family history of psychiatric illness (Santos et al. 2011). The treatment of poststroke mania is similar to treatment of bipolar mania, with evidence supporting the use of valproic acid, carbamazepine, and lithium (Bernardo et al. 2008). The use of antipsychotics for poststroke mania, especially in the elderly, is recommended only for short-term use in acute episodes to reduce risk of imminent harm to the patient.

Anxiety

Like depression, anxiety is a common comorbid condition poststroke, affecting 29% of patients (Hoffmann et al. 2015), that may respond to antidepressant therapy. One RCT from 2003 showed that nortriptyline was superior to placebo for poststroke anxiety with comorbid depression (Kimura et al. 2003). Another trial indicated that duloxetine was more effective than either sertraline or citalopram in the management of poststroke anxiety, and all three agents were equally efficacious in addressing poststroke depression, although there was no placebo control (Karaiskos et al. 2012). As in vascular dementia, the use of benzodiazepines should be avoided because of cognitive dulling and risk of delirium, falls, or further ischemic events due to hypotension.

Aggression and Irritability

The degree of aggression and irritability in patients poststroke depends on many factors, including prestroke psychiatric illness and extent of cerebral involvement. There have been small studies on the prevalence and treatment of poststroke aggression and irritability, which indicate that the prevalence may be as high as 25% (Chan et al. 2006). Data for the treatment of poststroke aggression and irritability are limited to antidepressants; for example, fluoxetine has been found to be effective in treating poststroke aggression and irritability (Choi-Kwon et al. 2006).

Traumatic Brain Injury

Traumatic brain injury (TBI) has become a major focus in the practice of neurological and psychiatric health care, with attention being drawn to the long-term effects of TBI by members of the military and professional athletes. Neuropsychiatric symptoms of TBI include impaired cognition, depression, mania, psychosis, mood lability, irritability, and anxiety (Warden et al. 2006).

Cognitive Deficits

The cognitive deficits seen as a result of TBI span multiple domains, including arousal, attention, concentration, memory, language, sleep, and executive functioning. An increasing body of data suggests that stimulants (including dextroamphetamine, methylphenidate, modafinil, armodafinil, and lisdexamfetamine) have utility in the treatment of post-TBI cognitive deficits (Johansson et al. 2015; Menn et al. 2014; Tramontana et al. 2014). A recent RCT demonstrated significant dose-dependent improvement of long-lasting mental fatigue and processing speed with methylphenidate (Johansson et al. 2015). Dopamine agonists (including amantadine, levodopa or carbidopa, and bromocriptine) have also shown improvement in reducing the cognitive deficits associated with TBI (Warden et al. 2006). The AchEIs have moderate data suggesting improvements in memory, concentration, attention, and data processing (Silver et al. 2009a; Tenovuo 2005; Zhang et al. 2004). Preliminary investigations of the use of lithium and valproic acid in patients who have experienced a TBI have shown promising data supporting a neuroprotective effect, which may lead to long-term improvement of neuropsychiatric sequelae of TBI, although clinical trials have yet to be completed (Chen et al. 2014; Leeds et al. 2014).

Depression

SSRIs are considered first-line agents for post-TBI depression. Citalopram and escitalopram have been found to be effective (Rapoport et al. 2008), with escitalopram having fewer drug-drug interactions. Serotonin-norepinephrine reuptake inhibitors (SNRIs), including venlafaxine and duloxetine, have been shown to be effective in the treatment of post-TBI depression (Silver et al. 2009b). If the SSRI or SNRI classes prove ineffective, psychostimulants or dopamine agents can be used for augmentation. Caution is advised with the use of bupropion because of its potential to reduce seizure threshold at higher doses.

Mania

Mania is a less common but clinically significant result of TBI. Literature regarding the treatment of mania in TBI is composed mainly of case reports, but a small case series suggests the effectiveness of the mood stabilizers lithium, carbamazepine, and valproic acid (Kim and Humaran 2002).

Psychosis

Psychosis can be a complicating adverse effect after TBI, and little literature is available regarding treatment. In general, the atypical antipsychotics are preferred over typical agents because of lower rates of extrapyramidal side effects. Case reports compose the majority of current data, describing positive results reported with olanzapine and risperidone (Guerreiro et al. 2009; Schreiber et al. 1998). Clozapine was found to be mildly effective; however, two of nine patients developed seizures (Michals et al. 1993), and thus clozapine should be used with caution in patients with neurological insult. It is important to keep in mind that unusual or treatment-resistant symptoms of psychosis in the setting of a neurological injury may be due to subclinical seizure activity, specifically partial complex seizures.

Aggression and Irritability

Aggression and irritability are common among patients post-TBI and may be transient, may resolve with neurological improvement, or may be persistent. Management of aggression and irritability in this population is similar to management of aggression and irritability after stroke, with judicious use of neuroleptics to avoid exacerbating neurological fragility. Unlike in patients with concern for ischemia, such as risk factors for stroke or vascular dementia, β-blockers can be safely used for agitation in patients with TBI (Fleminger et al. 2006). Anticonvulsants, including lithium, valproate, and carbamazepine, have shown modest effect of decreasing mood lability (Chiu et al. 2013), and the investigation of the neuroprotective features of lithium and valproate discussed in the section "Traumatic Brain Injury" may support their use as disease-modifying agents. Amantadine administered in the morning and at noon has been shown to decrease the intensity and frequency of post-TBI irritability and aggression (Hammond et al. 2014).

Benzodiazepines can be useful in short-term abortive therapy for aggression. However, a conservative risk-benefit calculus should be used because long-term benzodiazepine use can perpetuate cognitive dulling, delirium, or a cycle of dose escalation.

Multiple Sclerosis

Multiple sclerosis can result in motor, cognitive, and psychiatric disturbances, which may occur together or independently, as described in a thorough review (Feinstein et al. 2013). The neuropsychiatric disturbances of multiple sclerosis (which include cognitive deficits, depression, mania, psychosis, and fatigue) may occur only during acute exacerbations or as a chronic feature of the disease.

Cognitive Deficits

Cognitive impairments, including deficits of attention and memory, executive dysfunction, and information processing speed, may be present in almost 70% of patients with multiple sclerosis, and they may be present as early as the time of initial diagnosis (Achiron and Barak 2003; Chiaravalloti and DeLuca 2008). Disease-modifying agents such as interferon-β-a1 can prevent or reduce the progression of cognitive deficits in patients with multiple sclerosis (Fischer et al. 2000). In an RCT, cholinesterase inhibitors, specifically donepezil, have been found to improve memory (Christodoulou et al. 2006). However, a Cochrane review performed by He et al. (2013) concluded that because of the limited quality of available RCTs, there is currently no convincing evidence to support the efficacy of pharmacological symptomatic treatment for multiple sclerosis–associated memory disorder.

Depression and Fatigue

About 30% of patients with multiple sclerosis report depression (Beiske et al. 2008), and these patients carry an increased risk of suicide (Siegert and Abernethy 2005). The SSRIs escitalopram, citalopram, and sertraline are considered first-line agents because of their lower drug interaction profile (Kaplin 2007). The relatively small quantity of RCTs examining the treatment of depression in patients with multiple sclerosis have shown desipramine and sertraline to be effective pharmacological treatments, but they also indicate that there is a broadly heterogenous response to both antidepressants and psychotherapeutic interventions (Mohr et al. 2001; Schiffer and Wineman 1990). A small study suggests that paroxetine may be effective for the treatment of depression in patients with multiple sclerosis (Ehde et al. 2008). The management of depression in patients with multiple sclerosis can be tailored to treat concurrent somatic conditions. For example, TCAs can be used for depression co-occurring with incontinence, whereas SNRIs may be used in depression co-occurring with neuropathic pain.

Fatigue is common among patients with multiple sclerosis and can be an organic effect of the disease process or may occur as a neurovegetative symptom of an associated depression. For the management of concurrent depression and fatigue, bupropion may be a prudent choice, given the increased susceptibility to sexual dysfunction experienced with SSRIs in patients with multiple sclerosis who have extant impairment of spinal cord function (Kaplin 2007). Modafinil has been found to be effective for management of fatigue in a 2005 RCT (Kraft and Bowen 2005). Amantadine and carnitine have been evaluated for fatigue in patients with multiple sclerosis, but the efficacy is poorly documented, and more evidence is required to determine if there is any therapeutic advantage (Pucci et al. 2007; Tejani et al. 2012).

Mania

Mania is approximately twice as common in patients with multiple sclerosis as in the general population (Ghaffar and Feinstein 2007). However, there have been no clinical trials for the treatment of multiple sclerosis–associated mania. For management of mania, mood stabilizers, with adjunctive addition of antipsychotics or benzodiazepines for severe mania or the occurrence of psychotic features, have been found to be effective (Ameis et al. 2006).

Corticosteroids are a common necessary treatment for multiple sclerosis flares and can be a precipitant of mania. A 1979 chart review by Falk and colleagues found that none of the 27 patients who were pretreated with lithium prior to corticosteroid administration developed mania, compared with 6 of 44 patients who did not receive prophylactic lithium (Falk et al. 1979). If a patient develops mania during steroid therapy, lithium may be used to manage the mania in lieu of discontinuing the steroids (Feinstein 2007).

Psychosis

Psychosis is relatively rare in patients with multiple sclerosis, occurring in only 1%–3% of patients. There are no published trials regarding the treatment of psychosis in multiple sclerosis. Atypical antipsychotics are usually preferred in this patient population because of the lower risk of extrapyramidal side effects.

Parkinson's Disease

Parkinson's disease is characterized by motoric symptoms, including bradykinesia, resting tremor, rigidity, and postural and gait instability. The neuropsychiatric symptoms of Parkinson's disease are a significant cause of impairment in quality of life and increased caregiver burden. The pharmacological management of psychiatric disturbances in patients with Parkinson's disease is a delicate balance of neurotransmitter action and requires close longitudinal monitoring.

Cognitive Deficits

Cognitive symptoms, including psychomotor slowing, impaired verbal and working memory, executive dysfunction, and ultimately dementia, are common in patients with Parkinson's disease. Donepezil has shown efficacy in improving cognition and memory with little impact on motor function (Leroi et al. 2006), and rivastigmine has demonstrated moderate improvement in cognition but with increased rates of nausea and vomiting (Emre et al. 2004). Parkinson's disease–associated dementia has many of the clinical features of DLB. Some researchers have suggested that these two diagnoses are variant presentations of the same illness, which may indicate similar efficacies of treatment approaches to cognitive dysfunction (Dodel et al. 2008). For patients with executive dysfunction or inattention associated with Parkinson's disease, modafinil and atomoxetine can be beneficial (Bassett 2005). Rasagiline has shown marked improvement in cognitive domains of attention, executive functioning, and verbal fluency (Hanagasi et al. 2011).

The effect of dopamine agonists on cognition is not completely established, with some studies reporting certain ergot-derived dopamine agonists such as pergolide having no impact on cognition (Brusa et al. 2005), whereas some non-ergot-derived dopamine agonists, namely, pramipexole, have shown some impairment in verbal memory, executive functions, and attention (Brusa et al. 2003). The differences in receptor profile for dopamine agonists may explain the dichotomous outcomes. Newer studies continue to provide evidence that certain dopamine agonists can be used with little to no effect on cognition (Brusa et al. 2013).

Depression

Depression in patients with Parkinson's disease can exacerbate deficits of cognitive and motor function and is associated with a decreased quality of life. Clinical trials for treatment of depression in patients with Parkinson's disease are limited, and a 2003 Cochrane review found insufficient data on the safety and effectiveness of antidepressant therapy in patients with Parkinson's disease (Ghazi-Noori et al. 2003). In 2006, the American Academy of Neurology (AAN) produced a practice parameter from the six reviewed small randomized controlled trials that evaluated pharmacological treatment of depression in patients with Parkinson's disease (Miyasaki et al. 2006). The AAN subcommittee found insufficient information to support or refute the efficacy of antidepressants on the basis of the available data; however, SSRIs (specifically citalopram and paroxetine) and TCAs have some evidence supporting their use in the Parkinson's disease patient population. Reports of motor impairment with SSRIs in patients with Parkinson's disease have resulted in cautious use of these medications, although there is also evidence that fluoxetine can be used with no impact on motor movement (Kostić et al. 2012). Although use of the TCAs, specifically nortriptyline and desipramine, has evidence for efficacy (Devos et al. 2008; Menza et al. 2009), SSRIs have a lower side-effect profile. Dopamine agonists such as ropinirole and pramipexole also have evidence for effective treatment of depression (Barone et al. 2010). Although no rigorous evidence exists, SNRIs and bupropion may also be considered depending on the presentation of the individual patient.

Psychosis

Approximately 60% of patients with Parkinson's disease will experience psychosis at some point in their illness, with the common symptoms being visual hallucinations and persecutory delusions, most often occurring in patients also exhibiting symptoms of dementia (Forsaa et al. 2010). Treatment of psychosis in Parkinson's disease is complicated by the potential of antipsychotics to worsen motor symptoms via dopamine antagonism (Hasnain et al. 2009).

Management of psychosis in patients with Parkinson's disease should begin with titration of dopaminergic agents to the lowest effective dose, with antipsychotics added as adjunctive therapy if symptoms persist (Zahodne and Fernandez 2008). Clozapine remains the antipsychotic of choice, with low doses (6.25–50 mg daily) proven effective for control of psychotic symptoms without worsening motor function (Frieling et al. 2007). Unfortunately, clozapine continues to be underprescribed in patients with Parkinson's disease, in whom too frequent use of high-potency neuroleptics can worsen parkinsonism (Herrmann et al. 2013; Weintraub et al. 2011). Quetiapine has been found to be effective in controlling the symptoms of psychosis but has mixed evidence regarding impact on motor symptoms. Nevertheless, a 2011 review of prescribing practices reports an overall preference for quetiapine and more frequent use of aripiprazole for psychosis in patients with Parkinson's disease (Weintraub et al. 2011). Olanzapine, aripiprazole, and risperidone have been found to be ineffective and to worsen motor function in patients with Parkinson's disease, and they are not recommended (Ellis et al. 2000; Fernandez et al.

2003; Hasnain 2011). Information is limited regarding the use of ziprasidone and paliperidone.

The serotonin receptors 5-HT$_{2A}$ and 5-HT$_{2C}$ may be a large contributor to the evolution of Parkinson's disease psychosis. A case report noted improvement of psychosis with the addition of mirtazapine (Godschalx-Dekker and Siegers 2014). Rivastigmine is the only AchEI with data reporting significant improvement of hallucinations in a large RCT (Burn et al. 2006). Donepezil has repeatedly failed to show efficacy, and galantamine has little data to support its use. Pimavanserin is a novel 5-HT$_{2A}$ inverse agonist that has shown significant potential in Phase III trials for the treatment of Parkinson's disease–related psychosis with little to no impact on motor function (Broadstock et al. 2014).

Fatigue

Methylphenidate and modafinil have been shown to improve fatigue related to Parkinson's disease in two RCTs (Lou et al. 2007; Mendonça et al. 2007). Treatment with rasagiline has been shown to slow the progression of fatigue in Parkinson's disease in at least one RCT (Stocchi and ADAGIO investigators 2014).

Huntington's Disease

Huntington's disease is an autosomal dominant genetic disorder characterized by choreiform movements, dementia, and psychiatric symptoms, including depression, mania, obsessions and compulsions, and psychosis. Few controlled trials exist specifically for management of psychiatric symptoms in patients with Huntington's disease, and the approach typically mirrors that of other basal ganglia disorders. Pharmacological treatment of patients with Huntington's disease requires care because these patients are particularly susceptible to sedation, falls, cognitive impairment, and extrapyramidal symptoms (Rosenblatt 2007).

Depression

To date, there have been no RCTs for management of depression in patients with Huntington's disease. SSRIs have case reports for efficacy and are commonly used as first-line agents because they also reduce the irritability and anxiety commonly reported by patients with Huntington's disease (De Marchi et al. 2001). TCAs, MAOIs, and mirtazapine have been effective in case reports and small case series (Bonelli and Hofmann 2007). Given the autosomal dominant transmission of Huntington's disease, depression may precede the onset of symptoms if the individual is aware of the likelihood of developing the illness via either knowledge of a parental Huntington's disease diagnosis or confirmatory genetic testing.

Mania

Approximately 5%–10% of patients with Huntington's disease become manic, exhibiting grandiosity and elevated or irritable mood (Rosenblatt 2007). Patients with Huntington's disease may respond more positively to valproate or carbamazepine, with the available data indicating a less robust response to and more side effects with lithium (Rosenblatt 2007). Antipsychotics may be used as adjunctive treatment, but selection of a specific agent should be made with care as described in the following subsection.

Psychosis

Delusions are the most prominent symptom of psychosis in patients with Huntington's disease, followed by hallucinations. The choice of antipsychotic for Huntington's disease patients with psychosis (or requiring adjunctive medication for severe mania) should be determined by the severity of the choreiform movements. Haloperidol and other high-potency antipsychotics, which likely work by suppressing the oversupply of dopamine due to intrinsic striatal cell loss, are preferred in patients with severe chorea, and atypical antipsychotics are preferable in patients with minimal chorea (Chou et al. 2007). Substantial numbers of case reports suggest effectiveness of risperidone at low doses, with limited data available for the effectiveness of clozapine and quetiapine.

Epilepsy

Psychiatric disturbances in epilepsy include cognitive dysfunction, mood lability, impulsive behavior, and psychosis. These symptoms can be preictal, interictal, and postictal (for a thorough review, see LaFrance et al. 2008).

Cognitive Deficits

Cognitive disorders associated with epilepsy are common, and the most effective management depends on aggressive seizure control. Antiepileptic drugs with fewer cognitive side effects, specifically lamotrigine and levetiracetam, are generally preferred. Untreated depression can manifest as cognitive impairment, and treatment of comorbid depression can improve cognition (Shulman and Barr 2002). AchEIs have not been found to be effective for cognitive deficits in epilepsy (Hamberger et al. 2007). Memantine is not recommended because of a concern for increased seizure risk (Peltz et al. 2005).

Depression

Depression is very common in patients with epilepsy, with a prevalence of up to 10 times that of the general population and a risk of suicide of more than 3 times that of the general population (Hesdorffer et al. 2012). Despite this, a Cochrane Database meta-analysis of available data in 2014 concluded that no high-quality evidence is available to inform antidepressant selection in the context of epilepsy (Maguire et al. 2014). In general, depressive symptoms that are acutely temporally related to seizure activity (either ictal or peri-ictal) are best managed with improved seizure control. Interictal depressive symptoms can be managed using SSRIs as first-line agents because they have little effect on the seizure threshold. Conversely, bupropion and clomipramine are not recommended because of risk of lowering the seizure threshold.

Mania

Mania is rare in patients with epilepsy, with the exception of patients who have undergone disease-modifying surgeries, specifically lobectomies. The use of mood-stabilizing antiepileptic medications such as lamotrigine, valproate, and carbamazepine is considered first line, with cautious use of lithium as a second-line agent because of possible epileptogenic activity (Prueter and Norra 2005).

Anxiety

Anxiety can be present either as an ictal or peri-ictal symptom or may evolve as a chronic symptom as a result of anticipatory anxiety about a recurrence of seizure activity. No RCTs are available regarding the treatment of anxiety in patients with epilepsy. As with depression, SSRIs are the first-line agents because of minimal effect on seizure threshold. Benzodiazepines can be useful given their anxiolytic and anticonvulsant properties, but they require consideration of adverse motor and cognitive effects and the potential for dependence or abuse.

Psychosis

Patients with epilepsy have an eightfold risk of psychosis (Clancy et al. 2014). Psychosis in epilepsy may be classified as either ictal and postictal psychosis (psychoses closely linked to seizures), alternative psychosis (psychosis linked to seizure remission, also referred to as "forced normalization"), interictal psychosis (intermittent episodes of psychoses not associated with seizures), or iatrogenic psychosis (psychosis related to anticonvulsant drugs, most notoriously levetiracetam). Anticonvulsants are the primary treatment for ictal and postictal psychosis. The treatment of interictal psychosis includes both anticonvulsants and antipsychotics. Antipsychotics with a high risk of lowering seizure threshold, such as clozapine and low-potency typical agents, should be avoided.

Symptoms and Syndromes Common Across Neurological Disorders

Apathy

Scant data are available regarding the treatment of apathy. A Cochrane review of RCTs evaluating interventions for apathy in patients with TBI found no medication trials (Lane-Brown and Tate 2009). Methylphenidate has demonstrated safety and efficacy in treating apathy in patients with Alzheimer's disease (Rosenberg et al. 2013). Escitalopram has been shown to be effective in preventing apathy immediately after a stroke (within 3 months) (Mikami et al. 2013). Anecdotal evidence suggests that amantadine, bromocriptine, bupropion, modafinil, and AchEIs are effective in treating apathy (Galynker et al. 1997; Kraus and Maki 1997; Powell et al. 1996; Rodda et al. 2009).

Pseudobulbar Affect

A broad spectrum of neurological conditions have been associated with paroxysmal episodes of affective outbursts that are either exaggerated or grossly incongruent with the patient's internal mood state. This pathological separation of mood and affect has been referred to by a number of descriptors (including affective lability, emotional incontinence, pathological crying, or involuntary emotional expression disorder) but has most consistently been described by the term *pseudobulbar affect* (PBA). One study of patients with diagnoses of stroke, dementia, TBI, multiple sclerosis, Parkinson's disease, or amyotrophic lateral sclerosis found that more than one-third of these patients screened positive for symptoms of PBA (Brooks et al. 2013). PBA may be misdiagnosed as a primary mood disorder.

The sole current FDA-approved treatment for PBA is the combination of low-dose dextromethorphan and quinidine, based on data from a large double-blind, placebo-controlled trial. This formulation leverages inhibition of cytochrome P450 2D6 (CYP2D6) by quinidine to prevent metabolism of dextromethorphan to its active metabolite dextrorphan, increasing concentrations of the parent drug thirtyfold. Dextromethorphan is postulated to have antiglutamatergic activity in the CNS via activity at the NMDA and σ_1 receptors (Pioro et al. 2010). Patients should be monitored for adverse effects, including diarrhea and dizziness. Monitoring of the QTc may be indicated in patients with additional risk factors for arrhythmia. Patients receiving other medications that are metabolized by CYP2D6 should be observed for drug-drug interactions. SSRIs (which likely exert their effect in PBA by secondary modulation of glutamate by serotonin) and TCAs may be considered as second- and third-line approaches, with published studies limited by very small sample sizes (Andersen et al. 1993; Robinson et al. 1993; Wortzel et al. 2008).

Sexual Disinhibition

Sexual disinhibition is common in neurological patients with disturbances of frontal lobe function, particularly in men. A 2010 systematic literature review found no RCTs examining management of sexual disinhibition in dementia and no studies comparing efficacies of different agents (Tucker 2010). Small trials or case reports using SSRIs, gabapentin, pindolol, clomipramine, carbamazepine, cimetidine, and/or antipsychotics have reported some clinical benefit (Ozkan et al. 2008). Estrogen therapy was effective in a double-blind study (Kyomen et al. 1999), and Ozkan and colleagues reported effectiveness with leuprolide and cyproterone. Medroxyprogesterone acetate was reported as effective and well tolerated in a series of five geriatric patients with sexual disinhibition (Bardell et al. 2011). Dopamine agonists, discussed later in this chapter, have also been known to cause impulse-control issues, including the development of paraphilias.

Adverse Neurological Effects of Psychotropic Medications

Psychotropic medications have been associated with the potential to produce a number of adverse neurological effects, most notably extrapyramidal symptoms, including tardive dyskinesia, lowering of seizure threshold, cognitive impairment, delirium, and behavioral disinhibition (Table 9–1). Neuroleptic malignant syndrome and serotonin syndrome, which may develop in patients treated with antipsychotic drugs, are covered in Chapter 2, "Severe Drug Reactions."

Extrapyramidal Symptoms

Psychotropic-induced extrapyramidal symptoms include acute dyskinesias, tremor, dystonia, and akathisia. Patients with Parkinson's disease, DLB, vascular dementia, and multiple sclerosis are at greatest risk for developing these symptoms. Antipsychotics are the most common cause of extrapyramidal symptoms, with risk increasing as dopamine D_2 receptor blockade increases. High-potency first-generation antipsychotics such as haloperidol present the greatest risk, followed by phenothiazines and atypical antipsychotics. Among the atypical antipsychotics, the hierarchy of extrapyramidal symptom risk was evaluated on the basis of average extrapyramidal symptom presentation in patients with schizophrenia and bipolar disorder. The hierarchy (greater to lesser) is as follows: ziprasidone > aripiprazole > risperidone > paliperidone (estimated) > olanzapine > quetiapine > clozapine (Gao et al. 2008; Tandon 2002). Extrapyramidal symptoms have also been reported with antidepressants, including SSRIs, SNRIs, and bupropion. The symptoms are not dose related, and they can develop with short-term or long-term use (Madhusoodanan et al. 2010).

Tardive dyskinesia, characterized by repetitive, involuntary, purposeless movements, can be associated with chronic use or abrupt discontinuation of antipsychotic medications. It has also been reported with metoclopramide, phenothiazine antiemetics, and very rarely with SSRIs. Medical complications may include pain and impairment of gait, swallowing, and respiration. Neurologically ill and elderly patients are thought to be at increased risk. Tardive dystonia and tardive akathisia may also result from prolonged antipsychotic exposure. No cure for tardive dyskinesia has been found, but small open-label trials and RCTs suggest that clonazepam, donepezil (Caroff et al. 2001), low-

Table 9–1. Neurological adverse effects of psychotropic drugs

Medication	Neurological adverse effects
Antidepressants	
SSRIs or SNRIs	Tremor, parkinsonism, sedation, apathy
TCAs	Cognitive impairment (tertiary>secondary amines), seizure (particularly clomipramine), sedation (tertiary>secondary amines)
Amoxapine and maprotiline	Lower seizure threshold at therapeutic dosages
MAOIs	Sedation
Bupropion	Seizure (increased risk with doses exceeding 400 mg/day; however, the overall risk is low) (Ruffmann et al. 2006)
Antipsychotics	
Atypical and typical agents	Extrapyramidal symptoms and tardive dyskinesia, seizure (particularly clozapine, chlorpromazine, and loxapine), cognitive impairment (particularly low-potency typical agents), orthostatic hypotension, neuroleptic malignant syndrome
Mood stabilizers	
Carbamazepine	Dizziness, drowsiness, incoordination, blurred vision, nystagmus, ataxia
Lithium	Seizure, ataxia, delirium, slurred speech, dystonia, tics, tremor; deficits can be acute and chronic and are generally dose- and serum concentration–dependent
Valproate	Somnolence, dizziness, tremor, insomnia
Anticholinergics	
Benztropine and trihexyphenidyl	Delirium, visual hallucinations, cognitive impairment

Table 9–1.   Neurological adverse effects of psychotropic
                  drugs *(continued)*

Medication	Neurological adverse effects
Anxiolytics	
Benzodiazepines	Withdrawal seizures, delirium, disinhibition, cognitive impairment, sedation, dysarthria
Buspirone	Sedation, dizziness

Note.   MAOIs=monoamine oxidase inhibitors; SNRIs=serotonin-norepinephrine reuptake inhibitors; SSRIs=selective serotonin reuptake inhibitors; TCAs=tricyclic antidepressants.

dose clozapine (Spivak et al. 1997), olanzapine (Lucetti et al. 2002), and tetrabenazine may diminish the severity of these symptoms; however, a 2013 systematic literature review from the AAN indicates that data are insufficient to either support or refute the use of these medications (Bhidayasiri et al. 2013). Botulinum toxin type A has limited evidence for efficacy, and it may be clinically useful for localized tardive dyskinesia symptoms (Tarsy et al. 1997).

Seizures

Use of psychotropics for patients with epilepsy is generally regarded with caution. However, in a retrospective study assessing the impact of psychotropics on seizure frequency, Gross and colleagues (2000) found that seizure frequency decreased in 33% of patients, was unchanged in 44%, and increased in 23%. No significant difference in average seizure frequency was found between pretreatment and treatment periods. The authors concluded that psychotropic medications can be safely used in epilepsy patients with psychopathology if introduced slowly in low to moderate doses. However, certain psychotropics, such as chlorpromazine, clozapine, maprotiline, bupropion, and clomipramine, have been associated with increased seizure frequency and should be avoided in patients with epilepsy. Haloperidol and atypical antipsychotics other than clozapine have a lower risk of causing seizures than do the phenothiazine antipsychotics (Guarnieri et al. 2004). The rate of seizures with bupropion is dose related, with the greatest risk (about 0.4%) in patients without a co-occurring neurological diagnosis noted at dosages of 450 mg/day. Psychostimulants, including dextroamphetamine and methylphenidate, do not appear to increase seizure risk in patients with attention-deficit/hyperactivity disorder who have epilepsy and good seizure control (Kanner 2008). However, patients whose seizures are not well controlled may be at further risk with the addition of a stimulant medication (Gonzalez-Heydrich et al. 2007).

Cognitive Impairment and Delirium

The psychotropic medications most likely to cause or exacerbate cognitive impairment and delirium are benzodiazepines, medications with anticholinergic properties (e.g., benztropine, phenothiazines, tertiary-amine TCAs), lithium (especially at supratherapeutic levels), and topiramate. Behavioral disinhibition is often caused by benzodiazepines, particularly in patients with neurological illness, in children, and in older adults. Behavioral disinhibition often co-occurs with cognitive impairment and delirium. In general, benzodiazepines and lithium should be used with caution and monitored closely in patients with neurological conditions because each medication has a relatively low therapeutic index.

Adverse Psychiatric Effects of Neurological Medications

Dopamine Agonists

Dopamine agonists (Table 9–2), including levodopa, amantadine, pramipexole, and ropinirole, have been associated with hallucinations, delusions, and complex behavioral problems in patients with Parkinson's disease. Patients at greatest risk include those with advanced disease, prolonged treatment, cognitive impairment, and dyskinesias.

Complex behavioral problems associated with dopamine receptor stimulation in patients with Parkinson's disease include pathological gambling, hypersexuality, punding (intense fascination with repetitive handling, examining, sorting, and arranging of objects), compulsive shopping, and compulsive medication use (Weintraub et al. 2006). Paraphilias, defined as intense urges or behaviors involving nonnormative sexual interests, have been associated with dopamine agonist use (Solla et al. 2015). Sometimes described as

Table 9–2.   Psychiatric adverse effects of neurological drugs

Medication	Psychiatric adverse effects
Dopamine agonists	
Amantadine, levodopa/ carbidopa	Psychosis, agitation, insomnia, confusion
Pramipexole and ropinirole	Hallucinations, delusions, psychosis, agitation, somnolence, confusion, impulse-control disorders, paraphilias
Anticonvulsants	
Gabapentin	Sedation
Lamotrigine	Euphoria
Levetiracetam	Affective disorder, psychosis, aggressive behavior
Topiramate	Cognitive impairment, decreased appetite, affective disorder, psychosis, aggressive behavior
Valproate	Cognitive impairment, increased appetite
Interferons	
Interferon-β-1a/1b	Depression, affective lability, irritability
MAO-B inhibitors	
Selegiline	Dizziness, vivid dreams, agitation, insomnia; risk for hypertensive crisis and serotonin syndrome at dosages exceeding 10 mg/day
Rasagiline	Dizziness, vivid dreams, anxiety
COMT inhibitors	
Entacapone and tolcapone	Dyskinesia, sleep disorders, hallucinations, agitation
Immunomodulators	
Glatiramer, mitoxantrone, and natalizumab	Anxiety, agitation, delirium, depression

Table 9–2. Psychiatric adverse effects of neurological drugs *(continued)*

Medication	Psychiatric adverse effects
α₂ Adrenoceptor agonists	
Clonidine and guanfacine	Depression, anxiety, vivid dreams, restlessness, fatigue
Cholinesterase inhibitors	
Donepezil, rivastigmine, and galantamine	Insomnia, fatigue, anorexia, vivid dreams

Note. COMT = catechol-*O*-methyl transferase; MAO-B = monoamine oxidase B.

dopamine dysregulation syndrome, these behaviors affect up to 14% of patients with Parkinson's disease (Voon and Fox 2007). Management includes dopamine agonist dose reduction and treatment of secondary psychotic, manic, or behavioral symptoms.

Anticonvulsants

Adverse psychiatric effects (including affective disorder, psychosis, and aggressive behavior) were precipitated by the anticonvulsants topiramate in 24% (Mula et al. 2003a) and levetiracetam in 10%–16% (Mula et al. 2003b) of patients with epilepsy. Patients with a personal or family history of psychiatric disorder were found to be at increased risk for developing a psychiatric adverse effect with topiramate or levetiracetam.

Interferon-β-1a

Although interferon-α is commonly associated with depression, the risk of depression from interferon-β-1a, used for relapsing-remitting multiple sclerosis, is not well established. Interferon-β-1a is reported to have no depressive effect (Zephir et al. 2003) or may even have a benefit on mood and depression after prolonged treatment (Feinstein et al. 2002). Individuals with a prior history of major depression or psychosis may be at increased risk of depression; however, this has not been well defined. Psychosis and delirium have also been reported as adverse effects of this treatment (Goëb et al. 2003).

Drug-Drug Interactions

Pharmacokinetic and pharmacodynamic interactions between psychiatric and neurological medications are outlined in Tables 9–3 and 9–4. The pharmacokinetic interaction of greatest clinical significance is the induction of CYP1A2, CYP2C9, CYP2C19, and CYP3A4–mediated metabolism by phenytoin, phenobarbital, carbamazepine, and ethosuximide, resulting in decreased levels of many psychotropics. Valproate also may alter metabolism through hepatotoxicity and complex effects on induction and inhibition of several CYP enzymes. It is prudent to monitor (when possible) the levels of all coadministered medications with the potential for toxicity when prescribing anticonvulsant agents.

Many psychotropic medications (TCAs, bupropion [>450 mg/day], high-dose venlafaxine, maprotiline, lithium, low-potency typical antipsychotics, clozapine) have a lower seizure threshold, which can erode the therapeutic effects of anticonvulsants. Amantadine, fosphenytoin, and felbamate rarely may increase QTc prolongation when given with other QTc-prolonging psychotropic drugs such as antipsychotics, TCAs, and lithium (for a listing, see CredibleMeds 2016). Triptans and selegiline (inhibition of monoamine oxidase type A is significant at > 10 mg/day) increase the risk of serotonin syndrome when used in patients receiving SSRIs, SNRIs, mirtazapine, or TCAs. The risk of serotonin syndrome with rasagiline and serotonergic antidepressants is not known, but risk has been reported (Fernandes et al. 2011). Triptans have a black box warning of risk of serotonin syndrome in combination with serotonergic antidepressants; however, the frequency and clinical significance of this potential interaction has been questioned (Wenzel et al. 2008). Psychotogenic effects of dopamine agonists, topiramate, and levetiracetam may erode the therapeutic effects of antipsychotics in patients with schizophrenia.

Table 9–3.   Neurological medication–psychotropic medication interactions

Medication	Interaction mechanism	Effects on psychotropic drugs and management
Anticonvulsants		
Carbamazepine, phenobarbital, and phenytoin	Induction of CYP1A2, CYP2C9/19, and CYP3A4 and of UGT	Increased metabolism and decreased levels of clozapine, olanzapine, buspirone, benzodiazepines (except oxazepam, lorazepam, and temazepam), pimozide, trazodone, and zolpidem
Ethosuximide	Induction of CYP3A4	Increased metabolism and decreased levels of buspirone, benzodiazepines (except oxazepam, lorazepam, and temazepam), pimozide, trazodone, and zolpidem
Felbamate and fosphenytoin	QT prolongation	Increased risk of cardiac arrhythmias with other QT-prolonging agents, including TCAs, typical antipsychotics, pimozide, risperidone, paliperidone, iloperidone, quetiapine, ziprasidone, and lithium
Valproate	Inhibition of urea cycle	Hyperammonemia with topiramate (also a urea cycle inhibitor)
Antiparkinsonian medications		
Levodopa	Additive psychotogenic effect	Erosion of antipsychotic control of psychosis
Amantadine	QT prolongation	Increased risk of cardiac arrhythmias with other QT-prolonging agents, including TCAs, typical antipsychotics, pimozide, risperidone, paliperidone, iloperidone, quetiapine, ziprasidone, and lithium
	Additive psychotogenic effect	Erosion of antipsychotic control of psychosis

Table 9–3. Neurological medication–psychotropic medication interactions *(continued)*

Medication	Interaction mechanism	Effects on psychotropic drugs and management
Antiparkinsonian medications *(continued)*		
Selegiline and rasagiline	MAO-A inhibition at high dosage (selegiline >10 mg/day)	Increased risk of serotonin syndrome when combined with SSRIs, SNRIs, mirtazapine, MAOIs, lithium, or TCAs
Pramipexole and ropinirole	Additive hypotensive effects	Increased risk of hypotensive effects with antipsychotics, TCAs, and MAOIs
	Additive psychotogenic effect	Erosion of antipsychotic control of psychosis
Cognitive enhancers		
Donepezil, galantamine, and rivastigmine	Cholinesterase inhibition	Exacerbates extrapyramidal symptoms
Triptans	Serotonin receptor agonist	Serotonin syndrome (FDA black box warning)

Note. CYP=cytochrome P450; FDA=U.S. Food and Drug Administration; MAO-A=monoamine oxidase A; MAOIs=monoamine oxidase inhibitors; SNRIs=serotonin–norepinephrine reuptake inhibitors; SSRIs=selective serotonin reuptake inhibitors; TCAs=tricyclic antidepressants; UGT=uridine 5′-diphosphate glucuronosyltransferase.

Table 9–4. Psychotropic medication–neurological medication interactions

Medication	Interaction mechanism	Effects on neurological drugs and management
Antidepressants		
SSRIs		
Fluoxetine and fluvoxamine	Inhibits CYP1A2, CYP2C9/ 2C19, CYP3A4	Inhibited metabolism and increased levels and toxicities of CYP1A2 substrates (rasagiline, frovatriptan, zolmitriptan, ropinirole), CYP2C9 and CYP2C19 substrates (mephenytoin, phenytoin, tiagabine), and CYP3A4 substrates (ergotamine, carbamazepine, ethosuximide, phenytoin, phenobarbital, tiagabine, zonisamide).
SNRIs and novel-action agents		
Bupropion, venlafaxine, and desvenlafaxine	Reduced seizure threshold	Increased risk of seizures and erosion of therapeutic effect of anticonvulsants. Avoid bupropion at dosages >450 mg/day and high-dose venlafaxine.
TCAs	Reduced seizure threshold	Increased risk of seizures and erosion of therapeutic effect of anticonvulsants. Avoid clomipramine and maprotiline, especially at high dosages.
	QT prolongation	Additive QT prolongation in combination with amantadine, felbamate, and fosphenytoin. Consider QT-prolonging effects when selecting psychiatric and neurological medications.

Table 9–4.   Psychotropic medication–neurological medication interactions *(continued)*

Medication	Interaction mechanism	Effects on neurological drugs and management
Antidepressants *(continued)*		
MAOIs		
Moclobemide, phenelzine, tranylcypromine, and isocarboxazid	MAO inhibition	Inhibition of triptans metabolized by MAO, including sumatriptan, rizatriptan, and zolmitriptan. Avoid combining these triptans with MAOIs. Consider almotriptan, eletriptan, frovatriptan, or naratriptan, which are metabolized by CYP enzymes.
Mood stabilizers		
Valproic acid	CYP2C9 inhibition	Increased levels of phenytoin, carbamazepine, phenobarbital, and primidone.
	UGT inhibition	Reduced metabolism and increased levels of entacapone and tolcapone.
Lithium	Reduced seizure threshold	Increased risk of seizures and erosion of therapeutic effect of anticonvulsants.
	QT prolongation	Additive QT prolongation in combination with amantadine, felbamate, and fosphenytoin. Consider QT-prolonging effects when selecting psychiatric and neurological medications.

Table 9–4. Psychotropic medication–neurological medication interactions *(continued)*

Medication	Interaction mechanism	Effects on neurological drugs and management
Antipsychotics		
Atypical and typical agents	Dopamine receptor blockade	Extrapyramidal symptoms. Worsening of Parkinson's disease (except possibly with low-dose clozapine).
	Reduced seizure threshold	Increased risk of seizures and erosion of therapeutic effect of anticonvulsants. Avoid clozapine and low-potency typical agents.
Paliperidone, quetiapine, risperidone, thioridazine, and ziprasidone	QT prolongation	Additive QT prolongation in combination with amantadine, felbamate, and fosphenytoin. Consider QT-prolonging effects when selecting psychiatric and neurological medications.
Clozapine	Additive hematological toxicity	Increased risk of bone marrow suppression and agranulocytosis with carbamazepine.
	Reduced seizure threshold	Increased risk of seizures and erosion of therapeutic effect of anticonvulsants.
Psychostimulants		
Amphetamine and methylphenidate	Additive vasoconstriction	Excessive vasoconstriction, hypertension, and "ergotism" with triptans and ergot alkaloids.
	Dopamine receptor agonist	Increased risk of psychosis with levodopa, amantadine, pramipexole, and ropinirole.

Note.   CYP=cytochrome P450; MAO=monoamine oxidase; MAOIs=monoamine oxidase inhibitors; SNRIs=serotonin-norepinephrine reuptake inhibitors; SSRIs=selective serotonin reuptake inhibitors; TCAs=tricyclic antidepressants; UGT=uridine 5′-diphosphate glucuronosyltransferase.

Key Clinical Points

- Patient and family education improves medication compliance and side-effect reporting. Patients with cognitive impairment are at increased risk for noncompliance and often inaccurately report symptoms and side effects.

- A comprehensive neuropsychiatric evaluation should define the nature of the CNS disease, disease stage or time since injury, and any neuropsychiatric disturbances.

- Treatment selection should consider whether a single intervention could address disparate symptoms (e.g., dopaminergic agents for mild depression in Parkinson's disease, antiepileptic drugs for the treatment of ictal or peri-ictal psychiatric symptoms). Patients with neurological disease are often on multiple medications, and the "two birds, one stone" approach may help in lowering both the clinical and the financial burden of unnecessary polypharmacy.

- The "start low, go slow" approach should be used, especially when the agent being added may mechanistically exacerbate other symptoms. On occasion, consideration should be given to augmentation with a different agent rather than dose escalation in order to minimize exacerbation of extant neurological symptoms.

- Clinical response, side effects, and drug levels should be assessed frequently.

- Off-label use of medications in neuropsychiatry is the rule rather than the exception when addressing behavioral disturbances such as agitation, aggression, or sexual disinhibition. Mechanism of action and side-effect profile are often more pertinent considerations in a choice of agent than an approved indication.

- Clinicians should stay abreast of the latest developments in the treatment of primary neurological illnesses. New drugs and novel mechanisms of action continue to make their way to our pharmacological armamentarium.

References

Achiron A, Barak Y: Cognitive impairment in probable multiple sclerosis. J Neurol Neurosurg Psychiatry 74(4):443–446, 2003 12640060

Ameis SH, Feinstein A, Riis JO: Treatment of neuropsychiatric conditions associated with multiple sclerosis. Expert Rev Neurother 6(10):1555–1567, 2006 17078794

American Psychiatric Association: The American Psychiatric Association Practice Guideline on the Use of Antipsychotics to Treat Agitation or Psychosis in Patients With Dementia. Arlington, VA, American Psychiatric Association, 2016

American Psychiatric Association Work Group on Alzheimer's Disease and Other Dementias: American Psychiatric Association practice guideline for the treatment of patients with Alzheimer's disease and other dementias, second edition. Am J Psychiatry 164 (suppl 12):5–56, 2007 18340692

Andersen G, Vestergaard K, Riis JO: Citalopram for post-stroke pathological crying. Lancet 342:837–839, 1993 8104273

Ayerbe L, Ayis S, Wolfe CD, Rudd AG: Natural history, predictors and outcomes of depression after stroke: systematic review and meta-analysis. Br J Psychiatry 202(1):14–21, 2013 23284148

Ballard C, Holmes C, McKeith I, et al: Psychiatric morbidity in dementia with Lewy bodies: a prospective clinical and neuropathological comparative study with Alzheimer's disease. Am J Psychiatry 156(7):1039–1045, 1999 10401449

Ballard CG, Waite J, Birks J: Atypical antipsychotics for aggression and psychosis in Alzheimer's disease. Cochrane Database of Systematic Reviews, 2006 Issue 1. Art. No.: CD003476. DOI: 10.1002/14651858.CD003476.pub2 16437455

Banerjee S, Hellier J, Romeo R, et al: Study of the use of antidepressants for depression in dementia: the HTA-SADD trial—a multicentre, randomised, double-blind, placebo-controlled trial of the clinical effectiveness and cost-effectiveness of sertraline and mirtazapine. Health Technol Assess 17(7):1–166, 2013 23438937

Bardell A, Lau T, Fedoroff JP: Inappropriate sexual behavior in a geriatric population. Int Psychogeriatr 23(7):1182–1188, 2011 21554796

Barone P, Poewe W, Albrecht S, et al: Pramipexole for the treatment of depressive symptoms in patients with Parkinson's disease: a randomised, double-blind, placebo-controlled trial. Lancet Neurol 9(6):573–580, 2010 20452823

Bassett SS: Cognitive impairment in Parkinson's disease. Prim psychiatry 12:50–55, 2005

Beiske AG, Svensson E, Sandanger I, et al: Depression and anxiety amongst multiple sclerosis patients. Eur J Neurol 15(3):239–245, 2008 18215155

Bergh S, Selbaek G, Engedal K: Discontinuation of antidepressants in people with dementia and neuropsychiatric symptoms (DESEP study): double blind randomised, parallel group, placebo controlled trial. BMJ 344:e1566, 2012 22408266

Bernardo CG, Singh V, Thompson PM: Safety and efficacy of psychopharmacological agents used to treat the psychiatric sequelae of common neurological disorders. Expert Opin Drug Saf 7(4):435–445, 2008 18613807

Bhidayasiri R, Fahn S, Weiner WJ, et al; American Academy of Neurology: Evidence-based guideline: treatment of tardive syndromes: report of the Guideline Development Subcommittee of the American Academy of Neurology. Neurology 81(5):463–469, 2013 23897874

Birks JS, Chong LY, Grimley-Evans J: Rivastigmine for Alzheimer's disease. Cochrane Database of Systematic Reviews, 2015 Issue 9. Art. No.: CD001191. DOI: 10.1002/14651858.CD001191.pub2 26393402

Bonelli RM, Hofmann P: A systematic review of the treatment studies in Huntington's disease since 1990. Expert Opin Pharmacother 8(2):141–153, 2007 17257085

Boot BP, Chong LY, Grimley-Evans J: Comprehensive treatment of dementia with Lewy bodies. Alzheimers Res Ther 7(1):45, 2015 26029267

Boxer AL, Knopman DS, Kaufer DI, et al: Memantine in patients with frontotemporal lobar degeneration: a multicentre, randomised, double-blind, placebo-controlled trial. Lancet Neurol 12(2):149–156, 2013 23290598

Broadstock M, Ballard C, Corbett A: Novel pharmaceuticals in the treatment of psychosis in Parkinson's disease. Expert Rev Clin Pharmacol 7(6):779–786, 2014 25301532

Brooks BR, Crumpacker D, Fellus J, et al: PRISM: a novel research tool to assess the prevalence of pseudobulbar affect symptoms across neurological conditions. PLoS One 8(8):e72232, 2013 23991068

Brusa L, Bassi A, Stefani A, et al: Pramipexole in comparison to l-dopa: a neuropsychological study. J Neural Transm (Vienna) 110(4):373–380, 2003 12658365

Brusa L, Tiraboschi P, Koch G, et al: Pergolide effect on cognitive functions in early-mild Parkinson's disease. J Neural Transm (Vienna) 112(2):231–237, 2005 15365788

Brusa L, Pavino V, Massimetti MC, et al: The effect of dopamine agonists on cognitive functions in non-demented early-mild Parkinson's disease patients. Funct Neurol 28(1):13–17, 2013 23731911

Burn D, Emre M, McKeith I, et al: Effects of rivastigmine in patients with and without visual hallucinations in dementia associated with Parkinson's disease. Mov Disord 21(11):1899–1907, 2006 16960863

Caroff SN, Campbell EC, Havey J, et al: Treatment of tardive dyskinesia with donepezil: a pilot study. J Clin Psychiatry 62(10):772–775, 2001 11816865

Carson AJ, MacHale S, Allen K, et al: Depression after stroke and lesion location: a systematic review. Lancet 356(9224):122–126, 2000 10963248

Chan KL, Campayo A, Moser DJ, et al: Aggressive behavior in patients with stroke: association with psychopathology and results of antidepressant treatment on aggression. Arch Phys Med Rehabil 87(6):793–798, 2006 16731214

Chen S, Wu H, Klebe D, et al: Valproic acid: a new candidate of therapeutic application for the acute central nervous system injuries. Neurochem Res 39(9):1621–1633, 2014 24482021

Chiaravalloti ND, DeLuca J: Cognitive impairment in multiple sclerosis. Lancet Neurol 7(12):1139–1151, 2008 19007738

Chiu CT, Wang Z, Hunsberger JG, Chuang DM: Therapeutic potential of mood stabilizers lithium and valproic acid: beyond bipolar disorder. Pharmacol Rev 65(1):105–142, 2013 23300133

Choi-Kwon S, Han SW, Kwon SU, et al: Fluoxetine treatment in poststroke depression, emotional incontinence, and anger proneness: a double-blind, placebo-controlled study. Stroke 37(1):156–161, 2006 16306470

Chou KL, Borek LL, Friedman JH: The management of psychosis in movement disorder patients. Expert Opin Pharmacother 8(7):935–943, 2007 17472539

Christodoulou C, Melville P, Scherl WF, et al: Effects of donepezil on memory and cognition in multiple sclerosis. J Neurol Sci 245(1–2):127–136, 2006 16626752

Clancy MJ, Clarke MC, Connor DJ, et al: The prevalence of psychosis in epilepsy; a systematic review and meta-analysis. BMC Psychiatry 14:75, 2014 24625201

CredibleMeds: Combined list of drugs that prolong QT and/or cause torsades de pointes (TDP). June 15, 2016. Available at: https://crediblemeds.org. Accessed June 21, 2016.

Cummings J, Isaacson S, Mills R, et al: Pimavanserin for patients with Parkinson's disease psychosis: a randomised, placebo-controlled phase 3 trial. Lancet 383(9916):533–540, 2014 24183563

Cummings JL, Lyketsos CG, Peskind ER, et al: Effect of dextromethorphan-quinidine on agitation in patients with Alzheimer disease dementia. A randomized clinical trial. JAMA 314(12):1242–1254, 2015 26393847

De Marchi N, Daniele F, Ragone MA: Fluoxetine in the treatment of Huntington's disease. Psychopharmacology (Berl) 153(2):264–266, 2001 11205429

Devos D, Dujardin K, Poirot I, et al: Comparison of desipramine and citalopram treatments for depression in Parkinson's disease: a double-blind, randomized, placebo-controlled study. Mov Disord 23(6):850–857, 2008 18311826

Dodel R, Csoti I, Ebersbach G, et al: Lewy body dementia and Parkinson's disease with dementia. J Neurol 255 (suppl 5):39–47, 2008 18787881

Ehde DM, Kraft GH, Chwastiak L, et al: Efficacy of paroxetine in treating major depressive disorder in persons with multiple sclerosis. Gen Hosp Psychiatry 30(1):40–48, 2008 18164939

Ellis T, Cudkowicz ME, Sexton PM, Growdon JH: Clozapine and risperidone treatment of psychosis in Parkinson's disease. J Neuropsychiatry Clin Neurosci 12(3):364–369, 2000 10956570

Emre M, Aarsland D, Albanese A, et al: Rivastigmine for dementia associated with Parkinson's disease. N Engl J Med 351(24):2509–2518, 2004 15590953

Falk WE, Mahnke MW, Poskanzer DC: Lithium prophylaxis of corticotropin-induced psychosis. JAMA 241(10):1011–1012, 1979 216818

Farina N, Isaac MG, Clark AR, et al: Vitamin E for Alzheimer's dementia and mild cognitive impairment. Cochrane Database of Systematic Reviews 2012, Issue 11. Art. No.: CD002854. DOI: 10.1002/14651858.CD004854.pub3 23152215

Feinstein A: Neuropsychiatric syndromes associated with multiple sclerosis. J Neurol 254 (suppl 2):II73–II76, 2007 17503134

Feinstein A, O'Connor P, Feinstein K: Multiple sclerosis, interferon beta-1b and depression: a prospective investigation. J Neurol 249(7):815–820, 2002 12140662

Feinstein A, DeLuca J, Baune BT, et al: Cognitive and neuropsychiatric disease manifestations in MS. Mult Scler Relat Disord 2(1):4–12, 2013 25877449

Fernandes C, Reddy P, Kessel B: Rasagiline-induced serotonin syndrome. Mov Disord 26(4):766–767, 2011 21370275

Fernandez HH, Trieschmann ME, Friedman JH: Treatment of psychosis in Parkinson's disease: safety considerations. Drug Saf 26(9):643–659, 2003 12814332

Finger EC, MacKinley J, Blair M, et al: Oxytocin for frontotemporal dementia: a randomized dose-finding study of safety and tolerability. Neurology 84(2):174–181, 2015 25503617

Fischer JS, Priore RL, Jacobs LD, et al; Multiple Sclerosis Collaborative Research Group: Neuropsychological effects of interferon beta-1a in relapsing multiple sclerosis. Ann Neurol 48(6):885–892, 2000 11117545

Fleminger S, Greenwood RJ, Oliver DL: Pharmacological management for agitation and aggression in people with acquired brain injury. Cochrane Database of Systematic Reviews 2006, Issue 4. Art. No.: CD003299. DOI: 10.1002/14651858. CD003299.pub2 17054165

Forsaa EB, Larsen JP, Wentzel-Larsen T, et al: A 12-year population-based study of psychosis in Parkinson disease. Arch Neurol 67(8):996–1001, 2010 20697051

Frieling H, Hillemacher T, Ziegenbein M, et al: Treating dopamimetic psychosis in Parkinson's disease: structured review and meta-analysis. Eur Neuropsychopharmacol 17(3):165–171, 2007 17070675

Galynker I, Ieronimo C, Miner C, et al: Methylphenidate treatment of negative symptoms in patients with dementia. J Neuropsychiatry Clin Neurosci 9(2):231–239, 1997 9144102

Gao K, Kemp DE, Ganocy SJ, et al: Antipsychotic-induced extrapyramidal side effects in bipolar disorder and schizophrenia: a systematic review. J Clin Psychopharmacol 28(2):203–209, 2008 18344731

Ghaffar O, Feinstein A: The neuropsychiatry of multiple sclerosis: a review of recent developments. Curr Opin Psychiatry 20(3):278–285, 2007 17415083

Ghazi-Noori S, Chung TH, Deane K, et al: Therapies for depression in Parkinson's disease. Cochrane Database of Systematic Reviews 2003, Issue 2. Art. No.: CD003465. DOI: 10.1002/14651858.CD003465 12917968

Godschalx-Dekker JA, Siegers HP: Reduction of parkinsonism and psychosis with mirtazapine: a case report. Pharmacopsychiatry 47(3):81–83, 2014 24504487

Goëb JL, Cailleau A, Lainé P, et al: Acute delirium, delusion, and depression during IFN-beta-1a therapy for multiple sclerosis: a case report. Clin Neuropharmacol 26(1):5–7, 2003 12567157

Gonzalez-Heydrich J, Dodds A, Whitney J, et al: Psychiatric disorders and behavioral characteristics of pediatric patients with both epilepsy and attention-deficit hyperactivity disorder. Epilepsy Behav 10(3):384–388, 2007 17368109

Gross A, Devinsky O, Westbrook LE, et al: Psychotropic medication use in patients with epilepsy: effect on seizure frequency. J Neuropsychiatry Clin Neurosci 12(4):458–464, 2000 11083162

Guarnieri R, Hallak JE, Walz R, et al: Pharmacological treatment of psychosis in epilepsy [in Portuguese]. Rev Bras Psiquiatr 26(1):57–61, 2004 15057842

Guerreiro DF, Navarro R, Silva M, et al: Psychosis secondary to traumatic brain injury. Brain Inj 23(4):358–361, 2009 19274520

Hackett ML, Anderson CS, House A, Xia J: Interventions for treating depression after stroke. Cochrane Database of Systematic Reviews 2008, Issue 4. Art. No.: CD003437. DOI: 10.1002/14651858.CD003437.pub3 18843644

Hamberger MJ, Palmese CA, Scarmeas N, et al: A randomized, double-blind, placebo-controlled trial of donepezil to improve memory in epilepsy. Epilepsia 48(7):1283–1291, 2007 17484756

Hammond FM, Bickett AK, Norton JH, et al: Effectiveness of amantadine hydrochloride in the reduction of chronic traumatic brain injury irritability and aggression. J Head Trauma Rehabil 29(5):391–399, 2014 24263176

Hanagasi HA, Gurvit H, Unsalan P, et al: The effects of rasagiline on cognitive deficits in Parkinson's disease patients without dementia: a randomized, double-blind, placebo-controlled, multicenter study. Mov Disord 26(10):1851–1858, 2011 20280150

Hansen RA, Gartlehner G, Webb AP, et al: Efficacy and safety of donepezil, galantamine, and rivastigmine for the treatment of Alzheimer's disease: a systematic review and meta-analysis. Clin Interv Aging 3(2):211–225, 2008 18686744

Hasnain M: Psychosis in Parkinson's disease: therapeutic options. Drugs Today (Barc) 47(5):353–367, 2011 22013566

Hasnain M, Vieweg WV, Baron MS, et al: Pharmacological management of psychosis in elderly patients with parkinsonism. Am J Med 122(7):614–622, 2009 19559160

He D, Zhou H, Guo D, et al: Pharmacological treatment for memory disorder in multiple sclerosis. Cochrane Database of Systematic Reviews 2013, Issue 12. Art. No.: CD008876. DOI: 10.1002/14651858.CD008876.pub3 21975787

Herrmann N, Gauthier S, Boneva N, et al: A randomized, double-blind, placebo-controlled trial of memantine in a behaviorally enriched sample of patients with moderate-to-severe Alzheimer's disease. Int Psychogeriatr 25(6):919–927, 2013 23472619

Hesdorffer DC, Ishihara L, Mynepalli L, et al: Epilepsy, suicidality, and psychiatric disorders: a bidirectional association. Ann Neurol 72(2):184–191, 2012 22887468

Hoffmann T, Ownsworth T, Eames S, Shum D: Evaluation of brief interventions for managing depression and anxiety symptoms during early discharge period after stroke: a pilot randomized controlled trial. Top Stroke Rehabil 22(2):116–126, 2015 25936543

Hogervorst E, Yaffe K, Richards M, Huppert FA: Hormone replacement therapy to maintain cognitive function in women with dementia. Cochrane Database of Systematic Reviews 2009, Issue 1. Art. No.: CD003799. DOI: 10.1002/14651858.CD003799.pub2 19160224

Huey ED, Putnam KT, Grafman J: A systematic review of neurotransmitter deficits and treatments in frontotemporal dementia. Neurology 66(1):17–22, 2006 16401839

Jaturapatporn D, Isaac MG, McCleery J, Tabet N: Aspirin, steroidal and non-steroidal anti-inflammatory drugs for the treatment of Alzheimer's disease. Cochrane Database of Systematic Reviews 2012, Issue 2. Art. No.: CD006378. DOI: 10.1002/14651858.CD006378.pub2 22336816

Johansson B, Wentzel AP, Andréll P, et al: Methylphenidate reduces mental fatigue and improves processing speed in persons suffered a traumatic brain injury. Brain Inj 29(6):758–765, 2015 25794299

Kanner AM: The use of psychotropic drugs in epilepsy: what every neurologist should know. Semin Neurol 28(3):379–388, 2008 18777484

Kaplin A: Depression in multiple sclerosis, in Multiple Sclerosis Therapeutics. Edited by Cohen JA, Rudick R. London, Informa Healthcare, 2007, pp 823–840

Karaiskos D, Tzavellas E, Spengos K, et al: Duloxetine versus citalopram and sertraline in the treatment of poststroke depression, anxiety, and fatigue. J Neuropsychiatry Clin Neurosci 24(3):349–353, 2012 23037649

Kavirajan H, Schneider LS: Efficacy and adverse effects of cholinesterase inhibitors and memantine in vascular dementia: a meta-analysis of randomised controlled trials. Lancet Neurol 6(9):782–792, 2007 17689146

Kertesz A, Morlog D, Light M, et al: Galantamine in frontotemporal dementia and primary progressive aphasia. Dement Geriatr Cogn Disord 25(2):178–185, 2008 18196898

Kim E, Humaran TJ: Divalproex in the management of neuropsychiatric complications of remote acquired brain injury. J Neuropsychiatry Clin Neurosci 14(2):202–205, 2002 11983796

Kim JM, Stewart R, Kang HJ, et al: A prospective study of statin use and poststroke depression. J Clin Psychopharmacol 34(1):72–79, 2014 24304857

Kimura M, Tateno A, Robinson RG: Treatment of poststroke generalized anxiety disorder comorbid with poststroke depression: merged analysis of nortriptyline trials. Am J Geriatr Psychiatry 11(3):320–327, 2003 12724111

Kostić V, Dzoljić E, Todorović Z, et al: Fluoxetine does not impair motor function in patients with Parkinson's disease: correlation between mood and motor functions with plasma concentrations of fluoxetine/norfluoxetine. Vojnosanit Pregl 69(12):1067–1075, 2012 23424961

Kraft GH, Bowen J: Modafinil for fatigue in MS: a randomized placebo-controlled double-blind study. Neurology 65(12):1995–1997, author reply 1995–1997, 2005 16380634

Kraus MF, Maki PM: Effect of amantadine hydrochloride on symptoms of frontal lobe dysfunction in brain injury: case studies and review. J Neuropsychiatry Clin Neurosci 9(2):222–230, 1997 9144101

Kyomen HH, Satlin A, Hennen J, Wei JY: Estrogen therapy and aggressive behavior in elderly patients with moderate-to-severe dementia: results from a short-term, randomized, double-blind trial. Am J Geriatr Psychiatry 7(4):339–348, 1999 10521168

LaFrance WC Jr, Kanner AM, Hermann B: Psychiatric comorbidities in epilepsy. Int Rev Neurobiol 83:347–383, 2008 18929092

Lane-Brown A, Tate R: Interventions for apathy after traumatic brain injury. Cochrane Database of Systematic Reviews 2009, Issue 2. Art. No.: CD006341. DOI: 10.1002/14651858.CD006341.pub2 19370632

Lebert F, Stekke W, Hasenbroekx C, Pasquier F: Frontotemporal dementia: a randomised, controlled trial with trazodone. Dement Geriatr Cogn Disord 17(4):355–359, 2004 15178953

Leeds PR, Yu F, Wang Z, et al: A new avenue for lithium: intervention in traumatic brain injury. ACS Chem Neurosci 5(6):422–433, 2014 24697257

Leroi I, Collins D, Marsh L: Non-dopaminergic treatment of cognitive impairment and dementia in Parkinson's disease: a review. J Neurol Sci 248(1–2):104–114, 2006 16806271

Lou JS, Dimitrova DM, Johnson SC, et al: Modafinil reduces fatigue in PD: a double-blind, placebo-controlled pilot study (abstract). Ann Neurol 62 (suppl 11):S8, 2007

Lucetti C, Bellini G, Nuti A, et al: Treatment of patients with tardive dystonia with olanzapine. Clin Neuropharmacol 25(2):71–74, 2002 11981231

Madhusoodanan S, Alexeenko L, Sanders R, Brenner R: Extrapyramidal symptoms associated with antidepressants—a review of the literature and an analysis of spontaneous reports. Ann Clin Psychiatry 22:148–156, 2010

Maguire MJ, Weston J, Singh J, Marson AG: Antidepressants for people with epilepsy and depression. Cochrane Database of Systematic Reviews 2014, Issue 12. Art. No.: CD010682. DOI: 10.1002/14651858.CD010682.pub2 25464360

McCleery J, Cohen DA, Sharpley AL: Pharmacotherapies for sleep disturbances in Alzheimer's disease. Cochrane Database of Systematic Reviews 2014, Issue 3. Art. No.: CD009178. DOI: 10.1002/14651858.CD009178.pub2 24659320

McGuinness B, Craig D, Bullock R, et al: Statins for the treatment of dementia. Cochrane Database of Systematic Reviews 2014, Issue 7. Art. No.: CD007514. DOI: 10.1002/14651858.CD007514.pub3 25004278

Mendez MF, Shapira JS, McMurtray A, Licht E: Preliminary findings: behavioral worsening on donepezil in patients with frontotemporal dementia. Am J Geriatr Psychiatry 15(1):84–87, 2007 17194818

Mendonça DA, Menezes K, Jog MS: Methylphenidate improves fatigue scores in Parkinson's disease: a randomized controlled trial. Mov Disord 22:2070–2076, 2007 17674415

Menn SJ, Yang R, Lankford A: Armodafinil for the treatment of excessive sleepiness associated with mild or moderate closed traumatic brain injury: a 12-week, randomized, double-blind study followed by a 12-month open-label extension. J Clin Sleep Med 10(11):1181–1191, 2014 25325609

Menza M, Dobkin RD, Marin H, et al: A controlled trial of antidepressants in patients with Parkinson disease and depression. Neurology 72(10):886–892, 2009 19092112

Michals ML, Crismon ML, Roberts S, Childs A: Clozapine response and adverse effects in nine brain-injured patients. J Clin Psychopharmacol 13(3):198–203, 1993 8354736

Mikami K, Jorge RE, Moser DJ, et al: Prevention of poststroke apathy using escitalopram or problem-solving therapy. Am J Geriatr Psychiatry 21(9):855–862, 2013 23930743

Miyasaki JM, Shannon K, Voon V, et al; Quality Standards Subcommittee of the American Academy of Neurology: Practice Parameter: evaluation and treatment of depression, psychosis, and dementia in Parkinson disease (an evidence-based review): report of the Quality Standards Subcommittee of the American Academy of Neurology. Neurology 66(7):996–1002, 2006 16606910

Mohr DC, Boudewyn AC, Goodkin DE, et al: Comparative outcomes for individual cognitive-behavior therapy, supportive-expressive group psychotherapy, and sertraline for the treatment of depression in multiple sclerosis. J Consult Clin Psychol 69(6):942–949, 2001 11777121

Moretti R, Torre P, Antonello RM, et al: Frontotemporal dementia: paroxetine as a possible treatment of behavior symptoms. A randomized, controlled, open 14-month study. Eur Neurol 49(1):13–19, 2003 12464713

Moretti R, Torre P, Antonello RM, et al: Rivastigmine in frontotemporal dementia: an open-label study. Drugs Aging 21(14):931–937, 2004 15554751

Mori E, Ikeda M, Nagai R, et al: Long-term donepezil use for dementia with Lewy bodies: results from an open-label extension of Phase III trial. Alzheimers Res Ther 7(1):5, 2015 25713600

Mula M, Trimble MR, Lhatoo SD, Sander JW: Topiramate and psychiatric adverse events in patients with epilepsy. Epilepsia 44(5):659–663, 2003a 12752464

Mula M, Trimble MR, Yuen A, et al: Psychiatric adverse events during levetiracetam therapy. Neurology 61(5):704–706, 2003b 12963770

Niedermaier N, Bohrer E, Schulte K, et al: Prevention and treatment of poststroke depression with mirtazapine in patients with acute stroke. J Clin Psychiatry 65(12):1619–1623, 2004 15641866

Ozkan B, Wilkins K, Muralee S, Tampi RR: Pharmacotherapy for inappropriate sexual behaviors in dementia: a systematic review of literature. Am J Alzheimers Dis Other Demen 23(4):344–354, 2008 18509106

Peltz G, Pacific DM, Noviasky JA, et al: Seizures associated with memantine use. Am J Health Syst Pharm 62(4):420–421, 2005 15745897

Pioro EP, Brooks BR, Cummings J, et al; Safety, Tolerability, and Efficacy Results Trial of AVP-923 in PBA Investigators: Dextromethorphan plus ultra low-dose quinidine reduces pseudobulbar affect. Ann Neurol 68(5):693–702, 2010 20839238

Porsteinsson AP, Drye LT, Pollock BG, et al; CitAD Research Group: Effect of citalopram on agitation in Alzheimer disease: the CitAD randomized clinical trial. JAMA 311(7):682–691, 2014 24549548

Powell JH, al-Adawi S, Morgan J, Greenwood RJ: Motivational deficits after brain injury: effects of bromocriptine in 11 patients. J Neurol Neurosurg Psychiatry 60(4):416–421, 1996 8774407

Prueter C, Norra C: Mood disorders and their treatment in patients with epilepsy. J Neuropsychiatry Clin Neurosci 17(1):20–28, 2005 15746479

Pucci E, Branãs P, D'Amico R, et al: Amantadine for fatigue in multiple sclerosis. Cochrane Database of Systematic Reviews 2007, Issue 1. Art. No.: CD002818. DOI: 10.1002/14651858.CD002818.pub2 17253480

Rapoport MJ, Chan F, Lanctot K, et al: An open-label study of citalopram for major depression following traumatic brain injury. J Psychopharmacol 22(8):860–864, 2008 18208921

Robinson RG, Parikh RM, Lipsey JR, et al: Pathological laughing and crying following stroke: validation of a measurement scale and a double-blind treatment study. Am J Psychiatry 150(2):286–293, 1993 8422080

Robinson RG, Jorge RE, Moser DJ, et al: Escitalopram and problem-solving therapy for prevention of poststroke depression: a randomized controlled trial. JAMA 299(20):2391–2400, 2008 18505948

Rodda J, Morgan S, Walker Z: Are cholinesterase inhibitors effective in the management of the behavioral and psychological symptoms of dementia in Alzheimer's disease? A systematic review of randomized, placebo-controlled trials of donepezil, rivastigmine and galantamine. Int Psychogeriatr 21(5):813–824, 2009 19538824

Rosenberg PB, Drye LT, Martin BK, et al; DIADS-2 Research Group: Sertraline for the treatment of depression in Alzheimer disease. Am J Geriatr Psychiatry 18(2):136–145, 2010 20087081

Rosenberg PB, Lanctôt KL, Drye LT, et al; ADMET Investigators: Safety and efficacy of methylphenidate for apathy in Alzheimer's disease: a randomized, placebo-controlled trial. J Clin Psychiatry 74(8):810–816, 2013 24021498

Rosenblatt A: Neuropsychiatry of Huntington's disease. Dialogues Clin Neurosci 9(2):191–197, 2007 17726917

Ruffmann C, Bogliun G, Beghi E: Epileptogenic drugs: a systematic review. Expert Rev Neurother 6(4):575–589, 2006 16623656

Santos CO, Caeiro L, Ferro JM, Figueira ML: Mania and stroke: a systematic review. Cerebrovasc Dis 32(1):11–21, 2011 21576938

Schiffer RB, Wineman NM: Antidepressant pharmacotherapy of depression associated with multiple sclerosis. Am J Psychiatry 147(11):1493–1497, 1990 2221162

Schneider LS, Tariot PN, Dagerman KS, et al: Effectiveness of atypical antipsychotic drugs in patients with Alzheimer's disease. N Engl J Med 355(15):1525–1538, 2006 17035647

Schreiber S, Klag E, Gross Y, et al: Beneficial effect of risperidone on sleep disturbance and psychosis following traumatic brain injury. Int Clin Psychopharmacol 13(6):273–275, 1998 9861578

Seitz DP, Adunuri N, Gill SS, et al: Antidepressants for agitation and psychosis in dementia. Cochrane Database of Systematic Reviews 2011, Issue 2. Art. No.: CD008191, DOI: 10.1002/14651858.CD008191.pub2 21328305

Shulman MB, Barr W: Treatment of memory disorders in epilepsy. Epilepsy Behav 3(5S)(suppl):30–34, 2002 12609318

Siegert RJ, Abernethy DA: Depression in multiple sclerosis: a review. J Neurol Neurosurg Psychiatry 76(4):469–475, 2005 15774430

Silver JM, Koumaras B, Meng X, et al: Long-term effects of rivastigmine capsules in patients with traumatic brain injury. Brain Inj 23(2):123–132, 2009a 19191091

Silver JM, McAllister TW, Arciniegas DB: Depression and cognitive complaints following mild traumatic brain injury. Am J Psychiatry 166(6):653–661, 2009b 19487401

Sink KM, Holden KF, Yaffe K: Pharmacological treatment of neuropsychiatric symptoms of dementia: a review of the evidence. JAMA 293(5):596–608, 2005 15687315

Solla P, Bartolato M, Cannas A, et al: Paraphilias and paraphilic disorder in Parkinson's disease: a systematic review of the literature. Mov Disord 30(5):604–613, 2015 25759330

Spivak B, Mester R, Abesgaus J, et al: Clozapine treatment for neuroleptic-induced tardive dyskinesia, parkinsonism, and chronic akathisia in schizophrenic patients. J Clin Psychiatry 58(7):318–322, 1997 9269253

Stocchi F; ADAGIO investigators: Benefits of treatment with rasagiline for fatigue symptoms in patients with early Parkinson's disease. Eur J Neurol 21(2):357–360, 2014 23790011

Sultzer DL, Davis SM, Tariot PN, et al; CATIE-AD Study Group: Clinical symptom responses to atypical antipsychotic medications in Alzheimer's disease: phase 1 outcomes from the CATIE-AD effectiveness trial. Am J Psychiatry 165(7):844–854, 2008 18519523

Tandon R: Safety and tolerability: how do newer generation "atypical" antipsychotics compare? Psychiatr Q 73(4):297–311, 2002 12418358

Tarawneh R, Galvin JE: Distinguishing Lewy body dementias from Alzheimer's disease. Expert Rev Neurother 7(11):1499–1516, 2007 17997699

Tarsy D, Kaufman D, Sethi KD, et al: An open-label study of botulinum toxin A for treatment of tardive dystonia. Clin Neuropharmacol 20(1):90–93, 1997 9037579

Tejani AM, Wasdell M, Spiwak R, et al: Carnitine for fatigue in multiple sclerosis. Cochrane Database Systematic Reviews 2012, Issue 5. Art. No.: CD007280. DOI: 10.1002/14651858.CD007280.pub3 22592719

Tenovuo O: Central acetylcholinesterase inhibitors in the treatment of chronic traumatic brain injury—clinical experience in 111 patients. Prog Neuropsychopharmacol Biol Psychiatry 29(1):61–67, 2005 15610946

Tramontana MG, Cowan RL, Zald D, et al: Traumatic brain injury-related attention deficits: treatment outcomes with lisdexamfetamine dimesylate (Vyvanse). Brain Inj 28(11):1461–1472, 2014 24988121

Tucker I: Management of inappropriate sexual behaviors in dementia: a literature review. Int Psychogeriatr 22(5):683–692, 2010 20226113

Voon V, Fox SH: Medication-related impulse control and repetitive behaviors in Parkinson disease. Arch Neurol 64(8):1089–1096, 2007 17698698

Warden DL, Gordon B, McAllister TW, et al; Neurobehavioral Guidelines Working Group: Guidelines for the pharmacologic treatment of neurobehavioral sequelae of traumatic brain injury. J Neurotrauma 23(10):1468–1501, 2006 17020483

Weintraub D, Siderowf AD, Potenza MN, et al: Association of dopamine agonist use with impulse control disorders in Parkinson disease. Arch Neurol 63(7):969–973, 2006 16831966

Weintraub D, Rosenberg PB, Drye LT, et al: Sertraline for the treatment of depression in Alzheimer disease: week-24 outcomes. Am J Geriatr Psychiatry. 18(4):332–340, 2010 20220589

Weintraub D, Chen P, Ignacio RV, et al: Patterns and trends in antipsychotic prescribing for Parkinson disease patients. Arch Neurol 68(7):899–904, 2011 21747029

Wenzel RG, Tepper S, Korab WE, et al: Serotonin syndrome risks when combining SSRI/SNRI drugs and triptans: is the FDA's alert warranted? Ann Pharmacother 42:1692–1696, 2008 18957623

Wesnes KA, McKeith IG, Ferrara R, et al: Effects of rivastigmine on cognitive function in dementia with Lewy bodies: a randomised placebo-controlled international study using the cognitive drug research computerised assessment system. Dement Geriatr Cogn Disord 13(3):183–192, 2002 11893841

Wood LD, Neumiller JJ, Setter SM, Dobbins EK: Clinical review of treatment options for select nonmotor symptoms of Parkinson's disease. Am J Geriatr Pharmacother 8(4):294–315, 2010 20869620

Wortzel HS, Oster TJ, Anderson CA, Arciniegas DB: Pathological laughing and crying: epidemiology, pathophysiology and treatment. CNS Drugs 22(7):531–545, 2008 18547124

Yeh YC, Ouyang WC: Mood stabilizers for the treatment of behavioral and psychological symptoms of dementia: an update review. Kaohsiung J Med Sci 28(4):185–193, 2012 22453066

Zahodne LB, Fernandez HH: Pathophysiology and treatment of psychosis in Parkinson's disease: a review. Drugs Aging 25(8):665–682, 2008 18665659

Zephir H, De Seze J, Stojkovic T, et al: Multiple sclerosis and depression: influence of interferon beta therapy. Mult Scler 9(3):284–288, 2003 12814176

Zhang L, Plotkin RC, Wang G, et al: Cholinergic augmentation with donepezil enhances recovery in short-term memory and sustained attention after traumatic brain injury. Arch Phys Med Rehabil 85(7):1050–1055, 2004 15241749

Zheng L, Mack WJ, Dagerman KS, et al: Metabolic changes associated with second-generation antipsychotic use in Alzheimer's disease patients: the CATIE-AD study. Am J Psychiatry 166(5):583–590, 2009 19369318

10

Endocrine and Metabolic Disorders

Stephen J. Ferrando, M.D.

Sahi Munjal, M.D.

Jennifer Kraker, M.D., M.S.

Disorders of the endocrine system are well known for their prominent psychiatric manifestations due to their interrelationship with the nervous system. Generally, correction of the underlying endocrine disorder will lead to improvement in psychiatric symptoms; however, symptoms may persist beyond the restoration of normal serum hormone levels, in which case psychopharmacological agents are often prescribed.

Three important clinical dimensions are covered in this chapter: 1) primary endocrine disorders and their treatments may cause or exacerbate psychiatric symptoms via alterations of serum hormone levels (Table 10–1; see also Table 10–4 later in this chapter), 2) psychiatric disorders may play a role in endocrine dysregulation (e.g., depression exacerbates insulin resistance and

Table 10–1.　Psychiatric symptoms of endocrine and metabolic disorders

Endocrine/metabolic condition	Psychiatric symptoms
Acromegaly (overproduction of growth hormone)	Mood lability, personality change
Addison's disease	Apathy, depression, fatigue
Cushing's disease/syndrome	Depression, anxiety, mania, psychosis
Diabetes	Depression, anxiety, cognitive dysfunction
Hyperparathyroidism	Depression, apathy, psychosis, delirium
Hyperprolactinemia	Depression, anxiety, sexual dysfunction
Hyperthyroidism	Anxiety, irritability, mania, apathy, depression, psychosis
Hypogonadism	Decreased libido, low energy, low mood
Hypothyroidism	Depression, psychosis, delirium, "myxedema madness"
Pheochromocytoma	Anxiety, panic

impairs glycemic control in diabetes), and 3) psychiatric medications often cause endocrine side effects (see Table 10–2 later in this chapter).

In general, psychopharmacological treatment in the patient with endocrine dysfunction must accompany correction of the underlying hormone disorder. Psychopharmacological agents are generally prescribed when 1) psychiatric symptoms predate the endocrine disorder, 2) the patient presents with acute behavioral dysregulation as endocrine treatment is under way, or 3) psychiatric symptoms persist after the endocrine disorder is treated. No psychopharmacological treatment literature exists for several endocrine disorders with psychiatric manifestations; the psychiatric symptom treatment literature focuses on correction of the hormonal dysfunction. These disorders—Cushing's disease, Addison's disease, and growth hormone disorders—are not covered explicitly in this chapter, and the reader is referred to standard endocrinology texts.

Diabetes Mellitus

Diabetes has significant associations with psychiatric disorders. Although estimates vary, rates of overall mental disorders, particularly anxiety and depression, are 1.5–2 times higher among people with either type 1 or type 2 diabetes than in the general population (Das et al. 2007). Patients with schizophrenia, independent of antipsychotic medication use, are 2–3 times more likely than the general population to have type 2 diabetes (Smith et al. 2008; Stubbs et al. 2015), and up to 50% of patients with bipolar disorder and 26% of patients with schizoaffective disorder have type 2 diabetes (Regenold et al. 2002; Stubbs et al. 2015). Psychopharmacological treatments of psychiatric comorbidities may cause diabetes (see the subsection "Psychotropic-Induced Metabolic Syndrome" later in this chapter).

Differential diagnostic considerations for psychiatric symptoms in diabetes include prior history of psychiatric disorder, acute mood and cognitive effects of hyperglycemia and hypoglycemia, cognitive and behavioral impairment resulting from central nervous system microvascular disease, and common medical comorbidities and their treatments (e.g., cardiovascular, renal disease) that cause or exacerbate neuropsychiatric symptoms.

Depression

Depression in diabetes is associated with poor adherence to dietary and medication treatment; functional impairment; poor glycemic control; increased risk of diabetic complications, such as microvascular and macrovascular disease; increased medical costs; and mortality (Ciechanowski et al. 2000; de Groot et al. 2001; Plener et al. 2015). Studies have examined whether treatment of depression is associated with improved glycemic control, possibly through 1) improvement in adherence to diabetes treatment, 2) reversal of depression-induced physiological changes such as hypercortisolism, and/or 3) the potential direct euglycemic effects of antidepressant medication. There is conflicting evidence regarding the relationship of antidepressants to glycemic control. For instance, in a longitudinal study, antidepressant use did not influence the overall glycemic control in diabetes patients (Knol et al. 2008), but a retrospective cohort analysis found antidepressant use to be associated with an increased risk of diabetes (Khoza et al. 2012), and a meta-analysis found fluoxetine to be associated with improved glycemic control (Ye et al. 2011).

There has been some debate in the literature and among clinicians as to whether or not tricyclic antidepressants (TCAs) are prone to exacerbate glycemic control in diabetic patients compared with selective serotonin reuptake inhibitors (SSRIs). For instance, one early study found nortriptyline superior to placebo for depression, but nortriptyline was associated with poor glycemic control (Lustman et al. 1997). Overall, there are few data to support this contention. In general, TCAs may be helpful for patients with depression as well as painful diabetic peripheral neuropathy; however, the risks of weight gain and exacerbation of autonomic neuropathy (e.g., gastroparesis, postural hypotension) may bear important considerations, especially with tertiary-amine agents. In terms of SSRIs, a meta-analysis of five placebo-controlled trials of fluoxetine in adults with type 2 diabetes found fluoxetine to be more associated with weight loss (−4.3 kg) as well as improvement of fasting glucose and triglycerides compared with placebo in diabetic patients (Ye et al. 2011).

Maintenance antidepressant treatment is often necessary for depressed diabetic patients. In the acute treatment studies, as few as 4 in 10 diabetic patients with depression remained well after 1 year of successful treatment; approximately 15% had chronic treatment-resistant depression, and depression recurrence was associated with a decline in glycemic control (Lustman et al. 2006). In a multisite randomized controlled trial (RCT) comparing sertraline maintenance (after initial open-label response) with placebo in prevention of depression recurrence, sertraline-treated patients were half as likely to have a recurrence, time to recurrence was four times longer, and glycemic control was maintained when depression remained in remission (Lustman et al. 2006). However, in a multisite study, both sertraline and diabetes-specific cognitive-behavior therapy were effective for depression in only 46% of patients, and glycemic control was unchanged over the course of a year, suggesting that additional intervention is needed to both address depression and enhance glycemic control over time (Petrak et al. 2013).

The Pathways Study examined whether enhancing quality of care for depression in primary care improved both depression and diabetes outcomes

(Katon et al. 2004). Patients with diabetes and persistent depressive disorder (dysthymia) were randomly assigned to a stepped case management intervention or usual care. The intervention provided enhanced education and support of antidepressant medication treatment or problem-solving therapy. After 1 year, intervention patients showed greater improvement in adequacy of dosage of antidepressant medication treatment, less depression severity, a higher rating of patient-rated global improvement, and higher satisfaction with care, but glycemic control did not differ between the two groups. A subsequent study found that coordinated care management of depression and diabetes improved both outcomes in these patients. The intervention involved proactive follow-up by nurse care managers working closely with physicians, integrating the management of medical and psychological illnesses, and using individualized antidepressant treatment regimens guided by treat-to-target principles (Katon et al. 2010).

Anxiety

The association between diabetes and anxiety has been studied less thoroughly than that between diabetes and depression, even though anxiety symptoms and disorders may be more prevalent in patients with diabetes. A review of 18 studies (N= 4,076) found that 27% of individuals with diabetes had an anxiety disorder, and 40% reported subclinical anxiety symptoms (Grigsby et al. 2002). Like depression in patients with diabetes, anxiety is associated with poor glucose control and an increase in the reporting of symptoms (Roberts et al. 2015). A 3-month RCT of alprazolam (maximum 2 mg/day) treatment of generalized anxiety disorder showed a clinically significant reduction in anxiety symptoms and decreased hemoglobin A1c levels (Lustman et al. 1995).

Thyroid Disorders

Hypothyroidism

Clinical hypothyroidism is often associated with depressive symptoms, including depressed mood, fatigue, hypersomnolence, cognitive impairment, difficulty concentrating, and weight gain. However, the relationship between clinical depression and hypothyroidism remains unclear, with some studies finding an association and others not (Dayan and Panicker 2013; Demartini et al. 2014). An association between depression and subclinical hypothyroidism (defined biochemically as a normal serum free thyroxine [T_4] concentration in the presence of an elevated serum thyroid-stimulating hormone [TSH] concentration) is even less clear (Almeida et al. 2011; Blum et al. 2016; de Jongh et al. 2011). Subclinical thyroid dysfunction is largely a laboratory diagnosis that merits observation but not necessarily treatment. Watchful waiting is preferable in patients ages ≥65 years with mild subclinical hypothyroidism (TSH < 10 mU/L) unless they have prominent mood, cognitive, or medical conditions—such as congestive heart failure or hyperlipidemia—that could benefit from early thyroid replacement. In adults ages < 65 years, consider TSH 4.5–10 mU/L as a threshold for initiating thyroid replacement, particularly if anti–thyroid peroxidase antibodies are present (although prevailing recommendations still favor the watchful waiting approach) (Surks et al. 2004). Multiple studies have shown no evidence to support an association between subclinical hypothyroidism and cognitive impairment in relatively healthy older adults (Akintola et al. 2015; Parsaik et al. 2014). Profound hypothyroidism can produce psychosis ("myxedema madness"), delirium, and catatonia. A corticosteroid-responsive encephalopathy has been reported with Hashimoto's thyroiditis, persistent antithyroid antibodies, and adequate T_4 therapy (Fatourechi 2005). Symptomatic management with psychotropics may be required in these conditions; however, there is no guidance in the literature.

Some patients with treated hypothyroidism experience residual symptoms of low mood, fatigue, and cognitive impairment while on stable T_4 monotherapy. Some debate exists over the benefit of supplementing T_4 with low doses of triiodothyronine (T_3). Most guidelines show no additional benefit to combination $T_4 + T_3$ treatment, with the additional disadvantage of thyrotoxic side effects (most commonly palpitations and anxiety) (Garber et al. 2012; Jonklaas et al. 2014; Okosieme et al. 2016).

Little literature is available on antidepressant treatment of patients with hypothyroidism. One case series of psychiatrically hospitalized depressed hypothyroid patients compellingly documented poor response to antidepressants and electroconvulsive therapy without correction of serum T_4 (Russ and Ackerman 1989). Rapid cycling and lithium refractoriness have been associated with clinical and subclinical hypothyroidism in patients with bipolar disorder, underscoring the need for thyroid monitoring and treatment (see the subsection "Lithium-Induced Hypothyroidism" later in this chapter).

Hyperthyroidism

Psychiatric symptoms of overt and subclinical hyperthyroidism include heightened anxiety and mood symptoms and diminished quality of life (Gulseren et al. 2006). Patients with hyperthyroidism have significant psychiatric comorbidity. A population-based study reported 33% and 39% of patients were treated with antidepressants and anxiolytics, respectively, and hyperthyroid patients had an increased risk of psychiatric hospitalization (Brandt et al. 2013). Hyperthyroidism has also been shown to increase the risk of developing bipolar disorder (Hu et al. 2013). A population-based study reported that persons with subclinical hyperthyroidism (suppressed TSH with normal T_4) appear to have a modest increased risk of depression (Kvetny et al. 2015). Apathetic hyperthyroidism, characterized by apathy, somnolence, psychomotor retardation, and cognitive impairment, has also been reported, particularly in elderly patients (Wagle et al. 1998). Finally, psychosis and acute encephalopathy can occur, perhaps related to high antithyroid antibody concentrations in the central nervous system (Barker et al. 1996).

Anxiety, affective, and cognitive symptoms usually remit within weeks to months after normalization of thyroid function (Kathol and Delahunt 1986). Some studies, however, report residual symptoms that require psychopharmacological treatment (Fahrenfort et al. 2000).

β-Blockers, particularly propranolol, are part of standard therapy for hyperthyroidism, targeting adrenergic symptoms of anxiety, tremor, palpitations, and tachycardia. High-dose propranolol (and perhaps some other, but not all, β-blockers) reduces the transformation of T_4 to T_3 (Wiersinga and Touber 1977), but this is probably not a major contribution to the drug's clinical benefits. Lithium is an effective adjunct to antithyroid drugs and propranolol in the treatment of hyperthyroid-induced mania (Brownlie et al. 2000). Benzodiazepines are not recommended for long-term use, but one study documented benefit from the addition of the long-acting benzodiazepine bromazepam to antithyroid agents and propranolol for acute hyperthyroid symptoms (Benvenga 1996). Antipsychotic medications are used for severe agitation, mania, and psychosis, but no systematic data are available regarding their use in thyrotoxicosis. Antidepressants for patients with Graves' disease have received little attention and should likely be reserved for persistent anxiety and depression after antithyroid treatment with normal serum thyroid levels.

Hyperparathyroidism

Psychiatric symptoms associated with hyperparathyroidism include fatigue, depression, and cognitive impairment; in rare cases, delirium, psychosis, and mania occur (Brown et al. 2007; Das et al. 2007; Roman and Sosa 2007). Some studies of parathyroidectomy for patients with asymptomatic hyperparathyroidism documented improvements in health-related quality of life, depression, and neuropsychological testing (Roman and Sosa 2007; Roman et al. 2005; Wilhelm et al. 2004). Pooled data from randomized trials suggest that surgical treatment is superior to surveillance in the domain of emotional role functioning in patients with primary asymptomatic hyperparathyroidism (Cheng et al. 2015). In one study, 27% of patients taking antidepressants presurgically were able to discontinue antidepressant treatment, suggesting that although some patients improve, a substantial number continue to require antidepressant treatment after surgery (Wilhelm et al. 2004). Lithium can also induce hyperparathyroidism, as discussed later in the chapter.

Pheochromocytoma

Pheochromocytoma has been associated with anxiety and panic symptoms; however, development of anxiety disorders per se is rare (Starkman et al. 1990). Both TCAs and SSRIs have unmasked silent pheochromocytomas (Korzets et al. 1997; Lefebvre et al. 1995). The presumed mechanism of TCAs is via inhibition of neuronal uptake of the high circulating levels of catecholamines (Korzets et al. 1997). Monoamine oxidase inhibitors (MAOIs) would be expected to be even more hazardous. The mechanism with SSRIs is less clear (Seelen et al. 1997). However, antidepressants that increase norepinephrine can result in false positive laboratory tests for pheochromocytoma (Neary et al. 2011).

Antidiuretic Hormone

The syndrome of inappropriate antidiuretic hormone (vasopressin) secretion is discussed in Chapter 2, "Severe Drug Reactions," and Chapter 5, "Renal and Urological Disorders." A discussion of lithium-induced nephrogenic diabetes insipidus appears in the section "Endocrinological Side Effects of Psychiatric Medications" later in this chapter and in Chapter 5.

Reproductive Endocrine System Disorders

Disorders of the female reproductive endocrine system are discussed in Chapter 11, "Obstetrics and Gynecology." Hyperprolactinemia is discussed in the section "Endocrinological Side Effects of Psychiatric Medications" later in this chapter.

Hypogonadal Disorders

Low serum testosterone, or hypogonadism, in men is associated with aging and many chronic illnesses. Hypogonadism may cause depressed mood, low energy, and sexual and cognitive dysfunction. Testosterone replacement in aging men is controversial; however, it has become commonplace in some illnesses, such as HIV/AIDS (see Chapter 12, "Infectious Diseases").

In randomized and open-label extension trials in hypogonadal men, transdermal testosterone and 1% testosterone gel replacement therapy were associated with positive effects on fatigue, mood (increased wellness, sociability, decreased anger, anxiety, irritability), and sexual function, as well as with significant increases in sexual activity (Burris et al. 1992; McNicholas et al. 2003; Sih et al. 1997; Wang et al. 2004). Two RCTs demonstrated efficacy for testosterone gel and intramuscular injection augmentation of SSRIs in men with SSRI-refractory major depression (Pope et al. 2003; Seidman et al. 2005). In one RCT of depressed men with low or low-normal testosterone levels who continued to take serotonergic antidepressants, treatment with exogenous testosterone was associated with a significant improvement in sexual function, particularly including ejaculatory ability (Amiaz et al. 2011). In an open-label trial in men with congestive heart failure and hypogonadism, depot testosterone (100 mg every other week) resulted in delayed time to ischemia, improvements in mood, and reductions in total cholesterol and tumor necrosis factor alpha (Malkin et al. 2004). However, this group of researchers observed contrasting results in a subsequent placebo-controlled trial of testosterone transdermal patch therapy for exercise capacity and heart failure symptom improvement (Malkin et al. 2006). Overall, in a meta-analysis, testosterone replacement therapy has been shown to have modest beneficial effects on mood in men younger than 60 years but not in men older than 60 years (Amanatkar et al. 2014).

Testosterone replacement therapy has also been shown to have modest positive effects on various measures of cognitive function in hypogonadal men (Borst et al. 2014; Cherrier et al. 2015; Thilers et al. 2006). Psychiatric adverse effects of testosterone therapy are covered in the section "Psychiatric Side Effects of Endocrine Treatments" later in this chapter.

Endocrinological Side Effects of Psychiatric Medications

The endocrinological adverse effects of psychotropic medications, including antidepressants, antipsychotics, and mood stabilizers, are summarized in Table 10–2.

Lithium Effects on the Thyroid

Lithium has multifaceted effects on the thyroid axis. Lithium interferes with thyroid uptake of iodine and the iodination of tyrosine, alters thyroglobulin structure, and inhibits release of T_4 (Lazarus 1998). These effects of lithium have been used clinically, albeit rarely, to enhance the effectiveness of radioactive iodine when treating thyrotoxicosis (Bogazzi et al. 1999). Lithium increases TSH by decreasing T_4 and T_3 and by independently evoking an exaggerated TSH response to thyrotropin-releasing hormone. Exaggerated elevation of TSH is probably the main cause of goiter formation, reported in 3%–60% of lithium-treated patients (Lazarus 1998). Lithum-associated thyrotoxicosis and thyromegaly are rare but important adverse effects of lithium therapy. Surgery is an effective and preferred treatment for thyroid enlargement that causes airway compression, especially for substernal goiter (Verma et al. 2012).

Lithium-Induced Hypothyroidism

Lithium has been shown to increase the risk of developing hypothyroidism, up to sixfold in a recent meta-analysis (McKnight et al. 2012). However, most such patients are asymptomatic, and the diagnosis is purely biochemical. There is no evidence as to whether stopping lithium tends to lead to a recovery of thyroid function when function is abnormal (McKnight et al. 2012). Individuals taking lithium, those older than 60 years, women, and people with diabetes all had a significantly raised risk of hypothyroidism (Shine et al. 2015).

Table 10–2. Endocrinological adverse effects of psychotropic drugs

Medication	Endocrinological adverse effects
Antidepressants	
SSRIs or SNRIs	Hyperprolactinemia, hypoglycemia (rare), hypothyroidism (rare)
TCAs	Hyperglycemia
Tertiary-amine TCAs (e.g., imipramine, amitriptyline, clomipramine)	Hyperprolactinemia
Antipsychotics	
Atypical and typical antipsychotics	Hyperglycemia, hyperprolactinemia, hypogonadism
Mood stabilizers	
Lithium	Hypothyroidism, hyperthyroidism, hyperparathyroidism, nephrogenic diabetes insipidus
Carbamazepine	Hypothyroidism, decreased FSH and LH, hypogonadism
Valproic acid	Hypothyroidism, decreased FSH and LH, hyperandrogenism (women)

Note. FSH = follicle-stimulating hormone; LH = luteinizing hormone; SNRIs = serotonin-norepinephrine reuptake inhibitors; SSRIs = selective serotonin reuptake inhibitors; TCAs = tricyclic antidepressants.

There are various risk factors for the development of lithium-induced hypothyroidism, including female sex (Ahmadi-Abhari et al. 2003), preexisting vulnerability to autoimmune thyroiditis (Baethge et al. 2005), first-degree relatives with thyroid anomalies (Kusalic and Engelsmann 1999), increased duration of treatment, age older than 50 years (Ozpoyraz et al. 2002), and weight gain of more than 5 kg while receiving treatment (Cayköylü et al. 2002).

In one study, lithium-induced hypothyroidism developed in 38% of patients treated for bipolar disorder and was also correlated with a slower response to acute treatment and poorer quality of long-term remission (Fagiolini et al. 2006). It is controversial whether subclinical hypothyroidism is more prevalent than clinical hypothyroidism in patients undergoing lithium therapy. In one study of 132 outpatients receiving lithium therapy, 39% had subclinical hypothyroidism versus 3% with clinical hypothyroidism (Deodhar et al. 1999). However, in a study of 79 patients taking lithium, 11% developed subclinical hypothyroidism versus 24% with clinical hypothyroidism (van Melick et al. 2010).

Thyroid function tests (serum TSH, free thyroid hormone T_4 and T_3 concentrations, and thyroid autoantibodies) and clinical assessment of thyroid size are recommended for patients initiating lithium therapy at baseline and annually thereafter (Kibirige et al. 2013). A mild increase in TSH and a decrease in T_4 may be seen during the first few months of treatment; these effects are usually self-limited, and T_4 replacement is unwarranted (Maarbjerg et al. 1987). If clinically significant hypothyroidism develops or subclinical effects persist after 4 months of lithium treatment, T_4 replacement or a switch to an alternative mood stabilizer (e.g., valproate) is recommended (Kleiner et al. 1999).

Lithium-Induced Hyperthyroidism

Cases of hyperthyroidism have occurred with lithium treatment (Brownlie et al. 1976) but much less commonly than have cases of hypothyroidism and goiter. This phenomenon is documented primarily in case reports (Bogazzi et al. 1999). One study with 15-year follow-up found only one case of hyperthyroidism in 976 patients (Bocchetta et al. 2007). Because lithium is best known for inducing hypothyroidism and has even been used to treat refractory hyperthyroidism (Kessler et al. 2014), it seems paradoxical that it can induce hyperthyroidism. An observational trial demonstrated significant improvement in the cure rate of hyperthyroidism when lithium was added to radioactive iodine (Kessler et al. 2014). Lithium-induced hyperthyroidism may be missed because it is often transient, asymptomatic, and followed by hypothyroidism (Stowell and Barnhill 2005).

Lithium-induced or exacerbated autoimmune thyroiditis is the likely explanation for hyperthyroidism. Also, because lithium is concentrated within the thyroid, it is postulated that lithium might directly damage thyroid follicular cells, triggering temporary release of thyroglobulin into the circulation and causing thyrotoxicosis (Mizukami et al. 1995).

Although no treatment guidelines are available for lithium-induced hyperthyroidism, a switch from lithium to an alternative mood stabilizer is generally necessary. In the interim, sedative-hypnotics, benzodiazepines, β-blockers, and antipsychotic medications may be employed to treat the spectrum of activation symptoms.

Lithium and Hyperparathyroidism

Hyperparathyroidism is an underrecognized and frequent side effect of long-term lithium therapy. Primary hyperparathyroidism in patients receiving lithium has an absolute risk of 10% (vs. 0.1% of the general population). The risk of hyperparathyroidism is probably attributable to lithium's inactivation of the calcium-sensing receptor and interference with intracellular second messenger signaling. This effect leads to an increased release of parathyroid hormone, which raises calcium concentrations in serum (McKnight et al. 2012; Szalat et al. 2009). Considering that thyroid and parathyroid abnormalities can occur in about 25% of patients receiving lithium therapy, clinical monitoring should reflect this finding, and routine screening for hypercalcemia should be done along with the thyroid tests (McKnight et al. 2012; Saunders et al. 2009). However, although increases in parathyroid hormone during lithium treatment are common (14% of patients during the first 18 months in a recent study), clinically significant increases in calcium are much less common (Albert et al. 2015). Other studies have found higher rates of hyperparathyroidism with elevated calcium levels, especially in patients who were also vitamin D deficient (Meehan et al. 2015). Cessation of lithium often does not correct the hyperparathyroidism, necessitating parathyroidectomy. Although hyperparathyroidism is a risk factor for osteoporosis, patients taking lithium who have normal calcium and parathyroid hormone levels do not have an increased risk of osteoporosis. One study even found that maintenance therapy with lithium carbonate may actually preserve or enhance bone mass (Zamani et al. 2009).

Lithium and Nephrogenic Diabetes Insipidus

Lithium impairs antidiuretic hormone–induced water reabsorption in the cortical and medullary collecting tubules of the kidney, resulting in nephrogenic diabetes insipidus (NDI). Lithium-induced NDI occurs in upward of 15% of lithium-treated patients and is more prone to occur with higher dosages and longer treatment duration. Polydipsia and polyuria are observed clinically. In severe cases, dehydration, renal failure, and lithium toxicity may occur because of a combination of water diuresis and lithium-induced natriuresis. Confirmation of NDI requires a water deprivation test, followed by a vasopressin challenge. Inability to concentrate urine (greater than twofold increase in urine osmolality following 8-hour water deprivation) is suggestive of diabetes insipidus. NDI is confirmed by no change in urine osmolality over 1–2 hours following subcutaneous administration of 5 U vasopressin. The syndrome generally remits from days to weeks after discontinuation of lithium. If lithium is continued, ample fluid intake is indicated. The potassium-sparing diuretic amiloride may be used to treat lithium-induced NDI (Rej et al. 2012). In addition to sparing potassium, amiloride causes less natriuresis, lithium reabsorption, and volume contraction compared with other diuretics, thus reducing the risks for lithium toxicity, dehydration, and renal failure (Boton et al. 1987).

Psychotropic-Induced Metabolic Syndrome

Antipsychotics, both typical and atypical, are associated with metabolic syndrome, with prevalence rates around 30%–50% (Centorrino et al. 2012; Ko et al. 2013; Kraemer et al. 2011). TCAs, valproic acid, and lithium have also been implicated. Metabolic syndrome is defined by five criteria: abdominal obesity, triglycerides >150 mg/dL (>1.7 mmol/L), high-density lipoprotein (HDL) <40 mg/dL (<1.03 mmol/L) for men or <50 mg/dL (<1.28 mmol/L) for women, blood pressure >130/85 mm Hg, and fasting glucose >110 mg/dL (>6.0 mmol/L) (Expert Panel on Detection, Evaluation, and Treatment of High Blood Cholesterol in Adults 2001). Metabolic syndrome is an independent risk factor for diabetes (including ketoacidosis) and for cardiovascular, cerebrovascular, and peripheral vascular disease (Wilson et al. 2003).

All typical and atypical antipsychotics have a U.S. Food and Drug Administration black box warning that they may cause metabolic syndrome. The extent to which metabolic syndrome is solely a function of antipsychotic treatment is controversial. Compared with the general population, risk for metabolic syndrome is similarly elevated in the diagnostic subgroups with severe mental illness (Vancampfort et al. 2015). Overall, the development of metabolic syndrome is likely caused by inherent susceptibility, lifestyle, diet, and medication effects.

Generally, antipsychotic-induced metabolic changes are proportional to weight gain, which has been related to blockade of histamine H_2 and 5-hydroxytryptamine (serotonin; 5-HT) 2C receptors and to increased levels of insulin and leptin (Nasrallah 2003). Prospective data show mean weight increases during the first year of therapy of 6–12 kg for patients taking clozapine, 3–12 kg for olanzapine, 2–4 kg for quetiapine, and 2–3 kg for risperidone. Aripiprazole and ziprasidone are weight neutral. Elevations in serum triglycerides and low-density lipoprotein cholesterol as well as diminished HDL cholesterol usually occur in parallel, but these changes may exist in the absence of weight gain.

Patients taking antipsychotics should be monitored for weight gain, hypertension, glucose intolerance, and lipid derangements. Guidelines for patient monitoring are summarized in Table 10–3.

Treatment of metabolic syndrome begins with dosage adjustment when this has been shown to be beneficial (e.g., olanzapine) or cross-tapering to a more weight-neutral medication (e.g., aripiprazole, ziprasidone, molindone). Techniques including dietary education, exercise, and cognitive-behavioral interventions have been found in RCTs to be effective for either maintaining or losing weight in patients treated with an atypical antipsychotic. Meta-analysis suggests that adjunctive metformin (750 mg/day or even lower) is an effective, safe, and reasonable choice for antipsychotic-induced weight gain and metabolic abnormalities (Zheng et al. 2015).

Hyperprolactinemia

Hyperprolactinemia is a relatively common side effect of antipsychotics. The main physiological action of prolactin is to initiate and maintain lactation. Dopamine D_2 receptors of the pituitary lactotrophs, when activated by dopamine, suppress prolactin gene expression and lactotroph proliferation. Normal ranges of serum prolactin have an upper limit of 10 ng/mL for men and 15 ng/mL for women. Hyperprolactinemia is generally defined as prolactin>20 ng/mL (20 μg/L SI units) and may be physiological or pathogenic.

Hyperprolactinemia may cause impotence, menstrual dysregulation, infertility, and sexual dysfunction, primarily via inhibition of the pulsatile secretion of gonadotropin-releasing hormone (Bostwick et al. 2009). Symptoms of sexual dysfunction for men include loss of libido and erectile and ejaculatory dysfunction (Holtmann et al. 2003); for women, symptoms include loss of libido and anorgasmia (Canuso et al. 2002). Elevated prolactin may also give rise to galactorrhea and gynecomastia (Windgassen et al. 1996). Emerging evidence suggests long-term sequelae, including loss of bone mineral density, increasing the

Table 10–3.   Consensus guidelines for monitoring metabolic status in patients taking antipsychotic medications

Metabolic risk parameter	Baseline	4 weeks	8 weeks	12 weeks	Quarterly	Annually	Every 5 years
Personal or family history of DM or CVD	X					X	
Weight (BMI)	X	X	X	X	X		
Waist circumference	X					X	
Blood pressure	X			X		X	
Fasting plasma glucose	X			X		X	
Fasting lipid profile	X			X			X

Note.   BMI=body mass index (weight in kg/[height in m^2]); CVD=cardiovascular disease; DM=diabetes mellitus.
Source.   Adapted from American Diabetes Association et al. 2004.

risk for osteoporosis (Crews and Howes 2012; O'Keane and Meaney 2005); breast cancer (Tworoger and Hankinson 2006); and cardiovascular disease (Serri et al. 2006). Because bone loss may occur because of hyperprolactinemia-mediated hypogonadism, bone mineral density should be evaluated in patients with persistent high prolactin and reproductive dysfunction (Ajmal et al. 2014).

Antipsychotics are the most common drug-induced cause of hyperprolactinemia, but antidepressants, opioids, antiemetics, and antihypertensives may also be causal. An increase in serum prolactin usually occurs within hours of initiation of antipsychotic medication (Goode et al. 1981). There is recent evidence that hyperprolactinemia may be present in up to 39% of patients with schizophrenia independent of antipsychotic medication (Riecher-Rössler et al. 2013). Although there are reports of drug-induced hyperprolactinemia with serum concentrations of prolactin exceeding 200 ng/mL, this degree of elevation is rare, and other causes of hyperprolactinemia should be explored. Risk factors for drug-induced hyperprolactinemia include increased potency of D_2 blockade (Tsuboi et al. 2013), female sex, and increased age (Kinon et al. 2003) and perhaps schizophrenia itself (Riecher-Rössler et al. 2013). Additionally, an increased risk is identified in those with the cytochrome P450 (CYP) 2D6*10 allele (Ozdemir et al. 2007).

Risk for hyperprolactinemia with antipsychotics and antiemetics is proportional to potency of D_2 receptor blockade. Generally, the phenothiazine and butyrophenone antipsychotics and risperidone carry the greatest risk (Bushe and Shaw 2007). Haloperidol raises the serum prolactin concentration by an average of 17 ng/mL, whereas risperidone may raise it by 45–80 ng/mL, with larger increases in women than in men (David et al. 2000). The atypical antipsychotics olanzapine and quetiapine carry modest risk, and ziprasidone and aripiprazole are low risk (Crawford et al. 1997; Zhong et al. 2006). Antiemetics, such as prochlorperazine, metoclopramide, and trimethobenzamide, have also been reported to cause hyperprolactinemia and galactorrhea. Serotonergic antidepressants, including SSRIs, serotonin-norepinephrine reuptake inhibitors, trazodone, tertiary-amine TCAs, and MAOIs, have also been reported to cause hyperprolactinemia and galactorrhea, likely due to serotonin-mediated dopamine antagonism (Molitch 2008).

Little emphasis has been placed on monitoring and management of psychotropic-induced hyperprolactinemia. American Psychiatric Association guidelines recommend routine monitoring of prolactin serum levels only in symptomatic patients (Lehman et al. 2004). However, patients may not be aware of their symptoms or may be reluctant to address them. Studies have shown a high prevalence of osteoporosis in patients with schizophrenia on long-term conventional antipsychotic medication due to increased prolactin (Wang et al. 2014). In light of emerging evidence of long-term risk for breast cancer, osteoporosis, and cardiovascular disease, the prudent course is to monitor chronically treated patients for symptoms and serological evidence of hyperprolactinemia, perhaps in conjunction with other metabolic parameters, as outlined earlier in the subsection "Psychotropic-Induced Metabolic Syndrome."

Currently, limited data are available to offer insight on an optimal approach to the management of hyperprolactinemia. Treatment strategies include 1) decreasing the dosage of the offending agent, 2) changing medication to an agent less likely to affect prolactin, 3) using a dopamine agonist such as bromocriptine or a partial agonist such as aripiprazole, and 4) preventing long-term complications of hyperprolactinemia such as bone demineralization. Meng et al. (2015) systematically reviewed and evaluated all relevant RCTs and found that adjunctive aripiprazole is effective and safe to use in the treatment of antipsychotic-induced hyperprolactinemia. Treatment with a dopamine agonist such as bromocriptine (5–10 mg/day) is controversial because of risk for exacerbation of psychosis and questionable efficacy (Smith 1992). There is recent evidence indicating that adjunctive metformin lowered prolactin level and relieved prolactin-related symptoms in patients with antipsychotic-induced hyperprolactinemia (Bo et al. 2016). No reports have been published on the effects of hormone replacement on bone mineral density in patients taking antipsychotics long term, but preliminary data suggest that active management of bone loss in those with antipsychotic-associated bone disease may halt or even reverse this process (O'Keane 2008).

Psychiatric Side Effects of Endocrine Treatments

Psychiatric symptoms of endocrine disorders are manifestations of hormone toxicity or deficiency syndromes described previously in this chapter. However, hormone treatments used for reasons other than mere correction of deficiency (e.g., corticosteroids, nonhormonal medications that treat endocrine disorders) may also cause psychiatric side effects (Table 10–4).

Table 10–4.   Psychiatric adverse effects of endocrinological/ hormonal treatments

Medication	Psychiatric adverse effects
Steroid hormones	
Corticosteroids	Mania, anxiety, irritability, psychosis (acute), depression (chronic), delirium, suicidal ideation
Testosterone and other anabolic/ androgenic steroids (especially supraphysiological levels)	Irritability, mania, psychosis
Oral hypoglycemics	
Sulfonylureas, biguanides, α-glucosidase inhibitors, thiazolidinediones, and meglitinides	Anxiety, depression, irritability, cognitive impairment (secondary to hypoglycemia)
Antithyroid medications	
Carbimazole, methimazole, and propylthiouracil	None reported
Dopamine agonists	
Bromocriptine and cabergoline	Psychosis, hallucinations
Growth hormone–inhibiting hormones	
Somatostatin, octreotide, and lanreotide	Sleep disruption
Pegvisomant	None reported
Growth hormone	
Recombinant human growth hormone	Insomnia, fatigue

Oral Hypoglycemic Medications

The psychiatric side effects of oral hypoglycemic medications are secondary to their hypoglycemic effect. Psychiatric symptoms include most prominently anxiety, dysphoria, irritability, and confusion. Such effects can be exacerbated in severely depressed patients with anorexia.

Antithyroid Medications

Carbimazole, methimazole, and propylthiouracil have *not* been documented to cause psychiatric side effects.

Corticosteroids

Exogenous corticosteroids (e.g., hydrocortisone, cortisone, prednisone, methylprednisolone, dexamethasone) and adrenocorticotropic hormone are well known to cause a range of neuropsychiatric side effects (Warrington and Bostwick 2006). Adverse psychiatric reactions to corticosteroids have been reported in children as young as neonates (Drozdowicz and Bostwick 2014). Approximately 13%–62% of patients experience transient mild to moderate symptoms that do not reach severity or duration criteria for psychiatric disorder (Lewis and Smith 1983). These include activation symptoms, such as anxiety, insomnia, and irritability, and mood symptoms, such as dysphoria, euphoria, and lability.

Severe neuropsychiatric consequences have been reported to occur in 15.7 per 100 person-years at risk for all glucocorticoid courses and 22.2 per 100 person-years at risk for first courses (Judd et al. 2014). Greater risk of glucocorticoid-induced neuropsychiatric problems is associated with higher dosage, long-term treatment, greater patient age, and past history of a neuropsychiatric disorder during glucocorticoid treatment. Although mood disorders are most common, about 1 in 6 patients seen psychiatrically experiences delirium or psychosis (Dubovsky et al. 2012). Suicidal ideation can occur. High-dose, short-term administration is most often associated with mania and hypomania, whereas chronic therapy is most often associated with depression (Bolanos et al. 2004). Impairments in long-term recall of verbal information have been reported in patients with optic neuritis and multiple sclerosis receiving high-dose glucocorticoids; however, attentional and working memory function remain intact, and impairments reverse within 5 days of cessation of treatment (Brunner et al.

2005). Discontinuation of long-term glucocorticoid therapy is associated with an increased risk of both depression and delirium or confusion (Fardet et al. 2013). People treated with long-acting glucocorticoids are particularly at risk. Although prior psychiatric history, particularly mania, and prior steroid-induced psychiatric disorders are generally considered clinical risk factors, these have not been adequately addressed in the literature.

Successful prophylaxis against steroid-induced neuropsychiatric reactions has been reported for lithium (Falk et al. 1979), valproic acid (Abbas and Styra 1994), lamotrigine (Preda et al. 1999), and chlorpromazine (Bloch et al. 1994). Falk et al. (1979) initiated lithium carbonate (serum levels 0.8–1.2 mEq/L) concurrently with adrenocorticotropic hormone in 27 patients with multiple sclerosis and optic neuritis. None experienced affective or psychotic symptoms, but 14% of a matched sample of 44 patients had severe mood disorder with psychosis. The existing evidence is not sufficient to recommend prophylaxis for all patients receiving high-dose corticosteroids; however, prophylaxis may be warranted for patients with prior adverse psychiatric reactions to steroids.

In a patient with an active corticosteroid-induced mood disorder, tapered discontinuation or reduction to minimal effective dosage is recommended on the basis of status of the underlying illness (Dubovsky et al. 2012; Judd et al. 2014). Literature on psychopharmacological treatment of corticosteroid-induced mood and psychotic disorders has focused on TCAs, SSRIs, mood stabilizers, and antipsychotics. In case reports or series, imipramine, amitriptyline, and doxepin benefited depressive symptoms (Warrington and Bostwick 2006); however, caution may be warranted because agitation and psychosis have been reported (Malinow and Dorsch 1984). Fluoxetine, sertraline, and venlafaxine have also been reported to be beneficial in case series (Beshay and Pumariega 1998; Ismail and Lyster 2002; Ros 2004; Wyszynski and Wyszynski 1993).

For corticosteroid-induced depression and mania, case reports have supported use of antipsychotics, lithium, valproic acid, and carbamazepine (Judd et al. 2014; Kenna et al. 2011; Roxanas and Hunt 2012). Corticosteroid-treated patients taking lithium should be monitored closely for fluid and electrolyte status and lithium levels because of mineralocorticoid effects.

In a systematic review, steroid-induced manic and psychotic symptoms responded to low-dose typical antipsychotics with cessation of symptoms in 83% of patients, 60% of whom responded in less than 1 week and 80% in less than 2 weeks. Olanzapine at dosages of 2.5–15 mg/day has been reported in a case series (Goldman and Goveas 2002) and an open-label trial (Brown et al. 2004) to be beneficial for patients with multiple underlying illnesses and steroid-induced mixed and manic episodes. Olanzapine and other antipsychotic exacerbation of weight gain and insulin resistance in conjunction with corticosteroid use should be monitored. A case series showed that sodium valproate rapidly and safely reversed manic-like symptoms within a few days without corticosteroids needing to be stopped, thus allowing the medical treatment to continue (Roxanas and Hunt 2012). Prophylactic lamotrigine can reduce memory problems, and prophylactic treatment should also be considered for patients with neurological disorders involving mood or cognitive disturbance (Judd et al. 2014).

Rapid tapering or discontinuation of corticosteroids can also induce corticosteroid-withdrawal syndrome. Corticosteroid-withdrawal syndrome is manifested by headache, fever, myalgias, arthralgias, weakness, anorexia, nausea, weight loss, and orthostatic hypotension and sometimes by depression, anxiety, agitation, or psychosis (Wolkowitz 1989). Symptoms respond to an increase or resumption of corticosteroid dosage. Adjunctive treatment with antipsychotics, antidepressants, and mood stabilizers can be helpful, depending on the particular psychiatric symptom constellation.

Testosterone

The most common adverse effects of testosterone replacement therapy (TRT) are acne and mild activation symptoms. Chronic administration may result in testicular atrophy and watery ejaculate. Although aggression ("steroid rage") is a highly publicized effect of androgenic steroid administration, it most often occurs in the context of supraphysiological dosing common among athletes (Pope and Katz 1994). Only a small portion of eugonadal and hypogonadal men receiving TRT develop aggression (O'Connor et al. 2001). Furthermore, increased aggressiveness in the depressed, treatment-refractory hypogonadal male may reflect positive effects on vigor and energy (O'Connor et al. 2002). Rare cases of TRT-induced psychosis have been reported (Weiss et al. 1999).

Although not an adverse psychiatric effect, prostate cancer risk is a theoretical concern among aging men receiving TRT. In a meta-analysis, TRT did not increase prostate-specific androgen levels in men being treated for hypogonadism, except when it was given intramuscularly, and even then the increase was minimal (Kang and Li 2015). Further, in three studies that assessed incidence of prostate cancer, rates of prostate cancer were similar between subjects who received testosterone and controls. In women, there is concern regarding androgenic side effects and elevation of breast and endometrial cancer risk. In general, these adverse effects have not been supported by the literature and are found only with sustained supraphysiological levels (Bitzer et al. 2008; Dimitrakakis et al. 2004).

Growth Hormone (Somatotropin)

Psychiatric adverse effects with growth hormone treatment are infrequent. Pooled data from trials of growth hormone in HIV-associated adipose redistribution syndrome indicate higher rates of insomnia and fatigue compared with placebo (Serono EMD 2016).

Growth Hormone–Inhibiting Hormones

Both somatostatin and its long-acting analogue, octreotide, have been found to reduce total sleep time and rapid eye movement sleep, particularly in elderly patients (Frieboes et al. 1997; Ziegenbein et al. 2004).

Dopamine Agonists

The dopamine agonists bromocriptine and cabergoline may cause psychosis and hallucinations. This topic is covered in Chapter 9, "Central Nervous System Disorders" (see especially Table 9–4).

Drug-Drug Interactions

Potential clinically significant interactions between psychotropic drugs and medications used for endocrine disorders are listed in Tables 10–5 and 10–6. Clinically significant drug interactions are rarely reported in the literature, and many are speculative in nature (e.g., DeVane and Markowitz 2002). Data presented are largely derived from information in product monographs.

Table 10–5.   Psychotropic drug–endocrine drug interactions

Psychotropic drug	Mechanism of interaction	Endocrine drugs/classes affected	Clinical effects
Antidepressants			
Fluvoxamine and sertraline	CYP2C9 inhibition	Glimepiride, glipizide, glyburide, nateglinide, rosiglitazone, and tolbutamide	Reduced clearance of oral hypoglycemics; potential enhanced hypoglycemic effect
Fluoxetine, fluvoxamine, and nefazodone	CYP3A4 inhibition	Nateglinide, pioglitazone, and repaglinide	Reduced clearance of oral hypoglycemics; potential enhanced hypoglycemic effect
MAOIs	Stimulation of insulin release	Corticosteroids	Increased steroid levels and adverse effects
TCAs	Weight gain, insulin resistance	Insulin and oral hypoglycemics	Possibly enhanced hyperglycemic effect
	Unknown mechanism	Augmentation of vasopressin effects	Enhanced antidiuretic effect
All antidepressants	Increased receptor sensitivity to catecholamines	T_3 and T_4 supplementation	Increased activation, sympathetic autonomic symptoms

Table 10–5. Psychotropic drug–endocrine drug interactions (*continued*)

Psychotropic drug	Mechanism of interaction	Endocrine drugs/classes affected	Clinical effects
Mood stabilizers			
Lithium	Nephrogenic diabetes insipidus via ADH inhibition in kidney	Corticosteroids, mineralocorticoids, and vasopressin	Increased urination, serum osmolality, sodium, thirst
	Antithyroid effects	Thyroid hormone	Undercorrection of hypothyroidism
Carbamazepine, phenobarbital, and phenytoin	CYP2C9 induction	Glimepiride, glipizide, glyburide, nateglinide, rosiglitazone, and tolbutamide	Possibly reduced levels and effectiveness of oral hypoglycemics
	CYP3A4 induction	Nateglinide, pioglitazone, and repaglinide	Possibly reduced levels and effectiveness of oral hypoglycemics
	Induction of Phase 2 metabolism (UGT-sulfation)	T_4	Increased hepatic T_4 metabolism and decreased effect
	Unknown mechanism	Augmentation of vasopressin effects	Enhanced antidiuretic effect

Table 10–5.   Psychotropic drug–endocrine drug interactions *(continued)*

Psychotropic drug	Mechanism of interaction	Endocrine drugs/classes affected	Clinical effects
Antipsychotics			
Typical and atypical	Weight gain, insulin resistance	Antagonism of insulin and oral hypoglycemic	Possibly enhanced hyperglycemic effects
	Blockade of dopamine D_2 receptors	Hyperprolactinemia	Sexual dysfunction, galactorrhea, gynomastia
Opioids	Unknown mechanism	Pegvisomant	Reduced pegvisomant levels and clinical effect; increase dose with concurrent opioids

Note.   ADH=antidiuretic hormone; CYP=cytochrome P450; MAOIs=monoamine oxidase inhibitors; TCAs=tricyclic antidepressants; T_3=triiodothyronine; T_4=thyroxine; UGT=uridine 5′-diphosphate glucuronosyltransferase.

Table 10–6. Endocrine drug–psychotropic drug interactions

Endocrine drug	Mechanism of interaction	Psychotropic drugs/ classes affected	Clinical effects
Growth hormone			
Recombinant human growth hormone	CYP3A4 induction	Anticonvulsants, antidepressants, antipsychotics, benzodiazepines, and opioids	Possibly reduced serum psychotropic levels and reduced therapeutic effects
Growth hormone inhibitors			
Octreotide	General reduction in CYP-mediated metabolism via growth hormone inhibition	All drugs undergoing oxidative metabolism	Possibly increased serum psychotropic levels and increased aftereffects

Note. CYP = cytochrome P450.

Key Clinical Points

- Hormone deficiency and excess states are most likely to be associated with depression, anxiety, and cognitive impairment.
- Mania and hypomania occur predominantly with hyperthyroidism and with acute, high-dose corticosteroid therapy.
- Although psychosis is rare, it occurs with severe hypothyroidism and hyperthyroidism, hyperparathyroidism, and acute high-dose corticosteroid therapy.
- For many endocrinological disorders, correction of the underlying hormone deficiency or excess generally improves psychiatric symptoms.
- Psychiatric symptoms may persist beyond normalization of laboratory parameters.
- Successful psychopharmacological treatment generally requires prior or concurrent correction of the underlying endocrinological disorder.
- Psychotropic-induced endocrinological dysfunction is common and should be routinely screened via symptom assessment and laboratory testing. Examples of such dysfunction include lithium-induced hypothyroidism or nephrogenic diabetes insipidus and antipsychotic-induced metabolic syndrome or hyperprolactinemia.
- Because clinically significant psychotropic drug–endocrine drug or hormone interactions occur infrequently, these agents can generally be combined safely.

References

Abbas A, Styra R: Valproate prophylaxis against steroid induced psychosis. Can J Psychiatry 39(3):188–189, 1994 8033028

Ahmadi-Abhari SA, Ghaeli P, Fahimi F, et al: Risk factors of thyroid abnormalities in bipolar patients receiving lithium: a case control study. BMC Psychiatry 3:4, 2003 12740023

Ajmal A, Joffe H, Nachtigall LB: Psychotropic-induced hyperprolactinemia: a clinical review. Psychosomatics 55(1):29–36, 2014 24140188

Akintola AA, Jansen SW, van Bodegom D, et al: Subclinical hypothyroidism and cognitive function in people over 60 years: a systematic review and meta-analysis. Front Aging Neurosci 7:150, 2015 26321946

Albert U, De Cori D, Aguglia A, et al: Effects of maintenance lithium treatment on serum parathyroid hormone and calcium levels: a retrospective longitudinal naturalistic study. Neuropsychiatr Dis Treat 11:1785–1791, 2015 26229473

Almeida OP, Alfonso H, Flicker L, et al: Thyroid hormones and depression: the Health in Men study. Am J Geriatr Psychiatry 19(9):763–770, 2011 21873831

Amanatkar HR, Chibnall JT, Seo BW, et al: Impact of exogenous testosterone on mood: a systematic review and meta-analysis of randomized placebo-controlled trials. Ann Clin Psychiatry 26(1):19–32, 2014 24501728

American Diabetes Association; American Psychiatric Association; American Association of Clinical Endocrinologists; North American Association for the Study of Obesity: Consensus development conference on antipsychotic drugs and obesity and diabetes. Diabetes Care 27(2):596–601, 2004 14747245

Amiaz R, Pope HG Jr, Mahne T, et al: Testosterone gel replacement improves sexual function in depressed men taking serotonergic antidepressants: a randomized, placebo-controlled clinical trial. J Sex Marital Ther 37(4):243–254, 2011 21707327

Baethge C, Blumentritt H, Berghöfer A, et al: Long-term lithium treatment and thyroid antibodies: a controlled study. J Psychiatry Neurosci 30(6):423–427, 2005 16327876

Barker R, Zajicek J, Wilkinson I: Thyrotoxic Hashimoto's encephalopathy. J Neurol Neurosurg Psychiatry 60(2):234, 1996 8708668

Benvenga S: Benzodiazepine and remission of Graves' disease. Thyroid 6(6):659–660, 1996 9001204

Beshay H, Pumariega AJ: Sertraline treatment of mood disorder associated with prednisone: a case report. J Child Adolesc Psychopharmacol 8(3):187–193, 1998 9853693

Bitzer J, Kenemans P, Mueck AO; FSDeducation Group: Breast cancer risk in postmenopausal women using testosterone in combination with hormone replacement therapy. Maturitas 59(3):209–218, 2008 18343056

Bloch M, Gur E, Shalev A: Chlorpromazine prophylaxis of steroid-induced psychosis. Gen Hosp Psychiatry 16(1):42–44, 1994 8039683

Blum MR, Wijsman LW, Virgini VS, et al: Subclinical thyroid dysfunction and depressive symptoms among the elderly: a prospective cohort study. Neuroendocrinology 103(3–4):291–299, 2016 26202797

Bo Q-J, Wang ZM, Li XB, et al: Adjunctive metformin for antipsychotic-induced hyperprolactinemia: a systematic review. Psychiatry Res 237:257–263, 2016 26822064

Bocchetta A, Cocco F, Velluzzi F, et al: Fifteen-year follow-up of thyroid function in lithium patients. J Endocrinol Invest 30(5):363–366, 2007 17598966

Bogazzi F, Bartalena L, Brogioni S, et al: Comparison of radioiodine with radioiodine plus lithium in the treatment of Graves' hyperthyroidism. J Clin Endocrinol Metab 84(2):499–503, 1999 10022407

Bolanos SH, Khan DA, Hanczyc M, et al: Assessment of mood states in patients receiving long-term corticosteroid therapy and in controls with patient-rated and clinician-rated scales. Ann Allergy Asthma Immunol 92(5):500–505, 2004 15191017

Borst SE, Yarrow JF, Fernanez C, et al: Cognitive effects of testosterone and finasteride administration in older hypogonadal men. Clin Inter Aging 9:1327–1333, 2014 25143719

Bostwick JR, Guthrie SK, Ellingrod VL: Antipsychotic-induced hyperprolactinemia. Pharmacotherapy 29(1):64–73, 2009 19113797

Boton R, Gaviria M, Batlle DC: Prevalence, pathogenesis, and treatment of renal dysfunction associated with chronic lithium therapy. Am J Kidney Dis 10(5):329–345, 1987 3314489

Brandt F, Thvilum M, Almind D, et al: Hyperthyroidism and psychiatric morbidity: evidence from a Danish nationwide register study. Eur J Endocrinol 170(2):341–348, 2013 24282192

Brown ES, Chamberlain W, Dhanani N, et al: An open-label trial of olanzapine for corticosteroid-induced mood symptoms. J Affect Disord 83(2–3):277–281, 2004 15555725

Brown SW, Vyas BV, Spiegel DR: Mania in a case of hyperparathyroidism. Psychosomatics 48(3):265–268, 2007 17478597

Brownlie BE, Chambers ST, Sadler WA, Donald RA: Lithium associated thyroid disease—a report of 14 cases of hypothyroidism and 4 cases of thyrotoxicosis. Aust N Z J Med 6(3):223–229, 1976 1067821

Brownlie BE, Rae AM, Walshe JW, Wells JE: Psychoses associated with thyrotoxicosis—'thyrotoxic psychosis': a report of 18 cases, with statistical analysis of incidence. Eur J Endocrinol 142(5):438–444, 2000 10802519

Brunner R, Schaefer D, Hess K, et al: Effect of corticosteroids on short-term and long-term memory. Neurology 64(2):335–337, 2005 15668434

Burris AS, Banks SM, Carter CS, et al: A long-term, prospective study of the physiologic and behavioral effects of hormone replacement in untreated hypogonadal men. J Androl 13(4):297–304, 1992 1399830

Bushe C, Shaw M: Prevalence of hyperprolactinaemia in a naturalistic cohort of schizophrenia and bipolar outpatients during treatment with typical and atypical antipsychotics. J Psychopharmacol 21(7):768–773, 2007 17606473

Canuso CM, Goldstein JM, Wojcik J, et al: Antipsychotic medication, prolactin elevation, and ovarian function in women with schizophrenia and schizoaffective disorder. Psychiatry Res 111(1):11–20, 2002 12140115

Cayköylü A, Capoğlu I, Unüvar N, et al: Thyroid abnormalities in lithium-treated patients with bipolar affective disorder. J Int Med Res 30(1):80–84, 2002 11921503

Centorrino F, Masters GA, Talamo A, et al: Metabolic syndrome in psychiatrically hospitalized patients treated with antipsychotics and other psychotropics. Hum Psychopharmacol 27(5):521–526, 2012 22996619

Cheng SP, Lee JJ, Liu TP, et al: Quality of life after surgery or surveillance for asymptomatic primary hyperparathyroidism: a meta-analysis of randomized controlled trials. Medicine (Baltimore) 94(23):e931, 2015 26061318

Cherrier MM, Anderson K, Shofer J, et al: Testosterone treatment of men with mild cognitive impairment and low testosterone levels. Am J Alzheimers Dis Other Demen 30(4):421–430, 2015 25392187

Ciechanowski PS, Katon WJ, Russo JE: Depression and diabetes: impact of depressive symptoms on adherence, function, and costs. Arch Intern Med 160(21):3278–3285, 2000 11088090

Crawford AM, Beasley CM Jr, Tollefson GD: The acute and long-term effect of olanzapine compared with placebo and haloperidol on serum prolactin concentrations. Schizophr Res 26(1):41–54, 1997 9376336

Crews MP, Howes OD: Is antipsychotic treatment linked to low bone mineral density and osteoporosis? A review of the evidence and the clinical implications. Hum Psychopharmacol 27(1):15–23, 2012 22228316

Das PP, Sharan P, Grover S, Behera A: Parathyroid adenoma presenting as bipolar affective disorder. Psychosomatics 48(6):532–533, 2007 18071102

David SR, Taylor CC, Kinon BJ, Breier A: The effects of olanzapine, risperidone, and haloperidol on plasma prolactin levels in patients with schizophrenia. Clin Ther 22(9):1085–1096, 2000 11048906

Dayan CM, Panicker V: Hypothyroidism and depression. Eur Thyroid J 2(3):168–179, 2013 24847450

de Groot M, Anderson R, Freedland KE, et al: Association of depression and diabetes complications: a meta-analysis. Psychosom Med 63(4):619–630, 2001 11485116

de Jongh RT, Lips P, van Schoor NM, et al: Endogenous subclinical thyroid disorders, physical and cognitive function, depression, and mortality in older individuals. Eur J Endocrinol 165(4):545–554, 2011 21768248

Demartini B, Ranieri R, Masu A, et al: Depressive symptoms and major depressive disorder in patients affected by subclinical hypothyroidism: a cross-sectional study. J Nerv Ment Dis 202(8):603–607, 2014 25010109

Deodhar SD, Singh B, Pathak CM, et al: Thyroid functions in lithium-treated psychiatric patients: a cross-sectional study. Biol Trace Elem Res 67(2):151–163, 1999 10073421

DeVane CL, Markowitz JS: Psychoactive drug interactions with pharmacotherapy for diabetes. Psychopharmacol Bull 36(2):40–52, 2002 12397839

Dimitrakakis C, Jones RA, Liu A, Bondy CA: Breast cancer incidence in postmenopausal women using testosterone in addition to usual hormone therapy. Menopause 11(5):531–535, 2004 15356405

Drozdowicz LB, Bostwick JM: Psychiatric adverse effects of pediatric corticosteroid use. Mayo Clin Proc 89(6):817–834, 2014 24943696

Dubovsky AN, Arvikar S, Stern TA, Axelrod L: The neuropsychiatric complications of glucocorticoid use: steroid psychosis revisited. Psychosomatics 53(2):103–115, 2012 22424158

Expert Panel on Detection, Evaluation, and Treatment of High Blood Cholesterol in Adults: Executive summary of The Third Report of The National Cholesterol Education Program (NCEP) Expert Panel on Detection, Evaluation, and Treatment of High Blood Cholesterol In Adults (Adult Treatment Panel III). JAMA 285(19):2486–2497, 2001 11368702

Fagiolini A, Kupfer DJ, Scott J, et al: Hypothyroidism in patients with bipolar I disorder treated primarily with lithium. Epidemiol Psichiatr Soc 15(2):123–127, 2006 16865933

Fahrenfort JJ, Wilterdink AM, van der Veen EA: Long-term residual complaints and psychosocial sequelae after remission of hyperthyroidism. Psychoneuroendocrinology 25(2):201–211, 2000 10674283

Falk WE, Mahnke MW, Poskanzer DC: Lithium prophylaxis of corticotropin-induced psychosis. JAMA 241(10):1011–1012, 1979 216818

Fardet L, Nazareth I, Whitaker HJ, Petersen I: Severe neuropsychiatric outcomes following discontinuation of long-term glucocorticoid therapy: a cohort study. J Clin Psychiatry 74(4):e281–e286, 2013 23656853

Fatourechi V: Hashimoto's encephalopathy: myth or reality? An endocrinologist's perspective. Best Pract Res Clin Endocrinol Metab 19(1):53–66, 2005 15826922

Frieboes RM, Murck H, Schier T, et al: Somatostatin impairs sleep in elderly human subjects. Neuropsychopharmacology 16(5):339–345, 1997 9109105

Garber JR, Cobin RH, Gharib H, et al: Clinical practice guidelines for hypothyroidism in adults: cosponsored by the American Association of Clinical Endocrinologists and the American Thyroid Association. Endocr Pract 18(6):988–1028, 2012 23246686 Erratum in Endocr Pract 19(1):175, 2013

Goldman LS, Goveas J: Olanzapine treatment of corticosteroid-induced mood disorders. Psychosomatics 43(6):495–497, 2002 12444234

Goode DJ, Meltzer HY, Fang VS: Daytime variation in serum prolactin level in patients receiving oral and depot antipsychotic medication. Biol Psychiatry 16(7):653–662, 1981 7196775

Grigsby AB, Anderson RJ, Freedland KE, et al: Prevalence of anxiety in adults with diabetes: a systematic review. J Psychosom Res 53(6):1053–1060, 2002 12479986

Gulseren S, Gulseren L, Hekimsoy Z, et al: Depression, anxiety, health-related quality of life, and disability in patients with overt and subclinical thyroid dysfunction. Arch Med Res 37(1):133–139, 2006 16314199

Holtmann M, Gerstner S, Schmidt MH: Risperidone-associated ejaculatory and urinary dysfunction in male adolescents. J Child Adolesc Psychopharmacol 13(1):107–109, 2003 12804132

Hu LY, Shen CC, Hu YW, et al: Hyperthyroidism and risk for bipolar disorders: a nationwide population-based study. PLoS One 8(8):e73057, 2013 24023669

Ismail M, Lyster G: Treatment of psychotic depression associated with steroid therapy in Churg-Strauss syndrome. Ir Med J 95(1):18–19, 2002 11928783

Jonklaas J, Bianco AC, Bauer AJ, et al; American Thyroid Association Task Force on Thyroid Hormone Replacement: Guidelines for the treatment of hypothyroidism: prepared by the American Thyroid Association Task Force on Thyroid Hormone Replacement. Thyroid 24(12):1670–1751, 2014 25266247

Judd LL, Schettler PJ, Brown ES, et al: Adverse consequences of glucocorticoid medication: psychological, cognitive, and behavioral effects. Am J Psychiatry 171(10):1045–1051, 2014 25272344

Kang DY, Li HJ: The effect of testosterone replacement therapy on prostate-specific antigen (PSA) levels in men being treated for hypogonadism: a systematic review and meta-analysis. Medicine (Baltimore) 94(3):e410, 2015 25621688

Kathol RG, Delahunt JW: The relationship of anxiety and depression to symptoms of hyperthyroidism using operational criteria. Gen Hosp Psychiatry 8(1):23–28, 1986 3943712

Katon WJ, Von Korff M, Lin EH, et al: The Pathways Study: a randomized trial of collaborative care in patients with diabetes and depression. Arch Gen Psychiatry 61(10):1042–1049, 2004 15466678

Katon WJ, Lin EH, Von Korff M, et al: Collaborative care for patients with depression and chronic illnesses. N Engl J Med 363(27):2611–2620, 2010 21190455

Kenna HA, Poon AW, de los Angeles CP, Koran LM: Psychiatric complications of treatment with corticosteroids: review with case report. Psychiatry Clin Neurosci 65(6):549–560, 2011 22003987

Kessler L, Palla J, Baru JS, et al: Lithium as an adjunct to radioactive iodine for the treatment of hyperthyroidism: a systematic review and meta-analysis. Endocr Pract 20(7):737–745, 2014 24793920

Khoza S, Barner JC, Bohman TM, et al: Use of antidepressant agents and the risk of type 2 diabetes. Eur J Clin Pharmacol 68(9):1295–1302, 2012 22120432

Kibirige D, Luzinda K, Ssekitoleko R: Spectrum of lithium induced thyroid abnormalities: a current perspective. Thyroid Res 6(1):3, 2013 23391071

Kinon BJ, Gilmore JA, Liu H, Halbreich UM: Prevalence of hyperprolactinemia in schizophrenic patients treated with conventional antipsychotic medications or risperidone. Psychoneuroendocrinology 28 (suppl 2):55–68, 2003 12650681

Kleiner J, Altshuler L, Hendrick V, Hershman JM: Lithium-induced subclinical hypothyroidism: review of the literature and guidelines for treatment. J Clin Psychiatry 60(4):249–255, 1999 10221287

Knol MJ, Derijks HJ, Geerlings MI, et al: Influence of antidepressants on glycaemic control in patients with diabetes mellitus. Pharmacoepidemiol Drug Saf 17(6):577–586, 2008 18449949

Ko Y-K, Soh MA, Kang SH, Lee JI: The prevalence of metabolic syndrome in schizophrenic patients using antipsychotics. Clin Psychopharmacol Neurosci 11(2):80–88, 2013 24023552

Korzets A, Floro S, Ori Y, et al: Clomipramine-induced pheochromocytoma crisis: a near fatal complication of a tricyclic antidepressant. J Clin Psychopharmacol 17(5):428–430, 1997 9315999

Kraemer S, Minarzyk A, Forst T, et al: Prevalence of metabolic syndrome in patients with schizophrenia, and metabolic changes after 3 months of treatment with antipsychotics—results from a German observational study. BMC Psychiatry 11:173, 2011 22044502

Kusalic M, Engelsmann F: Effect of lithium maintenance therapy on thyroid and parathyroid function. J Psychiatry Neurosci 24(3):227–233, 1999 10354657

Kvetny J, Ellervik C, Bech P: Is suppressed thyroid-stimulating hormone (TSH) associated with subclinical depression in the Danish General Suburban Population Study? Nord J Psychiatry 69(4):282–286, 2015 25377023

Lazarus JH: The effects of lithium therapy on thyroid and thyrotropin-releasing hormone. Thyroid 8(10):909–913, 1998 9827658

Lefebvre H, Noblet C, Moore N, Wolf LM: Pseudo-phaeochromocytoma after multiple drug interactions involving the selective monoamine oxidase inhibitor selegiline. Clin Endocrinol (Oxf) 42(1):95–98, discussion 98–99, 1995 7889639

Lehman AF, Lieberman JA, Dixon LB, et al; American Psychiatric Association; Steering Committee on Practice Guidelines: Practice guideline for the treatment of patients with schizophrenia, second edition. Am J Psychiatry 161 (suppl 2):1–56, 2004 15000267

Lewis DA, Smith RE: Steroid-induced psychiatric syndromes: a report of 14 cases and a review of the literature. J Affect Disord 5(4):319–332, 1983 6319464

Lustman PJ, Griffith LS, Clouse RE, et al: Effects of alprazolam on glucose regulation in diabetes: results of double-blind, placebo-controlled trial. Diabetes Care 18(8):1133–1139, 1995 7587848

Lustman PJ, Griffith LS, Clouse RE, et al: Effects of nortriptyline on depression and glycemic control in diabetes: results of a double-blind, placebo-controlled trial. Psychosom Med 59(3):241–250, 1997 9178335

Lustman PJ, Clouse RE, Nix BD, et al: Sertraline for prevention of depression recurrence in diabetes mellitus: a randomized, double-blind, placebo-controlled trial. Arch Gen Psychiatry 63(5):521–529, 2006 16651509

Maarbjerg K, Vestergaard P, Schou M: Changes in serum thyroxine (T4) and serum thyroid stimulating hormone (TSH) during prolonged lithium treatment. Acta Psychiatr Scand 75(2):217–221, 1987 3565069

Malinow KL, Dorsch C: Tricyclic precipitation of steroid psychosis. Psychiatr Med 2(4):351–354, 1984 6599906

Malkin CJ, Pugh PJ, Morris PD, et al: Testosterone replacement in hypogonadal men with angina improves ischaemic threshold and quality of life. Heart 90(8):871–876, 2004 15253956

Malkin CJ, Pugh PJ, West JN, et al: Testosterone therapy in men with moderate severity heart failure: a double-blind randomized placebo controlled trial. Eur Heart J 27(1):57–64, 2006 16093267

McNicholas TA, Dean JD, Mulder H, et al: A novel testosterone gel formulation normalizes androgen levels in hypogonadal men, with improvements in body composition and sexual function. BJU Int 91(1):69–74, 2003 12614254

McKnight RF, Adida M, Budge K, et al: Lithium toxicity profile: a systematic review and meta-analysis. Lancet 379(9817):721–728, 2012 22265699

Meehan AD, Humble MB, Yazarloo P, et al: The prevalence of lithium-associated hyperparathyroidism in a large Swedish population attending psychiatric outpatient units. J Clin Psychopharmacol 35(3):279–285, 2015 25853371

Meng M, Li W, Zhang S, et al: Using aripiprazole to reduce antipsychotic-induced hyperprolactinemia: meta-analysis of currently available randomized controlled trials. Shanghai Arch Psychiatry 27:4–17, 2015 25852251

Mizukami Y, Michigishi T, Nonomura A, et al: Histological features of the thyroid gland in a patient with lithium induced thyrotoxicosis. J Clin Pathol 48(6):582–584, 1995 7665708

Molitch ME: Drugs and prolactin. Pituitary 11(2):209–218, 2008 18404390

Nasrallah H: A review of the effect of atypical antipsychotics on weight. Psychoneuroendocrinology 28 (suppl 1):83–96, 2003 12504074

National Institute for Health and Care Excellence (UK): Bipolar disorder: assessment and management, published September 2014 and updated February 2016. Available at: https://www.nice.org.uk/guidance/cg185. Accessed July 10, 2016.

Neary NM, King KS, Pacak K: Drugs and pheochromocytoma—don't be fooled by every elevated metanephrine. N Engl J Med 364(23):2268–2270, 2011 21651412

O'Connor DB, Archer J, Hair WM, Wu FC: Activational effects of testosterone on cognitive function in men. Neuropsychologia 39(13):1385–1394, 2001 11585606

O'Connor DB, Archer J, Hair WM, Wu FC: Exogenous testosterone, aggression, and mood in eugonadal and hypogonadal men. Physiol Behav 75(4):557–566, 2002 12062320

O'Keane V: Antipsychotic-induced hyperprolactinaemia, hypogonadism and osteoporosis in the treatment of schizophrenia. J Psychopharmacol 22(2)(suppl):70–75, 2008 18477623

O'Keane V, Meaney AM: Antipsychotic drugs: a new risk factor for osteoporosis in young women with schizophrenia? J Clin Psychopharmacol 25(1):26–31, 2005 15643097

Okosieme O, Gilbert J, Abraham P, et al: Management of primary hypothyroidism: statement by the British Thyroid Association Executive Committee. Clin Endocrinol (Oxf) 84(6):799–808, 2016 26010808

Ozdemir V, Bertilsson L, Miura J, et al: CYP2D6 genotype in relation to perphenazine concentration and pituitary pharmacodynamic tissue sensitivity in Asians: CYP2D6-serotonin-dopamine crosstalk revisited. Pharmacogenet Genomics 17(5):339–347, 2007 17429316

Ozpoyraz N, Tamam L, Kulan E: Thyroid abnormalities in lithium-treated patients. Adv Ther 19(4):176–184, 2002 12431043

Parsaik AK, Singh B, Roberts RO, et al: Hypothyroidism and risk of mild cognitive impairment in elderly persons. JAMA Neurology 71(2):201–207, 2014 24378475

Petrak F, Herpertz S, Albus C, et al: Study protocol of the Diabetes and Depression Study (DAD): a multi-center randomized controlled trial to compare the efficacy of a diabetes-specific cognitive behavioral group therapy versus sertraline in patients with major depression and poorly controlled diabetes mellitus. BMC Psychiatry 13:206, 2013 23915015

Plener PL, Molz E, Berger G, et al: Depression, metabolic control, and antidepressant medication in young patients with type 1 diabetes. Pediatr Diabetes 16(1):58–66, 2015 24636613

Pope HG Jr, Katz DL: Psychiatric and medical effects of anabolic-androgenic steroid use. A controlled study of 160 athletes. Arch Gen Psychiatry 51(5):375–382, 1994 8179461

Pope HG Jr, Cohane GH, Kanayama G, et al: Testosterone gel supplementation for men with refractory depression: a randomized, placebo-controlled trial. Am J Psychiatry 160(1):105–111, 2003 12505808

Preda A, Fazeli A, McKay BG, et al: Lamotrigine as prophylaxis against steroid-induced mania. J Clin Psychiatry 60(10):708–709, 1999 10549692

Regenold WT, Thapar RK, Marano C, et al: Increased prevalence of type 2 diabetes mellitus among psychiatric inpatients with bipolar I affective and schizoaffective disorders independent of psychotropic drug use. J Affect Disord 70(1):19–26, 2002 12113916

Rej S, Herrmann N, Shulman K: The effects of lithium on renal function in older adults—a systematic review. J Geriatr Psychiatry Neurol 25(1):51–61, 2012 22467847

Riecher-Rössler A, Rybakowski JK, Pflueger MO, et al; EUFEST Study Group: Hyperprolactinemia in antipsychotic-naive patients with first-episode psychosis. Psychol Med 43(12):2571–2582, 2013 23590895

Roberts AL, Agnew-Blais JC, Spiegelman D, et al: Posttraumatic stress disorder and incidence of type 2 diabetes mellitus in a sample of women: a 22-year longitudinal study. JAMA Psychiatry 72(3):203–210, 2015 25565410

Roman S, Sosa JA: Psychiatric and cognitive aspects of primary hyperparathyroidism. Curr Opin Oncol 19(1):1–5, 2007 17133104

Roman SA, Sosa JA, Mayes L, et al: Parathyroidectomy improves neurocognitive deficits in patients with primary hyperparathyroidism. Surgery 138(6):1121–1128, discussion 1128–1129, 2005 16360399

Ros LT: Symptomatic depression after long-term steroid treatment: a case report. Afr J Med Med Sci 33(3):263–265, 2004 15819475

Roxanas MG, Hunt GE: Rapid reversal of corticosteroid-induced mania with sodium valproate: a case series of 20 patients. Psychosomatics 53(6):575–581, 2012 23157995

Russ MJ, Ackerman SH: Antidepressant treatment response in depressed hypothyroid patients. Hosp Community Psychiatry 40(9):954–956, 1989 2793101

Saunders BD, Saunders EF, Gauger PG: Lithium therapy and hyperparathyroidism: an evidence-based assessment. World J Surg 33(11):2314–2323, 2009 19252941

Seelen MA, de Meijer PH, Meinders AE: Serotonin reuptake inhibitor unmasks a pheochromocytoma. Ann Intern Med 126(4):333, 1997 9036813

Seidman SN, Miyazaki M, Roose SP: Intramuscular testosterone supplementation to selective serotonin reuptake inhibitor in treatment-resistant depressed men: randomized placebo-controlled clinical trial. J Clin Psychopharmacol 25(6):584–588, 2005 16282843

Serono EMD: Serostim (somatropin). 2016. Available at: https://serostim.com/hcp/. Accessed April 19, 2016.

Serri O, Li L, Mamputu JC, et al: The influences of hyperprolactinemia and obesity on cardiovascular risk markers: effects of cabergoline therapy. Clin Endocrinol (Oxf) 64(4):366–370, 2006 16584506

Sih R, Morley JE, Kaiser FE, et al: Testosterone replacement in older hypogonadal men: a 12-month randomized controlled trial. J Clin Endocrinol Metab 82(6):1661–1667, 1997 9177359

Shine B, McKnight RF, Leaver L, Geddes JR: Long-term effects of lithium on renal, thyroid, and parathyroid function: a retrospective analysis of laboratory data. Lancet 386(9992):461–468, 2015 26003379

Smith M, Hopkins D, Peveler RC, et al: First- v second-generation antipsychotics and risk for diabetes in schizophrenia: systematic review and meta-analysis. Br J Psychiatry 192(6):406–411, 2008 18515889

Smith S: Neuroleptic-associated hyperprolactinemia: can it be treated with bromocriptine? J Reprod Med 37(8):737–740, 1992 1359137

Starkman MN, Cameron OG, Nesse RM, Zelnik T: Peripheral catecholamine levels and the symptoms of anxiety: studies in patients with and without pheochromocytoma. Psychosom Med 52(2):129–142, 1990 2330387

Stowell CP, Barnhill JW: Acute mania in the setting of severe hypothyroidism. Psychosomatics 46(3):259–261, 2005 15883148

Stubbs B, Vancampfort D, De Hert M, Mitchell AJ: The prevalence and predictors of type two diabetes mellitus in people with schizophrenia: a systematic review and comparative meta-analysis. Acta Psychiatr Scand 132(2):144–157, 2015 25943829

Surks MI, Ortiz E, Daniels GH, et al: Subclinical thyroid disease: scientific review and guidelines for diagnosis and management. JAMA 291(2):228–238, 2004 14722150

Szalat A, Mazeh H, Freund HR: Lithium-associated hyperparathyroidism: report of four cases and review of the literature. Eur J Endocrinol 160(2):317–323, 2009 19001061

Thilers PP, Macdonald SW, Herlitz A: The association between endogenous free testosterone and cognitive performance: a population-based study in 35 to 90 year-old men and women. Psychoneuroendocrinology 31(5):565–576, 2006 16487665

Tsuboi T, Bies RR, Suzuki T, et al: Hyperprolactinemia and estimated dopamine D2 receptor occupancy in patients with schizophrenia: analysis of the CATIE data. Prog Neuropsychopharmacol Biol Psychiatry 45:178–182, 2013 23727135

Tworoger SS, Hankinson SE: Prolactin and breast cancer risk. Cancer Lett 243(2):160–169, 2006 16530327

Vancampfort D, Stubbs B, Mitchell AJ, et al: Risk of metabolic syndrome and its components in people with schizophrenia and related psychotic disorders, bipolar disorder and major depressive disorder: a systematic review and meta-analysis. World Psychiatry 14(3):339–347, 2015 26407790

van Melick EJM, Wilting I, Meinders AE, Egberts TC: Prevalence and determinants of thyroid disorders in elderly patients with affective disorders: lithium and nonlithium patients. Am J Geriatr Psychiatry 18(5):395–403, 2010 20429083

Verma A, Wartak S, Tidswell M: Lithium-associated thyromegaly: an unusual cause of airway obstruction. Case Rep Med 2012:627415, 2012 DOI: 10.1155/2012/627415 22991519

Wada K, Yamada N, Sato T, et al: Corticosteroid-induced psychotic and mood disorders: diagnosis defined by DSM-IV and clinical pictures. Psychosomatics 42(6):461–466, 2001 11815680

Wagle AC, Wagle SA, Patel AG: Apathetic form of thyrotoxicosis. Can J Psychiatry 43(7):747–748, 1998 9773226

Wang C, Cunningham G, Dobs A, et al: Long-term testosterone gel (AndroGel) treatment maintains beneficial effects on sexual function and mood, lean and fat mass, and bone mineral density in hypogonadal men. J Clin Endocrinol Metab 89(5):2085–2098, 2004 15126525

Wang M, Hou R, Jian J, et al: Effects of antipsychotics on bone mineral density and prolactin levels in patients with schizophrenia: a 12-month prospective study. Hum Psychopharmacol 29(2):183–189, 2014 24738111

Warrington TP, Bostwick JM: Psychiatric adverse effects of corticosteroids. Mayo Clin Proc 81(10):1361–1367, 2006 17036562

Weiss EL, Bowers MBJ Jr, Mazure CM: Testosterone-patch-induced psychotic mania. Am J Psychiatry 156(6):969, 1999 10360145

Wiersinga WM, Touber JL: The influence of beta-adrenoceptor blocking agents on plasma thyroxine and triiodothyronine. J Clin Endocrinol Metab 45(2):293–298, 1977 885993

Wilhelm SM, Lee J, Prinz RA: Major depression due to primary hyperparathyroidism: a frequent and correctable disorder. Am Surg 70(2):175–179, discussion 179–180, 2004 15011923

Wilson DR, D'Souza L, Sarkar N, et al: New-onset diabetes and ketoacidosis with atypical antipsychotics. Schizophr Res 59(1):1–6, 2003 12413635

Windgassen K, Wesselmann U, Schulze Mönking H: Galactorrhea and hyperprolactinemia in schizophrenic patients on neuroleptics: frequency and etiology. Neuropsychobiology 33(3):142–146, 1996 8776743

Wolkowitz OM: Long-lasting behavioral changes following prednisone withdrawal. JAMA 261(12):1731–1732, 1989 2918667

Wyszynski AA, Wyszynski B: Treatment of depression with fluoxetine in corticosteroid-dependent central nervous system Sjögren's syndrome. Psychosomatics 34(2):173–177, 1993 8456162

Ye Z, Chen L, Yang Z, et al: Metabolic effects of fluoxetine in adults with type 2 diabetes mellitus: a meta-analysis of randomized placebo-controlled trials. PLoS One 6(7):e21551, 2011 21829436

Zamani A, Omrani GR, Nasab MM: Lithium's effect on bone mineral density. Bone 44(2):331–334, 2009 18992857

Zheng W, Li XB, Tang YL, et al: Metformin for weight gain and metabolic abnormalities associated with antipsychotic treatment: meta-analysis of randomized placebo-controlled trials. J Clin Psychopharmacol 35(5):499–509, 2015 26280837

Zhong KX, Sweitzer DE, Hamer RM, Lieberman JA: Comparison of quetiapine and risperidone in the treatment of schizophrenia: a randomized, double-blind, flexible-dose, 8-week study. J Clin Psychiatry 67(7):1093–1103, 2006 16889453

Ziegenbein M, Held K, Kuenzel HE, et al: The somatostatin analogue octreotide impairs sleep and decreases EEG sigma power in young male subjects. Neuropsychopharmacology 29(1):146–151, 2004 12955096

11

Obstetrics and Gynecology

Margaret Altemus, M.D.
Mallay Occhiogrosso, M.D.

The course of psychiatric illnesses in women is often modulated by reproductive events, including the menstrual cycle, pregnancy, lactation, and menopause. In addition, physiological changes during pregnancy, the postpartum period, and menopause can mimic psychiatric symptoms and should be considered in a differential diagnosis. Several gynecological disorders and treatments can also affect psychiatric status. Conversely, psychiatric disorders and psychopharmacological treatments can have an impact on reproductive functions. Because half of pregnancies are unintended and organ development occurs during the first trimester, it is often too late to avoid teratogenic drug effects before the pregnancy is identified. Treatment of any woman of reproductive age should include a plan for birth control and consideration of possible drug effects in the event of pregnancy.

Differential Diagnosis

Psychiatric Manifestations of Reproductive Conditions and Disorders

Psychiatric Manifestations of Menstrual Cycle and Fertility Disorders

Premenstrual dysphoric disorder (PMDD), which affects 3%–8% of menstruating women, is diagnosed if distinct mood and physical symptoms appear only during the luteal phase of the menstrual cycle and cause significant impairment. PMDD must be distinguished from premenstrual exacerbation of another psychiatric disorder. Depression, obsessive-compulsive disorder, and bulimia symptoms are thought to intensify during the luteal phase, but schizophrenia symptoms seem to be exacerbated in the early follicular phase of the cycle (Bergemann et al. 2007).

Polycystic ovarian syndrome, which affects 5%–10% of women of reproductive age, is associated with a three- to fourfold increased risk of depression and an increased risk of anxiety disorders and binge-eating disorder (Hollinrake et al. 2007; Månsson et al. 2008). In women with comorbid polycystic ovarian syndrome and affective illness, treatment of hyperandrogenism and insulin resistance should be considered, particularly if the affective illness is treatment resistant. It is not known whether depression will resolve without psychiatric treatment if hormonal abnormalities are corrected. However, one recent controlled trial found that pioglitazone had antidepressant effects.

Psychiatric Issues Related to Pregnancy

It is unclear whether rates of major and minor depression are increased during pregnancy or postpartum, but the postpartum period is associated with increased risk of onset or relapse of panic disorder (Sholomskas et al. 1993) and bipolar disorder (Viguera et al. 2000). Because of the increased risk of bipolar manic and depressive relapse postpartum, it is crucial to carefully manage perinatal bipolar illness, avoiding antidepressant monotherapy and sleep disruption and more frequently monitoring serum medication levels. Careful screening for prior episodes of mania or hypomania is valuable for identifying women with previously undiagnosed bipolar disorder.

Postpartum psychosis typically initiates in the first 6 weeks postpartum. It is characterized by insomnia, agitation, paranoia, manic symptoms, and, in some cases, delirium. Risk factors include antithyroid antibodies and a personal and family history of postpartum psychosis. It is a psychiatric emergency and usually requires hospitalization. There is generally a favorable prognosis for rapid remission following treatment with mood stabilizers, antipsychotics, benzodiazepines, or a combination of these agents. However, in the longer term it has a high association with chronic affective or psychotic disorder, as well as a 50% incidence of recurrence following future episodes of childbirth (Blackmore et al. 2013). Prophylactic treatment with mood stabilizers, either atypical neuroleptics or lithium, after parturition is recommended for patients with a history of postpartum psychosis (Bergink et al. 2012).

Women with antithyroid antibodies (up to 15% of reproductive-age women) have a 33%–50% risk of postpartum thyroiditis (Nicholson et al. 2006), which manifests as hyperthyroidism or hypothyroidism and can precipitate or worsen symptoms of depression and anxiety. Free thyroxine and thyroid-stimulating hormone (TSH) should be checked in women presenting with postpartum onset or worsening of depression or anxiety. Restless legs syndrome, in which patients present with insomnia and daytime fatigue, often begins or worsens during pregnancy and is associated with increased risk of depression during pregnancy and postpartum (Wesström et al. 2014).

Hyperemesis occurs in up to 2% of pregnant women. No psychiatric risk factors have been identified, but the condition itself is a severe stressor, causing insomnia, fatigue, anticipatory anxiety, and elevated risk for depression, even in the setting of no prior history (Aksoy et al. 2015). Anecdotal evidence suggests that mirtazapine may relieve severe nausea during pregnancy (Guclu et al. 2005). Benzodiazepines and tricyclic antidepressants (TCAs) have been suggested to target the associated anticipatory anxiety, but there is little or no evidence of efficacy.

Psychiatric Manifestations of Menopause

There is an increased risk of first-onset depression (approximately twofold) (Cohen et al. 2006b; Freeman et al. 2006) and recurrent depression (approximately four- to eightfold) (Freeman et al. 2014) during perimenopause but not after menopause. No controlled studies have been done on the effect of the menopausal transition on bipolar disorder or anxiety disorders; however, cross-sectional studies suggest these disorders may also be exacerbated (Marsh et al. 2015; Wittchen et al. 1994).

Obstetric and Gynecological Manifestations of Psychiatric Disorders

Effects of Psychiatric Disorders on Menstrual Cycle and Fertility

Eating disorders disrupt menstrual cyclicity in proportion to energy deficits brought on by dieting and exercise. Perceived stress has been shown to reduce estradiol and progesterone levels and to increase risk of anovulatory cycles (Schliep et al. 2015), but one meta-analysis found no effect of emotional distress on outcome of in vitro fertilization (Boivin et al. 2011).

Among major psychiatric disorders, autism spectrum disorder, schizophrenia, bipolar disorder, anorexia nervosa, and substance use disorders have been associated with having fewer children, but no effect was seen for depression (Power et al. 2013). Factors contributing to reduced fertility in major psychiatric disorders also include social isolation and medication side effects that have an impact on the gonadal hormone axis and sexual function. A retrospective study found no effect of selective serotonin reuptake inhibitors (SSRIs) on success of in vitro fertilization once the cycle was initiated (Friedman et al. 2009).

Effects of Psychiatric Disorders on Pregnancy and Fetus

Untreated mental illness can lead to maternal behaviors that can have adverse impacts on the fetus, including substance use, insomnia, poor nutrition, poor compliance with prenatal care, and ambivalence about the pregnancy. Reduced fetal weight gain and shortened gestation, as well as maternal stress and anxiety during pregnancy, have long-term impacts on the endocrine system, cognition, and mental health of offspring (Kingston et al. 2015; Malaspina et al. 2008; O'Donnell et al. 2014; Wadhwa 2005).

Depression during pregnancy seems to increase the risk of premature birth two- to threefold (Li et al. 2009; Wisner et al. 2009) and increases the likelihood of postpartum depression. Posttraumatic stress disorder also has been associated with shortened gestation (Yonkers et al. 2014). Compared with pregnant women without a psychiatric diagnosis, pregnant women with schizophrenia show increased rates of fetal death (almost twofold), placental abruption, interventions during labor and delivery, offspring with congenital anomalies, and neonatal complications (Jablensky et al. 2005; Webb et al. 2005). Eating disorders and dieting during the first trimester have been associated with neural tube defects (Carmichael et al. 2003).

Effects of Psychiatric Disorders on Perimenopause

Premorbid anxiety predicts increased risk of vasomotor symptoms during the menopausal transition (Freeman et al. 2005; Gold et al. 2006). A history of depression may predict earlier onset of menopause (Harlow et al. 2003).

Pharmacotherapy of Premenstrual Mood Symptoms

Premenstrual Dysphoric Disorder

SSRIs and serotonin-norepinephrine reuptake inhibitors (SNRIs) are first-line agents for treatment of PMDD and have been shown to be effective when taken either throughout the cycle or during the 2 weeks preceding menstruation and when administered during only symptomatic premenstrual days (Marjoribanks et al. 2013; Yonkers et al. 2015). Luteal phase dosing of alprazolam also has been effective in controlled trials (Williams et al. 2007). Yaz-24, an oral contraceptive containing the progestin drospirenone, has demonstrated efficacy for treatment of PMDD (Lopez et al. 2012). However, drospirenone-containing oral contraceptives have a U.S. Food and Drug Administration black box warning because of a relatively increased risk of serious cardiovascular events compared with other hormonal contraceptives. The relative efficacy of these oral contraceptives for treatment of PMDD compared with oral contraceptives containing other progestins is unclear (Lopez et al. 2012). Continuous dosing of oral contraceptives is commonly used for control of PMDD symptoms, but this is as yet not supported by controlled trials. Although some women experience reduction in premenstrual mood symptoms during oral contraceptive treatment, other women experience exacerbation of mood symptoms (Kulkarni 2007). Gonadotropin-releasing hormone agonists, which shut down the gonadal axis, are effective treatments for PMDD, but use is complicated by menopausal side effects.

Premenstrual Exacerbations of Depression and Anxiety

Despite strong evidence of premenstrual exacerbation of affective illness, limited studies have been done of potential changes in psychotropic drug metabolism across the menstrual cycle. A common approach to premenstrual exacerbation of affective illness is to increase doses of antidepressants and lithium premenstrually, but as yet only limited evidence of efficacy has been shown for this approach (Miller et al. 2008).

Pharmacotherapy of Menopause-Related Depression, Anxiety, and Insomnia

Studies of the effects of combined hormone replacement therapy (HRT) or estradiol treatment on mood in community samples of perimenopausal women without clinically diagnosed depression do not support a beneficial effect on mood (Rubinow et al. 2015). There is limited evidence that short-term transdermal estradiol treatment can relieve unipolar major depression in perimenopausal but not postmenopausal women (Morrison et al. 2004). Transdermal estradiol has been found to be effective for major and minor depression at doses of 50–100 μg/day for 8–12 weeks; response rate was independent of comorbid hot flashes (Joffe et al. 2011; Schmidt et al. 2000; Soares et al. 2001). Estrogen augmentation of antidepressant medication also may be effective during perimenopause (Morgan et al. 2005). One study reported that bipolar women who used HRT had less worsening of mood during perimenopause (Freeman et al. 2002).

Vasomotor symptoms are associated with increased risk for depression and insomnia, although insomnia is also exacerbated in perimenopausal women who do not experience hot flashes. Several psychotropic agents, including venlafaxine (75–150 mg/day) (Archer et al. 2009), paroxetine (7.5–10 mg/day) (Stearns et al. 2005), escitalopram (10–20 mg/day), and gabapentin (900–2,400 mg/day) (Toulis et al. 2009), can relieve hot flashes, and efficacy is similar to that seen with low-dose estrogen treatment (0.5 mg oral 17-β-estradiol) (Guthrie et al. 2015). Higher doses of estrogen treatments are more effective. Treatment with the nonbenzodiazepine hypnotics zolpidem and eszopiclone improved sleep and in one of two studies also produced improvement in subclinical depression symptoms and vasomotor symptoms (Dorsey et al. 2004; Soares et al. 2006). In a recent multicenter trial, yoga, exercise, and omega-3 fatty acid supplements did not relieve hot flashes more than placebo (Guthrie et al. 2015).

Psychopharmacology in Pregnancy and Breastfeeding

Approach to Pharmacotherapy During Pregnancy and Postpartum Period

Management of any psychiatric disorder during pregnancy and lactation is complicated by the need to consider the effects of psychiatric medication on the fetus and newborn (Table 11–1) as well as the potential effects of untreated illness on fetal development. Pregnant and lactating women should use the minimal number of medications at the lowest effective dosage. Current reviews of the reproductive safety of different classes of medication as well as of specific drugs are available online at the Massachusetts General Hospital Center for Women's Mental Health (https://womensmental health.org), and a compilation of relevant recent scientific articles is maintained in the U.S. National Library of Medicine's Developmental and Reproductive Toxicology (DART) database (http://toxnet.nlm.nih.gov/newtoxnet/dart.htm).

In 2015, the U.S. Food and Drug Administration published a new pregnancy and lactation labeling rule that removes the letter rating system (A, B, C, D, X), replacing it with more detailed summaries of available evidence regarding risks of drug exposure during pregnancy and lactation (www.fda.gov/Drugs/DevelopmentApprovalProcess/DevelopmentResources/Labeling/ucm093307.htm). The rule will be phased in gradually for existing medications and applies to all new medications. Under the letter system, some drugs received more favorable ratings because fewer data were available, and some drugs received less favorable ratings because of similarities to drugs with reported risks.

Prospective studies have found that 68% of pregnant women with recurrent depression who discontinued antidepressant use because of pregnancy relapsed during the first or second trimester (Cohen et al. 2006a), and 80% of bipolar women who discontinued mood stabilizers relapsed during pregnancy (Viguera et al. 2007b). No increased risk of relapse was seen in a community sample of women who discontinued antidepressant medication during pregnancy (Yonkers et al. 2011). Women with severe disease should continue their mood stabilizer or antidepressant treatments during the first trimester and throughout pregnancy (ACOG Committee on Practice Bulletins—Obstetrics

Table 11–1.   Effects of psychiatric medications on the fetus or infant

Medication	Pregnancy	Neonatal	Lactation
Anxiolytics			
Benzodiazepines	Teratogenic risk low.	Sedation and withdrawal symptoms possible.	Little information. Use short-half-life agents (e.g., oxazepam).
Antidepressants			
SSRIs	Two- to threefold increased risk of prematurity. Teratogenic risk low. Pulmonary hypertension risk increased by 30% but still very low. Placental transfer lowest for sertraline and paroxetine and highest for citalopram, escitalopram, and fluoxetine.	Neonatal syndrome (irritability, high-pitched cry) for 2–7 days postpartum in up to 30% (more likely with paroxetine and fluoxetine). Transient respiratory difficulty (rare).	Infant generally has low exposure to SSRIs. Lowest infant blood levels with paroxetine and sertraline. Fluoxetine produces infant serum levels >10% of maternal in 10% of infants.
SNRIs	Venlafaxine: limited data show no teratogenic risk. Duloxetine: limited data show no teratogenic risk.	Neonatal syndrome.	Active venlafaxine metabolite present in infant serum at up to 30% of maternal levels.

Table 11–1. Effects of psychiatric medications on the fetus or infant *(continued)*

Medication	Pregnancy	Neonatal	Lactation
Antidepressants *(continued)*			
Bupropion	No evidence of teratogenicity.		Generally undetectable levels in infant serum, but cases of infant seizures have been reported.
TCAs	Less data. No evidence of teratogenicity.	Neonatal syndrome with clomipramine.	Low infant serum levels with nortriptyline.
Electroconvulsive therapy	Case reports of premature labor and placental abruption in third trimester.		
Antipsychotics	Teratogenic risk likely low. Limited evidence. Increased risk of preterm birth and other birth complications. Cesarean section more likely.	Extrapyramidal symptoms; may be prolonged. Low birth weight Infant sedation. Abnormal muscle tone (transient).	Little evidence; olanzapine and risperidone preferred because of case reports of low infant serum levels.

Table 11–1.   Effects of psychiatric medications on the fetus or infant *(continued)*

Medication	Pregnancy	Neonatal	Lactation
Mood stabilizers			
Lithium	Increased risk of heart defect: 2%–8% for any heart defect, 0.1% for Ebstein's anomaly. Lower Apgar scores and increased CNS and neuromuscular complications with lithium level >0.64 mEq/L at delivery.	Case reports of neonatal hypothyroidism and hyperhydramnios.	Infant serum levels 30%–50% of maternal; monitor for dehydration and thyroid function.
Carbamazepine	Increased risk of neural tube defects, facial dysmorphism, and fingernail hypoplasia but less than with valproate.		Infant serum levels about 30% of maternal.
Lamotrigine	Moderate evidence of no increased risk.		Infant serum levels 18%–33% of maternal.
Valproic acid	Dose-dependent (1%–4%) risk of neural tube defect. Increased risk of other abnormalities, including cardiac defects, limb defects, craniofacial abnormalities, and cognitive impairment.	Risk of neonatal hepatic toxicity.	Low concentration in breast milk.

Table 11–1. Effects of psychiatric medications on the fetus or infant *(continued)*

Medication	Pregnancy	Neonatal	Lactation
Psychostimulants	Limited data. No evidence of teratogenicity.		Concentrates in breast milk; infant serum levels 10% of maternal.

Note. CNS = central nervous system; SNRIs = serotonin-norepinephrine reuptake inhibitors; SSRIs = selective serotonin reuptake inhibitors; TCAs = tricyclic antidepressants.

2008). In women with mild disease and low relapse risk, the mood stabilizer or antidepressant may be tapered off entirely or continued until pregnancy is achieved.

Use of the lowest effective dose of psychotropics will lessen the adverse effects of an abrupt taper. Abrupt cessation of mood stabilizers greatly increases the risk of relapse (50% within 2 weeks) compared with a gradual taper (Viguera et al. 2007b). In women with moderate disease and/or relapse risk who respond best to lithium, which has teratogenic risk, an option is to slowly discontinue lithium for conception and then restart lithium at 12 weeks, after the structural development of the fetal heart is complete. Monitoring of maternal serum levels and dosage adjustment of medication is advised as pregnancy progresses and during the early postpartum period because serum levels of lithium, TCAs, lamotrigine, and other psychotropics fall with pregnancy-related increases in volume of distribution, metabolic capacity, and renal filtration (Koren 2006). These changes reverse in the postpartum period, but timing is variable.

Electroconvulsive therapy is a safe, effective, and generally well-tolerated treatment option for acute episodes of mania and severe depression during pregnancy. During pregnancy, electroconvulsive therapy requires some modification of standard techniques (Anderson and Reti 2009).

Anxiolytics and Sedative-Hypnotics

Teratogenicity.   Benzodiazepine prescribing practices in pregnancy vary widely from country to country, from as low as 0.001% in one sample to 3% in another, making benzodiazepines in some countries among the most commonly prescribed type of psychotropic agent (Bellantuono et al. 2013). Despite their common usage, there are limited data to guide clinicians regarding the safety of the use of benzodiazepines in pregnancy and even less regarding use of nonbenzodiazepine sedative-hypnotics.

Several small retrospective case-control studies from the 1970s raised concerns that first-trimester exposure to benzodiazepines may be associated with an increased risk of cleft lip or cleft palate. Retrospective case-control studies are subject to recall bias, and any finding likely will overestimate risk. Furthermore, these studies were significantly underpowered. To get a truer sense of risk, the data from these studies were pooled and reanalyzed in a 1998 meta-analysis by Dolovich et al. They found that the pooled data showed a modestly increased odds ratio (OR) of 1.79 (95% confidence interval [CI] 1.13–2.82) for facial cleft. Cohort studies from that era were also pooled and reanalyzed by Dolovich in the same meta-analysis and did not suggest any rise in risk of facial cleft (Dolovich et al. 1998). Subjects in these early studies were predominantly using the long-acting benzodiazepines diazepam and chlordiazepoxide.

More recently undertaken cohort studies have drawn on large administrative databases to study teratogenicity. Shorter-acting benzodiazepines predominate in these studies. Ban et al. (2014) undertook a cohort study of U.K. general practice records, looking at both benzodiazepine and nonbenzodiazepine hypnotics. They found no evidence of an increase in major congenital malformations in children exposed to either class of medication in the first trimester of pregnancy. In a 2007 study using the Swedish birth registry, Wikner et al. looked at infants exposed to benzodiazepines and/or nonbenzodiazepine hypnotics and found a slight increase in the rate of major congenital malformations (OR=1.24, 95% CI 1.00–1.55) (Wikner et al. 2007). Wikner and Källén (2011) later used additional data from the same birth registry to ascertain whether nonbenzodiazepine hypnotics specifically were safe to use in pregnancy. They did not find evidence linking use with an increased rate of congenital malformations.

For treatment of insomnia during pregnancy, the over-the-counter antihistamine diphenhydramine is frequently recommended. Extremely limited research exists on safety, but a recent study of North American case-control registry data found no associated rise in malformation risk with first-trimester exposure to antihistamines (Li et al. 2013).

Restless legs syndrome develops in up to 30% of pregnant women (Wesström et al. 2014). If iron deficiency is not a factor, treatment options include opioids, gabapentin, and benzodiazepines (Djokanovic et al. 2008). Several small recent database studies on gabapentin have been reassuring with regard to its safety profile (e.g., Fujii et al. 2013; Holmes and Hernandez-Diaz 2012). Dopamine agonists, normally a first-line treatment for restless legs syndrome, should be avoided during pregnancy because little is known about potential effects on the fetus.

Neonatal symptoms.   If benzodiazepines are used late in pregnancy, infants should be closely monitored for neonatal adverse effects, including irritability, tremor, withdrawal seizures, floppy baby syndrome, and apnea and other respiratory difficulties, although there have been few case reports of these potential adverse effects. Patients who wish to discontinue benzodiazepines during pregnancy should taper gradually to avoid withdrawal effects on mother and fetus. Withdrawal symptoms could be long lasting in newborns. Short-half-life agents with no active metabolites, such as lorazepam and oxazepam, are less likely to accumulate in the fetus.

Postnatal development.   Hartz et al. (1975) found no differences in behavior at 8 months or IQ at 4 years in children exposed to chlordiazepoxide during gestation compared with children who were not. However, because little is known regarding the effects of in utero benzodiazepine exposure on neurobehavioral development, low doses and time-limited use are recommended during pregnancy. In addition, the combination of benzodiazepines and SSRIs should be avoided if possible, in light of evidence that the combination has greater adverse effects on infant arousal and regulation across the first month postpartum (Salisbury et al. 2016).

Antidepressants

Teratogenicity.   SSRIs are the most extensively studied class of medication regarding safety in pregnancy. Nonetheless, controversy persists regarding whether there may be a minor increased risk of cardiac malformation in infants exposed to SSRIs in the first trimester. A very small rise in increased risk above baseline has been found in some studies of paroxetine and fluoxetine (see, e.g., Reefhuis et al. 2015), although not in others (see, e.g., Huybrechts et al. 2014; Wichman et al. 2009). In December 2005, the U.S. Food and Drug Administration published an advisory warning of the potential risk of using paroxetine in pregnancy (U.S. Food and Drug Administration 2005), although there is still lack of clarity regarding the exact level of risk. One difficulty in clarifying the risk is the fact that the SSRI exposure may be a confounder by indication, as was in fact shown to be the case in a reanalysis of registry data in a study by Furu et al. (2015). By using a sibling pair analysis, Furu's team found that what had in an initial analysis looked like an increased cardiac and other malformation risk attributable to SSRI exposure was, in fact, a rise in risk attributable to previously unknown familial and environmental factors (Furu et al. 2015).

Risk of cardiac malformations may be increased if SSRIs are combined with benzodiazepines (Oberlander et al. 2008; Wikner et al. 2007). Teratogenic effects have not been found for venlafaxine, nefazodone, trazodone, or mirtazapine, but sample sizes have been underpowered (Einarson et al. 2009). Data on bupropion are limited, but its use appears to be safe in terms of cardiac defects (Huybrechts et al. 2014). Data on duloxetine are similarly sparse, but data appear to be reassuring in terms of cardiac risk (Andrade 2014; Einarson et al. 2012; Hoog et al. 2013). In addition, the rate of spontaneous abortion with duloxetine exposure was not significantly elevated relative to the general population (Hoog et al. 2013; Kjaersgaard et al. 2013). Although less formally studied, TCAs do not seem to be associated with birth defects. Little is known about the newer antidepressant agents vortioxetine and vilazodone, so their use in pregnancy should be avoided if possible.

In utero development.   Treatment of maternal psychiatric disorders with SSRIs in pregnancy appears to be protective of preterm birth and cesarean section relative to the offspring of mothers with psychiatric disorders who are unexposed to medications. However, SSRI exposure raises the risk of other complications, including neonatal abstinence syndrome (see the following subsection) and stay in the intensive care unit (Malm et al. 2015). Exposure to SSRIs in the third trimester of pregnancy, when lung maturation occurs, also appears to slightly increase the risk of persistent pulmonary hypertension of the newborn (PPHN). This condition occurs when pulmonary blood vessels fail to relax to allow increased blood flow after delivery. The most common risk factors are meconium aspiration and premature delivery, and the condition can range from transient to persistent pulmonary function deficits to fatal. Baseline risk of PPHN is estimated at 1.9 per 1,000 live births. To date, there have been no reported cases of PPHN associated with SSRI exposure resulting in death of an infant. With SSRI exposure, risk has been estimated to rise 1.2- to 3.5-fold, depending on the analysis methods (Grigoriadis et al. 2014; Huybrechts et al. 2015). Several risk factors for PPHN, including obesity, premature delivery, and cesarean section, are also associated with depression, making it difficult to sort out the degree of risk associated with SSRI exposure and depression itself (Occhiogrosso et al. 2012). Among the TCAs, nortriptyline and desipramine are preferred in order to minimize risk of maternal orthostatic hypotension, which could compromise placental perfusion.

Neonatal syndromes.   A neonatal syndrome has been associated with SSRI exposure in the third trimester. Symptoms can include difficulty feeding, tremor, high-pitched cry, irritability, muscle rigidity or low muscle tone, respiratory distress, tachypnea, jitteriness, and convulsions. This syndrome, most common with paroxetine and fluoxetine, occurs in approximately 20% of SSRI-exposed infants but usually lasts only a few days (Moses-Kolko et al. 2005; Oberlander et al. 2006; Sanz et al. 2005), although a recent study found that symptoms of hyperarousal persisted for up to 14 days postpartum (Salisbury et al. 2016). A similar neonatal syndrome has been described with in utero clomipramine exposure but not with exposure to other TCAs.

Postnatal development.   Infants exposed to SSRIs in utero appear to have normal neurocognitive outcomes, although data are limited. Cognitive function, temperament, and general behavior were similar in children exposed prenatally to TCAs or fluoxetine and in unexposed comparison children in two studies (Nulman et al. 1997, 2002).

Small studies seem to indicate that infants exposed to SSRIs in utero may have mild transient motor delays in the first year of life (e.g., Pedersen et al. 2010). However, these do not appear to be clinically significant (Santucci et al. 2014). SSRI exposure was not found to be linked with an increased risk of autism spectrum disorder in two Scandinavian registry studies when maternal psychiatric illness and other potential confounders were controlled for (Hviid et al. 2013; Sørensen et al. 2013).

Summary.   Sertraline is a first-line antidepressant for use during pregnancy, as supported by a large amount of reassuring teratogenicity data for SSRIs (Huybrechts et al. 2014; Reefhuis et al. 2015), evidence of less placental transfer for sertraline than other SSRIs (Hendrick et al. 2003; Loughhead et al. 2006), lower risk for neonatal withdrawal syndrome, and benign safety profile during lactation (see later subsection "Approach to Psychopharmacotherapy During Breastfeeding").

Antipsychotics

Few adequately powered studies exist to give a clear sense of the relative safety of the use of either first-generation antipsychotics (FGAs) or second-generation antipsychotics (SGAs) in pregnancy. A prospective cohort study by Habermann et al. (2013) of the use of SGAs in pregnancy showed a twofold increased risk of malformations, although this may have reflected a detection bias toward minor, transient cardiac defects. The rate of spontaneous abortions and stillbirths was not increased relative to baseline. Pooled data from smaller studies of exposure to both FGAs and SGAs in pregnancy also suggest a very small rise in risk of major malformations (Coughlin et al. 2015). One study suggested that although all SGAs examined passed into the placental circulation, quetiapine had the least and olanzapine the most placental transfer (Newport et al. 2007).

In utero development.   Antipsychotic use during pregnancy may be associated with other adverse birth outcomes. One study found that exposure to antipsychotics in pregnancy was associated with a predisposition to preterm birth and small-for-gestational-age birth weight (Coughlin et al. 2015). Habermann et al. (2013) found that exposure to FGAs but not SGAs was associated with preterm birth and low birth weight. The effect of atypical antipsychotics on weight gain in pregnancy is not known but is of concern because obesity is associated with an increased rate of multiple birth defects, eclampsia, insulin resistance, and high birth weight (Newham et al. 2008; Waller et al. 2007).

Mood Stabilizers

Teratogenicity.   Use of lithium in the pregnant patient has been associated with an overall 1.2- to 7.7-fold increase in fetal cardiac defects (Diav-Citrin et al. 2014; Yonkers et al. 2004), most of which are correctable and many of which resolve spontaneously. The risk for the potentially severe Ebstein's anomaly is increased twentyfold but is still low (1 in 1,000 infants) (Giles and Bannigan 2006). With fetal exposure to lithium in the first trimester, ultrasonography or fetal echocardiography to assess fetal cardiac development is advised. Use of sustained-release lithium preparations minimizes peak lithium levels, which may be protective (Yonkers et al. 2004). Another antimanic agent with more limited but positive efficacy and safety data is verapamil (Wisner et al. 2002).

Use of antiepileptic agents in pregnancy has been studied mainly in patients with epilepsy. Valproic acid is associated with a significantly increased risk of incomplete neural tube closure (1%–4%), cardiac defects, craniofacial abnormalities, and limb defects. Valproate exposure increases the rate of any congenital malformation to 9.3%. It has also been associated with neurodevelopmental delays and increased risk of autism. Risk increases with dosage and with combined anticonvulsant therapy. Carbamazepine is also terato-genic, increasing the risk of neural tube defects, facial dysmorphism, and fin-gernail hypoplasia, but the risk of malformations is much lower, at 3% in a large database study, than with valproate (Hernández-Díaz et al. 2012). Folate supplementation decreases the incidence of neural tube defects in carbamaze-pine-exposed pregnancies (Hernández-Díaz et al. 2001) but not in valproate-exposed pregnancies (Wyszynski et al. 2005).

Lamotrigine registry data to date indicate no increased risk of congenital malformations, although some database studies have found a risk of oral clefts slightly above population baseline (Hernández-Díaz et al. 2012). Topiramate was not associated with any structural abnormalities in a small prospective study of 52 women (Ornoy et al. 2008), but several recent studies have reported an increased risk of oral cleft (Hernández-Díaz et al. 2012). Insufficient data are available to assess teratogenicity of levetiracetam, gabapentin, or oxcarbaze-pine, but the small amount of existing data is reassuring (Hernández-Díaz et al. 2012).

In utero development.   Valproic acid exposure is associated with fetal growth restriction. Preliminary evidence suggests that topiramate reduces birth weight but does not increase the risk of prematurity (Ornoy et al. 2008).

Neonatal syndromes.   Lithium completely equilibrates across the placenta. Significantly lower Apgar scores, longer hospital stays, and higher rates of cen-tral nervous system and neuromuscular complications were observed in infants with higher lithium concentrations (>0.64 mEq/L) at delivery. Withholding lithium therapy for 24–48 hours before delivery reduces maternal lithium lev-els by more than one-third (Newport et al. 2005). Symptoms of neonatal lith-ium toxicity include flaccidity, lethargy, and poor reflexes. For the mother, intravenous fluids are indicated at delivery to counterbalance maternal blood volume contraction during delivery. Following delivery, the prepregnancy dosage should be resumed, with close monitoring for dosage adjustments as maternal fluid volume contracts.

Postnatal development.   A 5-year follow-up of 60 children exposed to lith-ium in utero did not find evidence of neurobehavioral toxicity (Schou 1976). In utero valproic acid exposure has been clearly linked to dose-dependent cog-nitive impairment, with IQ at 3 years reduced by 9 points and 6 points compared with children exposed to lamotrigine and carbamazepine, respectively (Meador et al. 2009).

Summary.   Because of the significant risks to the fetus of valproic acid exposure, a switch to lithium, lamotrigine, or an antipsychotic should be considered.

Psychostimulants

Insufficient data are available to evaluate the teratogenic effects of the therapeutic use of amphetamine, methylphenidate, modafinil, or atomoxetine during pregnancy. Two cohort studies of amphetamine administration for weight control during pregnancy did not show an increase in the rate of malformations. Another cohort study of first-trimester exposure to methylphenidate did not find any statistically significant increase in major malformations (Pottegård et al. 2014).

Approach to Psychopharmacotherapy During Breastfeeding

Concern about the exposure of breastfeeding infants to maternal medications leads women and their physicians to avoid medications, at times unnecessarily, and to avoid lactation. The clinician should put breastfeeding in context, giving the mother permission to forgo lactation if she requires a medication that poses a risk to the infant or if the demands of breastfeeding are impeding her recovery. Long-term outcome data from medication exposure during lactation are not available, but the long-term risks of maternal depression on infants and older siblings are substantial and well documented (Pilowsky et al. 2008). In general, infant exposure to medication can be reduced by replacing breast milk with formula at some feedings.

Although the quantitative data on infant exposure to drugs through breast milk are limited, the exposure is, with some exceptions, orders of magnitude less than exposure during pregnancy. In general, breast milk concentrations of medications and active metabolites are in equilibrium with maternal serum concentrations. Infant exposure is also determined by maturation of the infant's metabolic systems, gut-blood barrier, and blood-brain barrier. For example, lamotrigine levels are relatively high in infant serum because the glucuronidation metabolic pathway is inefficient in infants. For medications taken infrequently on an as-needed basis, half-life is an important consideration. Maternal serum and milk concentrations will be reduced by 75% after

two half-lives. Therapeutic drug level monitoring in infants is of limited clinical use because serum levels associated with toxicity have not been established
for infants. Online resources, including the U.S. National Library of Medicine's Drugs and Lactation Database (LactMed; U.S. National Library of
Medicine 2016), can provide more detailed, up-to-date information for specific drugs (see also Hospital for Sick Children 2016).

Anxiolytics and Sedative-Hypnotics

Limited information is available on the safety of benzodiazepines and the
newer nonbenzodiazepine hypnotics in lactating women, and no long-term
exposure data are available. However, case reports of exposure to clonazepam
suggest low infant serum levels (Birnbaum et al. 1999). Exposed infants
should be monitored for sedation and withdrawal. If sleep aids are necessary
for mothers, agents with short half-lives (e.g., zolpidem, oxazepam) are preferred. Nortriptyline and mirtazapine, which have minimal serum levels in
breast-fed infants, also can be used to promote sleep in lactating women.

Antidepressants

Paroxetine, sertraline, citalopram, mirtazapine, and nortriptyline have minimal or undetectable circulating levels in breast-fed infants. A few medications,
including venlafaxine, fluoxetine, and doxepin, frequently produce infant serum levels of parent drug plus active metabolites that are greater than 10% of
maternal serum levels, although these higher levels have not been linked to adverse outcomes (Weissman et al. 2004). One study found that infants exposed
to fluoxetine during pregnancy and lactation had less weight gain after birth
(Chambers et al. 1996). Although infant levels of bupropion and its active
metabolite are reportedly low (Baab et al. 2002; Briggs et al. 1993), authors of
two case reports described seizures in infants exposed to bupropion ("Bupropion" 2005; Chaudron and Schoenecker 2004). Little is known about newer
antidepressant agents vortioxetine and vilazodone, so their use in pregnancy
should be avoided if possible.

Antipsychotics

Little research has focused on infants exposed to antipsychotic medications
through breastfeeding. On the basis of case reports of infant serum levels, the
LactMed database (U.S. National Library of Medicine 2016) notes that olan-

zapine and risperidone have the best, although limited, evidence of low or undetectable infant serum levels and lack of adverse effects in the infant. A controlled study comparing outcomes up to 1 year among infants exposed to olanzapine through breast milk found no increase in adverse events compared with nonexposed infants whose mothers were taking olanzapine and infants of mothers not taking olanzapine (Gilad et al. 2011). Avoid, if possible, the use of newer antipsychotics such as lurasidone, paliperidone, and asenapine, whose effects on nursing infants still have not been studied.

Mood Stabilizers

Lithium levels in breast-fed infants average 30%–50% of maternal levels, raising concerns of lithium toxicity should the infant become dehydrated or febrile (Viguera et al. 2007a). Signs of lithium toxicity in an infant are lethargy, poor feeding, and hypotonia. Monitoring of lithium levels, blood urea nitrogen, creatinine, and TSH is indicated in exposed infants at 6-week intervals after the in utero contribution has been cleared. Use of infant blood sampling equipment containing lithium heparin may produce spuriously high lithium levels.

Studies suggest very limited diffusion of valproic acid into breast milk, although one case of thrombocytopenia and anemia, which resolved after cessation of breastfeeding, has been reported (Stahl et al. 1997). Liver function, platelets, and valproic acid levels should be monitored in exposed infants.

Carbamazepine is present in infant plasma at concentrations averaging 31% of maternal levels, and a few reports describe adverse events, including hepatic toxicity and poor feeding, in breast-fed infants (U.S. National Library of Medicine 2016). Use of carbamazepine while breastfeeding should be approached with caution, and infant serum levels, liver function, and complete blood count should be monitored.

Infant serum levels of lamotrigine have been found to be 18%–33% of maternal concentrations. No adverse effects, other than a case of mild thrombocytopenia, have been reported in infants (Newport et al. 2008). Complete blood count and liver function should be monitored.

Psychostimulants

Amphetamine or methylphenidate can suppress prolactin release and thus may inhibit lactation. Few data are available to evaluate infant exposure to methylphenidate or other stimulants through breast milk. Case reports indicate that dextroamphetamine and racemic amphetamine preferentially pass into breast milk, with threefold higher levels in milk than in maternal plasma, consistent with distribution of a weak base. Infant serum levels are approximately 10% of maternal serum levels (Öhman et al. 2015). No data have been published to guide use of modafinil or atomoxetine during lactation.

Adverse Obstetric and Gynecological Reactions to Psychotropic Drugs

Hyperprolactinemia

Hyperprolactinemia is a relatively common side effect of psychotropic drugs and can interfere with the menstrual cycle and fertility. A full discussion of this topic is provided in Chapter 10, "Endocrine and Metabolic Disorders."

Polycystic Ovarian Syndrome

Women receiving valproate have a 10% risk of developing polycystic ovarian syndrome, which often corrects on medication discontinuation (Joffe 2007). For premenopausal women starting to take valproate, menstrual cycle pattern, hirsutism, acne, and weight should be assessed at baseline and monitored closely, particularly during the first year of treatment, to detect development of polycystic ovarian syndrome.

Effects of Psychotropic Drugs on Sexual Function

SSRIs and SNRIs produce sexual side effects in 30%–70% of users. Women experience impairments in libido, genital sensitivity, and the ability to experience orgasm. The biological mechanism responsible for these side effects is not clear, but recent data suggest use of the phosphodiesterase type 5 inhibitor sildenafil on an as-needed basis to enhance ability to reach orgasm and sexual satisfaction (Nurnberg et al. 2008). There is also evidence in women, consistent with studies in men, that bupropion can enhance desire, lubrication, and ability to reach orgasm in women with SSRI-induced sexual dysfunction (Safarinejad 2011). Antipsychotics, TCAs, and monoamine oxidase inhibitors (MAOIs) also can impair sexual function. No pharmacological antidotes for these agents have been identified in controlled studies.

Psychiatric Effects of Obstetric and Gynecological Agents and Procedures

As discussed in the following subsections, a variety of obstetric and gynecological medications and procedures have negative psychiatric effects. Table 11–2 lists the psychiatric adverse effects of the medications.

Hormonal Contraceptives

Little systematic study has been done on the effects of hormonal contraceptives on mood, but estimates suggest that 10%–21% of patients experience adverse mood symptoms (Segebladh et al. 2009). A history of mood disorders or premenstrual mood symptoms has been linked to increased mood lability and depressive symptoms during oral contraceptive use (Kurshan and Neill Epperson 2006; Segebladh et al. 2009). Hormonal contraceptives lower free testosterone levels and may thereby reduce libido (Greco et al. 2007). Progestin-only contraceptives, recommended for lactating women because estrogen can reduce milk supply, have been reported to cause psychiatric adverse effects, more commonly with subdermal and injectable formulations than with oral formulations.

Infertility Treatment

Often during the course of artificial insemination, intrauterine insemination, and in vitro fertilization, medications are administered to stimulate ovarian follicle development, producing supraphysiological levels of circulating estrogen. Almost no systematic study has been done of the effects of ovarian stimulation on psychiatric disorders. Women with a history of depression or anxiety are more likely to have exacerbation of anxiety and depression symptoms during in vitro fertilization treatment than women with no history of affective disorders (Zaig et al. 2013). In a retrospective survey, 40%–60% of women treated with clomiphene or gonadotropins reported mood swings and irritability (Choi et al. 2005). In addition, there are case reports of manic and psychotic reactions to clomiphene and gonadotropins, often in women with preexisting mood disorders (Choi et al. 2005; Grimm and Hubrich 2008; Persaud and Lam 1998). Gonadotropin-releasing hormone agonists, often used to stop endogenous cycling for treatment of endometriosis and for in vitro fertilization protocols, also can cause depression (Warnock et al. 2000). However, depression

Table 11–2.   Psychiatric adverse effects of obstetric and gynecological drugs

Medication	Psychiatric adverse effects
Hormonal contraceptives	Increased mood lability and depressive symptoms
β-Adrenergic agonists (systemic)	
Terbutaline, salbutamol, and ritodrine	Anxiety
Galactogogues	
Metoclopramide	Anxiety, depression, extrapyramidal symptoms
Gonadotropins	Mood lability and irritability
Estrogen receptor modulators	
Clomiphene	Mood lability, irritability
Gonadotropin-releasing hormone agonists	
Buserelin, goserelin, histrelin, leuprolide, and nafarelin	Depression

induction is much rarer in women who have no history of psychiatric illness (Ben Dor et al. 2013). In light of these reports, women prone to mood destabilization who are undergoing gonadal suppression or ovarian stimulation may consider remaining on antidepressant medication or a mood stabilizer at least until pregnancy is achieved.

Tocolytics

β-Adrenergic agonists prescribed to halt premature labor can be anxiogenic, and among these, salbutamol is most likely to cause anxiety (Neilson et al. 2014).

Galactogogues

Agents commonly used to increase breast milk production include the herbal supplement fenugreek and the dopamine antagonists metoclopramide and domperidone, both of which enhance lactation by increasing prolactin release.

Domperidone (not available in the United States) has very limited central nervous system access and is without psychoactive effects (Osadchy et al. 2012). Metoclopramide acts centrally and peripherally and may cause clinically significant anxiety and depression and extrapyramidal symptoms (Anfinson 2002; Kluge et al. 2007).

Surgical or Medication-Induced Menopause

Ovariectomy or medical precipitation of menopause during treatment of endometriosis, fibroids, or breast cancer increases risk for hot flashes, depression, anxiety, pain, and sexual dysfunction compared with natural menopause and its more gradual drop in hormone levels (Aziz et al. 2005). Surgical menopause increases lifelong risk for anxiety, depression, and dementia (Faubion et al. 2015), likely due to a longer lifetime exposure to reduced hormone levels. Estrogen replacement therapy and the estrogen agonist tibolone improve anxiety in surgically menopausal women (Baksu et al. 2005). Menopausal phenomenology and treatment were also discussed earlier in the section "Pharmacotherapy of Menopause-Related Depression, Anxiety, and Insomnia."

Hormone Replacement Therapy

Estrogen and progesterone are often administered at menopause for a range of physical symptoms, including hot flashes, osteoporosis, and vaginal dryness. A proportion of healthy women have adverse mood reactions to HRT, particularly the progestin components, and premorbid anxiety is a risk factor for adverse mood reactions to combined HRT (Björn et al. 2006). Cessation of HRT may also adversely affect mood in some women, but this possibility has not been well studied. The increased risk of dementia in women with surgical menopause may be attenuated by HRT initiated prior to age 50 (Faubion et al. 2015). These findings are in contrast to the National Institutes of Health–sponsored Women's Health Initiative (WHI) study, which found that women initiating hormone therapy 10–15 years after menopause had increased risk for dementia (Shumaker et al. 2003). Although multiple trials have found increased risk of breast cancer, heart disease, stroke, and pulmonary embolism with HRT, there is evidence that these risks are lower in women who start HRT within 10 years of menopause (Boardman et al. 2015).

Testosterone supplementation can improve sexual desire in menopausal women. However, because available formulations have much higher doses intended for men, low-dose preparations must be specially compounded for women (see also Chapter 10, "Endocrine and Metabolic Disorders"). Flibanserin, a 5-hydroxytryptamine type 1A agonist and 2A antagonist, was approved in 2015 for treatment of low libido in premenopausal women.

Drug-Drug Interactions

A number of complex pharmacokinetic and pharmacodynamic interactions can occur between psychotropic drugs and obstetric and gynecological drugs (see Tables 11–3 and 11–4). See Chapter 1, "Pharmacokinetics, Pharmacodynamics, and Principles of Drug-Drug Interactions," for a comprehensive discussion.

Pharmacokinetic Interactions

A number of psychotropics, including carbamazepine, phenytoin, oxcarbazepine, topiramate, armodafinil, modafinil, and St. John's wort, induce cytochrome P450 3A4 (CYP3A4), the principal enzyme involved in sex steroid metabolism. This increased metabolism may reduce the effect of oral contraceptives and the vaginal ring (Thorneycroft et al. 2006). A survey and case series suggest an increase in contraceptive failure in the presence of anticonvulsant medications (Krauss et al. 1996). Estrogen, in turn, increases glucuronidation reactions through induction of uridine 5′-diphosphate glucuronosyltransferase. For psychotropic drugs eliminated primarily through conjugation (lamotrigine, oxazepam, lorazepam, temazepam, desvenlafaxine, and olanzapine), increased clearance and reduced therapeutic effects have been observed with estrogen coexposure. Estrogen-containing hormonal contraceptives reduce serum levels of lamotrigine by approximately 50%. Lamotrigine dosage adjustments are also required with the onset or cessation of HRT (Harden et al. 2006). By increasing estrogen, treatments that stimulate ovulation may also enhance glucuronidation (Reimers et al. 2005; Thorneycroft et al. 2006).

Pharmacodynamic Interactions

Several drugs used in obstetrics and gynecology, including terbutaline and domperidone, prolong QT interval (CredibleMeds 2016). These agents should be

Table 11–3. Obstetric and gynecological drug–psychotropic drug interactions

Medication	Interaction mechanism	Effects on psychotropic drugs and management
β-Adrenergic agonists (systemic) Terbutaline	Additive hypertensive effect	Increased risk of hypertension with MAOIs; avoid concurrent use.
Estrogen-containing preparations	Induction of UGT	Increased clearance and reduced therapeutic effect of drugs primarily eliminated through conjugation (e.g., desvenlafaxine, lamotrigine, lorazepam, olanzapine, oxazepam, temazepam). Estradiol in hormonal contraceptives reduces lamotrigine levels by 50%.
Domperidone and terbutaline	QT prolongation	Increased QT prolongation in combination with other QT-prolonging drugs such as TCAs, typical antipsychotics, lithium, pimozide, iloperidone, paliperidone, quetiapine, risperidone, and ziprasidone.
Domperidone	Peripheral dopamine receptor antagonism	Increased hyperprolactinemia and galactorrhea with antipsychotics.
Metoclopramide	Peripheral and central dopamine receptor antagonism	Increased EPS with antipsychotics, SNRIs, or SSRIs. Increased hyperprolactinemia and galactorrhea with antipsychotics.
Tamoxifen	Inhibits CYP2C9	Reduced phenytoin metabolism.

Note. CYP=cytochrome P450; EPS=extrapyramidal symptoms; MAOIs=monoamine oxidase inhibitors; SNRIs=serotonin-norepinephrine reuptake inhibitors; SSRIs=selective serotonin reuptake inhibitors; TCAs=tricyclic antidepressants; UGT=uridine 5′-diphosphate glucuronosyltransferase.

Table 11–4.   Psychotropic drug–obstetric and gynecological drug interactions

Medication	Interaction mechanism	Effects on obstetric and gynecological drugs and management
Carbamazepine, oxcarbazepine, phenytoin, and topiramate; armodafinil and modafinil; and St. John's wort	Induction of CYP3A4	Increased metabolism of sex steroids and reduced effect of oral contraceptives and vaginal ring. Surveys suggest increased risk of contraceptive failure.
Atomoxetine, bupropion, duloxetine, fluoxetine, moclobemide, and paroxetine	Inhibition of CYP2D6	Reduced bioactivation of prodrug tamoxifen and decreased therapeutic effect.
Atypical antipsychotics iloperidone, paliperidone, quetiapine, risperidone, and ziprasidone; lithium; pimozide; TCAs; and typical antipsychotics	QT prolongation	Increased QT prolongation in combination with other QT-prolonging drugs such as terbutaline and domperidone.

Note.   CYP = cytochrome P450; TCAs = tricyclic antidepressants.

used with caution in the presence of other drugs that have QT-prolonging effects, such as TCAs, typical antipsychotics, pimozide, risperidone, paliperidone, iloperidone, quetiapine, ziprasidone, and lithium (Kane et al. 2008; van Noord et al. 2009). Systemic β-adrenergic agonist tocolytics, such as terbutaline, may precipitate a hypertensive crisis in combination with MAOIs. Metoclopramide may increase extrapyramidal symptoms when coadministered with antipsychotics, SSRIs, or SNRIs.

Key Clinical Points

Menstruating Women

- All psychotropic medications must be selected assuming the possibility of pregnancy, and patients should be counseled regarding the risks and benefits of medication (and untreated psychopathology) for all aspects of reproduction.
- To distinguish PMDD from premenstrual exacerbation of another psychiatric disorder, PMDD should be diagnosed with two cycles of prospective ratings and a diagnostic interview prior to initiating treatment.
- SSRIs and the drospirenone-containing oral contraceptives are effective treatments for PMDD.

Pregnant Women

- Untreated psychiatric illness carries a risk to mother and fetus.
- Monotherapy with agents that have short half-lives is preferred.
- The clinician should maximize use of alternative therapies to pharmacotherapy, including psychotherapy and sleep hygiene.
- Valproic acid should be avoided if possible because of teratogenic and neurodevelopmental effects.

Lactating Women

- Generally, infant exposure to psychotropic drugs through breast milk is substantially lower than levels of exposure in utero. Lithium, carbamazepine, and lamotrigine are exceptions.
- Among antidepressants, sertraline and paroxetine have the most data supportive of safety during lactation.

Perimenopausal Women

- Risk of first-onset depression and relapse of depression is increased during perimenopause but not after menopause.
- Short-term hormone replacement therapy can relieve depression during perimenopause but not after menopause.
- Vasomotor symptoms respond to venlafaxine, paroxetine, and gabapentin in some women, but response rates are lower than with estradiol treatment.

References

ACOG Committee on Practice Bulletins—Obstetrics: ACOG Practice Bulletin: clinical management guidelines for obstetrician-gynecologists number 92, April 2008 (replaces practice bulletin number 87, November 2007). Use of psychiatric medications during pregnancy and lactation. Obstet Gynecol 111(4):1001–1020, 2008 18378767

Aksoy H, Aksoy Ü, Karadağ OI, et al: Depression levels in patients with hyperemesis gravidarum: a prospective case-control study. Springerplus 4:34, 2015 25646155

Anderson EL, Reti IM: ECT in pregnancy: a review of the literature from 1941 to 2007. Psychosom Med 71(2):235–242, 2009 19073751

Andrade C: The safety of duloxetine during pregnancy and lactation. J Clin Psychiatry 75(12):e1423–e1427, 2014 25551238

Anfinson TJ: Akathisia, panic, agoraphobia, and major depression following brief exposure to metoclopramide. Psychopharmacol Bull 36(1):82–93, 2002 12397849

Archer DF, Dupont CM, Constantine GD, et al; Study 319 Investigators: Desvenlafaxine for the treatment of vasomotor symptoms associated with menopause: a double-blind, randomized, placebo-controlled trial of efficacy and safety. Am J Obstet Gynecol 200(3):238.e1–238.e10, 2009 19167693

Aziz A, Bergquist C, Nordholm L, et al: Prophylactic oophorectomy at elective hysterectomy. Effects on psychological well-being at 1-year follow-up and its correlations to sexuality. Maturitas 51(4):349–357, 2005 16039407

Baab SW, Peindl KS, Piontek CM, Wisner KL: Serum bupropion levels in 2 breastfeeding mother-infant pairs. J Clin Psychiatry 63(10):910–911, 2002 12416600

Baksu A, Ayas B, Citak S, et al: Efficacy of tibolone and transdermal estrogen therapy on psychological symptoms in women following surgical menopause. Int J Gynaecol Obstet 91(1):58–62, 2005 15970290

Ban L, West J, Gibson JE, et al: First trimester exposure to anxiolytic and hypnotic drugs and the risks of major congenital anomalies: a United Kingdom population-based cohort study. PLoS One 9(6):e100996, 2014 24963627

Bellantuono C, Tofani S, Di Sciascio G, Santone G: Benzodiazepine exposure in pregnancy and risk of major malformations: a critical overview. Gen Hosp Psychiatry 35(1):3–8, 2013 23044244

Ben Dor R, Harsh VL, Fortinsky P, et al: Effects of pharmacologically induced hypogonadism on mood and behavior in healthy young women. Am J Psychiatry 170(4):426–433, 2013 23545794

Bergemann N, Parzer P, Runnebaum B, et al: Estrogen, menstrual cycle phases, and psychopathology in women suffering from schizophrenia. Psychol Med 37(10):1427–1436, 2007 17451629

Bergink V, Bouvy PF, Vervoort JS, et al: Prevention of postpartum psychosis and mania in women at high risk. Am J Psychiatry 169(6):609–615, 2012 22407083

Birnbaum CS, Cohen LS, Bailey JW, et al: Serum concentrations of antidepressants and benzodiazepines in nursing infants: a case series. Pediatrics 104(1):e11, 1999 10390297

Björn I, Bäckström T, Lalos A, Sundström-Poromaa I: Adverse mood effects during postmenopausal hormone treatment in relation to personality traits. Climacteric 9(4):290–297, 2006 16857659

Blackmore ER, Rubinow DR, O'Connor TG, et al: Reproductive outcomes and risk of subsequent illness in women diagnosed with postpartum psychosis. Bipolar Disord 15(4):394–404, 2013 23651079

Boardman HM, Hartley L, Eisinga A, et al: Hormone therapy for preventing cardiovascular disease in post-menopausal women. Cochrane Database of Systematic Reviews, 2015, Issue 3. Art. No.: CD002229. DOI: 10.1002/14651858.CD002229.pub4 25754617

Boivin J, Griffiths E, Venetis CA: Emotional distress in infertile women and failure of assisted reproductive technologies: meta-analysis of prospective psychosocial studies. BMJ 342:d223, 2011 21345903

Briggs GG, Samson JH, Ambrose PJ, Schroeder DH: Excretion of bupropion in breast milk. Ann Pharmacother 27(4):431–433, 1993 8477117

Bupropion: seizures in an infant exposed through breast-feeding. Prescrire Int 14(78):144, 2005 16108101

Carmichael SL, Shaw GM, Schaffer DM, et al: Dieting behaviors and risk of neural tube defects. Am J Epidemiol 158(12):1127–1131, 2003 14652296

Chambers CD, Johnson KA, Dick LM, et al: Birth outcomes in pregnant women taking fluoxetine. N Engl J Med 335(14):1010–1015, 1996 8793924

Chambers CD, Hernandez-Diaz S, Van Marter LJ, et al: Selective serotonin-reuptake inhibitors and risk of persistent pulmonary hypertension of the newborn. N Engl J Med 354(6):579–587, 2006 16467545

Chaudron LH, Schoenecker CJ: Bupropion and breastfeeding: a case of a possible infant seizure. J Clin Psychiatry 65(6):881–882, 2004 15291673

Choi SH, Shapiro H, Robinson GE, et al: Psychological side-effects of clomiphene citrate and human menopausal gonadotrophin. J Psychosom Obstet Gynaecol 26(2):93–100, 2005 16050534

Cohen LS, Altshuler LL, Harlow BL, et al: Relapse of major depression during pregnancy in women who maintain or discontinue antidepressant treatment. JAMA 295(5):499–507, 2006a 16449615

Cohen LS, Soares CN, Vitonis AF, et al: Risk for new onset of depression during the menopausal transition: the Harvard study of moods and cycles. Arch Gen Psychiatry 63(4):385–390, 2006b 16585467

Coughlin CG, Blackwell KA, Bartley C, et al: Obstetric and neonatal outcomes after antipsychotic medication exposure in pregnancy. Obstet Gynecol 125(5):1224–1235, 2015 25932852

CredibleMeds: Risk categories for drugs that prolong QT and induce torsades de pointes (TdP), June 15, 2016. Available at: https://crediblemeds.org. Accessed July 7, 2016.

Diav-Citrin O, Shechtman S, Tahover E, et al: Pregnancy outcome following in utero prospective, comparative, observational study. Am J Psychiatry 171(7):785–794, 2014 24781368

Djokanovic N, Garcia-Bournissen F, Koren G: Medications for restless legs syndrome in pregnancy. J Obstet Gynaecol Can 30(6):505–507, 2008 18611302

Dolovich LR, Addis A, Vaillancourt JM, et al: Benzodiazepine use in pregnancy and major malformations or oral cleft: meta-analysis of cohort and case-control studies. BMJ 317(7162):839–843, 1998 9748174

Dorsey CM, Lee KA, Scharf MB: Effect of zolpidem on sleep in women with perimenopausal and postmenopausal insomnia: a 4-week, randomized, multicenter, double-blind, placebo-controlled study. Clin Ther 26(10):1578–1586, 2004 15598474

Einarson A, Choi J, Einarson TR, Koren G: Incidence of major malformations in infants following antidepressant exposure in pregnancy: results of a large prospective cohort study. Can J Psychiatry 54(4):242–246, 2009 19321030

Einarson A, Smart K, Vial T, et al: Rates of major malformations in infants following exposure to duloxetine during pregnancy: a preliminary report. J Clin Psychiatry 73(11):1471, 2012 23218163

Ernst CL, Goldberg JF: The reproductive safety profile of mood stabilizers, atypical antipsychotics, and broad-spectrum psychotropics. J Clin Psychiatry 63 (suppl 4):42–55, 2002 11913676

Faubion SS, Kuhle CL, Shuster LT, Rocca WA: Long-term health consequences of premature or early menopause and considerations for management. Climacteric 18(4):483–491, 2015 25845383

Freeman EW, Sammel MD, Lin H, et al: The role of anxiety and hormonal changes in menopausal hot flashes. Menopause 12(3):258–266, 2005 15879914

Freeman EW, Sammel MD, Lin H, Nelson DB: Associations of hormones and menopausal status with depressed mood in women with no history of depression. Arch Gen Psychiatry 63(4):375–382, 2006 16585466

Freeman EW, Sammel MD, Boorman DW, Zhang R: Longitudinal pattern of depressive symptoms around natural menopause. JAMA Psychiatry 71(1):36–43, 2014 24227182

Freeman MP, Smith KW, Freeman SA, et al: The impact of reproductive events on the course of bipolar disorder in women. J Clin Psychiatry 63(4):284–287, 2002 12004800

Friedman BE, Rogers JL, Shahine LK, et al: Effect of selective serotonin reuptake inhibitors on in vitro fertilization outcome. Fertil Steril 92(4):1312–1314, 2009 19423105

Fujii H, Goel A, Bernard N, et al: Pregnancy outcomes following gabapentin use: results of a prospective comparative cohort study. Neurology 80(17):1565–1570, 2013 23553472

Furu K, Kieler H, Haglund B, et al: Selective serotonin reuptake inhibitors and venlafaxine in early pregnancy and risk of birth defects: population based cohort study and sibling design. BMJ 350:h1798, 2015 25888213

Gilad O, Merlob P, Stahl B, Klinger G: Outcome of infants exposed to olanzapine during breastfeeding. Breastfeed Med 6(2):55–58, 2011 21034242

Giles JJ, Bannigan JG: Teratogenic and developmental effects of lithium. Curr Pharm Des 12(12):1531–1541, 2006 16611133

Gold EB, Colvin A, Avis N, et al: Longitudinal analysis of the association between vasomotor symptoms and race/ethnicity across the menopausal transition: study of women's health across the nation. Am J Public Health 96(7):1226–1235, 2006 16735636

Greco T, Graham CA, Bancroft J, et al: The effects of oral contraceptives on androgen levels and their relevance to premenstrual mood and sexual interest: a comparison of two triphasic formulations containing norgestimate and either 35 or 25 microg of ethinyl estradiol. Contraception 76(1):8–17, 2007 17586130

Grigoriadis S, Vonderporten EH, Mamisashvili L, et al: Prenatal exposure to antidepressants and persistent pulmonary hypertension of the newborn: systematic review and meta-analysis. BMJ 348:f6932, 2014 24429387

Grimm O, Hubrich P: Delusional belief induced by clomiphene treatment. Prog Neuropsychopharmacol Biol Psychiatry 32(5):1338–1339, 2008 18538909

Guclu S, Gol M, Dogan E, Saygili U: Mirtazapine use in resistant hyperemesis gravidarum: report of three cases and review of the literature. Arch Gynecol Obstet 272(4):298–300, 2005 16007504

Guthrie KA, LaCroix AZ, Ensrud KE, et al: Pooled analysis of six pharmacologic and nonpharmacologic interventions for vasomotor symptoms. Obstet Gynecol 126(2):413–422, 2015 26241433

Habermann F, Fritzsche J, Fuhlbrück F, et al: Atypical antipsychotic drugs and pregnancy outcome: a prospective, cohort study. J Clin Psychopharmacol 33(4):453–462, 2013 23764684

Harden CL, Herzog AG, Nikolov BG, et al: Hormone replacement therapy in women with epilepsy: a randomized, double-blind, placebo-controlled study. Epilepsia 47(9):1447–1451, 2006 16981859

Harlow BL, Wise LA, Otto MW, et al: Depression and its influence on reproductive endocrine and menstrual cycle markers associated with perimenopause: the Harvard Study of Moods and Cycles. Arch Gen Psychiatry 60(1):29–36, 2003 12511170

Hartz SC, Heinonen OP, Shapiro S, et al: Antenatal exposure to meprobamate and chlordiazepoxide in relation to malformations, mental development, and childhood mortality. N Engl J Med 292(14):726–728, 1975 1113782

Hendrick V, Stowe ZN, Altshuler LL, et al: Placental passage of antidepressant medications. Am J Psychiatry 160(5):993–996, 2003 12727706

Hernández-Díaz S, Werler MM, Walker AM, Mitchell AA: Neural tube defects in relation to use of folic acid antagonists during pregnancy. Am J Epidemiol 153(10):961–968, 2001 11384952

Hernández-Díaz S, Smith CR, Shen A, et al; North American AED Pregnancy Registry: Comparative safety of antiepileptic drugs during pregnancy. Neurology 78(21):1692–1699, 2012 22551726

Hollinrake E, Abreu A, Maifeld M, et al: Increased risk of depressive disorders in women with polycystic ovary syndrome. Fertil Steril 87(6):1369–1376, 2007 17397839

Holmes LB, Hernandez-Diaz S: Newer anticonvulsants: lamotrigine, topiramate and gabapentin. Birth Defects Res A Clin Mol Teratol 94(8):599–606, 2012 22730257

Hoog SL, Cheng Y, Elpers J, Dowsett SA: Duloxetine and pregnancy outcomes: safety surveillance findings. Int J Med Sci 10(4):413–419, 2013 23471302

Hospital for Sick Children: Motherisk: Pregnancy & breastfeeding resources. Available at: www.motherisk.org. Accessed April 8, 2016.

Huybrechts KF, Palmsten K, Avorn J, et al: Antidepressant use in pregnancy and the risk of cardiac defects. N Engl J Med 370(25):2397–2407, 2014 24941178

Huybrechts KF, Bateman BT, Palmsten K, et al: Antidepressant use late in pregnancy and risk of persistent pulmonary hypertension of the newborn. JAMA 313(21):2142–2151, 2015 26034955

Hviid A, Melbye M, Pasternak B: Use of selective serotonin reuptake inhibitors during pregnancy and risk of autism. N Engl J Med 369(25):2406–2415, 2013 24350950

Jablensky AV, Morgan V, Zubrick SR, et al: Pregnancy, delivery, and neonatal complications in a population cohort of women with schizophrenia and major affective disorders. Am J Psychiatry 162(1):79–91, 2005 15625205

Joffe H: Reproductive biology and psychotropic treatments in premenopausal women with bipolar disorder. J Clin Psychiatry 68 (suppl 9):10–15, 2007 17764379

Joffe H, Petrillo LF, Koukopoulos A, et al: Increased estradiol and improved sleep, but not hot flashes, predict enhanced mood during the menopausal transition. J Clin Endocrinol Metab 96(7):E1044–E1054, 2011 21525161

Kane JM, Lauriello J, Laska E, et al: Long-term efficacy and safety of iloperidone: results from 3 clinical trials for the treatment of schizophrenia. J Clin Psychopharmacol 28(2) (suppl 1):S29–S35, 2008 18334910

Kingston D, McDonald S, Austin MP, Tough S: Association between prenatal and postnatal psychological distress and toddler cognitive development: a systemic review. PLoS One 10(5):e0126929, 2015 25996151

Kjaersgaard MI, Parner ET, Vestergaard M, et al: Prenatal antidepressant exposure and risk of spontaneous abortion: a population-based study. PLoS One 8(8):e72095, 2013 24015208

Kluge M, Schüssler P, Steiger A: Persistent generalized anxiety after brief exposure to the dopamine antagonist metoclopramide. Psychiatry Clin Neurosci 61(2):193–195, 2007 17362439

Koren G: Changes in drug handling during pregnancy: what it might mean for your patients. Can Fam Physician 52(10):1214–1215, 2006 17279178

Krauss GL, Brandt J, Campbell M, et al: Antiepileptic medication and oral contraceptive interactions: a national survey of neurologists and obstetricians. Neurology 46(6):1534–1539, 1996 8649543

Kulkarni J: Depression as a side effect of the contraceptive pill. Expert Opin Drug Saf 6(4):371–374, 2007 17688380

Kurshan N, Neill Epperson C: Oral contraceptives and mood in women with and without premenstrual dysphoria: a theoretical model. Arch Women Ment Health 9(1):1–14, 2006 16206030

Li D, Liu L, Odouli R: Presence of depressive symptoms during early pregnancy and the risk of preterm delivery: a prospective cohort study. Hum Reprod 24(1):146–153, 2009 18948314

Li Q, Mitchell AA, Werler MM, et al: Assessment of antihistamine use in early pregnancy and birth defects. J Allergy Clin Immunol Pract 1(6):666–74.e1, 2013 24565715

Lopez LM Kaptien AA, Helmerhorst FM: Oral contraceptives containing drospirenone for premenstrual syndrome. Cochrane Database of Systematic Reviews, 2012, Issue 2. Art. No.: CD006586. DOI: 10.1002/14651858.CD006586.pub4 22336820

Loughhead AM, Stowe ZN, Newport DJ, et al: Placental passage of tricyclic antidepressants. Biol Psychiatry 59(3):287–290, 2006 16271264

Malaspina D, Corcoran C, Kleinhaus KR, et al: Acute maternal stress in pregnancy and schizophrenia in offspring: a cohort prospective study. BMC Psychiatry 8:71–79, 2008 18717990

Malm H, Sourander A, Gissler M, et al: Pregnancy complications following prenatal exposure to SSRIs or maternal psychiatric disorders: results from population-based national register data. Am J Psychiatry 172(12):1224–1232, 2015 26238606

Månsson M, Holte J, Landin-Wilhelmsen K, et al: Women with polycystic ovary syndrome are often depressed or anxious—a case control study. Psychoneuroendocrinology 33(8):1132–1138, 2008 18672334

Marjoribanks J, Brown J, O'Brien PM, Wyatt K: Selective serotonin reuptake inhibitors for premenstrual syndrome. Cochrane Database of Systematic Reviews, 2013, Issue 6. Art. No.: CD001396. DOI: 10.1002/14651858.CD001396.pub3 23744611

Marsh WK, Gershenson B, Rothschild AJ: Symptom severity of bipolar disorder during the menopausal transition. Int J Bipolar Disord 3:35, 2015

Meador KJ, Baker GA, Browning N, et al; NEAD Study Group: Cognitive function at 3 years of age after fetal exposure to antiepileptic drugs. N Engl J Med 360(16):1597–1605, 2009 19369666

Miller MN, Newell CL, Miller BE, et al: Variable dosing of sertraline for premenstrual exacerbation of depression: a pilot study. J Womens Health (Larchmt) 17(6):993–997, 2008 18681820

Morgan ML, Cook IA, Rapkin AJ, Leuchter AF: Estrogen augmentation of antidepressants in perimenopausal depression: a pilot study. J Clin Psychiatry 66(6):774–780, 2005 15960574

Morrison MF, Kallan MJ, Ten Have T, et al: Lack of efficacy of estradiol for depression in postmenopausal women: a randomized, controlled trial. Biol Psychiatry 55(4):406–412, 2004 14960294

Moses-Kolko EL, Bogen D, Perel J, et al: Neonatal signs after late in utero exposure to serotonin reuptake inhibitors: literature review and implications for clinical applications. JAMA 293(19):2372–2383, 2005 15900008

Neilson JP, West HM, Dowswell T: Betamimetics for inhibiting preterm labour. Cochrane Database of Systematic Reviews, 2014, Issue 2. Art. No.: CD004352. DOI: 10.1002/14651858.CD004352.pub3 24500892

Newham JJ, Thomas SH, MacRitchie K, et al: Birth weight of infants after maternal exposure to typical and atypical antipsychotics: prospective comparison study. Br J Psychiatry 192(5):333–337, 2008 18450655

Newport DJ, Viguera AC, Beach AJ, et al: Lithium placental passage and obstetrical outcome: implications for clinical management during late pregnancy. Am J Psychiatry 162(11):2162–2170, 2005 16263858

Newport DJ, Calamaras MR, DeVane CL, et al: Atypical antipsychotic administration during late pregnancy: placental passage and obstetrical outcomes. Am J Psychiatry 164(8):1214–1220, 2007 17671284

Newport DJ, Pennell PB, Calamaras MR, et al: Lamotrigine in breast milk and nursing infants: determination of exposure. Pediatrics 122(1):e223–e231, 2008 18591203

Nicholson WK, Robinson KA, Smallridge RC, et al: Prevalence of postpartum thyroid dysfunction: a quantitative review. Thyroid 16(6):573–582, 2006 16839259

Nulman I, Rovet J, Stewart DE, et al: Neurodevelopment of children exposed in utero to antidepressant drugs. N Engl J Med 336(4):258–262, 1997 8995088

Nulman I, Rovet J, Stewart DE, et al: Child development following exposure to tricyclic antidepressants or fluoxetine throughout fetal life: a prospective, controlled study. Am J Psychiatry 159(11):1889–1895, 2002 12411224

Nurnberg HG, Hensley PL, Heiman JR, et al: Sildenafil treatment of women with antidepressant-associated sexual dysfunction: a randomized controlled trial. JAMA 300(4):395–404, 2008 18647982

Oberlander TF, Warburton W, Misri S, et al: Neonatal outcomes after prenatal exposure to selective serotonin reuptake inhibitor antidepressants and maternal depression using population-based linked health data. Arch Gen Psychiatry 63(8):898–906, 2006 16894066

Oberlander TF, Warburton W, Misri S, et al: Major congenital malformations following prenatal exposure to serotonin reuptake inhibitors and benzodiazepines using population-based health data. Birth Defects Res B Dev Reprod Toxicol 83(1):68–76, 2008 18293409

Occhiogrosso M, Omran SS, Altemus M: Persistent pulmonary hypertension of the newborn and selective serotonin reuptake inhibitors: lessons from clinical and translational studies. Am J Psychiatry 169(2):134–140, 2012 22420034

O'Donnell KJ, Glover V, Barker ED, O'Connor TG: The persisting effect of maternal mood in pregnancy on childhood psychopathology. Dev Psychopathol 26(2):393–403, 2014 24621564

Öhman I, Wikner BN, Beck O, Sarman I: Narcolepsy treated with racemic amphetamine during pregnancy and breastfeeding. J Hum Lact 31(3):374–376, 2015 25948577

Ornoy A, Zvi N, Arnon J, et al: The outcome of pregnancy following topiramate treatment: a study on 52 pregnancies. Reprod Toxicol 25(3):388–389, 2008 18424066

Osadchy A, Moretti ME, Koren G: Effect of domperidone on insufficient lactation in puerperal women: a systematic review and meta-analysis of randomized controlled trials. Obstet Gynecol Int 2012:642893, 2012 22461793

Pedersen LH, Henriksen TB, Olsen J: Fetal exposure to antidepressants and normal milestone development at 6 and 19 months of age. Pediatrics 125(3):e600–e608, 2010 20176667

Persaud RN, Lam RW: Manic reaction after induction of ovulation with gonadotropins. Am J Psychiatry 155(3):447–448, 1998 9501764

Pilowsky DJ, Wickramaratne P, Talati A, et al: Children of depressed mothers 1 year after the initiation of maternal treatment: findings from the STAR*D-Child Study. Am J Psychiatry 165(9):1136–1147, 2008 18558646

Pottegård A, Hallas J, Andersen JT, et al: First-trimester exposure to methylphenidate: a population-based cohort study. J Clin Psychiatry 75(1):e88–e93, 2014 24502866

Power RA, Kyaga S, Uher R, et al: Fecundity of patients with schizophrenia, autism, bipolar disorder, depression, anorexia nervosa, or substance abuse vs their unaffected siblings. JAMA Psychiatry 70(1):22–30, 2013 23147713

Reefhuis J, Devine O, Friedman JM, et al; National Birth Defects Prevention Study: Specific SSRIs and birth defects: Bayesian analysis to interpret new data in the context of previous reports. BMJ 351:h3190, 2015 26156519

Reimers A, Helde G, Brodtkorb E: Ethinyl estradiol, not progestogens, reduces lamotrigine serum concentrations. Epilepsia 46(9):1414–1417, 2005 16146436

Reis M, Källén B: Maternal use of antipsychotics in early pregnancy and delivery outcome. J Clin Psychopharmacol 28(3):279–288, 2008 18480684

Rubinow DR, Johnson SL, Schmidt PJ, et al: Efficacy of estradiol in perimenopausal depression: so much promise and so few answers. Depress Anxiety 32(8):539–549, 2015 26130315

Safarinejad MR: Reversal of SSRI-induced female sexual dysfunction by adjunctive bupropion in menstruating women: a double-blind, placebo-controlled and randomized study. J Psychopharmacol 25(3):370–378, 2011 20080928

Salisbury AL, O'Grady KE, Battle CL, et al: The roles of maternal depression, serotonin reuptake inhibitor treatment, and concomitant benzodiazepine use on infant neurobehavioral functioning over the first postnatal month. Am J Psychiatry 173(2):147–157, 2016 26514656

Sanz EJ, De-las-Cuevas C, Kiuru A, et al: Selective serotonin reuptake inhibitors in pregnant women and neonatal withdrawal syndrome: a database analysis. Lancet 365(9458):482–487, 2005 15705457

Santucci AK, Singer LT, Wisniewski SR, et al: Impact of prenatal exposure to serotonin reuptake inhibitors or maternal major depressive disorder on infant developmental outcomes. J Clin Psychiatry 75(10):1088–1095, 2014 25373117

Schliep KC, Mumford SL, Vladutiu CJ, et al: Perceived stress, reproductive hormones, and ovulatory function: a prospective cohort study. Epidemiology 26(2):177–184, 2015 25643098

Schmidt PJ, Nieman L, Danaceau MA, et al: Estrogen replacement in perimenopause-related depression: a preliminary report. Am J Obstet Gynecol 183(2):414–420, 2000 10942479

Schou M: What happened later to the lithium babies? A follow-up study of children born without malformations. Acta Psychiatr Scand 54(3):193–197, 1976 970196

Segebladh B, Borgström A, Odlind V, et al: Prevalence of psychiatric disorders and premenstrual dysphoric symptoms in patients with experience of adverse mood during treatment with combined oral contraceptives. Contraception 79(1):50–55, 2009 19041441

Sholomskas DE, Wickamaratne PJ, Dogolo L, et al: Postpartum onset of panic disorder: a coincidental event? J Clin Psychiatry 54(12):476–480, 1993 8276738

Shumaker SA, Legault C, Rapp SR, et al; WHIMS Investigators: Estrogen plus progestin and the incidence of dementia and mild cognitive impairment in postmenopausal women: the Women's Health Initiative Memory Study: a randomized controlled trial. JAMA 289(20):2651–2662, 2003 12771112

Soares CN, Almeida OP, Joffe H, Cohen LS: Efficacy of estradiol for the treatment of depressive disorders in perimenopausal women: a double-blind, randomized, placebo-controlled trial. Arch Gen Psychiatry 58(6):529–534, 2001 11386980

Soares CN, Arsenio H, Joffe H, et al: Escitalopram versus ethinyl estradiol and norethindrone acetate for symptomatic peri- and postmenopausal women: impact on depression, vasomotor symptoms, sleep, and quality of life. Menopause 13(5):780–786, 2006 16894334

Sørensen MJ, Grønborg TK, Christensen J, et al: Antidepressant exposure in pregnancy and risk of autism spectrum disorders. Clin Epidemiol 5:449–459, 2013 24255601

Stahl MMS, Neiderud J, Vinge E: Thrombocytopenic purpura and anemia in a breast-fed infant whose mother was treated with valproic acid. J Pediatr 130(6):1001–1003, 1997 9202628

Stearns V, Slack R, Greep N, et al: Paroxetine is an effective treatment for hot flashes: results from a prospective randomized clinical trial. J Clin Oncol 23(28):6919–6930, 2005 16192581

Thorneycroft I, Klein P, Simon J: The impact of antiepileptic drug therapy on steroidal contraceptive efficacy. Epilepsy Behav 9(1):31–39, 2006 16766231

Toulis KA, Tzellos T, Kouvelas D, Goulis DG: Gabapentin for the treatment of hot flashes in women with natural or tamoxifen-induced menopause: a systematic review and meta-analysis. Clin Ther 31(2):221–235, 2009 19302896

U.S. Food and Drug Administration: FDA advising of risk of birth defects with Paxil. Dec 8, 2005. Available at: www.fda.gov/NewsEvents/Newsroom/PressAnnouncements/2005/ucm108527.htm. Accessed April 20, 2016.

U.S. National Library of Medicine: TOXNET databases. 2016. Available at: www.toxnet.nlm.nih.gov. Accessed April 20, 2016.

van Noord C, Straus SM, Sturkenboom MC, et al: Psychotropic drugs associated with corrected QT interval prolongation. J Clin Psychopharmacol 29(1):9–15, 2009 19142100

Viguera AC, Nonacs R, Cohen LS, et al: Risk of recurrence of bipolar disorder in pregnant and nonpregnant women after discontinuing lithium maintenance. Am J Psychiatry 157(2):179–184, 2000 10671384

Viguera AC, Newport DJ, Ritchie J, et al: Lithium in breast milk and nursing infants: clinical implications. Am J Psychiatry 164(2):342–345, 2007a 17267800

Viguera AC, Whitfield T, Baldessarini RJ, et al: Risk of recurrence in women with bipolar disorder during pregnancy: prospective study of mood stabilizer discontinuation. Am J Psychiatry 164(12):1817–1824, quiz 1923, 2007b 18056236

Wadhwa PD: Psychoneuroendocrine processes in human pregnancy influence fetal development and health. Psychoneuroendocrinology 30(8):724–743, 2005 15919579

Waller DK, Shaw GM, Rasmussen SA, et al; National Birth Defects Prevention Study: Prepregnancy obesity as a risk factor for structural birth defects. Arch Pediatr Adolesc Med 161(8):745–750, 2007 17679655

Warnock JK, Bundren JC, Morris DW: Depressive mood symptoms associated with ovarian suppression. Fertil Steril 74(5):984–986, 2000 11056245

Webb R, Abel K, Pickles A, Appleby L: Mortality in offspring of parents with psychotic disorders: a critical review and meta-analysis. Am J Psychiatry 162(6):1045–1056, 2005 15930050

Weissman AM, Levy BT, Hartz AJ, et al: Pooled analysis of antidepressant levels in lactating mothers, breast milk, and nursing infants. Am J Psychiatry 161(6):1066–1078, 2004 15169695

Wesström J, Skalkidou A, Manconi M, et al: Pre-pregnancy restless legs syndrome (Willis-Ekbom disease) is associated with perinatal depression. J Clin Sleep Med 10(5):527–533, 2014 24812538

Wichman CL, Moore KM, Lang TR, et al: Congenital heart disease associated with selective serotonin reuptake inhibitor use during pregnancy. Mayo Clin Proc 84(1):23–27, 2009 19121250

Wikner BN, Källén B: Are hypnotic benzodiazepine receptor agonists teratogenic in humans? J Clin Psychopharmacol 31(3):356–359, 2011 21508851

Wikner BN, Stiller CO, Bergman U, et al: Use of benzodiazepines and benzodiazepine receptor agonists during pregnancy: neonatal outcome and congenital malformations. Pharmacoepidemiol Drug Saf 16(11):1203–1210, 2007 17894421

Williams KE, Marsh WK, Rasgon NL: Mood disorders and fertility in women: a critical review of the literature and implications for future research. Hum Reprod Update 13(6):607–616, 2007 17895237

Wisner KL, Peindl KS, Perel JM, et al: Verapamil treatment for women with bipolar disorder. Biol Psychiatry 51(9):745–752, 2002 11983188

Wisner KL, Sit DK, Hanusa BH, et al: Major depression and antidepressant treatment: impact on pregnancy and neonatal outcomes. Am J Psychiatry 166(5):557–566, 2009 19289451

Wittchen HU, Zhao S, Kessler RC, Eaton WW: DSM-III-R generalized anxiety disorder in the National Comorbidity Survey. Arch Gen Psychiatry 51(5):355–364, 1994 8179459

Wyszynski DF, Nambisan M, Surve T, et al; Antiepileptic Drug Pregnancy Registry: Increased rate of major malformations in offspring exposed to valproate during pregnancy. Neurology 64(6):961–965, 2005 15781808

Yonkers KA, Wisner KL, Stowe Z, et al: Management of bipolar disorder during pregnancy and the postpartum period. Am J Psychiatry 161(4):608–620, 2004 15056503

Yonkers KA, Gotman N, Smith MV, et al: Does antidepressant use attenuate the risk of a major depressive episode in pregnancy? Epidemiology 22(6):848–854, 2011 21900825

Yonkers KA, Norwitz ER, Smith MV, et al: Depression and serotonin reuptake inhibitor treatment as risk factors for preterm birth. Epidemiology 23(5):677–685, 2012 22627901

Yonkers KA, Smith MV, Forray A, et al: Pregnant women with posttraumatic stress disorder and risk of preterm birth. JAMA Psychiatry 71(8):897–904, 2014 24920287

Yonkers KA, Kornstein SG, Gueorguieva R, et al: Symptom-onset dosing of sertraline for the treatment of premenstrual dysphoric disorder: a randomized clinical trial. JAMA Psychiatry 72(10):1037–1044, 2015 26351969

Zaig I, Azem F, Schreiber S, et al: Psychological response and cortisol reactivity to in vitro fertilization treatment in women with a lifetime anxiety or unipolar mood disorder diagnosis. J Clin Psychiatry 74(4):386–392, 2013 23656846

12

Infectious Diseases

Christopher P. Kogut, M.D.

Stephen J. Ferrando, M.D.

James L. Levenson, M.D.

James A. Owen, Ph.D.

Psychiatric symptoms are part of many systemic and central nervous system (CNS) infections. Even limited infections may cause neuropsychiatric symptoms in vulnerable patients, such as those who are elderly or who have preexisting brain disease. In this chapter, we discuss bacterial, viral, and parasitic infections with prominent neuropsychiatric involvement, with a focus on HIV and AIDS. (Hepatitis C is covered in Chapter 4, "Gastrointestinal Disorders.") Neuropsychiatric side effects of commonly used antibiotics, as well as drug-disease and drug-drug interactions, are reviewed (see also Chapter 1, "Pharmacokinetics, Pharmacodynamics, and Principles of Drug-Drug Interactions").

Bacterial Infections

Pediatric Autoimmune Neuropsychiatric Disorders Associated With Streptococcal Infections

Pediatric autoimmune neuropsychiatric disorders associated with streptococcal infections (PANDAS) refer to a subset of obsessive-compulsive and tic disorders that appear to have been triggered by an infection with group A β-hemolytic streptococci (GABHS). PANDAS are defined by onset of symptoms during early childhood; an episodic course characterized by abrupt onset of symptoms with frequent relapses and remissions; associated neurological signs, especially tics; and temporal association with GABHS infections (most commonly pharyngitis). Children with uncomplicated strep infections treated with antibiotics appear to have no increased risk for PANDAS (Perrin et al. 2004).

Although PANDAS are conceptualized as autoimmune disorders, antibiotics active against GABHS may be beneficial in reducing current symptoms (Snider et al. 2005). In children with recurrent streptococcal infections, antibiotic prophylaxis to prevent neuropsychiatric exacerbations has yielded mixed results. Whereas one double-blind, placebo-controlled trial found no benefit of penicillin over placebo in preventing PANDAS exacerbations (Garvey et al. 1999), another trial found that either penicillin or azithromycin was able to lower rates of recurrent streptococcal infections and to decrease PANDAS symptom exacerbations (Snider et al. 2005). Improvements in PANDAS symptoms have also been demonstrated in patients following use of plasma exchange and intravenous immunoglobulin (IVIG). In one study, severity of obsessive-compulsive disorder symptoms diminished by 45%–58% following treatment with either plasma exchange or IVIG (Perlmutter et al. 1999). A recent series of 12 cases with long follow-up also supported the potential of IVIG as part of a multimodal treatment approach (Kovacevic et al. 2015). However, immunomodulatory therapies have not been recommended as a routine treatment for PANDAS.

Neuroborreliosis

Lyme disease is caused by the spirochete *Borrelia burgdorferi*. If untreated, patients may develop chronic neuroborreliosis, including a mild sensory radiculopathy, difficulty with concentration and memory, fatigue, daytime hypersomnolence, irritability, and depression. These chronic symptoms are not distinctive but are almost always preceded by the classic early symptoms of Lyme disease. The differential diagnosis of neuroborreliosis in a patient presenting with poorly explained fatigue, depression, and/or impaired cognition includes fibromyalgia, chronic fatigue syndrome, other infections, somatoform disorders, depression, autoimmune diseases, and multiple sclerosis.

Neither serological testing nor antibiotic treatment is cost effective in patients who have a low probability of having the disease (i.e., nonspecific symptoms, low-incidence region). Meta-analysis of antibiotic treatment for acute Lyme disease found no differences between doxycycline and β-lactam antibiotics regarding residual neurological symptoms at 4–12 months (Dersch et al. 2015). Multiple controlled trials have found no benefit of extended intravenous or oral antibiotics in patients with well-documented previously treated Lyme disease who had persistent pain, neurocognitive symptoms, dysesthesia, or fatigue (Dersch et al. 2015; Kaplan et al. 2003; Klempner et al. 2001; Krupp et al. 2003; Oksi et al. 2007). The only exception is a very small ($N=37$) placebo-controlled trial of 10 weeks of intravenous ceftriaxone in patients with at least 3 weeks of prior intravenous antibiotics; moderate generalized cognitive improvement was seen at week 12 but was not sustained to week 24 (Fallon et al. 2008). Although there has been some reappraisal of the findings of these studies, the consensus of experts is that chronic antibiotic therapy is not indicated for persistent neuropsychiatric symptoms in patients previously adequately treated for Lyme disease (Delong et al. 2012; Fallon et al. 2012; Feder et al. 2007; Klempner et al. 2013). A double-blind, randomized controlled trial is in progress to clarify the role of prolonged antibiotic treatment (Berende et al. 2014).

Neurosyphilis

Neurosyphilis is now the predominant form of tertiary syphilis and most frequently occurs in immunocompromised patients. Symptoms include cognitive dysfunction, including dementia, changes in personality, psychosis, and seizures. Intravenous penicillin G is the recommended treatment for all forms of neurosyphilis (Jay 2006). In some patients with dementia due to neurosyphilis, the infection appears to have "burned out," and they show no clinical response to penicillin G. A recent review found insufficient data to support the long-term benefit of penicillin therapy on cognitive function (Moulton and Koychev 2015). Multiple case reports but no controlled trials have addressed treatment of psychiatric symptoms associated with neurosyphilis. One review recommended treatment of psychosis in neurosyphilis patients using the typical antipsychotic haloperidol or the atypical agents quetiapine or risperidone (Sanchez and Zisselman 2007). An anticonvulsant such as divalproex sodium was also recommended for agitation and mood stabilization. Case reports have supported atypical antipsychotics, such as olanzapine and quetiapine, in treatment of neurosyphilis-associated psychosis (Taycan et al. 2006; Turan et al. 2007), electroconvulsive therapy in treatment-refractory cases (Pecenak et al. 2015), and donepezil for residual neurocognitive symptoms (Wu et al. 2015).

Tuberculosis in the Central Nervous System

Tuberculosis of the brain, spinal cord, or meninges (CNS TB) is caused primarily by *Mycobacterium tuberculosis* and most often occurs in immunocompromised patients. CNS TB may manifest with meningitis, cerebritis, tuberculomas, and abscesses. Seizures are common, and psychiatric symptoms include delirium, delusions, hallucinations, and affective lability. Corticosteroids used to reduce inflammation and edema may exacerbate these symptoms (see Chapter 10, "Endocrine and Metabolic Disorders"). Antitubercular agents have been reported to cause multiple psychiatric adverse effects (see Table 12–1) and may be associated with significant interactions with psychotropic drugs (see Table 12–2). Literature on psychopharmacological treatment of CNS TB is scant. Anticonvulsants are used for seizures and may treat affective instability, whereas antipsychotics may be used for psychotic symptoms, with caution exercised because of the risk of developing extrapyramidal side effects (EPS) and lowering of the seizure threshold (Woodroof and Gleason 2002).

Viral Infections

HIV/AIDS

Substantial research data demonstrate the safety and efficacy of psychopharmacological treatments in patients with HIV/AIDS. Knowledge about differential diagnosis, neuropsychiatric adverse effects of antiretrovirals, and drug-drug interactions are particularly important in the psychopharmacological management of these patients.

Table 12–1. Psychiatric adverse effects of antibiotic therapy

Medication	Neuropsychiatric adverse effects
Antibacterials	
Aminoglycosides	Delirium, psychosis
Antitubercular agents	
Cycloserine	Agitated depression, mania, psychosis, delirium, confusion, insomnia, anxiety
Ethambutol	Confusion, psychosis
Ethionamide (thiocarbamides)	Depression, psychosis, sedation
Isoniazid (hydrazides)	Insomnia, cognitive dysfunction, hallucinations, delusions, obsessive-compulsive symptoms, depression, agitation, anxiety, mania, suicidal ideation and behavior
Rifampin	Drowsiness, cognitive dysfunction, delusions, hallucinations, dizziness
β-*Lactam agents*	
Cephalosporins	Euphoria, delusions, depersonalization, visual illusions
Imipenem	Encephalopathy
Lactam antibiotics	Confusion, paranoia, hallucinations, mania
Penicillins	Anxiety, illusions and hallucinations, depersonalization, agitation, insomnia, delirium, mania (amoxicillin), psychosis and delirium (procaine penicillin)
Fluoroquinolones	
Ciprofloxacin, levofloxacin, moxifloxacin, and ofloxacin	Class effects: psychosis, insomnia, delirium, mania, depression

Table 12–1. Psychiatric adverse effects of antibiotic
therapy *(continued)*

Medication	Neuropsychiatric adverse effects
Antibacterials *(continued)*	
Macrolides	
Clarithromycin and erythromycin	Nightmares, confusion, anxiety, mood lability, psychosis, mania
Metronidazole	Agitated depression, insomnia, confusion, panic, delusions, hallucinations, mania, disulfiram-like reaction
Quinolones	Class effects: restlessness, hallucinations, delusions, irritability, delirium, anxiety, insomnia, depression, psychosis
Sulfonamides	
Trimethoprim/ sulfamethoxazole, dapsone	Class effects: depression, mania, restlessness, irritability, panic, hallucinations, delusions, delirium, confusion, anorexia
Tetracyclines	Class effects: memory disturbance
Antivirals	
Nucleoside reverse transcriptase inhibitors	
Abacavir	Depression, mania, suicidal ideation, anxiety, psychosis, insomnia, nightmares, fatigue
Didanosine	Nervousness, agitation, mania, insomnia, dizziness, lethargy
Emtricitabine	Depression, abnormal dreams, insomnia, dizziness, confusion, irritability
Interferon-α-2a	Depression, suicidal ideation, anxiety, mania, psychosis, sleep disturbance, fatigue, delirium, cognitive dysfunction
Lamivudine	Depression, insomnia, dizziness, dystonia
Zidovudine	Anxiety, agitation, restlessness, insomnia, mild confusion, mania, psychosis

Table 12–1. Psychiatric adverse effects of antibiotic therapy *(continued)*

Medication	Neuropsychiatric adverse effects
Nonnucleoside reverse transcriptase inhibitors (continued)	
Delavirdine	Anxiety, agitation, amnesia, confusion, dizziness
Efavirenz	Anxiety, insomnia, irritability, depression, suicidal ideation and behavior, psychosis, vivid dreams/nightmares, cognitive dysfunction, dizziness
Nevirapine	Vivid dreams or nightmares, visual hallucinations, delusions, mood changes
Etravirine	Sleep changes, dizziness
Rilpivirine	Abnormal dreams, insomnia, dizziness
Protease inhibitors	
Atazanavir	Depression, insomnia
Fosamprenavir	Depression
Indinavir	Anxiety, agitation, insomnia
Lopinavir and ritonavir	Insomnia
Nelfinavir	Depression, anxiety, insomnia
Ritonavir	Anxiety, agitation, insomnia, confusion, amnesia, emotional lability, euphoria, hallucinations, decreased libido, metallic taste
Saquinavir	Anxiety, agitation, irritability, depression, excessive dreaming, hallucinations, euphoria, confusion, amnesia
Tipranavir	Depression

Table 12–1.   Psychiatric adverse effects of antibiotic
therapy *(continued)*

Medication	Neuropsychiatric adverse effects
Antivirals *(continued)*	
Integrase inhibitors	
Raltegravir	Depression, suicidal ideation, psychosis, vivid dreams or nightmares, vertigo, dizziness
Elvitegravir	Depression, insomnia, suicidal ideation
Dolutegravir	Insomnia, fatigue
Fusion inhibitors	
Enfuvirtide	Depression, insomnia
Maraviroc	Dizziness, insomnia
Antiherpetics	
Acyclovir and valacyclovir	Visual hallucinations, depersonalization, mood lability, delusions, insomnia, lethargy, agitation, delirium
Other antivirals	
Amantadine	Insomnia, anxiety, irritability, nightmares, depression, confusion, psychosis
Foscarnet	Irritability, hallucinations
Ganciclovir	Nightmares, hallucinations, agitation
Antifungals	
Amphotericin B	Delirium, lethargy
Ketoconazole	Somnolence, dizziness, asthenia, hallucinations
Pentamidine	Confusion, anxiety, mood lability, hallucinations

Table 12–1. Psychiatric adverse effects of antibiotic therapy *(continued)*

Medication	Neuropsychiatric adverse effects
Antihelmintics	
Thiabendazole	Hallucinations

Source. Compiled in part from Abers et al. 2014; Abouesh et al. 2002; Celano et al. 2011; "Drugs That May Cause Psychiatric Symptoms" 2002; Sternbach and State 1997; Warnke et al. 2007; Witkowski et al. 2007.

Differential Diagnosis

The differential diagnosis of psychiatric symptoms in HIV/AIDS patients is extensive. HIV-infected patients have a higher prevalence of psychiatric disorders than the general population, with mood and anxiety disorders, substance abuse, and cognitive disorders predominating (Bing et al. 2001; Ferrando 2000). Delirium, dementia, and manic spectrum disorders are commonplace in the medically hospitalized patient with HIV/AIDS (Ferrando and Lyketsos 2006).

Even though 60%–70% of patients with HIV have a history of psychiatric disorder prior to contracting HIV illness (Williams et al. 1991) and HIV diagnosis or disease exacerbation may trigger relapse, it is essential to consider potential medical etiologies. HIV-associated neuropsychiatric disorders can have multiple cognitive as well as behavioral symptoms, including apathy, depression, sleep disturbances, mania, and psychosis (Ferrando 2000). Patients with CNS opportunistic infections (including cryptococcal meningitis, toxoplasmosis, progressive multifocal leukoencephalopathy) and cancers can also present with a wide range of behavioral symptoms, as a result of focal or generalized neuropathological processes. Substance intoxication and withdrawal states are also common, and preexisting psychopathology may be exacerbated by ongoing substance use (Batki et al. 1996). The high rate of polysubstance abuse complicates the assessment of behavioral symptoms and presents the challenge of treating mixed withdrawal states.

Antiretroviral and other medications used in the context of HIV have been associated with neuropsychiatric adverse effects (see Table 12–1). Most of these effects are infrequent, and causal relationships are often difficult to establish. Clinical concern resulted from early reports of sudden-onset depression and suicidal ideation associated with interferon-α-2a (see Chapter 4) and neuropsychi-

Table 12–2.   Antibiotic drug–psychotropic drug interactions

Medication	Mechanism of interaction	Effects on psychotropic drug levels	Potential clinical effects
Antibacterials			
Antitubercular agents			
Isoniazid	Inhibition of MAO-A	Increased potential for serotonin syndrome with SSRIs, SNRIs	Serotonin syndrome
		Hypertensive crisis possible with TCAs, meperidine, tyramine-containing foods, OTC sympathomimetics, and stimulants	Hypertensive crisis
		Hypertensive crisis	
	Inhibition of CYP2C19 and CYP3A4	Phenytoin levels increased	Increased phenytoin effects and adverse effects
		Carbamazepine levels increased	Increased carbamazepine adverse effects
		Benzodiazepine serum levels increased, except for oxazepam, lorazepam, and temazepam	May increase benzodiazepine effects
Rifampin and rifabutin (to a lesser degree)	Induction of CYP3A4	Risperidone levels reduced	Reduced risperidone effect
		Sertraline levels reduced	Sertraline withdrawal symptoms
		Benzodiazepine (especially midazolam and triazolam) serum levels reduced, except for oxazepam, lorazepam, and temazepam	May reduce benzodiazepine effects

Table 12–2. Antibiotic drug–psychotropic drug interactions *(continued)*

Medication	Mechanism of interaction	Effects on psychotropic drug levels	Potential clinical effects
Antitubercular agents (continued)			
Rifampin and rifabutin (to a lesser degree) *(continued)*		Phenytoin levels reduced	Reduced phenytoin effects
		Methadone levels reduced	Reduced methadone effects and opioid withdrawal
		Clozapine levels reduced	Reduced clozapine therapeutic effects
		Morphine and codeine levels reduced	Reduced analgesic effect
		Zolpidem levels reduced (AUC reduced 73%)	Reduced hypnotic effect
		Carbamazepine induces its own metabolism; coadministration can significantly reduce carbamazepine levels	Diminished therapeutic effect

Table 12–2.   Antibiotic drug–psychotropic drug interactions *(continued)*

Medication	Mechanism of interaction	Effects on psychotropic drug levels	Potential clinical effects
Antibacterials *(continued)*			
Clarithromycin, erythromycin, telithromycin, and troleandomycin	Inhibition of CYP3A4	Benzodiazepine serum levels may increase, except for oxazepam, lorazepam, and temazepam	May increase benzodiazepine levels and effects (sedation, confusion, respiratory depression)
		Buspirone levels increased (AUC increased sixfold)	May increase psychomotor impairment and buspirone adverse effects
		Carbamazepine levels increased	Increased carbamazepine adverse effects
		Pimozide, haloperidol, aripiprazole, and quetiapine levels increased	Increased drug effects, including hypotension, arrhythmias, sedation
Ciprofloxacin and norfloxacin	Inhibition of CYP1A2 and CYP3A4	Benzodiazepine serum levels increased, except for oxazepam, lorazepam, and temazepam	May increase benzodiazepine levels and effects (sedation, confusion, respiratory depression)
		Methadone levels increased	Increased methadone effects (sedation, respiratory depression)

Table 12–2. Antibiotic drug–psychotropic drug interactions (*continued*)

Medication	Mechanism of interaction	Effects on psychotropic drug levels	Potential clinical effects
Antibacterials (*continued*)			
Ciprofloxacin and norfloxacin (*continued*)		Clozapine levels increased	Increased clozapine effects
		Olanzapine levels increased	Increased olanzapine effects
Enoxacin	Inhibition of CYP1A2	Clozapine levels increased	Increased clozapine effects
		Olanzapine levels increased	Increased olanzapine effects
Linezolid	Inhibition of MAO-A	Increased potential for serotonin syndrome with SSRIs and SNRIs	Serotonin syndrome
		Hypertensive crisis possible with TCAs, meperidine, tyramine-containing foods, OTC sympathomimetics, and stimulants	Hypertensive crisis
Antivirals			
Delavirdine	Inhibition of CYP3A4 and CYP2C9	Benzodiazepine serum levels increased, except for oxazepam, lorazepam, and temazepam	May increase benzodiazepine levels and effects (sedation, confusion, respiratory depression)

Table 12–2.   Antibiotic drug–psychotropic drug interactions *(continued)*

Medication	Mechanism of interaction	Effects on psychotropic drug levels	Potential clinical effects
Antivirals *(continued)*			
Efavirenz	Induction of CYP2B6	Bupropion levels reduced (AUC reduced 55%)	Reduced bupropion effects
	Induction of CYP3A4	Phenytoin levels reduced	Reduced phenytoin effects
		Carbamazepine levels reduced (AUC reduced 26%)	Reduced carbamazepine efficacy
		Buprenorphine levels reduced (AUC reduced 49%)	Possible reduced buprenorphine effects
		Methadone levels reduced 30%–60%	Reduced methadone effects and opioid withdrawal
Nevirapine	Induction of CYP3A4	Carbamazepine levels reduced	Reduced carbamazepine efficacy
		Methadone levels reduced 30%–60%	Reduced methadone effects and opioid withdrawal

Table 12–2. Antibiotic drug–psychotropic drug interactions (*continued*)

Medication	Mechanism of interaction	Effects on psychotropic drug levels	Potential clinical effects
Antivirals (continued)			
General protease inhibitor interactions	Most protease inhibitors inhibit CYP2D6 and CYP3A4.	Benzodiazepine serum levels increased, except for oxazepam, lorazepam, and temazepam	Increased benzodiazepine levels and effects (sedation, confusion, respiratory depression)
	Exceptions include darunavir, fosamprenavir, and ritonavir, which induce CYP2D6 and inhibit CYP3A4, and tipranavir, which in itself is a CYP3A4 inducer (see below)	Pimozide levels increased	Increased pimozide effects, including hypotension, arrhythmias
		Clozapine levels increased	Increased clozapine effects and adverse effects
		Methadone levels reduced 16%–53%	Reduced methadone effects and opioid withdrawal
Amprenavir	Inhibition of CYP3A4	Carbamazepine levels increased	Increased carbamazepine adverse effects
Darunavir	Mechanism unclear	Paroxetine levels reduced (AUC reduced 39%)	Reduced paroxetine effects
		Sertraline levels reduced (AUC reduced 49%)	Reduced sertraline effects

Table 12–2.   Antibiotic drug–psychotropic drug interactions (*continued*)

Medication	Mechanism of interaction	Effects on psychotropic drug levels	Potential clinical effects
Antivirals (*continued*)			
Darunavir (*continued*)	Inhibition of CYP3A4	Trazodone levels increased (AUC increased 240%)	Increased trazodone adverse effects (nausea, dizziness, hypotension, syncope)
Fosamprenavir	Induction of CYP3A4 Inhibition of CYP3A4	Paroxetine levels reduced (AUC reduced 55%)	Reduced paroxetine effect
Indinavir	Inhibition of CYP3A4	Trazodone levels increased	Increased trazodone adverse effects (nausea, dizziness, hypotension, syncope)
		Carbamazepine levels increased	Increased carbamazepine adverse effects
Lopinavir	Inhibition of CYP3A4	Trazodone levels increased (AUC increased 240%)	Increased trazodone adverse effects (nausea, dizziness, hypotension, syncope)
	Possible induction of CYP2C9	Phenytoin levels reduced	Reduced phenytoin effects
	Possible induction of UGT-mediated glucuronidation by lopinavir + ritonavir	Lamotrigine levels reduced (AUC reduced 50%)	Reduced lamotrigine effects
Nelfinavir	Inhibition of CYP2D6 and CYP3A4	Carbamazepine levels increased	Increased carbamazepine adverse effects

Table 12–2. Antibiotic drug–psychotropic drug interactions (*continued*)

Medication	Mechanism of interaction	Effects on psychotropic drug levels	Potential clinical effects
Antivirals (*continued*)			
Ritonavir	Inhibition of CYP3A4	Trazodone levels increased (AUC increased 240%)	Increased trazodone adverse effects (nausea, dizziness, hypotension, syncope)
		Carbamazepine levels increased	Increased carbamazepine adverse effects
		Quetiapine levels increased	Increased quetiapine adverse effects
	Induction of CYP1A2	Olanzapine levels reduced (AUC reduced 53%)	Reduced olanzapine effects
		Clozapine levels reduced	Reduced clozapine effects
	Induction of CYP2B6	Bupropion levels reduced	Reduced bupropion effects
Tipranavir	Alone, tipranavir is an inducer of CYP3A4; however, the combination with ritonavir is a CYP3A4 inhibitor	Tipranavir alone: reduced bupropion (AUC reduced 46%) and carbamazepine levels	Increased or reduced bupropion and carbamazepine effects and adverse effects
		Tipranavir and ritonavir combination: increased bupropion and carbamazepine (AUC increased 24%) levels	

Table 12–2.   Antibiotic drug–psychotropic drug interactions *(continued)*

Medication	Mechanism of interaction	Effects on psychotropic drug levels	Potential clinical effects
Antivirals *(continued)*			
Fluconazole	Inhibition of CYP2C19	Amitriptyline and nortriptyline levels increased	Increased adverse effects (behavioral changes and toxicity)
		Phenytoin levels increased	Increased phenytoin effects and adverse effects
		Triazolam and midazolam serum levels increased	Increased triazolam and midazolam levels and effects, including adverse effects (sedation, confusion, respiratory depression)
Itraconazole	Inhibition of CYP3A4	Benzodiazepine serum levels increased, except for oxazepam, lorazepam, and temazepam	Increased benzodiazepine levels and effects (sedation, confusion, respiratory depression)

Table 12–2. Antibiotic drug–psychotropic drug interactions (*continued*)

Medication	Mechanism of interaction	Effects on psychotropic drug levels	Potential clinical effects
Antivirals (*continued*)			
Ketoconazole	Inhibition of CYP3A4	Benzodiazepine serum levels increased, except for oxazepam, lorazepam, and temazepam	Increased benzodiazepine levels and effects (sedation, confusion, respiratory depression)
		Buspirone levels possibly increased	May increase psychomotor impairment and buspirone adverse effects
Miconazole and sulfamethoxazole	Inhibition of CYP2C9	Phenytoin levels increased	Increased phenytoin effects and adverse effects

Note. AUC=area under the curve; CYP=cytochrome P450; MAO-A=monoamine oxidase type A; OTC=over the counter; SNRIs=serotonin–norepinephrine reuptake inhibitors; SSRIs=selective serotonin reuptake inhibitors; TCAs=tricyclic antidepressants; UGT=uridine 5′-diphosphate glucuronosyltransferase.

Source. Compiled in part from Bruce et al. 2006; Cozza et al. 2003; Desta et al. 2001; Finch et al. 2002; Flockhart et al. 2000; Jacobs et al. 2014; Kharasch et al. 2008; Kuper and D'Aprile 2000; Ma et al. 2005; Mahatthanatrakul et al. 2007; Repetto and Petitto 2008; Venkatakrishnan et al. 2000; Warnke et al. 2007; Witkowski et al. 2007; Yew 2002.

atric adverse effects of efavirenz in more than 50% of patients (Staszewski et al. 1999). Although it seems that the overall rate of severe neuropsychiatric adverse effects of efavirenz is low (Ford et al. 2015), symptoms have been shown to decrease after switching to an alternative regimen (Mothapo et al. 2015).

HIV/AIDS patients often experience endocrinopathies that may produce psychiatric symptoms. These include clinical and subclinical hypothyroidism (16% of patients) (Beltran et al. 2003; Chen et al. 2005), hypogonadism (50% of males) (Mylonakis et al. 2001; Rabkin et al. 1999b, Rochira and Guaraldi 2014), and hypothalamic-pituitary-adrenal axis dysfunction (Chrousos and Zapanti 2014), including adrenal insufficiency (50% of patients) (Marik et al. 2002; Mayo et al. 2002). These endocrinopathies can be associated with fatigue, low mood, low libido, and loss of lean body mass. Patients with Graves' disease (autoimmune thyroiditis) present with anxiety, irritability, insomnia, weight loss, mania, and agitation when the disease occurs in the setting of immune reconstitution (Chen et al. 2005).

Treatment of Psychiatric Symptoms in Patients With HIV/AIDS

Depression

Conventional Antidepressants

Multiple open-label and double-blind, placebo-controlled clinical trials of antidepressant treatment of depression in patients with HIV have been conducted. In general, women and injection drug users have been underrepresented in antidepressant studies.

Two early randomized controlled trials (RCTs) demonstrated the efficacy of imipramine for depression in patients with HIV (Manning et al. 1990; Rabkin et al. 1994a). However, in the imipramine-treated groups, anticholinergic, antihistaminic, and antiadrenergic side effects were common and contributed to significant attrition. Response rates and adverse effects did not vary as a function of CD4+lymphocyte count.

Early open-label trials (Ferrando et al. 1997, 1999a; Rabkin et al. 1994a, 1994b, 1994c) and more recent RCTs of selective serotonin reuptake inhibitors (SSRIs) alone or compared with tricyclic antidepressants (TCAs) and group therapy for patients with HIV have demonstrated efficacy of SSRIs with few adverse effects, supporting use of SSRIs as first-line treatment for depression in patients with HIV (Batki et al. 1993; Elliott et al. 1998; Rabkin et al. 1999a; Schwartz and McDaniel 1999; Zisook et al. 1998). However, fixed-dose escitalopram 10 mg daily was not more efficacious than placebo over 6 weeks (Hoare et al. 2014). Weekly directly observed fluoxetine 90 mg was found to be more efficacious in treating depression than standard care in homeless and marginally housed HIV/AIDS patients (Tsai et al. 2013).

Results from one study suggested that combining psychotherapy with medication may be the optimal approach to treating depression in patients with HIV (Markowitz et al. 1998). In a comparison of four treatment approaches, both interpersonal psychotherapy with imipramine and supportive therapy with imipramine were superior to supportive therapy alone or cognitive-behavioral therapy in ameliorating depressive symptoms and improving the patient's Karnofsky Performance Scale score (a measure of physical function).

Mirtazapine, nefazodone, venlafaxine, and sustained-release bupropion have been studied in small open-label trials in patients with major depression and HIV infection (Currier et al. 2003; Elliott and Roy-Byrne 2000; Elliott et al. 1998, 1999; Ferrando and Freyberg 2008). All of the medications were associated with favorable response rates (>60%–70%) and few adverse effects. One nefazodone-treated patient discontinued treatment because of a clinically significant interaction with ritonavir.

Psychostimulants and Wakefulness Agents

Psychostimulants have demonstrated efficacy in the treatment of depressed mood, fatigue, and cognitive impairment in both open-label (Holmes et al. 1989; Wagner et al. 1997) and placebo-controlled studies in patients with HIV (Breitbart et al. 2001; Wagner and Rabkin 2000). For patients in both RCTs, overstimulation was more common with psychostimulants than with placebo. Also, concern over abuse liability may limit the use of psychostimulants, particularly in substance abusers with early HIV infection. In two RCTs in which fatigue was the primary outcome measure, the wakefulness agents modafinil and armodafinil significantly improved depression compared with placebo only in the presence of improved fatigue (Rabkin et al. 2010, 2011).

Nonconventional Agents With Antidepressant Efficacy

Testosterone deficiency with clinical symptoms of hypogonadism (depressed mood, fatigue, diminished libido, decreased appetite, and loss of lean body mass) is present in up to 50% of men with symptomatic HIV or AIDS (Rabkin et al. 1999b). Deficiency of adrenal androgens, particularly dehydroepiandrosterone (DHEA), is also common in both men and women with HIV (Ferrando et al. 1999b). These abnormalities have led to clinical interest in administering anabolic androgenic steroids, most commonly testosterone, to patients with HIV infection.

Open-label trials and RCTs have demonstrated efficacy of weekly to biweekly testosterone decanoate injections for HIV-infected men with low serum testosterone and low libido, low energy, and subclinical depressive symptoms (Rabkin et al. 2000). A more recent prospective observational registry also confirmed efficacy of testosterone replacement in men with HIV (Blick et al. 2013). In these studies, fewer than 5% of patients dropped out of treatment because of adverse effects (irritability, tension, reduced energy, bossiness, hair loss, and acne). Extreme irritability and assaultiveness ("roid rage") did not occur at replacement dosages (usually 400 mg), unlike the supraphysiological dosing used illicitly for anabolic effects. Long-term adverse effects include testicular atrophy, decreased volume of ejaculate, and watery ejaculate. Long-term testosterone replacement was also efficacious for depression and body composition measures in HIV-infected women (Dolan Looby et al. 2009). No studies have reported serious hepatotoxicity or prostate cancer associated with chronic treatment.

Testosterone replacement preparations include esterified oral testosterone (undecanoate capsules, available in Canada only) and intramuscular depot testosterone (propionate, enanthate, and cypionate), skin patches, and testosterone gel. Intramuscular depot preparations are the least expensive and most studied. Patch and gel formulations may produce less variability in serum testosterone levels and, therefore, in target symptoms.

DHEA, an adrenal androgen, has mild androgenic and anabolic effects and is a precursor to testosterone. It has been studied in an RCT, and efficacy was demonstrated at dosages of 100–400 mg/day in HIV patients with dysthymia or subsyndromal depression (Rabkin et al. 2006). Other steroid hormones, including nandrolone and oxandrolone, are widely used but have not been studied for their mood effects in patients with HIV.

St. John's wort is not recommended for use by HIV patients because it is a cytochrome P450 3A4 (CYP3A4) inducer and may reduce levels of protease inhibitors. S-adenosylmethionine demonstrated mood improvement in an open-label trial in HIV-infected patients with major depression (Jones et al. 2002).

Anxiety

Anxiety is present in 11%–25% of patients with HIV, is often comorbid with depression, and is associated with fatigue and physical functional limitations (Sewell et al. 2000). The most common manifestations are posttraumatic stress disorder, social phobia, agoraphobia, generalized anxiety disorder, and panic disorder.

SSRIs are first-line agents for the treatment of chronic anxiety disorders; however, there are no published trials in patients with HIV. Buspirone has been shown to be effective for treating anxiety symptoms in asymptomatic gay men and intravenous drug users with HIV and is well tolerated, with a low risk for drug interactions (Batki 1990; Hirsch et al. 1990). Benzodiazepines should be used with caution because of their risk for drug interactions (see Table 12–2), excessive sedation, cognitive impairment, and abuse liability. Lorazepam has the advantage of having no active metabolites and nonoxidative metabolism, but disadvantages include a shorter half-life and more frequent dosing. Benzodiazepines should be avoided in HIV/AIDS patients with cognitive impairment and delirium (Breitbart et al. 1996). Nonaddictive alternatives to benzodiazepines for rapid anxiety relief include the antihistamines diphenhydramine and hydroxyzine, sedating TCAs, and trazodone. Excessive sedation and anticholinergic-induced cognitive impairment should be monitored.

Mania

Manic symptoms in patients with HIV may be found in conjunction with primary bipolar illness or with HIV infection of the brain (HIV-associated mania) (Lyketsos et al. 1997). HIV-associated mania is a secondary affective illness associated with HIV infection of the brain and, compared with primary bipolar mania, is less associated with a personal or family history of mood disorder and may include more irritability, less hypertalkativeness, and more cognitive impairment. Given that HIV-associated mania is directly related to HIV brain infection, antiretroviral agents that penetrate cerebrospinal fluid may offer some protection from incident mania (Mijch et al. 1999). Despite some reports of manic or hypomanic symptoms being associated with antiretroviral medications (Kieburtz et al. 1991), since the advent of highly active antiretroviral therapy, HIV-associated mania appears to be declining in incidence, consistent with the reduction in HIV-associated dementia.

Practice guidelines recommend lithium, valproic acid, or carbamazepine as standard therapy for bipolar mania (American Psychiatric Association 2002). However, there are concerns regarding their use in patients with HIV infection, especially those with later-stage illness. Lithium has a low therapeutic index and a risk for neurotoxicity. Valproate is associated with hepatotoxicity (Cozza et al. 2000) and has been found to stimulate HIV-1 replication in vitro (Jennings and Romanelli 1999). Carbamazepine may cause blood dyscrasias and may lower serum levels of protease inhibitors. Their use is further complicated by the requirement for serum drug level monitoring.

Relatively little research has been published on the psychopharmacological treatment of HIV-associated mania. A case report of lithium for HIV-associated mania in an AIDS patient showed control of symptoms at a dosage of 1,200 mg/day; however, significant neurotoxicity (cognitive slowing, fine tremor) occurred, leading to discontinuation (Tanquary 1993). One study showed that valproic acid, up to 1,750 mg/day, led to significant improvement in acute manic symptoms, with few adverse effects, at serum levels of 50–110 μg/L (Halman et al. 1993; RachBeisel and Weintraub 1997). There have been reports that valproic acid increases HIV replication in vitro in a dose-dependent manner (Jennings and Romanelli 1999) and that it both increases cytomegalovirus replication and reduces the effectiveness of antiviral drugs used to treat cytomegalovirus (Michaelis et al. 2008). The clinical relevance of these findings remains controversial, and, to date, no reports have been published of valproic acid causing elevations in viral load in vivo.

The anticonvulsant lamotrigine, which has been approved by the U.S. Food and Drug Administration for maintenance therapy in bipolar illness, particularly for patients with prominent depression, may also be useful for treating mania in patients with HIV. A study of lamotrigine treatment for peripheral neuropathy in patients with HIV suggests its safety; however, careful upward dose titration is required because of risk of severe hypersensitivity (Simpson et al. 2003). Gabapentin, an anticonvulsant commonly used to treat HIV-associated peripheral neuropathy, has not demonstrated mood-stabilizing properties in controlled trials (Evins 2003).

Atypical antipsychotics may improve HIV-associated mania. Risperidone treatment significantly decreased patients' Young Mania Rating Scale scores in a case report of four patients with HIV-related manic psychosis (Singh and Catalan 1994) and successfully treated mania with catatonia when used in conjunction with lorazepam (Prakash and Bagepally 2012). Ziprasidone was effective in treating acute mania in a series of HIV patients without a previous history of bipolar disorder (Spiegel et al. 2010).

A case report of clonazepam treatment of HIV-associated manic symptoms described rapid clinical response, reduction of concurrent antipsychotic dosage, and few adverse effects (Budman and Vandersall 1990). However, given the cognitive impairment associated with HIV mania, as well as comorbid substance abuse, benzodiazepines should be used only for acute stabilization.

Psychosis

New-onset psychosis in patients with HIV, which has a prevalence ranging from 0.5% to 15% (McDaniel 2000), is most often seen in neurocognitive disorders, such as delirium, HIV-associated dementia, or HIV-associated minor cognitive motor disorder. One study comparing new-onset psychotic to nonpsychotic HIV patients with similar demographic and illness profiles showed a trend toward greater global neuropsychological impairment, prior history of substance abuse, and higher mortality in the psychosis group (Sewell et al. 1994a). Psychosis presumed secondary to antiretroviral medications has been reported (Foster et al. 2003); however, as with HIV-associated mania, antiretrovirals are much more likely to be protective in this regard (de Ronchi et al. 2000).

Antipsychotic treatment is complicated by HIV-infected patients' susceptibility to drug-related EPS as a result of HIV-induced damage to the basal ganglia. Movement disorders (acute dystonia, parkinsonism, ataxia) can be seen in advanced HIV disease in the absence of antipsychotic exposure. General recommendations include avoidance of high-potency typical antipsychotics (e.g., haloperidol) and depot antipsychotics and brief treatment when possible.

Studies of treatment of psychosis in patients with HIV are rare and have generally focused on psychosis occurring in encephalopathic, schizophrenic, and manic patients. The typical antipsychotics haloperidol and thioridazine were effective in treating positive psychotic symptoms associated with HIV and schizophrenia. Haloperidol, but not thioridazine, was associated with a high incidence of EPS (Mauri et al. 1997; Sewell et al. 1994b). Similarly, molindone was beneficial for HIV-associated psychosis and agitation, with minimal EPS (Fernandez and Levy 1993).

Clozapine was found to be effective and generally safe in treating HIV-associated psychosis (including negative symptoms) in patients with prior drug-induced parkinsonism (Dettling et al. 1998; Lera and Zirulnik 1999) and in HIV-infected patients with schizophrenia (Nejad et al. 2009). However, clozapine must be used with caution in HIV-infected patients because of the risk of agranulocytosis, and it is contraindicated with ritonavir. Risperidone improved HIV-related psychotic and manic symptoms and was associated with mild sedation and sialorrhea but few EPS (Singh et al. 1997; Zilikis et al. 1998). Olanzapine treatment of a patient with AIDS and psychosis who developed EPS with risperidone and other antipsychotics is described in a case report; however, this patient experienced akathisia, requiring propranolol (Meyer et al. 1998). Adverse reactions have been reported from quetiapine in patients taking atazanavir or ritonavir, likely due to ritonavir's inhibition of CYP3A4 (Pollack et al. 2009). Lorazepam was reported to be useful in the treatment of AIDS-associated psychosis with catatonia (Scamvougeras and Rosebush 1992).

Delirium

Delirium is diagnosed in 11%–29% of hospitalized patients with HIV and AIDS, is generally multifactorial in etiology, and is often superimposed on HIV-associated neurocognitive disorders (Ferrando et al. 1998). In a study of delirium in AIDS, patients had an average of 12.6 medical complications, with the most common being hematological (anemia, leukopenia, thrombocytopenia) and infectious diseases (e.g., septicemia, systemic fungal infections, Pneumocystis carinii pneumonia, tuberculosis, disseminated viral infections) (Breitbart et al. 1996).

Pharmacological treatment of delirium in HIV is generally with atypical antipsychotics because of concern for EPS. However, the only double-blind clinical trial of delirium treatment in AIDS compared low-dose haloperidol, chlorpromazine, and lorazepam (Breitbart et al. 1996). There were three important findings in that study: 1) haloperidol and chlorpromazine were equally effective; 2) lorazepam worsened delirium symptoms, including oversedation, disinhibition, ataxia, and increased confusion; and 3) antipsychotic adverse effects were limited and included mild EPS. Benzodiazepines should be reserved for delirium secondary to the withdrawal of alcohol or another CNS-depressant agent or for severe agitation that fails to respond to antipsychotics.

Sleep Disorders

Sleep disorders, primarily insomnia, are prevalent in the HIV-infected population. In a survey study of 115 HIV clinic patients, 73% endorsed insomnia (Wiegand et al. 1991). Poor sleep quality in HIV-infected patients accompanies higher levels of depressive, anxiety, and physical symptoms; daytime sleepiness; and cognitive and functional impairment (Nokes and Kendrew 2001; Rubinstein and Selwyn 1998). High efavirenz serum levels have been associated with the development of insomnia (Núñez et al. 2001) and with transient vivid dreams and insomnia during the early stages of treatment (Clifford 2003).

Psychopharmacological treatment of insomnia should utilize a hierarchical approach based on safety, abuse liability, and chronicity of symptoms, similar to that of anxiety disorders. Generally, benzodiazepines are indicated for short-term use only and should be avoided in patients with substance abuse histories. The nonbenzodiazepine sedative-hypnotics eszopiclone, zopiclone (available in Canada), and zolpidem are preferred for long-term use. In general, they have less abuse potential; however, patients with substance use histories should be monitored because abuse of these drugs has been reported (Brunelle et al. 2005; Hajak et al. 2003; Jaffe et al. 2004). The melatonin receptor agonist ramelteon and the orexin antagonist suvorexant have not been studied in HIV. Other agents, such as sedating antidepressants, atypical antipsychotics, and anticonvulsants, may be used with comorbid psychiatric symptoms.

Viral Infections Other Than HIV

Viruses can produce psychiatric symptoms by primary CNS involvement, through secondary effects of immune activation, or indirectly from systemic effects. One serious sequela of several viral infections is acute disseminated encephalomyelitis, which can present with encephalopathy, acute psychosis, seizures, and other CNS dysfunction.

Systemic Viral Infections

Patients who have chronic viral infections (e.g., Epstein-Barr virus, cytomegalovirus) may report overwhelming fatigue, malaise, depression, low-grade fever, lymphadenopathy, and other nonspecific symptoms. Although viral infections may resemble chronic fatigue syndrome, only a small fraction of chronic fatigue symptoms are attributable to specific viral infection, and the differential diagnosis should also include depression and other common causes of fatigue. Epstein-Barr virus infection is most common in adolescents and young adults. Cytomegalovirus should be considered when acute depression or cognitive dysfunction appears in immunocompromised patients (e.g., during the first few months after transplantation). Although controlled trials are lacking, both antidepressants and stimulants have been reported as beneficial in patients with depressive symptoms and fatigue following recovery from acute viral infection or accompanying chronic viral infection.

Herpes Encephalitis

Herpes simplex virus type 1 causes herpes simplex encephalitis (HSE), which is the most common source of acute viral encephalitis in the United States and is the most common identified cause of viral encephalitis simulating a primary psychiatric disorder (Arciniegas and Anderson 2004; Caroff et al. 2001; Chaudhuri and Kennedy 2002). HSE can cause personality change, dysphasia, seizures, olfactory hallucinations, autonomic dysfunction, ataxia, delirium, psychosis, and focal neurological symptoms. One possible sequela is Klüver-Bucy syndrome, which includes oral touching compulsions, hypersexuality, amnesia, placidity, agnosia, and hyperphagia. Early antiviral treatment may ameliorate some of these symptoms; however, especially in the young and elderly, cognitive impairment secondary to HSE may lead to postencephalitic dementia.

HSE is treated with intravenous acyclovir. Recovery is related to the speed of treatment, with increased morbidity and mortality associated with delays in treatment. Acyclovir may cause neuropsychiatric adverse effects, including lethargy, agitation, delirium, and hallucinations (see Table 12–1) (Rashiq et al. 1993). These effects may be difficult to distinguish from HSE itself but are generally self-limited and dose dependent. Patients who are elderly, who have renal impairment, or who are taking other neurotoxic medications are at heightened risk for neuropsychiatric effects of acyclovir. Although there are no well-defined treatments for the associated cognitive and neuropsychiatric symptoms of HSE, case reports describe success with anticonvulsants, such as carbamazepine (Vallini and Burns 1987), atypical antipsychotics (Guaiana and Markova 2006), atypical antipsychotics combined with anticonvulsants (Vasconcelos-Moreno et al. 2011), SSRIs (Mendhekar and Duggal 2005), stimulants, clonidine (Begum et al. 2006), and cholinesterase inhibitors (Catsman-Berrevoets et al. 1986).

Parasitic Infections: Neurocysticercosis

Neurocysticercosis, caused by the tapeworm *Taenia solium* acquired from undercooked pork, is the most common parasitic disease of the CNS, particularly in Asia, Latin America, and Africa. It is now appearing more frequently in the southwestern United States. Neurocysticercosis is the major etiology for acquired epilepsy in affected areas, and patients are often left with chronic neurocognitive and psychiatric problems, most commonly depression, but psychosis and dementia are possible sequelae (Del Brutto 2005; Shah and Chakrabarti 2013; Srivastava et al. 2013). Neurocysticercosis is treated with antihelmintic agents, such as praziquantel and albendazole, which are relatively free of neuropsychiatric side effects and drug-drug interactions (Nash et al. 2006). Other agents given with these drugs include systemic corticosteroids (see Chapter 10) to treat pericystic inflammation and encephalitis, as well as anticonvulsants to treat seizures. Antipsychotics may be used to treat psychotic symptoms, but patients may be susceptible to EPS, including tardive dyskinesia (Bills and Symon 1992).

Adverse Psychiatric Effects of Antibiotics

Antimicrobials can cause a multitude of psychiatric symptoms. Although many of these adverse effects are rare, clinical suspicion is warranted with new onset or exacerbation of preexisting psychiatric symptoms when these drugs are initiated. The best documented psychiatric side effects of selected antibiotic drugs are listed in Table 12–1. Delirium and psychosis have been particularly associated with quinolones (e.g., ciprofloxacin), procaine penicillin, antimalarial and other antiparasitic drugs, and the antituberculous drug cycloserine. The most common adverse effect causing discontinuation of interferon is depression. Depression, anxiety, and insomnia are the most frequently reported neuropsychiatric adverse effects of antiretroviral medications for HIV infection.

Drug-Drug Interactions

Acute infection results in the downregulation of multiple CYP enzymes as well as of uridine 5′-diphosphate glucuronosyltransferase activity, potentially resulting in impaired drug metabolism and excretion and elevated toxicity

(Morgan et al. 2008; Renton 2005). This effect appears to be mediated by proinflammatory cytokines, including interferon, interleukin-1, tumor necrosis factor, and interleukin-6. Inhibition of CYP1A2 and CYP3A4 appears to have the most potential clinical significance in humans. For example, elevated levels of clozapine, a CYP1A2 substrate, have been reported in the setting of acute bacterial pneumonia (Raaska et al. 2002) and urinary tract infection (Jecel et al. 2005) in the absence of other causal factors. The clinical significance of this phenomenon for the metabolism of other psychotropic drugs is not known; however, in the setting of acute infection, careful dosage titration and serum level monitoring (when available) are prudent.

A number of pharmacokinetic drug interactions may occur between antibiotics and psychotropic drugs. Selected well-established interactions are described in Table 12–2. Drug interactions are discussed in more detail in Chapter 1. Many antibacterials, including macrolides and fluoroquinolones, conazole antifungals, and antiretrovirals, are potent inhibitors of one or more CYP isozymes, whereas the antitubercular agent rifampin and several nonnucleoside reverse transcriptase inhibitors and protease inhibitors induce multiple CYP enzymes. Isoniazid and linezolid are weak inhibitors of monoamine oxidase type A (MAO-A). Erythromycin (and similar macrolide antibiotics, such as clarithromycin) and ketoconazole (and similar antifungals) may cause QT interval prolongation and ventricular arrhythmias when given to a patient taking other QT-prolonging drugs, including TCAs and many antipsychotics.

Multiple case reports have described serotonin syndrome associated with coadministration of linezolid, a weak, reversible MAO-A inhibitor, indicated for the treatment of methicillin-resistant *Staphylococcus aureus*, and SSRIs and serotonin-norepinephrine reuptake inhibitors (SNRIs), with an incidence of 1.8%–3% in retrospective studies (Lorenz et al. 2008; Taylor et al. 2006). An observational matched comparison study in acutely ill hospitalized veterans did not find an increased risk for serotonin toxicity or serotonin syndrome in patients receiving linezolid compared with vancomycin (Lodise et al. 2013). The literature suggests that patients being treated with SSRIs and SNRIs can safely receive linezolid as long as there is clinical vigilance for signs and symptoms of serotonin toxicity. Coadministration of linezolid with direct or indirect sympathomimetic drugs (e.g., psychostimulants, meperidine) may precipitate hypertensive crisis.

Use of the anticonvulsants carbamazepine, phenytoin, and phenobarbital is of concern in HIV infection. In addition to possible anticonvulsant toxicity caused by protease inhibitor–mediated inhibition of anticonvulsant metabolism, these anticonvulsants also induce protease inhibitor metabolism, which reduces protease inhibitor serum levels and leads to virological failure (Bartt 1998; Repetto and Petitto 2008).

Potentially dangerous cardiovascular side effects have occurred because of increased levels of sildenafil, commonly used for sexual dysfunction, following concurrent administration of ritonavir, saquinavir, and indinavir (Merry et al. 1999; Muirhead et al. 2000). Illicit drugs may have dangerous clinical interactions with protease inhibitors. Fatalities have been reported with concurrent use of 3,4-methylenedioxymethamphetamine (MDMA; commonly called "ecstasy"), methamphetamine, and ritonavir (Hales et al. 2000; Mirken 1997).

Key Clinical Points

- Systemic and CNS infectious diseases may cause psychiatric and cognitive symptoms that persist despite antibiotic treatment and require psychopharmacological intervention.
- Acute infection may inhibit metabolism of psychotropic drugs, warranting caution with initial dosage and subsequent titration.
- There is significant potential for interaction between psychotropic drugs and antibiotics. Clinicians should query for potential interactions prior to combining these agents.
- Substantial evidence supports the efficacy of SSRIs and some novel agents for the treatment of depression in HIV/AIDS. However, the psychopharmacology literature is limited for other psychiatric disorders within the context of infectious diseases.
- Patients with HIV/AIDS and other infections with CNS involvement are susceptible to extrapyramidal side effects of antipsychotic drugs.

References

Abers MS, Shandera WX, Kass JS: Neurological and psychiatric adverse effects of antiretroviral drugs. CNS Drugs 28(2):131–145, 2014 24362768

Abouesh A, Stone C, Hobbs WR: Antimicrobial-induced mania (antibiomania): a review of spontaneous reports. J Clin Psychopharmacol 22(1):71–81, 2002 11799346

American Psychiatric Association: Practice guideline for the treatment of patients with bipolar disorder (revision). Am J Psychiatry 159(4)(suppl):1–50, 2002 11958165

Arciniegas DB, Anderson CA: Viral encephalitis: neuropsychiatric and neurobehavioral aspects. Curr Psychiatry Rep 6(5):372–379, 2004 15355760

Bartt R: An effect of anticonvulsants on antiretroviral therapy: neuroscience of HIV infection. J Neurovirol 4(suppl):340, 1998

Batki SL: Buspirone in drug users with AIDS or AIDS-related complex. J Clin Psychopharmacol 10(3)(suppl):111S–115S, 1990 2376626

Batki SL, Manfredi LB, Jacob P 3rd, Jones RT: Fluoxetine for cocaine dependence in methadone maintenance: quantitative plasma and urine cocaine/benzoylecgonine concentrations. J Clin Psychopharmacol 13(4):243–250, 1993 8376611

Batki S, Ferrando S, Manfredi L, et al: Psychiatric disorders, drug use, and HIV disease in 84 injection drug users. Am J Addict 5:249–258, 1996

Begum H, Nayek K, Khuntdar BK: Kluver-Bucy syndrome—a rare complication of herpes simplex encephalitis. J Indian Med Assoc 104(11):637–638, 2006 17444064

Beltran S, Lescure FX, Desailloud R, et al; Thyroid and VIH Group: Increased prevalence of hypothyroidism among human immunodeficiency virus–infected patients: a need for screening. Clin Infect Dis 37(4):579–583, 2003 12905143

Berende A, Ter Hofstede HJ, Donders AR, et al: Persistent Lyme Empiric Antibiotic Study Europe (PLEASE)—design of a randomized controlled trial of prolonged antibiotic treatment in patients with persistent symptoms attributed to Lyme borreliosis. BMC Infect Dis 14:543, 2014 25318999

Bills DC, Symon L: Cysticercosis producing various neurological presentations in a patient: case report. Br J Neurosurg 6(4):365–369, 1992 1388832

Bing EG, Burnam MA, Longshore D, et al: Psychiatric disorders and drug use among human immunodeficiency virus–infected adults in the United States. Arch Gen Psychiatry 58(8):721–728, 2001 11483137

Blick G, Khera M, Bhattacharya RK, et al: Testosterone replacement therapy in men with hypogonadism and HIV/AIDS: results from the TRiUS registry. Postgrad Med 125(2):19–29, 2013 23816768

Breitbart W, Marotta R, Platt MM, et al: A double-blind trial of haloperidol, chlorpromazine, and lorazepam in the treatment of delirium in hospitalized AIDS patients. Am J Psychiatry 153(2):231–237, 1996 8561204

Breitbart W, Rosenfeld B, Kaim M, Funesti-Esch J: A randomized, double-blind, placebo-controlled trial of psychostimulants for the treatment of fatigue in ambulatory patients with human immunodeficiency virus disease. Arch Intern Med 161(3):411–420, 2001 11176767

Bruce RD, McCance-Katz E, Kharasch ED, et al: Pharmacokinetic interactions between buprenorphine and antiretroviral medications. Clin Infect Dis 43 (suppl 4):S216–S223, 2006 17109308

Brunelle E, Rotily M, Lancon C, et al: Zolpidem: intravenous misuse in drug abusers. Addiction 100(9):1377–1378, 2005 16128733

Budman CL, Vandersall TA: Clonazepam treatment of acute mania in an AIDS patient. J Clin Psychiatry 51(5):212, 1990 2335499

Caroff SN, Mann SC, Glittoo MF, et al: Psychiatric manifestations of acute viral encephalitis. Psychiatr Ann 31:193–204, 2001

Catsman-Berrevoets CE, Van Harskamp F, Appelhof A: Beneficial effect of physostigmine on clinical amnesic behaviour and neuropsychological test results in a patient with a post-encephalitic amnesic syndrome. J Neurol Neurosurg Psychiatry 49(9):1088–1090, 1986 3760902

Celano CM, Freudenreich O, Fernandez-Robles C, et al: Depressogenic effects of medications: a review. Dialogues Clin Neurosci 13(1):109–125, 2011 21485751

Chaudhuri A, Kennedy PG: Diagnosis and treatment of viral encephalitis. Postgrad Med J 78(924):575–583, 2002 12415078

Chen F, Day SL, Metcalfe RA, et al: Characteristics of autoimmune thyroid disease occurring as a late complication of immune reconstitution in patients with advanced human immunodeficiency virus (HIV) disease. Medicine (Baltimore) 84(2):98–106, 2005 15758839

Chrousos GP, Zapanti ED: Hypothalamic-pituitary-adrenal axis in HIV infection and disease. Endocrinol Metab Clin North Am 43(3):791–806, 2014 25169568

Clifford DB; ACTG 5097 Team: Impact of EF on neuropsychological performance, mood and sleep behavior in HIV-positive individuals. Paper presented at 2nd International AIDS Society Conference on HIV Pathogenesis and Treatment, Paris, July 2003

Cozza KL, Swanton EJ, Humphreys CW: Hepatotoxicity with combination of valproic acid, ritonavir, and nevirapine: a case report. Psychosomatics 41(5):452–453, 2000 11015639

Cozza KL, Armstrong SC, Oesterheld JR: Concise Guide to the Cytochrome P450 System: Drug Interaction Principles for Medical Practice. Washington, DC, American Psychiatric Publishing, 2003

Currier MB, Molina G, Kato M: A prospective trial of sustained-release bupropion for depression in HIV-seropositive and AIDS patients. Psychosomatics 44(2):120–125, 2003 12618534

Del Brutto OH: Neurocysticercosis. Semin Neurol 25(3):243–251, 2005 16170737

Delong AK, Blossom B, Maloney EL, Phillips SE: Antibiotic retreatment of Lyme disease in patients with persistent symptoms: a biostatistical review of randomized, placebo-controlled, clinical trials. Contemp Clin Trials 33(6):1132–1142, 2012 22922244

de Ronchi D, Faranca I, Forti P, et al: Development of acute psychotic disorders and HIV-1 infection. Int J Psychiatry Med 30(2):173–183, 2000 11001280

Dersch R, Freitag MH, Schmidt S, et al: Efficacy and safety of pharmacological treatments for acute Lyme neuroborreliosis—a systematic review. Eur J Neurol 22(9):1249–1259, 2015 26058321

Desta Z, Soukhova NV, Flockhart DA: Inhibition of cytochrome P450 (CYP450) isoforms by isoniazid: potent inhibition of CYP2C19 and CYP3A. Antimicrob Agents Chemother 45(2):382–392, 2001 11158730

Dettling M, Müller-Oerlinghausen B, Britsch P: Clozapine treatment of HIV-associated psychosis—too much bone marrow toxicity? Pharmacopsychiatry 31(4):156–157, 1998 9754853

Dolan Looby SE, Collins M, Lee H, Grinspoon S: Effects of long-term testosterone administration in HIV-infected women: a randomized, placebo-controlled trial. AIDS 23(8):951–959, 2009 19287303

Drugs that may cause psychiatric symptoms. Med Lett Drugs Ther 44(1134):59–62, 2002 12138379

Elliott AJ, Roy-Byrne PP: Mirtazapine for depression in patients with human immunodeficiency virus. J Clin Psychopharmacol 20(2):265–267, 2000 10770469

Elliott AJ, Uldall KK, Bergam K, et al: Randomized, placebo-controlled trial of paroxetine versus imipramine in depressed HIV-positive outpatients. Am J Psychiatry 155(3):367–372, 1998 9501747

Elliott AJ, Russo J, Bergam K, et al: Antidepressant efficacy in HIV-seropositive outpatients with major depressive disorder: an open trial of nefazodone. J Clin Psychiatry 60(4):226–231, 1999 10221282

Evins AE: Efficacy of newer anticonvulsant medications in bipolar spectrum mood disorders. J Clin Psychiatry 64 (suppl 8):9–14, 2003 12892536

Fallon BA, Keilp JG, Corbera KM, et al: A randomized, placebo-controlled trial of repeated IV antibiotic therapy for Lyme encephalopathy. Neurology 70(13):992–1003, 2008 17928580

Fallon BA, Petkova E, Keilp JG, Britton CB: A reappraisal of the U.S. clinical trials of post-treatment Lyme disease syndrome. Open Neurol J 6:79–87, 2012 23091568

Feder HMJr, Johnson BJ, O'Connell S, et al; Ad Hoc International Lyme Disease Group: A critical appraisal of "chronic Lyme disease." N Engl J Med 357(14):1422–1430, 2007 17914043

Fernandez F, Levy JK: The use of molindone in the treatment of psychotic and delirious patients infected with the human immunodeficiency virus: case reports. Gen Hosp Psychiatry 15(1):31–35, 1993 8094699

Ferrando SJ: Diagnosis and treatment of HIV-associated neurocognitive disorders. New Dir Ment Health Serv 87(87):25–35, 2000 11031798

Ferrando SJ, Freyberg Z: Treatment of depression in HIV positive individuals: a critical review. Int Rev Psychiatry 20(1):61–71, 2008 18240063

Ferrando SJ, Lyketsos CG: Psychiatric comorbidities in medically ill patients with HIV/AIDS, in Psychiatric Aspects of HIV/AIDS. Edited by Fernandez F, Ruiz P. Philadelphia, PA, Lippincott Williams & Wilkins, 2006, pp 198–211

Ferrando SJ, Goldman JD, Charness WE: Selective serotonin reuptake inhibitor treatment of depression in symptomatic HIV infection and AIDS: improvements in affective and somatic symptoms. Gen Hosp Psychiatry 19(2):89–97, 1997 9097063

Ferrando SJ, Rabkin JG, Rothenberg J: Psychiatric disorders and adjustment in HIV and AIDS patients during and after medical hospitalization. Psychosomatics 39:214–215, 1998

Ferrando SJ, Rabkin JG, de Moore GM, Rabkin R: Antidepressant treatment of depression in HIV-seropositive women. J Clin Psychiatry 60(11):741–746, 1999a 10584761

Ferrando SJ, Rabkin JG, Poretsky L: Dehydroepiandrosterone sulfate (DHEAS) and testosterone: relation to HIV illness stage and progression over one year. J Acquir Immune Defic Syndr 22(2):146–154, 1999b 10843528

Finch CK, Chrisman CR, Baciewicz AM, Self TH: Rifampin and rifabutin drug interactions: an update. Arch Intern Med 162(9):985–992, 2002 11996607

Flockhart DA, Drici MD, Kerbusch T, et al: Studies on the mechanism of a fatal clarithromycin-pimozide interaction in a patient with Tourette syndrome. J Clin Psychopharmacol 20(3):317–324, 2000 10831018

Ford N, Shubber Z, Pozniak A, et al: Comparative safety and neuropsychiatric adverse events associated with efavirenz use in first-line antiretroviral therapy: a systematic review and meta-analysis of randomized trials. J Acquir Immune Defic Syndr 69(4):422–239, 2015 25850607

Foster R, Olajide D, Everall IP: Antiretroviral therapy–induced psychosis: case report and brief review of the literature. HIV Med 4(2):139–144, 2003 12702135

Garvey MA, Perlmutter SJ, Allen AJ, et al: A pilot study of penicillin prophylaxis for neuropsychiatric exacerbations triggered by streptococcal infections. Biol Psychiatry 45(12):1564–1571, 1999 10376116

Guaiana G, Markova I: Antipsychotic treatment improves outcome in herpes simplex encephalitis: a case report. J Neuropsychiatry Clin Neurosci 18(2):247, 2006 16720808

Hajak G, Müller WE, Wittchen HU, et al: Abuse and dependence potential for the non-benzodiazepine hypnotics zolpidem and zopiclone: a review of case reports and epidemiological data. Addiction 98(10):1371–1378, 2003 14519173

Hales G, Roth N, Smith D: Possible fatal interaction between protease inhibitors and methamphetamine. Antivir Ther 5(1):19, 2000 10846588

Halman MH, Worth JL, Sanders KM, et al: Anticonvulsant use in the treatment of manic syndromes in patients with HIV-1 infection. J Neuropsychiatry Clin Neurosci 5(4):430–434, 1993 8286943

Hirsch DA, Fishman J, Jacobsen P, et al: Treatment of anxiety in HIV positive asymptomatic men with buspirone. Paper presented at the 7th International Conference on AIDS, San Francisco, CA, June 1990

Hoare J, Carey P, Joska JA, et al: Escitalopram treatment of depression in human immunodeficiency virus/acquired immunodeficiency syndrome: a randomized, double-blind, placebo-controlled study. J Nerv Ment Dis 202(2):133–137, 2014 24469525

Holmes VF, Fernandez F, Levy JK: Psychostimulant response in AIDS-related complex patients. J Clin Psychiatry 50(1):5–8, 1989 2642894

Jacobs BS, Colbers AP, Velthoven-Graafland K, et al: Effect of fosamprenavir/ritonavir on the pharmacokinetics of single-dose olanzapine in healthy volunteers. Int J Antimicrob Agents 44(2):173–177, 2014 24929949

Jaffe JH, Bloor R, Crome I, et al: A postmarketing study of relative abuse liability of hypnotic sedative drugs. Addiction 99(2):165–173, 2004 14756709

Jay CA: Treatment of neurosyphilis. Curr Treat Options Neurol 8(3):185–192, 2006 16569377

Jecel J, Michel TM, Gutknecht L, et al: Toxic clozapine serum levels during acute urinary tract infection: a case report. Eur J Clin Pharmacol 60(12):909–910, 2005 15657777

Jennings HR, Romanelli F: The use of valproic acid in HIV-positive patients. Ann Pharmacother 33(10):1113–1116, 1999 10534224

Jones K, Goldenberg R, Cerngul I: An open-label trial of S-adenosylmethionine (SAM-e) for major depression in HIV patients. Paper presented at the 14th International AIDS Conference, Barcelona, Spain, July 2002

Kaplan RF, Trevino RP, Johnson GM, et al: Cognitive function in post-treatment Lyme disease: do additional antibiotics help? Neurology 60(12):1916–1922, 2003 12821733

Kharasch ED, Mitchell D, Coles R, Blanco R: Rapid clinical induction of hepatic cytochrome P4502B6 activity by ritonavir. Antimicrob Agents Chemother 52(5):1663–1669, 2008 18285471

Kieburtz K, Zettelmaier AE, Ketonen L, et al: Manic syndrome in AIDS. Am J Psychiatry 148(8):1068–1070, 1991 1853958

Klempner MS, Hu LT, Evans J, et al: Two controlled trials of antibiotic treatment in patients with persistent symptoms and a history of Lyme disease. N Engl J Med 345(2):85–92, 2001 11450676

Klempner MS, Baker PJ, Shapiro ED, et al: Treatment trials for post-Lyme disease symptoms revisited. Am J Med 126(8):665–669, 2013 23764268

Kovacevic M, Grant P, Swedo SE: Use of intravenous immunoglobulin in the treatment of twelve youths with pediatric autoimmune neuropsychiatric disorders associated with streptococcal infections. J Child Adolesc Psychopharmacol 25(1):65–69, 2015 25658609

Krupp LB, Hyman LG, Grimson R, et al: Study and treatment of post Lyme disease (STOP-LD): a randomized double masked clinical trial. Neurology 60(12):1923–1930, 2003 12821734

Kuper JI, D'Aprile M: Drug-drug interactions of clinical significance in the treatment of patients with Mycobacterium avium complex disease. Clin Pharmacokinet 39(3):203–214, 2000 11020135

Lera G, Zirulnik J: Pilot study with clozapine in patients with HIV-associated psychosis and drug-induced parkinsonism. Mov Disord 14(1):128–131, 1999 9918355

Lodise TP, Patel N, Rivera A, et al: Comparative evaluation of serotonin toxicity among veterans affairs patients receiving linezolid and vancomycin. Antimicrob Agents Chemother 57(12):5901–5911, 2013 24041888

Lorenz RA, Vandenberg AM, Canepa EA: Serotonergic antidepressants and linezolid: a retrospective chart review and presentation of cases. Int J Psychiatry Med 38(1):81–90, 2008 18624020

Lyketsos CG, Schwartz J, Fishman M, Treisman G: AIDS mania. J Neuropsychiatry Clin Neurosci 9(2):277–279, 1997 9144109

Ma Q, Okusanya OO, Smith PF, et al: Pharmacokinetic drug interactions with non-nucleoside reverse transcriptase inhibitors. Expert Opin Drug Metab Toxicol 1(3):473–485, 2005 16863456

Mahatthanatrakul W, Nontaput T, Ridtitid W, et al: Rifampin, a cytochrome P450 3A inducer, decreases plasma concentrations of antipsychotic risperidone in healthy volunteers. J Clin Pharm Ther 32(2):161–167, 2007 17381666

Manning D, Jacobsberg L, Erhart S, et al: The efficacy of imipramine in the treatment of HIV-related depression. Paper presented at the 7th International Conference on AIDS, San Francisco, CA, June 1990

Marik PE, Kiminyo K, Zaloga GP: Adrenal insufficiency in critically ill patients with human immunodeficiency virus. Crit Care Med 30(6):1267–1273, 2002 12072680

Markowitz JC, Kocsis JH, Fishman B, et al: Treatment of depressive symptoms in human immunodeficiency virus–positive patients. Arch Gen Psychiatry 55(5):452–457, 1998 9596048

Mauri MC, Fabiano L, Bravin S, et al: Schizophrenic patients before and after HIV infection: a case-control study. Encephale 23(6):437–441, 1997 9488926

Mayo J, Collazos J, Martínez E, Ibarra S: Adrenal function in the human immunodeficiency virus-infected patient. Arch Intern Med 162(10):1095–1098, 2002 12020177

McDaniel JS: Working Group on HIV/AIDS: Practice guideline for the treatment of patients with HIV/AIDS. Am J Psychiatry 157:1–62, 2000

Mendhekar DN, Duggal HS: Sertraline for Klüver-Bucy syndrome in an adolescent. Eur Psychiatry 20(4):355–356, 2005 16018931

Merry C, Barry MG, Ryan M, et al: Interaction of sildenafil and indinavir when co-administered to HIV-positive patients. AIDS 13(15):F101–F107, 1999 10546851

Meyer JM, Marsh J, Simpson G: Differential sensitivities to risperidone and olanzapine in a human immunodeficiency virus patient. Biol Psychiatry 44(8):791–794, 1998 9798086

Michaelis M, Ha TA, Doerr HW, Cinatl J Jr: Valproic acid interferes with antiviral treatment in human cytomegalovirus-infected endothelial cells. Cardiovasc Res 77(3):544–550, 2008 18006438

Mijch AM, Judd FK, Lyketsos CG, et al: Secondary mania in patients with HIV infection: are antiretrovirals protective? J Neuropsychiatry Clin Neurosci 11(4):475–480, 1999 10570761

Mirken B: Danger: possibly fatal interactions between ritonavir and "ecstasy," some other psychoactive drugs (abstract). AIDS Treat News 265(265):5, 1997 11364241

Morgan ET, Goralski KB, Piquette-Miller M, et al: Regulation of drug-metabolizing enzymes and transporters in infection, inflammation, and cancer. Drug Metab Dispos 36(2):205–216, 2008 18218849

Mothapo KM, Schellekens A, van Crevel R, et al: Improvement of depression and anxiety after discontinuation of long-term efavirenz treatment. CNS Neurol Disord Drug Targets 14(6):811–818, 2015 25808896

Moulton CD, Koychev I: The effect of penicillin therapy on cognitive outcomes in neurosyphilis: a systematic review of the literature. Gen Hosp Psychiatry 37(1):49–52, 2015 25468254

Muirhead GJ, Wulff MB, Fielding A, et al: Pharmacokinetic interactions between sildenafil and saquinavir/ritonavir. Br J Clin Pharmacol 50(2):99–107, 2000 10930961

Mylonakis E, Koutkia P, Grinspoon S: Diagnosis and treatment of androgen deficiency in human immunodeficiency virus–infected men and women. Clin Infect Dis 33(6):857–864, 2001 11512091

Nash TE, Singh G, White AC, et al: Treatment of neurocysticercosis: current status and future research needs. Neurology 67(7):1120–1127, 2006 17030744

Nejad SH, Gandhi RT, Freudenreich O: Clozapine use in HIV-infected schizophrenia patients: a case-based discussion and review. Psychosomatics 50(6):626–632, 2009 19996235

Nokes KM, Kendrew J: Correlates of sleep quality in persons with HIV disease. J Assoc Nurses AIDS Care 12(1):17–22, 2001 11211669

Núñez M, González de Requena D, Gallego L, et al: Higher efavirenz plasma levels correlate with development of insomnia. J Acquir Immune Defic Syndr 28(4):399–400, 2001 11707679

Oksi J, Nikoskelainen J, Hiekkanen H, et al: Duration of antibiotic treatment in disseminated Lyme borreliosis: a double-blind, randomized, placebo-controlled, multicenter clinical study. Eur J Clin Microbiol Infect Dis 26(8):571–581, 2007 17587070

Pecenak J, Janik P, Vaseckova B, Trebulova K: Electroconvulsive therapy treatment in a patient with neurosyphilis and psychotic disorder:ase report and literature review. J ECT 31(4):268–270, 2015 25634568

Perlmutter SJ, Leitman SF, Garvey MA, et al: Therapeutic plasma exchange and intravenous immunoglobulin for obsessive-compulsive disorder and tic disorders in childhood. Lancet 354(9185):1153–1158, 1999 10513708

Perrin EM, Murphy ML, Casey JR, et al: Does group A beta-hemolytic streptococcal infection increase risk for behavioral and neuropsychiatric symptoms in children? Arch Pediatr Adolesc Med 158(9):848–856, 2004 15351749

Pollack TM, McCoy C, Stead W: Clinically significant adverse events from a drug interaction between quetiapine and atazanavir-ritonavir in two patients. Pharmacotherapy 29(11):1386–1391, 2009 19857154

Prakash O, Bagepally BS: Catatonia and mania in patient with AIDS: treatment with lorazepam and risperidone. Gen Hosp Psychiatry 34(3):321.e5–321.e6, 2012 22361355

Raaska K, Raitasuo V, Arstila M, Neuvonen PJ: Bacterial pneumonia can increase serum concentration of clozapine. Eur J Clin Pharmacol 58(5):321–322, 2002 12185555

Rabkin JG, Rabkin R, Harrison W, Wagner G: Effect of imipramine on mood and enumerative measures of immune status in depressed patients with HIV illness. Am J Psychiatry 151(4):516–523, 1994a 7908501

Rabkin JG, Rabkin R, Wagner G: Effects of fluoxetine on mood and immune status in depressed patients with HIV illness. J Clin Psychiatry 55(3):92–97, 1994b 7915270

Rabkin JG, Wagner G, Rabkin R: Effects of sertraline on mood and immune status in patients with major depression and HIV illness: an open trial. J Clin Psychiatry 55(10):433–439, 1994c 7961520

Rabkin JG, Wagner GJ, Rabkin R: Fluoxetine treatment for depression in patients with HIV and AIDS: a randomized, placebo-controlled trial. Am J Psychiatry 156(1):101–107, 1999a 9892304

Rabkin JG, Wagner GJ, Rabkin R: Testosterone therapy for human immunodeficiency virus–positive men with and without hypogonadism. J Clin Psychopharmacol 19(1):19–27, 1999b 9934939

Rabkin JG, Wagner GJ, Rabkin R: A double-blind, placebo-controlled trial of testosterone therapy for HIV-positive men with hypogonadal symptoms. Arch Gen Psychiatry 57(2):141–147, discussion 155–156, 2000 10665616

Rabkin JG, McElhiney MC, Rabkin R, et al: Placebo-controlled trial of dehydroepiandrosterone (DHEA) for treatment of nonmajor depression in patients with HIV/AIDS. Am J Psychiatry 163(1):59–66, 2006 16390890

Rabkin JG, McElhiney MC, Rabkin R, McGrath PJ: Modafinil treatment for fatigue in HIV/AIDS: a randomized placebo-controlled trial. J Clin Psychiatry 71:707–715, 2010 20492840

Rabkin JG, McElhiney MC, Rabkin R: Treatment of HIV-related fatigue with armodafinil: a placebo-controlled randomized trial. Psychosomatics 52:328–336, 2011 21777715

RachBeisel JA, Weintraub E: Valproic acid treatment of AIDS-related mania. J Clin Psychiatry 58:406–407, 1997

Rashiq S, Briewa L, Mooney M, et al: Distinguishing acyclovir neurotoxicity from encephalomyelitis. J Intern Med 234(5):507–511, 1993 8228796

Renton KW: Regulation of drug metabolism and disposition during inflammation and infection. Expert Opin Drug Metab Toxicol 1(4):629–640, 2005 16863429

Repetto MJ, Petitto JM: Psychopharmacology in HIV-infected patients. Psychosom Med 70(5):585–592, 2008 18519881

Rochira V, Guaraldi G: Hypogonadism in the HIV-infected man. Endocrinol Metab Clin North Am 43(3):709–730, 2014 25169563

Rubinstein ML, Selwyn PA: High prevalence of insomnia in an outpatient population with HIV infection. J Acquir Immune Defic Syndr Hum Retrovirol 19(3):260–265, 1998 9803968

Sanchez FM, Zisselman MH: Treatment of psychiatric symptoms associated with neurosyphilis. Psychosomatics 48(5):440–445, 2007 17878505

Scamvougeras A, Rosebush PI: AIDS-related psychosis with catatonia responding to low-dose lorazepam. J Clin Psychiatry 53(11):414–415, 1992 1459974

Schwartz JA, McDaniel JS: Double-blind comparison of fluoxetine and desipramine in the treatment of depressed women with advanced HIV disease: a pilot study. Depress Anxiety 9(2):70–74, 1999 10207661

Sewell DD, Jeste DV, Atkinson JH, et al; San Diego HIV Neurobehavioral Research Center Group: HIV-associated psychosis: a study of 20 cases. Am J Psychiatry 151(2):237–242, 1994a 8296896

Sewell DD, Jeste DV, McAdams LA, et al: Neuroleptic treatment of HIV-associated psychosis. Neuropsychopharmacology 10(4):223–229, 1994b 7945732

Sewell MC, Goggin KJ, Rabkin JG, et al: Anxiety syndromes and symptoms among men with AIDS: a longitudinal controlled study. Psychosomatics 41(4):294–300, 2000 10906351

Shah R, Chakrabarti S: Neuropsychiatric manifestations and treatment of disseminated neurocysticercosis: a compilation of three cases. Asian J Psychiatr 6(4):344–346, 2013 23810145

Simpson DM, McArthur JC, Olney R, et al; Lamotrigine HIV Neuropathy Study Team: Lamotrigine for HIV-associated painful sensory neuropathies: a placebo-controlled trial. Neurology 60(9):1508–1514, 2003 12743240

Singh AN, Catalan J: Risperidone in HIV-related manic psychosis. Lancet 344(8928):1029–1030, 1994 7523809

Singh AN, Golledge H, Catalan J: Treatment of HIV-related psychotic disorders with risperidone: a series of 21 cases. J Psychosom Res 42(5):489–493, 1997 9194023

Snider LA, Lougee L, Slattery M, et al: Antibiotic prophylaxis with azithromycin or penicillin for childhood-onset neuropsychiatric disorders. Biol Psychiatry 57(7):788–792, 2005 15820236

Spiegel DR, Weller AL, Pennell K, Turner K: The successful treatment of mania due to acquired immunodeficiency syndrome using ziprasidone: a case series. J Neuropsychiatry Clin Neurosci 22(1):111–114, 2010 20160218

Srivastava S, Chadda RK, Bala K, Majumdar P: A study of neuropsychiatric manifestations in patients of neurocysticercosis. Indian J Psychiatry 55(3):264–267, 2013 24082247

Staszewski S, Morales-Ramirez J, Tashima KT, et al; Study 006 Team: Efavirenz plus zidovudine and lamivudine, efavirenz plus indinavir, and indinavir plus zidovudine and lamivudine in the treatment of HIV-1 infection in adults. N Engl J Med 341(25):1865–1873, 1999 10601505

Sternbach H, State R: Antibiotics: neuropsychiatric effects and psychotropic interactions. Harv Rev Psychiatry 5(4):214–226, 1997 9427014

Tanquary J: Lithium neurotoxicity at therapeutic levels in an AIDS patient. J Nerv Ment Dis 181(8):518–519, 1993 8360645

Taycan O, Ugur M, Ozmen M: Quetiapine vs. risperidone in treating psychosis in neurosyphilis: a case report. Gen Hosp Psychiatry 28(4):359–361, 2006 16814638

Taylor JJ, Wilson JW, Estes LL: Linezolid and serotonergic drug interactions: a retrospective survey. Clin Infect Dis 43(2):180–187, 2006 16779744

Tsai AC, Karasic DH, Hammer GP, et al: Directly observed antidepressant medication treatment and HIV outcomes among homeless and marginally housed HIV-positive adults: a randomized controlled trial. Am J Public Health 103(2):308–315, 2013 22720766

Turan S, Emul M, Duran A, et al: Effectiveness of olanzapine in neurosyphilis related organic psychosis: a case report. J Psychopharmacol 21(5):556–558, 2007 17092977

Vallini AD, Burns RL: Carbamazepine as therapy for psychiatric sequelae of herpes simplex encephalitis. South Med J 80(12):1590–1592, 1987 3423906

Vasconcelos-Moreno MP, Dargél AA, Goi PD, et al: Improvement of behavioural and manic-like symptoms secondary to herpes simplex virus encephalitis with mood stabilizers: a case report. Int J Neuropsychopharmacol 14(5):718–720, 2011 21294940

Venkatakrishnan K, von Moltke LL, Greenblatt DJ: Effects of the antifungal agents on oxidative drug metabolism: clinical relevance. Clin Pharmacokinet 38(2):111–180, 2000 10709776

Wagner GJ, Rabkin R: Effects of dextroamphetamine on depression and fatigue in men with HIV: a double-blind, placebo-controlled trial. J Clin Psychiatry 61(6):436–440, 2000 10901342

Wagner GJ, Rabkin JG, Rabkin R: Dextroamphetamine as a treatment for depression and low energy in AIDS patients: a pilot study. J Psychosom Res 42(4):407–411, 1997 9160280

Warnke D, Barreto J, Temesgen Z: Antiretroviral drugs. J Clin Pharmacol 47(12):1570–1579, 2007 18048575

Wiegand M, Möller AA, Schreiber W, et al: Alterations of nocturnal sleep in patients with HIV infection. Acta Neurol Scand 83(2):141–142, 1991 2017899

Williams JB, Rabkin JG, Remien RH, et al: Multidisciplinary baseline assessment of homosexual men with and without human immunodeficiency virus infection, II: standardized clinical assessment of current and lifetime psychopathology. Arch Gen Psychiatry 48(2):124–130, 1991 1671198

Witkowski AE, Manabat CG, Bourgeois JA: Isoniazid-associated psychosis. Gen Hosp Psychiatry 29(1):85–86, 2007 17189755

Woodroof A, Gleason O: Psychiatric symptoms in a case of intracranial tuberculosis (letter). Psychosomatics 43(1):82–84, 2002 11927766

Wu YS, Lane HY, Lin CH: Donepezil improved cognitive deficits in a patient with neurosyphilis. Clin Neuropharmacol 38(4):156–157, 2015 26166240

Yew WW: Clinically significant interactions with drugs used in the treatment of tuberculosis. Drug Saf 25(2):111–133, 2002 11888353

Zilikis N, Nimatoudis I, Kiosses V, Ierodiakonou C: Treatment with risperidone of an acute psychotic episode in a patient with AIDS. Gen Hosp Psychiatry 20(6):384–385, 1998 9854654

Zisook S, Peterkin J, Goggin KJ, et al; HIV Neurobehavioral Research Center Group: Treatment of major depression in HIV-seropositive men. J Clin Psychiatry 59(5):217–224, 1998 9632030

13

Dermatological Disorders

Madhulika A. Gupta, M.D., FRCPC

James L. Levenson, M.D.

Psychiatric and psychosocial comorbidity is present among 25%–30% of dermatology patients (Gupta and Gupta 1996), and effective management of the dermatological condition involves management of the associated psychiatric factors. The skin is both a source and a target of immunomodulatory mediators of psychological stress response (Arck et al. 2006). Acute psychological stress and sleep restriction adversely affect skin barrier function recovery and may exacerbate barrier-mediated dermatoses such as psoriasis and atopic dermatitis (Choi et al. 2005). Various skin-related factors show circadian rhythmicity, including the stratum corneum barrier of the skin, transepidermal water loss (TEWL), skin surface pH, and skin temperature at most anatomic sites, with skin permeability being higher in the evening and night than the morning (Yosipovitch et al. 1998). Higher TEWL in the evening suggests that the epidermal barrier function at this time is not optimal, and TEWL is associated with greater itch intensity, which typically tends to be higher in the evening before bedtime. These circadian rhythms are maintained during treatment with high-potency and medium-potency corticosteroids in healthy skin (Yosipovitch et al. 2004). Clinically, this could be an important consideration in the use of moisturizers and timing of topical drug application (Patel et al. 2007; Yosipovitch et al. 1998, 2004).

The skin is also a large sensory organ with afferent sensory nerves conveying sensations of itch, touch, pain, temperature, and other physical stimuli to the central nervous system (CNS) and the efferent autonomic nerves, which are mainly sympathetic and cholinergic, that regulate vasomotor and pilomotor functions and the activity of the apocrine and eccrine sweat glands. Unlike other organs, reactions of the skin therefore represent a primarily sympathetic nervous system response, a factor that can be very relevant in a range of psychiatric disorders (Gupta and Gupta 2014a). Manipulation of the skin and its appendages (skin picking, hair pulling, nail peeling, scratching) can be used to manage high levels of anxiety in dissociative and obsessive-compulsive states and can result in self-induced dermatoses (Gupta et al. 1987).

Psychodermatological disorders are generally classified into two major categories (Medansky and Handler 1981; Gupta and Gupta 1996): 1) dermatological symptoms of psychiatric disorders and 2) psychiatric symptoms of dermatological disorders. The first category includes two diagnoses in the DSM-5 (American Psychiatric Association 2013) chapter "Obsessive-Compulsive and Related Disorders": body-focused repetitive behaviors (BFRBs) consisting of excoriation (skin-picking) disorder, trichotillomania (hair-pulling disorder), and pathological onychophagia (nail biting) (Gupta and Gupta 2014a), as well as delusions of infestation or parasitosis, considered to be delusional disorder, somatic type.

The second category has been further subdivided into 1) disorders that have a primary dermatopathological basis but may be influenced in part by psychological factors (e.g., psoriasis; atopic dermatitis; urticaria and angioedema; alopecia areata; acne; and possibly lichen planus, vitiligo, viral warts, and rosacea), 2) disorders that represent an accentuated physiological response (e.g., hyperhidrosis, blushing), and 3) disorders that result in an emotional reaction primarily as a result of cosmetic disfigurement and/or the social stigma associated with the disease. These subcategories are not mutually exclusive.

The focus in this chapter is on psychopharmacological treatment of psychiatric comorbidity, including adverse dermatological reactions to psychotropic drugs, adverse psychiatric effects of dermatological drugs, and drug-drug interactions. Clinically, most patients require a comprehensive biopsychosocial approach that typically includes both psychopharmacological treatments and psychotherapeutic interventions (e.g., cognitive-behavioral therapy, including habit reversal therapy, and dialectical behavior therapy). In some dermatological patients with psychiatric comorbidities, certain biologics may also have a direct antidepressant effect; a study of medically stable patients with treatment-resistant major depression suggested that the tumor necrosis factor alpha antagonist infliximab improves depression only in patients with high baseline inflammatory biomarkers (Raison et al. 2013), which would theoretically be the case in inflammatory dermatoses such as psoriasis. Currently, no orally administered psychotropic agents are approved by the U.S. Food and Drug Administration (FDA) for the treatment of a primary dermatological disorder or a BFRB involving the skin; 5% topical doxepin cream is FDA approved for short-term management (up to 8 days) of moderate pruritus in adults with conditions such as atopic dermatitis.

Differential Diagnosis

Dermatological Manifestations of Psychiatric Disorders

Cutaneous Symptoms of Psychiatric Disorders

Delusional disorder, somatic type, classified in DSM-5 under the diagnostic class of schizophrenia spectrum and other psychotic disorders, can manifest as a delusion that there is an infestation on or in the skin (delusions of parasitosis) or that a foul odor is being emitted from the skin and/or mucous membranes (delusions of bromhidrosis). Tactile hallucinations are particularly frequent in delirium, drug intoxication, and drug withdrawal.

Flushing of the skin and profuse daytime perspiration may be the presenting features of panic attacks. Unexplained night sweats can be a feature of an exacerbation and sympathetic nervous arousal in posttraumatic stress disorder (PTSD; Gupta and Gupta 2014b). Dramatic unexplained cutaneous sensory symptoms may represent a conversion reaction or a posttraumatic flashback (Gupta 2013b). Excessive complaints about imagined or slight "flaws" are a common feature of body dysmorphic disorder, which is classified as an obsessive-compulsive and related disorder in DSM-5 and is encountered in 9%–15% of dermatology patients (American Psychiatric Association 2013).

In DSM-5, under associated features supporting diagnosis, it is noted that for trichotillomania (hair-pulling disorder), some individuals display "more automatic behavior (in which the hair pulling seems to occur without full awareness)" (American Psychiatric Association 2013, p. 252), and for excoriation disorder, some individuals "engage in more automatic skin-picking (i.e., when skin picking occurs without preceding tension and without full awareness)" (p. 255). However, DSM-5 does not specifically mention the possible role of dissociation. It is important to assess for dissociative symptoms in the BFRBs (Gupta et al. 2015) because patients with high dissociative symptoms are not likely to respond well to the standard treatments for obsessive-compulsive disorder.

Cutaneous and Mucosal Sensory Syndromes

The cutaneous and mucosal sensory syndromes represent a heterogeneous clinical situation in which the patient presents with a disagreeable sensation such as itching, burning, stinging, or pain or allodynia and/or negative sensory symptoms such as numbness and hypoaesthesia, with no apparently diagnosable dermatological or medical condition that explains the symptoms. Skin regions that normally have a greater density of epidermal innervation tend to be most susceptible, and generally, these syndromes tend to be confined to the face, scalp, and perineum and have been referred to in the literature with region-specific terms such as scalp dysesthesias, burning mouth syndrome or glossodynia, and vulvodynia (Gupta and Gupta 2013a). These sensory syndromes represent a complex and often poorly understood interplay between local dermatological and neurobiological factors associated with neuropathic pain, neuropathic itch, and neurological or neuropsychiatric states (e.g., radiculopathies, stroke, depression, PTSD) (Gupta and Gupta 2013a).

Psychiatric Manifestations of Dermatological Disorders

General Psychopathological Effects of Dermatological Diseases

Various studies have reported a high prevalence of suicidal ideation in psoriasis, atopic dermatitis, acne, other disfiguring skin conditions, and severe pruritus; there is a correlation between patient-rated severity of dermatological disease and suicidal ideation (Dalgard et al. 2015; Picardi et al. 2013). In some instances, the degree of suicidality may be severe and out of proportion to the clinical severity of the skin disorder, such as in some acne patients, or when the skin disorder is clinically mild but affects socially stigmatizing body regions (Gupta 2011); in such instances comorbid body dysmorphic disorder should also be ruled out. Stress and daily hassles from the impact of a cosmetically disfiguring dermatological disorder on quality of life can in turn lead to exacerbations of some of the stress-reactive dermatoses such as psoriasis (Gupta et al. 1989).

Pruritus, including nocturnal pruritus, is one of the most common symptoms of dermatological disease and can aggravate mood and anxiety disorders. Scratching during sleep, which has been shown to be proportional to the overall level of sympathetic nervous activity during the respective sleep stages, usually occurs most frequently during non–rapid eye movement stages N1 and N2 and in rapid eye movement or stage R, in which the severity of scratching is similar to stage N2, and least frequently in stage N3, when the sympathetic tone is the lowest (Gupta and Gupta 2013b). Benzodiazepines suppress stage N3 sleep, and their long-term use can be associated with autonomic dysregulation as a result of withdrawal symptoms. Benzodiazepines are not recommended as a treatment for sleep disturbance due to pruritus.

Psychopathology in Specific Dermatological Diseases

Atopic dermatitis or eczema.   Anxiety and depression are frequent consequences of atopic dermatitis (eczema), but they also aggravate it. Suicidal ideation has been reported at rates ranging from 2% in patients with mild to moderate atopic dermatitis (Gupta and Gupta 1998) to 20% in patients with severe atopic dermatitis (Picardi et al. 2013). Sleep disruption in children as a result of pruritus can stress the entire family, exacerbate the atopic dermatitis as a result of the itch-scratch cycle, affect cognitive functioning, and simulate attention-deficit/hyperactivity disorder (Camfferman et al. 2010).

Psoriasis.   Psoriasis is associated with a variety of psychiatric and psychological difficulties, including poor self-esteem, sexual dysfunction, anxiety, depression, and suicidal ideation in 2.5%–10% of patients (Levenson 2008a; Picardi et al. 2013). In a multicenter European study (Dalgard et al. 2015), suicidal ideation was significantly more common in dermatological patients versus control subjects (hospital employees) (adjusted odds ratio [OR] = 1.94, 95% confidence interval [CI] 1.33–2.82); among the individual dermatological disorders, only psoriasis had a significant association with suicidal ideation (Dalgard et al. 2015). A systematic review and meta-analysis (Dowlatshahi et al. 2014) reported a 28% prevalence of clinical depression among patients with psoriasis in studies using questionnaires and a 19% prevalence using DSM-IV criteria; population-based studies showed that psoriasis patients were more likely to experience depression (OR=1.57, 95% CI 1.40–1.76) and use more antidepressants (OR=4.24, 95% CI 1.53–11.76) than control subjects. Inpatients with severe psoriasis are almost 2.5 times more likely than the general population to be receiving psychotropic medications (Gerdes et al. 2008). In a cohort study, 25,691 psoriasis patients and 128,573 reference subjects were followed for >9 years (Dowlatshahi et al. 2013). The adjusted hazard ratio of first antidepressant use in psoriasis was 1.55 (95% CI 1.50–1.61); within the psoriasis cohort, the hazard ratio of receiving an antidepressant was significantly higher (1.07) after the first anti-psoriatic treatment (95% CI 1.02–1.12).

Clinically mild psoriasis that affects a small percentage of total body surface in socially visible regions or the genital area (emotionally charged body regions) can carry a significant psychosocial burden. Psoriasis-related stress, most often associated with psoriasis in emotionally charged body regions, can in turn lead to exacerbations of the psoriasis (Gupta et al. 1989). A review of the literature concluded that psoriasis patients suffer psychiatric and psychosocial morbidity that is not commensurate with the extent of cutaneous lesions (Rieder and Tausk 2012).

Urticaria and angioedema.   The underlying etiology of urticaria (hives) is typically not identifiable in about 70% of patients; psychogenic factors have been reported to be important in about 40% of cases, but their role is very difficult to assess (Gupta 2009). Stress can precipitate acute urticaria and perpetuate chronic urticaria (Gupta 2009). Urticarial reactions can occur as a conditioned response to a previously neutral stimulus that may come to have a specific negative psychological association for the patient (Gupta 2009). The frequency of psychiatric comorbidity is well established, with about half of patients with chronic urticaria having a comorbid psychiatric condition, especially obsessive-compulsive disorder and major depression (Staubach et al. 2006; Uguz et al. 2008). The role of chronic PTSD tends to be underrecognized as a factor in idiopathic and cholinergic urticaria (Gupta 2009; Hunkin and Chung 2012). Depression and insomnia resulting from pruritus aggravate chronic urticaria (Yang et al. 2005; Yosipovitch et al. 2002). Adrenergic urticaria is a rare stress-induced disorder that responds to propranolol (Hogan et al. 2014) and may be associated with PTSD.

Alopecia areata. A review of psychiatric comorbidities in children and adolescents with alopecia areata (hair loss) reported a 50% prevalence rate of depression, 39% rate of generalized anxiety disorder, and 35.7% rate of obsessive-compulsive disorder (Ghanizadeh and Ayoobzadehshirazi 2014). No clear correlation exists between severity of psychiatric symptoms and severity of alopecia, but cosmetic disfigurement can be a significant source of psychological distress. In an epidemiological study from Taiwan, a younger age at onset of alopecia areata was associated with greater psychiatric morbidity, and 50% of the psychiatric disorders were present prior to the onset of alopecia areata (Chu et al. 2012).

Acne. Severe acne has been associated with increased depression, anxiety, poor self-image, and poor self-esteem (Saitta et al. 2011a). Body image pathologies such as eating disorders and body dysmorphic disorder are commonly encountered in patients who are excessively preoccupied by clinically mild acne. In addition, frequent bingeing in eating disorders is associated with flare-ups of acne. Psychiatric comorbidity is often the most disabling feature of acne and is one of the considerations in deciding whether to institute dermatological therapies. Psychiatric morbidity in acne, including the 5%–7% prevalence rate of suicidal ideation (Gupta and Gupta 1998; Picardi et al. 2006), is not consistently related to the clinical severity of the skin condition; in such cases comorbid body dysmorphic disorder should be ruled out. Epidemiological studies of adolescents with acne suggest a higher prevalence of suicidal thoughts (25.5%–34%) and suicide attempts (13%) in adolescents who self-rated their acne as more substantial and problematic; the association of self-perceived acne with suicidal ideation was independent of anxiety and depressive symptoms (Halvorsen et al. 2011; Purvis et al. 2006).

Pharmacotherapy of Specific Disorders

Dermatological Manifestations of Psychiatric Disorders

Delusional Disorder, Somatic Type

The biggest challenge in the pharmacotherapy of delusions of infestation (parasitosis) is convincing patients to take a psychiatric drug, because they do not view themselves as having a psychiatric disorder. A strong therapeutic alliance is therefore an essential prerequisite for effective pharmacotherapy, and treatment has to be customized depending on the underlying cause of the delusion. In cases of secondary delusions of infestation (other psychiatric disorder, sensory deprivation, early dementia, effects of prescription medication or illicit drugs), the primary disorder has to be managed (Heller et al. 2013).

Selective serotonin reuptake inhibitors (SSRIs) have sometimes been helpful in patients with delusions of infestation whose parasite sensations are more obsessional than delusional. Pimozide has been referred to as the "gold standard" for treating delusions of infestation (Heller et al. 2013); however there is little evidence to substantiate its use. The recommended starting dosage for pimozide is 0.5 mg/day to a maximum of 4 mg/day, with a therapeutic range of 2–3 mg/day (Heller et al. 2013); this is not an FDA-approved indication for pimozide, and no clinical trials have demonstrated superiority of pimozide over other typical or atypical antipsychotics. It has been recommended by some researchers that pimozide not be used as a first-line drug because of its extensive side-effect profile (Lepping and Freudenmann 2008). Sudden unexpected deaths have been reported with pimozide, the possible mechanism being ventricular arrhythmias caused by QTc prolongation (see Table 13–1 in the section "Drug-Drug Interactions").

In a study of 17 consecutive patients with delusions of infestation, 88% were taking antipsychotics, and 71% reached full remission; the average duration of treatment was 3.8 years (Huber et al. 2011). Both first-generation (haloperidol) and second-generation (risperidone, olanzapine, quetiapine) antipsychotics and aripiprazole have been used in delusions of infestation (Heller et al. 2013); risperidone and olanzapine have been reported to be the most commonly used second-generation antipsychotics, with about a 70% efficacy with doses lower than those used in schizophrenia (Freudenmann and Lepping 2008).

Cutaneous and Mucosal Dysesthesias

The cutaneous and mucosal dysesthesias represent a heterogeneous group of disorders; treatments used and their efficacy depend largely on the etiology of the cutaneous sensory syndrome (Gupta and Gupta 2013a). Burning mouth syndrome (BMS) is a complex, chronic disorder of orofacial sensation that is difficult both to diagnose and to treat, with psychological or psychiatric factors present in up to 85% of patients with BMS (Charleston 2013). In a 10-week randomized controlled trial, clonazepam 0.5 mg/day was more effective than placebo in treating pain of idiopathic BMS (Heckmann et al. 2012). A retrospective chart review of 51 patients with BMS seen over a period of 10 years revealed that 42 patients (82.4%) had been prescribed antidepressants, and 31 (60.8%) had been prescribed SSRIs. SSRIs tended to be more effective in patients who reported that stress was the major factor aggravating their BMS (Fleuret et al. 2014). Some psychopharmacological agents reported to have beneficial effects in BMS include anxiolytics (RCTs using clonazepam and diazepam; open-label or case studies using ketazolam), anticonvulsants (RCTs using gabapentin; open-label or case studies of pregabalin), antidepressants (open-label or case studies using duloxetine, milnacipran, and moclobemide), atypical antipsychotics (open-label or case studies of amisulpride and olanzapine), histamine receptor antagonists (RCT using lafutidine), and dopamine agonists (open-label or case studies using pramipexole) (Charleston 2013).

Vulvodynia is a complex disorder, in which patients typically present with complaints of burning, stinging, irritation, or rawness that is difficult to treat (Stockdale and Lawson 2014). Treatment guidelines for vulvodynia based on expert consensus (Stockdale and Lawson 2014) include tricyclic antidepressants (TCAs), such as amitriptyline, nortriptyline, and desipramine, starting at 10–25 mg at bedtime, which may be increased to 100–150 mg depending on the response; other antidepressants, including venlafaxine and SSRIs; and some anticonvulsants (Haefner et al. 2005). Rapid resolution of symptoms in vulvodynia is unusual even with appropriate therapy, and no single treatment is successful in all women (Stockdale and Lawson 2014).

Case reports suggest that scalp dysesthesia may respond to low doses of antihistaminic TCAs, such as amitriptyline 10–50 mg/day and doxepin 20–50 mg/day (Hoss and Segal 1998), or pregabalin 75–150 mg/day (Sarifakioglu and Onur 2013). Idiopathic pruritic states, including prurigo nodularis, have been reported to respond to SSRIs, TCAs (amitriptyline, clomipramine, doxepin), and mirtazapine (Ständer et al. 2008).

Body-Focused Repetitive Behaviors

There are no medications that are specifically FDA approved for the treatment of BFRBs involving the integument (excoriation disorder, trichotillomania). Psychotherapeutic agents have been shown to be more effective when the BFRB is significantly mediated by underlying depression or anxiety. The BFRBs may further exacerbate an underlying dermatological disorder (e.g., acne excoriée).

Nonpharmacological interventions such as cognitive-behavioral therapy (including habit reversal therapy) tend to be more effective in the treatment of the behavioral component of the BFRB. Trichotillomania is associated with trichobezoars in up to 10% of cases, which can lead to bowel obstruction and require surgical removal. If the grooming behaviors in the patient are strictly to improve appearance, the patient may have body dysmorphic disorder; it is important to recognize comorbid body dysmorphic disorder because it responds more favorably to SSRIs than do the BFRBs.

Excoriation disorder is present in up to 30% of patients with body dysmorphic disorder (Odlaug and Grant 2012). Excoriation disorder represents a heterogeneous group of disorders, from the typical patient who picks benign irregularities, pimples, or scabs to cases of dermatitis artefacta, in which the lesions are wholly self-inflicted. The latter patients typically deny the self-inflicted nature of their lesions, which are often bizarre looking and surrounded by normal-looking skin. Presentation of these lesions (e.g., blisters, purpura, ulcers, erythema, edema, sinuses, nodules) depends on the means employed to create them, such as deep excoriation by fingernails or sharp object or chemical and thermal burns (Gupta et al. 1987). Dermatitis artefacta can result in full-thickness skin loss and severe scarring, necessitating extensive plastic surgery and even amputations (Gupta et al. 1987). Clinical evaluation of excoriation disorder ideally involves an interdisciplinary approach that assesses both physical and psychiatric factors (Grant et al. 2012).

Various approaches to the treatment of excoriation disorder include cognitive-behavioral therapy (including habit reversal therapy), SSRIs (fluoxetine average dose of 55 mg/day, citalopram 20 mg/day), N-acetylcysteine (Grant et al. 2009), and naltrexone. Lamotrigine 25–300 mg/day was shown to be effective in excoriation disorder in a 12-week open-label trial (Grant et al. 2007) but failed to demonstrate greater benefit than placebo in excoriation disorder in a follow-up double-blind, placebo-controlled trial (Grant et al. 2010). A Cochrane review (Rothbart et al. 2013) identified a large degree of heterogeneity in the literature in the treatment of trichotillomania and identified single studies that point to the beneficial effect of clomipramine (Ninan 2000; Swedo et al. 1989), olanzapine (Van Ameringen et al. 2010), and N-acetylcysteine (Grant et al. 2009) and also noted lack of evidence for fluoxetine, sertraline, or naltrexone therapy. Aripiprazole has been reported to be effective in trichotillomania in a few case studies (Jefferys and Burrows 2008; Yasui-Furukori and Kaneko 2011) as well as in an open-label study (White and Koran 2011). An open-label study ($N=14$) of topiramate 50–250 mg/day in trichotillomania revealed a significant improvement in the primary outcome measure, the Massachusetts General Hospital Hair Pulling Scale score, at 16 weeks in the 9 trichotillomania patients who completed the study; other clinician-rated measures did not show significant improvement (Lochner et al. 2006).

Dissociative states tend to be underrecognized in the BFRBs (Gupta et al. 2015); excoriation disorder manifesting as dermatitis artefacta typically is associated with high levels of dissociation. Case studies suggest that mood stabilizers (lamotrigine, divalproex) are effective in managing both the anxiety and manipulation of the integument when high levels of dissociation are present (Gupta 2013a). High dissociation levels in patients with obsessive-compulsive-related disorders tend to be associated with a poor response to standard therapies (Belli et al. 2012; Semiz et al. 2014). Studies of mood stabilizers in the BFRBs—lamotrigine in excoriation disorder (Grant et al. 2007, 2010) and topiramate in trichotillomania (Lochner et al. 2006)—have reported essentially negative results; these studies included all patients with BFRBs and did not consider only the subgroup with high dissociation levels.

Psychiatric Manifestations of Dermatological Disorders

Atopic Dermatitis or Eczema

The management of atopic dermatitis requires a multifaceted approach that takes into consideration the psychiatric and psychosocial dimensions of the condition (Senra and Wollenberg 2014; Sidbury et al. 2014). An important goal in the pharmacotherapy of atopic dermatitis is the interruption of the itch-scratch cycle and optimization of nighttime sleep (Levenson 2008a). Topical doxepin (5% cream) is effective in the treatment of pruritus in atopic dermatitis (Drake et al. 1995) and is FDA approved for short-term (up to 8 days) treatment of moderate pruritus in adults with atopic dermatitis but not in children because of the greater risk of systemic side effects such as drowsiness. Low-dose oral doxepin (e.g., starting at 10 mg at bedtime and titrated on the basis of efficacy and side effects) is helpful in adults because of its antihistaminic sedative properties (Kelsay 2006). Sedating antidepressants may be beneficial in part through promoting sleep. Furthermore, the strongly antihistaminic antidepressants doxepin, trimipramine, and amitriptyline may also be effective because of their strong anticholinergic properties because the eccrine sweat glands in atopic dermatitis have been found to be hypersensitive to acetylcholine. In an earlier double-blind, placebo-controlled study of adult patients with atopic dermatitis (Savin et al. 1979), the phenothiazine trimeprazine 20 mg was compared with the TCA trimipramine 50 mg and placebo over 3 nights; both trimipramine and trimeprazine were associated with a decrease in nocturnal scratching, and trimipramine was associated with greater improvement in sleep architecture. Bupropion has been reported to be beneficial in atopic dermatitis in case reports (González et al. 2006) and a small open-label study of bupropion SR 150 mg/day for 3 weeks, followed by 150 mg twice a day for 3 weeks (Modell et al. 2002). There are also case reports of benefits from dextroamphetamine (Check and Chan 2014), mirtazapine 15 mg /day (Hundley and Yosipovitch 2004), and mirtazapine 30 mg/day with olanzapine up to 7.5 mg at bedtime (Mahtani et al. 2005). No guidelines have been established for the treatment of sleep disturbance in atopic dermatitis (Kelsay 2006). In a small short-term, double-blind, placebo-controlled crossover trial, the benzodiazepine nitrazepam did not significantly reduce nocturnal scratching (Ebata et al. 1998). The lack of response of pruritus to nitrazepam is consistent with the observation that scratching from pruritus is least likely to occur during stage N3 sleep, which is suppressed by benzodiazepines (Gupta and Gupta 2013b). For anxiety in atopic dermatitis, an antihistaminic TCA such as doxepin starting at 10 mg/day is recommended over benzodiazepines because benzodiazepine withdrawal may further exacerbate pruritus.

Psoriasis

Improvement in the clinical severity of psoriasis is generally associated with an improvement in psychiatric comorbidity. In a study of 414 psoriasis patients, dermatological improvement was less likely to be associated with psychological improvement in female patients and those with localization of the psoriasis on the face (Sampogna et al. 2007). SSRI antidepressant use in psoriasis has been associated with a decreased need for systemic psoriasis treatments. A Swedish population-based cohort study of 1,282 plaque psoriasis patients (89% with mild psoriasis) who also had prescriptions of SSRIs twice during a 6-month period and 1,282 psoriasis patients matched for demographics and psoriasis severity who were not exposed to SSRIs revealed that the risk of switching from less aggressive topical therapies to systemic psoriasis treatments was significantly decreased in the SSRI-exposed group (OR = 0.44,

95% CI 0.28–0.68) (Thorslund et al. 2013). The authors discuss various possible factors, including an improvement in the SSRI-exposed subjects' mood, which increased compliance with nonsystemic psoriasis treatments, and a direct anti-inflammatory effect from the SSRIs (Thorslund et al. 2013). Several studies have reported a significant improvement in psychiatric comorbidity in patients with psoriasis who are treated with biological drugs ("biologics"), specifically infliximab (Bassukas et al. 2008), ustekinumab (Langley et al. 2010), and etanercept (Tyring et al. 2006).

Meditation, relaxation training, and cognitive-behavioral stress management are some psychological therapies that have been reported to be effective for patients with psoriasis (Levenson 2008b). Obesity, moderately heavy alcohol use, and tobacco smoking should be addressed in the management of psoriasis because they have been associated with poor response to dermatological therapies (Gottlieb et al. 2008). The association between psoriasis and metabolic syndrome, obesity, hyperlipidemia, hypertension, and cardiovascular mortality (Armstrong et al. 2013a, 2013b; Gottlieb et al. 2008) has important implications in the choice of psychopharmacological agents, which may also be associated with glycemic dysregulation, dyslipidemias, and metabolic syndrome.

Treatment of depressive symptoms may reduce pruritus and insomnia in patients with psoriasis. In a placebo-controlled trial, the reversible monoamine oxidase inhibitor (MAOI) moclobemide reduced psoriasis severity and anxiety (Alpsoy et al. 1998). In a small open-label trial, bupropion induced improvement in psoriasis, with return to baseline levels after its discontinuation (Modell et al. 2002), and paroxetine was reported to be effective in two patients with both depression and psoriasis (Luis Blay 2006). Overall, the evidence base is limited, and antidepressants, including bupropion (Cox et al. 2002), sometimes have been reported to cause or aggravate psoriasis (Warnock and Morris 2002a). There is a case study of improvement of psoriasis with pregabalin or gabapentin (Boyd et al. 2008). A case series of seven psoriasis patients (six of whom also had a mood disorder) treated with topiramate for a minimum of 4 months at an average dosage of 56 mg/day demonstrated significant improvement in their psoriasis (Ryback 2002).

Urticaria

In interpreting the chronic idiopathic urticaria (CIU) treatment literature, one must take into consideration the very high rate of response to placebo

(Rudzki et al. 1970). A low dose of a sedating antihistaminic antidepressant, such as doxepin, is helpful in the management of pruritus in CIU, especially when pruritus interferes with sleep (Yosipovitch et al. 2002). Doxepin may provide more than symptomatic relief, reducing the urticarial reaction itself (Greene et al. 1985; Goldsobel et al. 1986; Rao et al. 1988). Potent histaminic H_1 plus H_2 blockers, such as doxepin, trimipramine, and amitriptyline, are more effective than H_1 antihistamines alone for urticaria (Levenson 2008b). There are also case reports of the benefits of mirtazapine (Bigatà et al. 2005) and SSRIs (Gupta and Gupta 1995). A small open-label study ($N=16$) of recalcitrant CIU reported a significant reduction in urticarial activity scores with reserpine 0.3–0.4 mg/day as an add-on therapy to antihistamines at 1–2 weeks and 4–8 weeks (Demitsu et al. 2010). A mood stabilizer may be used when urticaria is a feature of the physiological effect of severe emotional dysregulation in PTSD (Gupta and Gupta 2012), including cases of cholinergic urticaria.

Alopecia Areata

The literature on the use of psychotropic agents in treating alopecia areata is inconclusive and further confounded by the fact that patients may experience spontaneous remission of their alopecia in the absence of any treatments (Levenson 2008b). In a study of 60 patients with alopecia areata (with <25% scalp involvement), 30 who were also diagnosed with major depression received citalopram 20 mg/day plus triamcinolone injections every 4 weeks, compared with 30 patients without depression who received triamcinolone injections alone. After 6 months of therapy, the citalopram group had greater improvement in alopecia than the triamcinolone alone group, suggesting that antidepressant treatment might help in improving alopecia areata in those patients who also have major depression (Abedini et al. 2014). Small double-blind, placebo-controlled trials have reported benefit from imipramine ($N=13$) (Perini et al. 1994) and paroxetine ($N=13$) (Cipriani et al. 2001).

Acne

The focus of psychiatric drug treatment for patients with acne should be on any underlying psychiatric disorder (e.g., major depressive disorder, body dysmorphic disorder, bulimia nervosa). Various antidepressants (clomipramine, fluoxetine, paroxetine) have been shown to be effective in treating depression in acne (Saitta et al. 2011a, 2011b). The patient should be evaluated for acne excoriée because the excoriation of the acne lesion can exacerbate the under-lying inflammation in acne. Case studies suggest efficacy of olanzapine in treating self-excoriative behavior in acne excoriée (Gupta and Gupta 2000). Isotretinoin, which is indicated for the treatment of nodulocystic acne, has been associated with suicide attempts and suicide, in addition to other side ef-fects, including teratogenicity. There is an extensive literature on suicide and suicide attempts with isotretinoin, but a causal relationship has not been proven; this highlights the importance of assessing and monitoring every pa-tient taking isotretinoin for suicide risk (refer to the section "Adverse Psychi-atric Effects of Dermatological Agents"). In some case studies, hormonal contraceptives have failed in patients who self-medicated their depression with St. John's wort (Hall et al. 2003). St. John's wort is a cytochrome P450 3A4 (CYP3A4) inducer that increases the metabolism of some hormonal con-traceptives and decreases their efficacy; patients taking isotretinoin and hor-monal contraceptives should be advised of this interaction.

Adverse Cutaneous Drug Reactions to Psychotropic Agents

Adverse cutaneous drug reactions (ACDRs; Litt 2013; Warnock and Morris 2002a, 2002b, 2003) can be divided into common (usually relatively benign) reactions, rare life-threatening reactions, and precipitation or aggravation of a primary dermatological disorder. ACDRs are reported to affect 2%–3% of hospitalized patients, and 2% of these cutaneous reactions are severe and life threatening. Approximately 2%–5% of patients receiving psychotropic med-ications will develop ACDRs, which remain the most common allergic reac-tion to these agents (Kimyai-Asadi et al. 1999).

Mild Adverse Cutaneous Drug Reactions

Common ACDRs include pruritus, exanthematous rashes, urticaria with or without angioedema, fixed drug eruptions, photosensitivity reactions, drug-induced pigmentation, and alopecia. *Pruritus* is the most common ACDR, encountered with all antipsychotics, antidepressants, and mood stabilizers, and is usually secondary to other ACDRs.

Exanthematous rashes (morbilliform or maculopapular eruptions) can oc-cur with all antipsychotics, antidepressants, and mood stabilizers. The rash usually occurs within the first 3–14 days of starting the drug and may subside without discontinuation of the causative agent. In some cases, the rash, especially if it includes painful lesions, may represent the early stages of one of the more severe and life-threatening ACDRs, such as Stevens-Johnson syndrome.

Urticaria, with or without angioedema, is the second most common ACDR after pruritus. It occurs within minutes to a few hours but sometimes as late as several days after starting the drug and can lead to laryngeal angioedema and anaphylaxis. Urticaria can occur with all antipsychotics, antidepressants, and anticonvulsants.

Fixed drug eruptions can theoretically occur with any drug. They characteristically appear as sharply demarcated, solitary, or occasionally multiple lesions that occur within a few to 24 hours after ingestion of the drug and resolve within several weeks of drug discontinuation.

Photosensitivity reactions are the result of an interaction of the drug with ultraviolet radiation and are limited to body regions exposed to light. Such reactions can be caused by any of the antipsychotics but are much more frequently associated with chlorpromazine (3% incidence) (Warnock and Morris 2002b). Photosensitivity also occurs with antidepressants, including the TCAs and SSRIs; some mood stabilizers, including carbamazepine, valproic acid, topiramate, gabapentin, and oxcarbazepine; and some sedatives and hypnotics, including amobarbital, phenobarbital, pentobarbital, alprazolam, estazolam, chlordiazepoxide, eszopiclone, zaleplon and zolpidem. The incidence of photosensitivity for each of the medications from the three classes of drugs is 1% or less (Litt 2013). Patients should be advised regarding the use of sunscreen and minimization of sun exposure in those instances in which the medication has to be continued. Photosensitivity caused by psychotropic drugs may interfere with psoralen plus ultraviolet A and ultraviolet B light therapy for psoriasis and other pruritic dermatoses.

Drug-induced pigmentation, which may involve the skin and eyes (retina, lens, and cornea), has been reported after long-term (>6 months), high-dose (>500 mg/day) use of low-potency typical antipsychotics, especially chlorpromazine and thioridazine. The cutaneous discoloration in some instances is secondary to dermal granules containing melanin bound to the drug or its metabolites; the discoloration can take months to years to completely resolve after discontinuation of the drug. Pigmentary changes have been associated with some antidepressants, including various TCAs, all SSRIs, and venlafaxine (hypopigmentation), and with some anticonvulsants, including lamotrigine (also associated with leukoderma), carbamazepine, topiramate, gabapentin, and valproic acid (also associated with changes in hair color and texture).

Alopecia, which typically appears as diffuse, nonscarring, and localized or generalized hair loss from the scalp, is usually reversible after discontinuation of the offending drug. Hair loss may occur rapidly or a few months after the drug has been started, with recovery generally 2–5 months after drug discontinuation. Alopecia has been reported frequently with lithium (> 5%) and valproic acid (> 5%) and less frequently with the other mood stabilizers. Alopecia has also been associated with most antidepressants, including all SSRIs, bupropion, venlafaxine, and duloxetine, and with several antipsychotics, including olanzapine, risperidone, ziprasidone, loxapine, and haloperidol.

Severe Adverse Cutaneous Drug Reactions

Severe and life-threatening skin reactions are most frequently associated with anticonvulsants and include erythema multiforme (EM), Stevens-Johnson syndrome (SJS), toxic epidermal necrolysis (TEN or Lyell's syndrome), drug hypersensitivity syndrome or drug rash (or reaction) with eosinophilia and systemic symptoms (DRESS), exfoliative dermatitis, and vasculitis (Litt 2013; Warnock and Morris 2002a, 2002b, 2003). EM, SJS, and TEN lie on a continuum of increasing severity. About 16% of cases of SJS or TEN have been associated with short-term use of anticonvulsant drugs, with greatest risk for development of TEN within the first 8 weeks of initiating therapy. Use of multiple anticonvulsants and administration of higher doses increase the risk. Treatment of severe reactions should include immediate discontinuation of the drug and an emergency dermatology consultation. Patients typically require fluid and nutritional support, as well as infection and pain control, which may involve management in an intensive care or burn unit. Increased risk is associated with immunosuppression, especially when accompanied by primary or viral reactivation of herpesviruses (e.g., human herpesviruses 6 and 7) or infection with Epstein-Barr virus or HIV (Dodiuk-Gad et al. 2014; Husain et al. 2013). Adequate psychiatric supervision should also be provided when mood stabilizer anticonvulsants are abruptly discontinued because significant relapse of psychiatric symptoms may occur (Bliss and Warnock 2013).

Increased risk of developing SJS/TEN because of use of anticonvulsants, most commonly carbamazepine, has been attributed to several human leukocyte antigen (HLA) allele variants (Cheng et al. 2014; Grover and Kukreti 2014), specifically, *HLA-B*1502* and *HLA-A*3101*. The *B*1502* variant is seen more often in Asian populations. The FDA suggests that individuals of Asian (including south Asian Indian) ancestry be screened for the *B*1502* variant prior to commencing carbamazepine or phenytoin therapy (U.S. Food and Drug Administration 2007). This variant has also been associated with SJS/TEN induced by other anticonvulsants (Hung et al. 2010). The *A*3101* variant is seen in numerous populations, including whites, and is associated with a number of ACDRs, including SJS/TEN and DRESS. At the present time, the FDA does not explicitly suggest genotyping for the *A*3101* variant prior to commencing carbamazepine; however, some investigators (Amstutz et al. 2014) have recommended screening for the *A*3101* allele among all carbamazepine-naïve patients.

Erythema multiforme occurs within days of starting the drug and may present as a polymorphous eruption, with pathognomonic "target lesions" typically involving the extremities and palmoplantar surfaces. Progression of EM to more serious SJS and TEN should always be considered a possibility. Although EM is most commonly associated with carbamazepine, valproic acid, lamotrigine, gabapentin, and oxcarbazepine, it has also (albeit rarely) been associated with antipsychotics (e.g., clozapine, risperidone) and antidepressants (e.g., fluoxetine, paroxetine, bupropion) and occasionally with sedative-hypnotics (including barbiturates, some benzodiazepines, and eszopiclone).

Stevens-Johnson syndrome usually occurs within the first few weeks after drug exposure. Patients present with flu-like symptoms, followed by mucocutaneous lesions and a mortality rate as high as 5% due to loss of the cutaneous barrier and sepsis. Bullous lesions can involve mucosal surfaces, including the eyes, mouth, and genital tract. SJS is most frequently associated with the same anticonvulsants as EM.

Toxic epidermal necrolysis is considered to be an extreme variant of SJS, resulting in epidermal detachment in more than 30% of patients, occurring within the first 2 months of treatment, with a mortality rate as high as 45% due to sepsis. In 80% of TEN cases, a strong association is made with specific medications (vs. a 50% association with specific medications in SJS), most often anticonvulsants (Litt 2013; Warnock and Morris 2002a, 2002b, 2003). Use of more than one anticonvulsant increases the risk of SJS/TEN. For lamotrigine the risk of a serious rash may be increased by coadministration with divalproex sodium, exceeding the initial recommended dosage, or exceeding the recommended dosage escalation. Benign rashes also occur with lamotrigine, and it is not possible to reliably predict which rash will prove to be serious or life-threatening. Therefore, lamotrigine should be discontinued at the first sign of a rash unless the rash is clearly benign or not drug related.

Drug hypersensitivity syndrome, or DRESS, characteristically occurs 1–8 weeks after the start of drug treatment and manifests as a drug eruption, most commonly a morbilliform rash, with fever, eosinophilia, lymphadenopathy, and multiple organ involvement (including liver, kidney, lungs, and brain). Treatment involves immediate discontinuation of the suspected drug. Antihistamines and systemic corticosteroids may be required. The mortality rate is 10% if symptoms are unrecognized or untreated. The rash can range from a simple exanthem to TEN. DRESS is most commonly associated with anticonvulsants and has been reported with bupropion and fluoxetine (Husain et al. 2013).

Exfoliative dermatitis appears as a widespread rash characterized by desquamation, pruritic erythema, fever, and lymphadenopathy within the first few weeks of drug therapy, with a good prognosis if the causative agent is withdrawn immediately. It has been reported with antipsychotics, most TCAs and other antidepressants, mood stabilizers, lithium, sedatives, and hypnotics.

Drug hypersensitivity vasculitis is characterized by inflammation and necrosis of the walls of blood vessels within a few weeks of starting a drug. Lesions (e.g., palpable purpura) are localized primarily on the lower third of the legs and ankles. It has been associated with clozapine, maprotiline, trazodone, carbamazepine, lithium, phenobarbital, pentobarbital, diazepam, and chlordiazepoxide.

Exacerbation of Dermatological Disorders by Psychotropic Medications

Psychotropic drugs may precipitate or exacerbate a number of primary dermatological disorders (Litt 2013; Warnock and Morris 2002a, 2002b, 2003), including acne, psoriasis, seborrheic dermatitis, hyperhidrosis, and porphyria. *Acne* has been associated with most TCAs, all SSRIs, and other antidepressants such as venlafaxine, duloxetine, and bupropion; lithium carbonate and occasionally other anticonvulsant mood stabilizers, including topiramate, lamotrigine, gabapentin, and oxcarbazepine; and antipsychotics such as quetiapine and haloperidol.

Lithium is well known to precipitate or exacerbate *psoriasis* (Brauchli et al. 2009). Lithium-induced psoriasis can occur within a few months but usually occurs within the first few years of treatment. Lithium has an inhibitory effect on intracellular cyclic adenosine monophosphate and the phosphoinositides. Inositol supplements have been shown to have a significant beneficial effect on psoriasis in patients taking lithium (Allan et al. 2004). The β-blocker propranolol, which is often used to treat lithium-induced tremors, has also been associated with psoriasis, but a population-based study by Brauchli et al. (2008) does not support this. Psoriasis precipitated or exacerbated by lithium is typically resistant to conventional antipsoriatic treatments, and usually there is no family history of psoriasis. When psoriasis becomes intractable, lithium must be discontinued, and remission usually follows within a few months. Anticonvulsants, atypical antipsychotics, and SSRIs have been reported less commonly to precipitate or aggravate psoriasis. Results of an epidemiological study suggest possible reduced psoriasis risk with atypical antipsychotics, mainly olanzapine (Brauchli et al. 2009), although case studies have reported onset or exacerbation of psoriasis by olanzapine (Latini and Carducci 2003).

Seborrheic dermatitis typically occurs in regions where the sebaceous glands are most active, such as the scalp, face, chest, and genitalia. Seborrheic dermatitis is very common in patients taking long-term phenothiazines and also has been reported with other antipsychotics, including olanzapine, quetiapine, and loxapine. Seborrheic eruptions have also been reported with lithium and anticonvulsants.

Hyperhidrosis, often manifested as night sweats, is common with SSRIs, serotonin-norepinephrine reuptake inhibitors, bupropion, and MAOIs. Sweating is mediated by the sympathetic cholinergic innervation of the eccrine sweat glands; however, the more anticholinergic TCAs have also caused hyperhidrosis, and therefore switching to a more anticholinergic antidepressant is not necessarily helpful. The mechanism underlying the antidepressant-mediated hyperhidrosis is believed to be centrally mediated but is unclear. Hyperhidrosis has also been reported with antipsychotics (e.g., olanzapine, quetiapine, pimozide) and mood stabilizers (e.g., carbamazepine, topiramate [1% of patients], lamotrigine [2%], gabapentin, oxcarbazepine [3%]) (Litt 2013; Warnock and Morris 2002a, 2002b, 2003).

Porphyria may be exacerbated by certain drugs, such as carbamazepine, valproic acid, and many sedative-hypnotics (especially barbiturates and other

sedative-hypnotics, excluding benzodiazepines), resulting in acute dermatological, neuropsychiatric, and abdominal pain symptoms. Chlorpromazine,
although photosensitizing, is considered to be safe and actually was approved
by the FDA for use in acute intermittent porphyria.

Adverse Psychiatric Effects of Dermatological Agents

Corticosteroids

Psychiatric side effects of systemic glucocorticoid therapy are reviewed in detail
in Chapter 7, "Respiratory Disorders," and Chapter 10, "Endocrine and Metabolic Disorders." Topical corticosteroids may cause psychiatric adverse effects,
especially in patients with extensive lesions who are using high-potency topical
steroids (Hughes et al. 1983).

Retinoids

Isotretinoin is generally used to treat nodulocystic acne or acne that is refractory to other therapies and has been associated with depression, psychosis, suicide attempts, and suicide (Azoulay et al. 2008; Borovaya et al. 2013; Jick et
al. 2000; Marqueling and Zane 2007; Marron et al. 2013; McGrath et al.
2010; Nevoralová and Dvořáková 2013; Rademaker 2010; Rehn et al. 2009;
Sundström et al. 2010; Thomas et al. 2014). In an analysis of reports of depression and suicide to the FDA from the initial marketing of isotretinoin
from 1982 to May 2000, the FDA received reports regarding 431 patients: 37
completed suicides (24 while using isotretinoin and 13 after stopping isotretinoin); 110 hospitalizations for depression, suicidal ideation, or suicide attempt; and 284 cases of nonhospitalized depression (Wysowski et al. 2001).
Factors suggesting a possible association between isotretinoin and depression included a temporal association between isotretinoin use and depression, positive
dechallenges (often requiring psychiatric treatment), and positive rechallenges.
Compared with all drugs in the FDA's Adverse Event Reporting System, isotretinoin ranked within the top 10 for number of reports of depression and suicide
(Wysowski et al. 2001). The study concluded that "additional studies are
needed to determine whether isotretinoin causes depression and to identify
susceptible persons" (Wysowski et al. 2001, p. 518). The general consensus is

that the research on the possible causal effect of isotretinoin use on psychiatric morbidity, including suicide risk, is inconclusive.

The guidelines for prescribing isotretinoin (earlier trade name Accutane; only generic brands have been marketed since 2009) (Physicians' Desk Reference 2009) include the following warning:

> Accutane may cause depression, psychosis and, rarely, suicidal ideation, suicide attempts, suicide, and aggressive and/or violent behaviors. No mechanism of action has been established for these events.... Therefore prior to initiation of Accutane therapy, patients and family members should be asked about any history of psychiatric disorder, and at each visit during therapy patients should be assessed for symptoms of depression, mood disturbance, psychosis, or aggression to determine if further evaluation may be necessary. (pp. 2607–2614)

The guidelines further indicate that if patients develop psychiatric symptoms, they should promptly stop the isotretinoin and contact the prescriber. Prescribing of isotrenoin must also follow an FDA-approved risk evaluation and mitigation strategy under the iPLEDGE Program, which closely monitors prescribing and dispensing of isotrenoin (U.S. Food and Drug Administration 2012). Discontinuation of isotretinoin does not always lead to remission of psychiatric symptoms, including suicide risk, and further evaluation and treatment may be necessary. The determination as to whether a patient should continue taking isotretinoin after having experienced a psychiatric reaction should be based on the risk-benefit ratio for that particular patient. Some investigators have proposed that the comorbidity of major psychiatric disorders (psychosis, affective disorders) and isotretinion-associated psychiatric effects suggests a genetic vulnerability in isotretinoin users who experience psychiatric reactions (Kontaxakis et al. 2010). However, it is important to note that serious psychiatric reactions associated with isotretinoin such as suicide attempt can occur in patients without a personal or family history of psychiatric disorders (Goldsmith et al. 2004). A 2010 statement from the American Academy of Dermatology has noted, "A correlation between isotretinoin use and depression/anxiety symptoms has been suggested but an evidence-based causal relationship has not been established" (American Academy of Dermatology 2010, p. 1). A study of 500 Israeli conscripts who were seen by a dermatologist for severe acne reported five cases of psychosis (two soldiers diagnosed with schizophreniform disorder and three with schizoaffective disorder) in individuals on receiving isotretinoin whose psychiatric histories were negative prior to recruitment, with a mean lag time from intake of isotretinoin to occurrence of psychosis of 7.6 ± 4.2 months (Barak et al. 2005). Other retinoids such as etretinate and acitretin have also been reported to cause depression and suicidal thoughts (Arican et al. 2006; Henderson and Highet 1989).

Antihistamines

Sedating first-generation H_1 histamine-receptor antagonists such as diphenhydramine and hydroxyzine readily cross the blood-brain barrier and have antianxiety and sedative effects. In diphenhydramine overdose, patients may present with a toxic psychosis with bizarre behavior and hallucinations (Jones et al. 1986) and a trend toward an increased risk of delirium (Clegg and Young 2011). The anticholinergic effects of these antihistamines may cause subtle cognitive impairment and, in overdose, an anticholinergic delirium. The H_2 histamine-receptor antagonists cimetidine, ranitidine, and famotidine have been associated with mania (von Einsiedel et al. 2002), depression, and delirium (Catalano et al. 1996).

Antifungal and Antimicrobial Agents

The antifungal agent voriconazole has been associated with visual hallucinations in about 17% of cases, accompanied by auditory hallucinations in about 5% of patients (Zonios et al. 2014), within the first week of treatment. The hallucinations, which are a sign of neurotoxicity, are more common in the slow metabolizer phenotype of CYP2C19, and patients with this phenotype achieve significantly higher blood levels of voriconazole. The hallucinations resolve with decrease or discontinuation of voriconazole.

Minocycline, which is used in the treatment of acne and rosacea, may have beneficial effects in the treatment of schizophrenia (Chaudhry et al. 2012; Dodd et al. 2013; Keller et al. 2013) and depression (Miyaoka et al. 2012; Soczynska et al. 2012). Other antimicrobials can cause a variety of psychiatric symptoms. These medications are discussed in Chapter 12, "Infectious Diseases."

Biologics

Several studies have reported significant improvement in comorbid psychiatric symptoms in psoriasis patients treated with biologics such as etanercept (Tyring et al. 2006), infliximab (Bassukas et al. 2008), and ustekinumab (Langley et al. 2010; O'Brien et al. 2004). There have been occasional case reports of adverse psychiatric side effects (psychosis, mania, depression, or suicide) of biologics such as etanercept (Atigari and Healy 2014), adalimumab (Ellard et al. 2014), and infliximab (Austin and Tan 2012; Elisa and Beny 2010; Eshuis et al. 2010), but causal relationships have not been clearly demonstrated.

Other Agents

Finasteride, used for alopecia, has been associated with long-lasting sexual dysfunction and depression (Altomare and Capella 2002; Irwig 2012a, 2012b). Cyclosporine, an immunosuppressant used in organ transplantation and also used in severe psoriasis, has been associated with organic mental disorders, with various symptoms—including mood disorders, anxiety disorders, hallucinations and delusions, cognitive difficulties, and delirium—usually observed within 2 weeks of beginning treatment (Craven 1991). Cyclosporine is covered in Chapter 16, "Organ Transplantation." Dapsone, used for a variety of dermatological conditions, has been associated with mania (Carmichael and Paul 1989) in several reports.

Drug-Drug Interactions

Most pharmacokinetic interactions (Litt 2013) between dermatological and psychotropic drugs result from inhibition of CYP-mediated drug metabolism, mainly the CYP2D6 and CYP3A4 isozymes. Some of the key interactions are listed in Table 13–1 (see also Chapter 1, "Pharmacokinetics, Pharmacodynamics, and Principles of Drug-Drug Interactions," for a comprehensive drug interaction listing; Chapter 12, "Infectious Diseases," for antimicrobials; and Chapter 10, "Endocrine and Metabolic Disorders," for corticosteroids).

Many drugs used in dermatological conditions are inhibitors of CYP3A4, including azole antifungals (e.g., itraconazole, ketoconazole), some macrolides (erythromycin, clarithromycin), and cyclosporine, which is also a CYP3A4 substrate. Use of these drugs can dramatically increase blood levels of psychotropic drugs that are CYP3A4 substrates, including anticonvulsants such as carbamazepine; antidepressants such as doxepin, amitriptyline, and imipramine; benzodiazepines such as alprazolam, triazolam, and diazepam;

Table 13–1. Some dermatological drug–psychotropic drug pharmacokinetic interactions

Medication	Interaction mechanism	Effects on psychotropic drug levels	Management
Azole antifungals (oral formulations only) Itraconazole Ketoconazole	Inhibition of CYP3A4	Benzodiazepine serum levels for agents undergoing hepatic oxidative metabolism, such as alprazolam and triazolam, may increase.	Consider alternative benzodiazepines, such as oxazepam, which is metabolized by glucuronidation.
Macrolide antibiotics Clarithromycin Erythromycin	Inhibition of CYP3A4	Buspirone levels increased. Carbamazepine levels increased.	Consider alternative anxiolytics. Use alternative anticonvulsants.
Cyclosporine	Substrate and inhibition of CYP3A4	Doxepin, amitriptyline, and imipramine levels increased, with risk of arrhythmias. Pimozide levels increased, with risk of arrhythmias.	Decrease dosage or use alternative antidepressants. Do not coadminister pimozide with these agents.[a]
Terbinafine	Inhibition of CYP2D6	Antidepressant serum level may increase for CYP2D6 substrates, including TCAs, paroxetine, venlafaxine, and atomoxetine.	Consider alternative agents such as citalopram or sertraline. Atomoxetine dosage usually needs to be reduced.

Table 13–1. Some dermatological drug–psychotropic drug pharmacokinetic interactions *(continued)*

Medication	Interaction mechanism	Effects on psychotropic drug levels	Management
Terbafine *(continued)*		Antipsychotic serum levels may increase for CYP2D6 substrates, including phenothiazines (risking arrhythmias), haloperidol, risperidone, olanzapine, clozapine, and aripiprazole.	Decrease dosage or consider alternatives such as paliperidone or quetiapine.
Antihistamines Chlorpheniramine Diphenhydramine Hydroxyzine	Substrate of CYP2D6	Potential for QTc prolongation at higher dosages if taken with CYP2D6 inhibitors (e.g., the SSRIs paroxetine, fluoxetine, sertraline).	Lower dosage of antihistamine or use alternative antidepressant (e.g., venlafaxine).

Note. CYP=cytochrome P450; SSRIs=selective serotonin reuptake inhibitors; TCAs=tricyclic antidepressants.
[a]Several atypical antipsychotics (e.g., clozapine, quetiapine, ziprasidone, aripiprazole) are also CYP3A4 substrates; if used with a CYP3A4 inhibitor, their dosage may need to be decreased.

and the antipsychotic pimozide. Elevated levels of certain drugs such as antidepressants and pimozide can result in prolongation of the QTc interval and cardiac arrhythmias (Beach et al. 2013). The clinical importance of this interaction is exemplified by the fact that the antihistamines terfenadine and astemizole, both CYP3A4 substrates, have been withdrawn from the market because of potentially fatal interactions with CYP3A4 inhibitors resulting in life-threatening ventricular arrhythmias.

The antifungal agent terbinafine is a CYP2D6 inhibitor and can result in drug toxicity, such as serious cardiac arrhythmias, when administered in conjunction with CYP2D6 substrates, such as the TCAs and the phenothiazine antipsychotics. Alternatively, elevated levels of the antihistamines chlorpheniramine, diphenhydramine, and hydoxyzine, all of which are CYP2D6 substrates, may occur when these drugs are used in conjunction with psychiatric agents that are CYP2D6 inhibitors (e.g., SSRI antidepressants; see Table 13–1).

In addition, significant adverse effects may occur as a result of elevated levels of CYP3A4 substrates such as cyclosporine and corticosteroids when they are coadministered with psychotropic agents that are CYP3A4 inhibitors, such as fluoxetine, fluvoxamine, and nefazodone. Cyclosporine is both substrate and inhibitor of CYP3A4, resulting in many potential drug-drug interactions. Carbamazepine and other CYP3A4 inducers lower cyclosporine and pimozide blood levels and may decrease their therapeutic effect.

The following dermatological medications are associated with a known risk of torsades de pointes (defined as "substantial evidence supports the conclusion that these drugs prolong the QTc interval and are clearly associated with a risk of torsades de pointes [TdP], even when taken as directed in official labelling"): fluconazole, azithromycin, ciprofloxacin, clarithromycin, erythromycin, levofloxacin, moxifloxacin or pentamidine (dermatological agents) (Woosley and Romero 2015). There may be a synergistic effect when two drugs that are known to produce torsades de pointes are taken together.

Key Clinical Points

- Standard psychopharmacological agents may be used with adequate clinical monitoring to treat psychiatric comorbidity in dermatological disorders.

- Pruritus and sleep difficulties contribute to dermatological and psychiatric morbidity, including increased suicide risk. Effective management of sleep difficulties and pruritus is important in the choice of a psychopharmacological agent.

- The strongly antihistaminic TCA doxepin is effective for pruritus and sleep difficulties in the pruritic dermatoses.

- Disease-related stress should be addressed in the treatment plan because it can increase psychiatric morbidity and contribute to stress-related exacerbations of certain disorders (e.g., atopic dermatitis, psoriasis).

- The high prevalence of suicidal ideation in dermatology patients is not always associated with more clinically severe skin disease (e.g., in the adolescent patient with acne). Covert body dysmorphic disorder or other psychiatric comorbidities (e.g., PTSD) can increase suicide risk and treatment resistance. Certain medications (e.g., isotretinoin) may also be associated with increased suicidal ideation.

- Severe and life-threatening dermatological reactions such as Stevens-Johnson syndrome (SJS), toxic epidermal necrolysis (TEN), and drug hypersensitivity syndrome are most frequently associated with the mood-stabilizer anticonvulsants, with greatest risk of development within the first 2 months of therapy.

- Increased risk of developing SJS/TEN due to anticonvulsants, most commonly carbamazepine, has been attributed to several HLA allele variants, specifically *HLA-B*1502*, in individuals of Asian (including south Asian Indian) descent. Individuals of Asian ancestry should be screened for the *B*1502* allele prior to commencing carbamazepine or phenytoin therapy (U.S. Food and Drug Administration 2007).

- Most important dermatological drug–psychotropic drug inter-actions involve the use of CYP3A4 inhibitors (e.g., azole antifun-gals, macrolide antibiotics) with CYP3A4 substrates such as pimozide, resulting in increased blood levels of these medica-tions and increased risk of cardiac side effects secondary to QTc prolongation.

References

Abedini H, Farshi S, Mirabzadeh A, Keshavarz S: Antidepressant effects of citalopram on treatment of alopecia areata in patients with major depressive disorder. J Dermatolog Treat 25(2):153–155, 2014 23339335

Allan SJ, Kavanagh GM, Herd RM, Savin JA: The effect of inositol supplements on the psoriasis of patients taking lithium: a randomized, placebo-controlled trial. Br J Dermatol 150(5):966–969, 2004 15149510

Alpsoy E, Ozcan E, Cetin L, et al: Is the efficacy of topical corticosteroid therapy for psoriasis vulgaris enhanced by concurrent moclobemide therapy? A double-blind, placebo-controlled study. J Am Acad Dermatol 38(2 Pt 1):197–200, 1998 9486674

Altomare G, Capella GL: Depression circumstantially related to the administration of finasteride for androgenetic alopecia. J Dermatol 29(10):665–669, 2002 12433001

American Academy of Dermatology: Position statement on isotretinoin, 2010. Available at: https://www.aad.org/Forms/Policies/Uploads/PS/PS-Isotretinoin.pdf. Accessed July 15, 2015.

American Psychiatric Association: Diagnostic and Statistical Manual of Mental Disorders, 5th Edition. Arlington, VA, American Psychiatric Association, 2013

Amstutz U, Shear NH, Rieder MJ, et al; CPNDS clinical recommendation group: Recommendations for HLA-B*15:02 and HLA-A*31:01 genetic testing to reduce the risk of carbamazepine-induced hypersensitivity reactions. Epilepsia 55(4):496–506, 2014 24597466

Arck PC, Slominski A, Theoharides TC, et al: Neuroimmunology of stress: skin takes center stage. J Invest Dermatol 126(8):1697–1704, 2006 16845409

Arican O, Sasmaz S, Ozbulut O: Increased suicidal tendency in a case of psoriasis vulgaris under acitretin treatment. J Eur Acad Dermatol Venereol 20(4):464–465, 2006 16643152

Armstrong AW, Harskamp CT, Armstrong EJ: Psoriasis and metabolic syndrome: a systematic review and meta-analysis of observational studies. J Am Acad Dermatol 68(4):654–662, 2013a 23360868

Armstrong EJ, Harskamp CT, Armstrong AW: Psoriasis and major adverse cardiovascular events: a systematic review and meta-analysis of observational studies. J Am Heart Assoc 2(2):e000062, 2013b 23557749

Atigari OV, Healy D: Schizophrenia-like disorder associated with etanercept treatment. BMJ Case Rep 2014:bcr2013200464, 2014 24419811

Austin M, Tan YC: Mania associated with infliximab. Aust N Z J Psychiatry 46(7):684–685, 2012 22735640

Azoulay L, Blais L, Koren G, et al: Isotretinoin and the risk of depression in patients with acne vulgaris: a case-crossover study. J Clin Psychiatry 69(4):526–532, 2008 18363422

Barak Y, Wohl Y, Greenberg Y, et al: Affective psychosis following Accutane (isotretinoin) treatment. Int Clin Psychopharmacol 20(1):39–41, 2005 15602115

Bassukas ID, Hyphantis T, Gamvroulia C, et al: Infliximab for patients with plaque psoriasis and severe psychiatric comorbidity. J Eur Acad Dermatol Venereol 22(2):257–258, 2008 18211435

Beach SR, Celano CM, Noseworthy PA, et al: QTc prolongation, torsades de pointes, and psychotropic medications. Psychosomatics 54(1):1–13, 2013 23295003

Belli H, Ural C, Vardar MK, et al: Dissociative symptoms and dissociative disorder comorbidity in patients with obsessive-compulsive disorder. Compr Psychiatry 53(7):975–980, 2012 22425531

Bigatà X, Sais G, Soler F: Severe chronic urticaria: response to mirtazapine. J Am Acad Dermatol 53(5):916–917, 2005 16243165

Bliss SA, Warnock JK: Psychiatric medications: adverse cutaneous drug reactions. Clin Dermatol 31(1):101–109, 2013 23245981

Borovaya A, Olisova O, Ruzicka T, Sárdy M: Does isotretinoin therapy of acne cure or cause depression? Int J Dermatol 52(9):1040–1052, 2013 23962262

Boyd ST, Mihm L, Causey NW: Improvement in psoriasis following treatment with gabapentin and pregabalin. Am J Clin Dermatol 9(6):419, 2008 18973412

Brauchli YB, Jick SS, Curtin F, Meier CR: Association between beta-blockers, other antihypertensive drugs and psoriasis: population-based case-control study. Br J Dermatol 158(6):1299–1307, 2008 18410416

Brauchli YB, Jick SS, Curtin F, Meier CR: Lithium, antipsychotics, and risk of psoriasis. J Clin Psychopharmacol 29(2):134–140, 2009 19512974

Camfferman D, Kennedy JD, Gold M, et al: Eczema and sleep and its relationship to daytime functioning in children. Sleep Med Rev 14(6):359–369, 2010 20392655

Carmichael AJ, Paul CJ: Idiosyncratic dapsone induced manic depression. BMJ 298(6686):1524, 1989 2503107

Catalano G, Catalano MC, Alberts VA: Famotidine-associated delirium: a series of six cases. Psychosomatics 37(4):349–355, 1996 8701013

Charleston L IV: Burning mouth syndrome: a review of recent literature. Curr Pain Headache Rep 17(6):336, 2013 23645183

Chaudhry IB, Hallak J, Husain N, et al: Minocycline benefits negative symptoms in early schizophrenia: a randomised double-blind placebo-controlled clinical trial in patients on standard treatment. J Psychopharmacol 26(9):1185–1193, 2012 22526685

Check JH, Chan S: Complete eradication of chronic long standing eczema and keratosis pilaris following treatment with dextroamphetamine sulfate. Clin Exp Obstet Gynecol 41(2):202–204, 2014 24779252

Cheng CY, Su SC, Chen CH, et al: HLA associations and clinical implications in T-cell mediated drug hypersensitivity reactions: an updated review. J Immunol Res 2014:565320, 2014 24901010

Choi EH, Brown BE, Crumrine D, et al: Mechanisms by which psychologic stress alters cutaneous permeability barrier homeostasis and stratum corneum integrity. J Invest Dermatol 124(3):587–595, 2005 15737200

Chu SY, Chen YJ, Tseng WC, et al: Psychiatric comorbidities in patients with alopecia areata in Taiwan: a case-control study. Br J Dermatol 166(3):525–531, 2012 22049923

Cipriani R, Perini GI, Rampinelli S: Paroxetine in alopecia areata. Int J Dermatol 40(9):600–601, 2001 11737460

Clegg A, Young JB: Which medications to avoid in people at risk of delirium: a systematic review. Age Ageing 40(1):23–29, 2011 21068014

Cox NH, Gordon PM, Dodd H: Generalized pustular and erythrodermic psoriasis associated with bupropion treatment. Br J Dermatol 146(6):1061–1063, 2002 12072078

Craven JL: Cyclosporine-associated organic mental disorders in liver transplant recipients. Psychosomatics 32(1):94–102, 1991 2003144

Dalgard FJ, Gieler U, Tomas-Aragones L, et al: The psychological burden of skin diseases: a cross-sectional multicenter study among dermatological out-patients in 13 European countries. J Invest Dermatol 135(4):984–991, 2015 25521458

Demitsu T, Yoneda K, Kakurai M, et al: Clinical efficacy of reserpine as "add-on therapy" to antihistamines in patients with recalcitrant chronic idiopathic urticaria and urticarial vasculitis. J Dermatol 37(9):827–829, 2010 20883370

Dodd S, Maes M, Anderson G, et al: Putative neuroprotective agents in neuropsychiatric disorders. Prog Neuropsychopharmacol Biol Psychiatry 42:135–145, 2013 23178231

Dodiuk-Gad RP, Laws PM, Shear NH: Epidemiology of severe drug hypersensitivity. Semin Cutan Med Surg 33(1):2–9, 2014 25037253

Dowlatshahi EA, Wakkee M, Herings RM, et al: Increased antidepressant drug exposure in psoriasis patients: a longitudinal population-based cohort study. Acta Derm Venereol 93(5):544–550, 2013 23529077

Dowlatshahi EA, Wakkee M, Arends LR, Nijsten T: The prevalence and odds of depressive symptoms and clinical depression in psoriasis patients: a systematic review and meta-analysis. J Invest Dermatol 134(6):1542–1551, 2014 24284419

Drake LA, Millikan LE; Doxepin Study Group: The antipruritic effect of 5% doxepin cream in patients with eczematous dermatitis. Arch Dermatol 131(12):1403–1408, 1995 7492129

Ebata T, Izumi H, Aizawa H, et al: Effects of nitrazepam on nocturnal scratching in adults with atopic dermatitis: a double-blind placebo-controlled crossover study. Br J Dermatol 138(4):631–634, 1998 9640368

Elisa B, Beny L: Induction of manic switch by the tumour necrosis factor–alpha antagonist infliximab. Psychiatry Clin Neurosci 64(4):442–443, 2010 20653912

Ellard R, Ahmed A, Shah R, Bewley A: Suicide and depression in a patient with psoriasis receiving adalimumab: the role of the dermatologist. Clin Exp Dermatol 39(5):624–627, 2014 24934916

Eshuis EJ, Magnin KM, Stokkers PC, et al: Suicide attempt in ulcerative colitis patient after 4 months of infliximab therapy—a case report. J Crohns Colitis 4(5):591–593, 2010 21122565

Fleuret C, Le Toux G, Morvan J, et al: Use of selective serotonin reuptake inhibitors in the treatment of burning mouth syndrome. Dermatology 228(2):172–176, 2014 24557331

Freudenmann RW, Lepping P: Second-generation antipsychotics in primary and secondary delusional parasitosis: outcome and efficacy. J Clin Psychopharmacol 28(5):500–508, 2008 18794644

Gerdes S, Zahl VA, Knopf H, et al: Comedication related to comorbidities: a study in 1203 hospitalized patients with severe psoriasis. Br J Dermatol 159(5):1116–1123, 2008 18717681

Ghanizadeh A, Ayoobzadehshirazi A: A review of psychiatric disorders comorbidities in patients with alopecia areata. Int J Trichology 6(1):2–4, 2014 25114444

Goldsmith LA, Bolognia JL, Callen JP, et al; American Academy of Dermatology: American Academy of Dermatology Consensus Conference on the safe and optimal use of isotretinoin: summary and recommendations. J Am Acad Dermatol 50(6):900–906, 2004 Correction in J Am Acad Dermatol 51(3):348, 2004 15153892

Goldsobel AB, Rohr AS, Siegel SC, et al: Efficacy of doxepin in the treatment of chronic idiopathic urticaria. J Allergy Clin Immunol 78(5 Pt 1):867–873, 1986 3782654

González E, Sanguino RM, Franco MA: Bupropion in atopic dermatitis. Pharmacopsychiatry 39(6):229, 2006 17124645

Gottlieb AB, Chao C, Dann F: Psoriasis comorbidities. J Dermatolog Treat 19(1):5–21, 2008 18273720

Grant JE, Odlaug BL, Kim SW: Lamotrigine treatment of pathologic skin picking: an open-label study. J Clin Psychiatry 68(9):1384–1391, 2007 17915977

Grant JE, Odlaug BL, Kim SW: N-acetylcysteine, a glutamate modulator, in the treatment of trichotillomania: a double-blind, placebo-controlled study. Arch Gen Psychiatry 66(7):756–763, 2009 19581567

Grant JE, Odlaug BL, Chamberlain SR, Kim SW: A double-blind, placebo-controlled trial of lamotrigine for pathological skin picking: treatment efficacy and neurocognitive predictors of response. J Clin Psychopharmacol 30(4):396–403, 2010 20531220

Grant JE, Odlaug BL, Chamberlain SR, et al: Skin picking disorder. Am J Psychiatry 169(11):1143–1149, 2012 23128921

Greene SL, Reed CE, Schroeter AL: Double-blind crossover study comparing doxepin with diphenhydramine for the treatment of chronic urticaria. J Am Acad Dermatol 12(4):669–675, 1985 3886724

Grover S, Kukreti R: HLA alleles and hypersensitivity to carbamazepine: an updated systematic review with meta-analysis. Pharmacogenet Genomics 24(2):94–112, 2014 24336023

Gupta MA: Stress and urticarial, in Neuroimmunology of the Skin: Basic Science to Clinical Practice. Edited by Granstein RD, Luger TA. Berlin, Springer-Verlag, 2009, pp 209–217

Gupta MA: Suicide risk and skin diseases, in Medical Conditions Associated With Suicide Risk. Edited by Berman J, Pompili M. Washington, DC, American Association of Suicidology, 2011, pp 667–690

Gupta MA: Emotional regulation, dissociation, and the self-induced dermatoses: clinical features and implications for treatment with mood stabilizers. Clin Dermatol 31(1):110–117, 2013a 23245982

Gupta MA: Review of somatic symptoms in post-traumatic stress disorder. Int Rev Psychiatry 25(1):86–99, 2013b 23383670

Gupta MA, Gupta AK: Chronic idiopathic urticaria associated with panic disorder: a syndrome responsive to selective serotonin reuptake inhibitor antidepressants? Cutis 56(1):53–54, 1995 7555104

Gupta MA, Gupta AK: Psychodermatology: an update. J Am Acad Dermatol 34(6):1030–1046, 1996 8647969

Gupta MA, Gupta AK: Depression and suicidal ideation in dermatology patients with acne, alopecia areata, atopic dermatitis and psoriasis. Br J Dermatol 139(5):846–850, 1998 9892952

Gupta MA, Gupta AK: Olanzapine is effective in the management of some self-induced dermatoses: three case reports. Cutis 66(2):143–146, 2000 10955197

Gupta MA, Gupta AK: Chronic idiopathic urticaria and post-traumatic stress disorder (PTSD): an under-recognized comorbidity. Clin Dermatol 30(3):351–354, 2012 22507051

Gupta MA, Gupta AK: Cutaneous sensory disorder. Semin Cutan Med Surg 32(2):110–118, 2013a 24049969

Gupta MA, Gupta AK: Sleep-wake disorders and dermatology. Clin Dermatol 31(1):118–126, 2013b 23245983

Gupta MA, Gupta AK: Current concepts in psychodermatology. Curr Psychiatry Rep 16(6):449, 2014a 24740235

Gupta MA, Gupta AK: Night sweating, daytime hyperhidrosis, autonomic nervous system (ANS) hyperarousal and suicidality in posttraumatic stress disorder (PTSD): clinical features and treatment implications (meeting abstract 1388). Biol Psychiatry 75(9, supplement S), 2014b

Gupta MA, Gupta AK, Haberman HF: The self-inflicted dermatoses: a critical review. Gen Hosp Psychiatry 9(1):45–52, 1987 3817460

Gupta MA, Gupta AK, Kirkby S, et al: A psychocutaneous profile of psoriasis patients who are stress reactors. A study of 127 patients. Gen Hosp Psychiatry 11(3):166–173, 1989 2721939

Gupta MA, Gupta AK, Vujcic B: Body-focused repetitive behaviors (hair-pulling, skin-picking, onychophagia) and dissociation: an under-recognized association (meeting abstract 131). Biol Psychiatry 99(9, supplement S):48S, 2015

Haefner HK, Collins ME, Davis GD, et al: The vulvodynia guideline. J Low Genit Tract Dis 9(1):40–51, 2005 15870521

Hall SD, Wang Z, Huang SM, et al: The interaction between St John's wort and an oral contraceptive. Clin Pharmacol Ther 74(6):525–535, 2003 14663455

Halvorsen JA, Stern RS, Dalgard F, et al: Suicidal ideation, mental health problems, and social impairment are increased in adolescents with acne: a population-based study. J Invest Dermatol 131(2):363–370, 2011 20844551

Heckmann SM, Kirchner E, Grushka M, et al: A double-blind study on clonazepam in patients with burning mouth syndrome. Laryngoscope 122(4):813–816, 2012 22344742

Heller MM, Wong JW, Lee ES, et al: Delusional infestations: clinical presentation, diagnosis and treatment. Int J Dermatol 52(7):775–783, 2013 23789596

Henderson CA, Highet AS: Depression induced by etretinate. BMJ 298(6678):964, 1989 2497882

Hogan SR, Mandrell J, Eilers D: Adrenergic urticaria: review of the literature and proposed mechanism. J Am Acad Dermatol 70(4):763–766, 2014 24373776

Hoss D, Segal S: Scalp dysesthesia. Arch Dermatol 134(3):327–330, 1998 9521031

Huber M, Lepping P, Pycha R, et al: Delusional infestation: treatment outcome with antipsychotics in 17 consecutive patients (using standardized reporting criteria). Gen Hosp Psychiatry 33(6):604–611, 2011 21762999

Hughes JE, Barraclough BM, Hamblin LG, White JE: Psychiatric symptoms in dermatology patients. Br J Psychiatry 143:51–54, 1983 6882992

Hundley JL, Yosipovitch G: Mirtazapine for reducing nocturnal itch in patients with chronic pruritus: a pilot study. J Am Acad Dermatol 50(6):889–891, 2004 15153889

Hung SI, Chung WH, Liu ZS, et al: Common risk allele in aromatic antiepileptic drug induced Stevens-Johnson syndrome and toxic epidermal necrolysis in Han Chinese. Pharmacogenomics 11(3):349–356, 2010 20235791

Hunkin V, Chung MC: Chronic idiopathic urticaria, psychological co-morbidity and posttraumatic stress: the impact of alexithymia and repression. Psychiatr Q 83(4):431–447, 2012 22362490

Husain Z, Reddy BY, Schwartz RA: DRESS syndrome, part I: clinical perspectives. J Am Acad Dermatol 68(5):693.e1–693.e14; quiz 706–698, 2013 23602182

Irwig MS: Depressive symptoms and suicidal thoughts among former users of finasteride with persistent sexual side effects. J Clin Psychiatry 73(9):1220–1223, 2012a 22939118

Irwig MS: Persistent sexual side effects of finasteride: could they be permanent? J Sex Med 9(11):2927–2932, 2012b 22789024

Jefferys D, Burrows G: Reversal of trichotillomania with aripiprazole. Depress Anxiety 25(6):E37–E40, 2008 17941109

Jick SS, Kremers HM, Vasilakis-Scaramozza C: Isotretinoin use and risk of depression, psychotic symptoms, suicide, and attempted suicide. Arch Dermatol 136(10):1231–1236, 2000 11030769

Jones J, Dougherty J, Cannon L: Diphenhydramine-induced toxic psychosis. Am J Emerg Med 4(4):369–371, 1986 3718632

Keller WR, Kum LM, Wehring HJ, et al: A review of anti-inflammatory agents for symptoms of schizophrenia. J Psychopharmacol 27(4):337–342, 2013 23151612

Kelsay K: Management of sleep disturbance associated with atopic dermatitis. J Allergy Clin Immunol 118(1):198–201, 2006 16815155

Kimyai-Asadi A, Harris JC, Nousari HC: Critical overview: adverse cutaneous reactions to psychotropic medications. J Clin Psychiatry 60(10):714–725, quiz 726, 1999 10549695

Kontaxakis VP, Ferentinos PP, Havaki-Kontaxaki BJ, Papadimitriou GN: Genetic vulnerability and isotretinoin-induced psychiatric adverse events. World J Biol Psychiatry 11(2):158–159, 2010 20109108

Langley RG, Feldman SR, Han C, et al: Ustekinumab significantly improves symptoms of anxiety, depression, and skin-related quality of life in patients with moderate-to-severe psoriasis: results from a randomized, double-blind, placebo-controlled phase III trial. J Am Acad Dermatol 63(3):457–465, 2010 20462664

Latini A, Carducci M: Psoriasis during therapy with olanzapine. Eur J Dermatol 13(4):404–405, 2003 12948926

Lepping P, Freudenmann RW: Delusional parasitosis: a new pathway for diagnosis and treatment. Clin Exp Dermatol 33(2):113–117, 2008 18205853

Levenson JL: Psychiatric issues in dermatology, part 1: atopic dermatitis and psoriasis. Prim psychiatry 15:31–34, 2008a

Levenson JL: Psychiatric issues in dermatology, part 2: alopecia areata, urticaria, and angioedema. Prim psychiatry 15:31–34, 2008b

Litt JZ: Litt's Drug Eruptions & Reactions Manual: D.E.R.M. Boca Raton, FL, CRC Press, 2013

Lochner C, Seedat S, Niehaus DJ, Stein DJ: Topiramate in the treatment of trichotillomania: an open-label pilot study. Int Clin Psychopharmacol 21(5):255–259, 2006 16877895

Luis Blay S: Depression and psoriasis comorbidity. Treatment with paroxetine: two case reports. Ann Clin Psychiatry 18(4):271–272, 2006 17162628

Mahtani R, Parekh N, Mangat I, Bhalerao S: Alleviating the itch-scratch cycle in atopic dermatitis. Psychosomatics 46(4):373–374, 2005 16000683

Marqueling AL, Zane LT: Depression and suicidal behavior in acne patients treated with isotretinoin: a systematic review. Semin Cutan Med Surg 26(4):210–220, 2007 18395669

Marron SE, Tomas-Aragones L, Boira S: Anxiety, depression, quality of life and patient satisfaction in acne patients treated with oral isotretinoin. Acta Derm Venereol 93(6):701–706, 2013 23727704

McGrath EJ, Lovell CR, Gillison F, et al: A prospective trial of the effects of isotretinoin on quality of life and depressive symptoms. Br J Dermatol 163(6):1323–1329, 2010 21137117

Medansky RS, Handler RM: Dermatopsychosomatics: classification, physiology, and therapeutic approaches. J Am Acad Dermatol 5(2):125–136, 1981 7021610

Miyaoka T, Wake R, Furuya M, et al: Minocycline as adjunctive therapy for patients with unipolar psychotic depression: an open-label study. Prog Neuropsychopharmacol Biol Psychiatry 37(2):222–226, 2012 22349578

Modell JG, Boyce S, Taylor E, Katholi C: Treatment of atopic dermatitis and psoriasis vulgaris with bupropion-SR: a pilot study. Psychosom Med 64(5):835–840, 2002 12271115

Nevoralová Z, Dvořáková D: Mood changes, depression and suicide risk during isotretinoin treatment: a prospective study. Int J Dermatol 52(2):163–168, 2013 23347302

Ninan PT: Conceptual issues in trichotillomania, a prototypical impulse control disorder. Curr Psychiatry Rep 2(1):72–75, 2000 11122936

O'Brien SM, Scott LV, Dinan TG: Cytokines: abnormalities in major depression and implications for pharmacological treatment. Hum Psychopharmacol 19(6):397–403, 2004 15303243

Odlaug BL, Grant JE: Pathological skin picking, in Trichotillomania, Skin Picking, and Other Body-Focused Repetitive Behaviors. Edited by Grant JE, Stein DJ, Woods DW, Keuthen NJ. Washington, DC, American Psychiatric Publishing, 2012, pp 21–41

Patel T, Ishiuji Y, Yosipovitch G: Nocturnal itch: why do we itch at night? Acta Derm Venereol 87(4):295–298, 2007 17598030

Perini G, Zara M, Cipriani R, et al: Imipramine in alopecia areata. A double-blind, placebo-controlled study. Psychother Psychosom 61(3-4):195–198, 1994 8066157

Physicians' Desk Reference: Physicians' Desk Reference, 63rd Edition. Montvale, NJ, Physicians' Desk Reference Inc, 2009

Picardi A, Mazzotti E, Pasquini P: Prevalence and correlates of suicidal ideation among patients with skin disease. J Am Acad Dermatol 54(3):420–426, 2006 16488292

Picardi A, Lega I, Tarolla E: Suicide risk in skin disorders. Clin Dermatol 31(1):47–56, 2013 23245973

Purvis D, Robinson E, Merry S, Watson P: Acne, anxiety, depression and suicide in teenagers: a cross-sectional survey of New Zealand secondary school students. J Paediatr Child Health 42(12):793–796, 2006 17096715

Rademaker M: Adverse effects of isotretinoin: A retrospective review of 1743 patients started on isotretinoin. Australas J Dermatol 51(4):248–253, 2010 21198520

Raison CL, Rutherford RE, Woolwine BJ, et al: A randomized controlled trial of the tumor necrosis factor antagonist infliximab for treatment-resistant depression: the role of baseline inflammatory biomarkers. JAMA Psychiatry 70(1):31–41, 2013 22945416

Rao KS, Menon PK, Hilman BC, et al: Duration of the suppressive effect of tricyclic antidepressants on histamine-induced wheal-and-flare reactions in human skin. J Allergy Clin Immunol 82(5 Pt 1):752–757, 1988 2903876

Rehn LM, Meririnne E, Höök-Nikanne J, et al: Depressive symptoms and suicidal ideation during isotretinoin treatment: a 12-week follow-up study of male Finnish military conscripts. J Eur Acad Dermatol Venereol 23(11):1294–1297, 2009 19522777

Rieder E, Tausk F: Psoriasis, a model of dermatologic psychosomatic disease: psychiatric implications and treatments. Int J Dermatol 51(1):12–26, 2012 22182372

Rothbart R, Amos T, Siegfried N, et al: Pharmacotherapy for trichotillomania. Cochrane Database of Systematic Reviews 2013, Issue 11. Art. No.: CD007662. DOI: 10.1002/14651858.CD007662.pub2 24214100

Rudzki E, Borkowski W, Czubalski K: The suggestive effect of placebo on the intensity of chronic urticaria. Acta Allergol 25(1):70–73, 1970 5468243

Ryback R: Topiramate in the treatment of psoriasis: a pilot study. Br J Dermatol 147(1):130–133, 2002 12100195

Saitta P, Keehan P, Yousif J, et al: An update on the presence of psychiatric comorbidities in acne patients, part 1: overview of prevalence. Cutis 88(1):33–40, 2011a 21877504

Saitta P, Keehan P, Yousif J, et al: An update on the presence of psychiatric comorbidities in acne patients, part 2: depression, anxiety, and suicide. Cutis 88(2):92–97, 2011b 21916276

Sampogna F, Tabolli S, Abeni D; IDI Multipurpose Psoriasis Research on Vital Experiences (IMPROVE) investigators: The impact of changes in clinical severity on psychiatric morbidity in patients with psoriasis: a follow-up study. Br J Dermatol 157(3):508–513, 2007 17627789

Sarifakioglu E, Onur O: Women with scalp dysesthesia treated with pregabalin. Int J Dermatol 52(11):1417–1418, 2013 23557491

Savin JA, Paterson WD, Adam K, Oswald I: Effects of trimeprazine and trimipramine on nocturnal scratching in patients with atopic eczema. Arch Dermatol 115(3):313–315, 1979 373632

Semiz UB, Inanc L, Bezgin CH: Are trauma and dissociation related to treatment resistance in patients with obsessive-compulsive disorder? Soc Psychiatry Psychiatr Epidemiol 49(8):1287–1296, 2014 24213522

Senra MS, Wollenberg A: Psychodermatological aspects of atopic dermatitis. Br J Dermatol 170 (suppl 1):38–43, 2014 24930567

Sidbury R, Tom WL, Bergman JN, et al: Guidelines of care for the management of atopic dermatitis, section 4: prevention of disease flares and use of adjunctive therapies and approaches. J Am Acad Dermatol 71(6):1218–1233, 2014 25264237

Soczynska JK, Mansur RB, Brietzke E, et al: Novel therapeutic targets in depression: minocycline as a candidate treatment. Behav Brain Res 235(2):302–317, 2012 22963995

Ständer S, Weisshaar E, Luger TA: Neurophysiological and neurochemical basis of modern pruritus treatment. Exp Dermatol 17(3):161–169, 2008 18070080

Staubach P, Eckhardt-Henn A, Dechene M, et al: Quality of life in patients with chronic urticaria is differentially impaired and determined by psychiatric comorbidity. Br J Dermatol 154(2):294–298, 2006 16433799

Stockdale CK, Lawson HW: 2013 Vulvodynia Guideline update. J Low Genit Tract Dis 18(2):93–100, 2014 24633161

Sundström A, Alfredsson L, Sjölin-Forsberg G, et al: Association of suicide attempts with acne and treatment with isotretinoin: retrospective Swedish cohort study. BMJ 341:c5812, 2010 21071484

Swedo SE, Leonard HL, Rapoport JL, et al: A double-blind comparison of clomipramine and desipramine in the treatment of trichotillomania (hair pulling). N Engl J Med 321(8):497–501, 1989 2761586

Thomas KH, Martin RM, Potokar J, et al: Reporting of drug induced depression and fatal and non-fatal suicidal behaviour in the UK from 1998 to 2011. BMC Pharmacol Toxicol 15:54, 2014 25266008

Thorslund K, Svensson T, Nordlind K, et al: Use of serotonin reuptake inhibitors in patients with psoriasis is associated with a decreased need for systemic psoriasis treatment: a population-based cohort study. J Intern Med 274(3):281–287, 2013 23711088

Tyring S, Gottlieb A, Papp K, et al: Etanercept and clinical outcomes, fatigue, and depression in psoriasis: double-blind placebo-controlled randomised phase III trial. Lancet 367(9504):29–35, 2006 16399150

Uguz F, Engin B, Yilmaz E: Axis I and Axis II diagnoses in patients with chronic idiopathic urticaria. J Psychosom Res 64(2):225–229, 2008 18222137

U.S. Food and Drug Administration: Information for Healthcare Professionals: Dangerous or Even Fatal Skin Reactions—Carbamazepine (Marketed as Carbatrol, Equetro, Tegretol and Generics), 2007. Washington, DC, U.S. Food and Drug Administration. Available at http://www.fda.gov/Drugs/DrugSafety/PostmarketDrugSafetyInformationforPatientsandProviders/ucm124718.htm. Accessed July 15, 2015.

U.S. Food and Drug Administration: Risk Evaluation and Mitigation Strategy (REMS). The iPLEDGE Program. Single shared system for isotretinoin, 2012. Washington, DC, U.S. Food and Drug Administration. Available at http://www.fda.gov/downloads/Drugs/DrugSafety/PostmarketDrugSafetyInformationforPatientsandProviders/UCM234639.pdf. Accessed July 30, 2015.

Van Ameringen M, Mancini C, Patterson B, et al: A randomized, double-blind, placebo-controlled trial of olanzapine in the treatment of trichotillomania. J Clin Psychiatry 71(10):1336–1343, 2010 20441724

von Einsiedel RW, Roesch-Ely D, Diebold K, et al: H(2)-histamine antagonist (famotidine) induced adverse CNS reactions with long-standing secondary mania and epileptic seizures. Pharmacopsychiatry 35(4):152–154, 2002 12163986

Warnock JK, Morris DW: Adverse cutaneous reactions to antidepressants. Am J Clin Dermatol 3(5):329–339, 2002a 12069639

Warnock JK, Morris DW: Adverse cutaneous reactions to antipsychotics. Am J Clin Dermatol 3(9):629–636, 2002b 12444805

Warnock JK, Morris DW: Adverse cutaneous reactions to mood stabilizers. Am J Clin Dermatol 4(1):21–30, 2003 12477370

White MP, Koran LM: Open-label trial of aripiprazole in the treatment of trichotillomania. J Clin Psychopharmacol 31(4):503–506, 2011 21694623

Woosley RL, Romero KA: QT Drugs List, 2015. Available at: www.crediblemeds.org. Accessed May 19, 2015.

Wysowski DK, Pitts M, Beitz J: An analysis of reports of depression and suicide in patients treated with isotretinoin. J Am Acad Dermatol 45(4):515–519, 2001 11568740

Yang HY, Sun CC, Wu YC, Wang JD: Stress, insomnia, and chronic idiopathic urticarial—a case-control study. J Formos Med Assoc 104(4):254–263, 2005 15909063

Yasui-Furukori N, Kaneko S: The efficacy of low-dose aripiprazole treatment for trichotillomania. Clin Neuropharmacol 34(6):258–259, 2011 22104636

Yosipovitch G, Xiong GL, Haus E, et al: Time-dependent variations of the skin barrier function in humans: transepidermal water loss, stratum corneum hydration, skin surface pH, and skin temperature. J Invest Dermatol 110(1):20–23, 1998 9424081

Yosipovitch G, Ansari N, Goon A, et al: Clinical characteristics of pruritus in chronic idiopathic urticaria. Br J Dermatol 147(1):32–36, 2002 12100181

Yosipovitch G, Sackett-Lundeen L, Goon A, et al: Circadian and ultradian (12 h) variations of skin blood flow and barrier function in non-irritated and irritated skin-effect of topical corticosteroids. J Invest Dermatol 122(3):824–829, 2004 15086571

Zonios D, Yamazaki H, Murayama N, et al: Voriconazole metabolism, toxicity, and the effect of cytochrome P450 2C19 genotype. J Infect Dis 209(12):1941–1948, 2014 24403552

14

Rheumatological Disorders

James L. Levenson, M.D.
Stephen J. Ferrando, M.D.

Neuropsychiatric disorders are common in patients with rheumatological disorders. On the basis of standardized research interviews, nearly one-fifth of patients with rheumatoid arthritis are estimated to have a psychiatric disorder, most often a depressive disorder (Levenson et al. 2011). Depressed patients with rheumatoid arthritis are more likely to report pain, are less likely to comply with medications, and have poorer quality of life than other patients with rheumatoid arthritis. However, rheumatologists underrecognize depression in their patients with rheumatoid arthritis (Rathbun et al. 2014). Research on depression in osteoarthritis has revealed similar findings, with high rates of depression associated with increased pain and poorer quality of life (Joshi et al. 2015). Studies of patients with systemic lupus erythematosus found that 30%–50% of the patients have depression, 13%–24% have anxiety, 3%–4% have mania or mixed episodes, and up to 5% have psychosis (Levenson et al. 2011). The differential diagnosis of psychiatric disorders in patients with rheumatological disorders includes primary psychiatric disorders, secondary syndromes (e.g., psychosis due to central nervous system [CNS] lupus), and side effects of rheumatological medications.

Treatment of Psychiatric Disorders

For the most part, treatment of depression, anxiety, mania, psychosis, delirium, and pain in patients with rheumatological disorders is similar to their treatment in patients with other medical diseases, following the principles covered in other chapters in this book. Few clinical trials have been done specifically in patients with rheumatological disorders. One study observed that sertraline had robust effects on depression outcomes in a group of depressed patients with rheumatoid arthritis, compared with a group of patients who were clinically followed but received no antidepressants (Parker et al. 2003). Similarly, sertraline 100 mg/day was effective with very few side effects (<4% of patients treated) in depressed patients with rheumatoid arthritis treated openly for up to 15 months (Slaughter et al. 2002). In an open-label trial, dothiepin, a sedating tertiary-amine tricyclic antidepressant (TCA) similar to doxepin, was found to be effective and well tolerated for depression and anxiety in patients with rheumatoid arthritis and major depression (Dhavale et al. 2005). With respect to the potential limitations of TCA treatment in depressed patients with rheumatoid arthritis, in a large randomized controlled trial (RCT) comparing paroxetine 20–40 mg/day with amitriptyline 75–150 mg/day, the two drugs were equally efficacious for depression and pain reports; however, paroxetine was better tolerated, with significantly fewer anticholinergic side effects (Bird and Broggini 2000). There is some suggestion from basic science that activation of serotonin receptors has potent anti-inflammatory effects (Yu et al. 2008), but the clinical implication of these findings for the treatment of depression in patients with rheumatoid arthritis is not known.

Despite the wide prevalence of depression in patients with osteoarthritis, fewer intervention studies have examined the efficacy of antidepressants in osteoarthritis. Duloxetine was effective in elderly patients with major depression and osteoarthritis (Wohlreich et al. 2009). Those studies that have been performed suggest that antidepressants are beneficial in the treatment of depression in patients with osteoarthritis and that improvement in depression is associated with reduced pain and disability (Lin et al. 2003). When pharmacotherapy of depression is part of a collaborative care approach, outcomes are improved over usual care (Lin et al. 2006).

Although current evidence indicates that all antidepressants have roughly equal efficacy in the treatment of depression, they differ in their analgesic efficacy, tolerability, and potential drug interactions. TCAs have long been recognized to have analgesic benefits, even at low dose (e.g., amitriptyline 25 mg) and independent of the presence of depression (see also Chapter 17, "Pain Management"). In higher doses, the tolerability and safety of TCAs are poor. Selective serotonin reuptake inhibitors (SSRIs) have comparable antidepressant efficacy but less analgesic efficacy. Serotonin-norepinephrine reuptake inhibitors (SNRIs) possess more analgesic potential than SSRIs. Most RCTs demonstrating analgesic efficacy of antidepressants in rheumatological disorders have been of TCAs (e.g., Ash et al. 1999; Grace et al. 1985). More recently, duloxetine (60–120 mg/day) has been shown to be efficacious in several randomized placebo-controlled trials (e.g., Chappell et al. 2009; Frakes et al. 2011; Micca et al. 2013). Drug interactions may occur, although this is generally not a problem with first- and second-line treatments for rheumatoid arthritis.

Psychopharmacological treatment of neuropsychiatric symptoms (particularly psychosis and mania) in patients with lupus cerebritis is a challenge, with no guidance from randomized trials (Tincani et al. 1996). Most recent reports have been in children and adolescents (e.g., Lim et al. 2013; Zuniga Zambrano et al. 2014). High-dose corticosteroids are considered first-line treatment to suppress CNS inflammation; however, they may exacerbate neuropsychiatric symptoms. Second-line agents include azathioprine and cyclophosphamide. Antipsychotics are frequently used for symptomatic treatment concurrent with corticosteroids. Clinically, agents with high potency at dopamine D_2 receptors appear generally the most effective, especially in severe cases. Patients with lupus cerebritis must be monitored closely for extrapyramidal symptoms and seizures. Anticonvulsant mood stabilizers are often used for prophylaxis or treatment of seizures, as well as for their mood-stabilizing properties. Benzodiazepines should be used with caution because of risk of confusion and behavioral disinhibition.

Psychiatric Side Effects of Rheumatological Medications

The differential diagnosis of psychiatric disorders in patients with rheumatological disorders includes side effects of rheumatological medications. Table 14–1 lists the reported psychiatric side effects of rheumatological medica-

Table 14–1. Psychiatric side effects of medications used in treating rheumatological disorders

Medication	Psychiatric side effects
Abatacept	None reported
Adalimumab	None reported
Azathioprine	Delirium
Belimumab	None reported
Corticosteroids	Mood lability, euphoria, irritability, anxiety, insomnia, mania, depression, psychosis, delirium, cognitive disturbance
Cyclophosphamide	Delirium (at high doses) (rare)
Cyclosporine	Anxiety, delirium, visual hallucinations
Etanercept	None reported
Gold	None reported
Hydroxychloroquine	Confusion, psychosis, mania, depression, nightmares, anxiety, aggression, delirium
Immunoglobulin (intravenous)	Delirium, agitation
Infliximab	None reported
Leflunomide	Anxiety
LJP394[a]	None reported
Methotrexate	Delirium (at high doses) (rare)
Mycophenolate mofetil	Anxiety, depression, sedation (all rare)
NSAIDs (high dose)	Depression, anxiety, paranoia, hallucinations, concentration, hostility, confusion, delirium
Penicillamine	None reported
Rituximab	None reported
Sulfasalazine	Insomnia, depression, hallucinations
Tacrolimus	Anxiety, delirium, insomnia, restlessness

Table 14–1.   Psychiatric side effects of medications used in treating rheumatological disorders *(continued)*

Medication	Psychiatric side effects
Tocilizumab	None reported
Tofacitinib	None reported

Note.   NSAIDs = nonsteroidal anti-inflammatory drugs.
[a]B-cell tolerogen–anti-anti-double-stranded DNA antibodies.

tions. Corticosteroid-induced psychiatric symptoms are reviewed in Chapter 10, "Endocrine and Metabolic Disorders."

Rheumatological Side Effects of Psychotropic Medications: Psychotropic Drug–Induced Lupus

Patients who are receiving antipsychotic drugs, particularly chlorpromazine, may have positive antinuclear and antiphospholipid antibodies, but most do not develop signs of an autoantibody-associated disease. Compared with other (nonpsychiatric) drugs known to cause a symptomatic lupus-like syndrome, chlorpromazine and carbamazepine carry low risk, and several other psychotropics (valproic acid, other anticonvulsants, phenelzine, and lithium) carry very low risk. There are isolated reports of lupus with sertraline and bupropion (Cassis and Callen 2005; Hussain and Zakaria 2008). Drug-induced lupus is actually more commonly caused by rheumatological drugs (most commonly with infliximab and adalimumab) than psychotropics. CNS involvement is usually absent in drug-induced lupus. Laboratory findings may include mild cytopenia, elevated erythrocyte sedimentation rate, and elevated antinuclear antibody titers. Antihistone antibodies are positive in up to 95% of patients but are not pathognomonic of drug-induced lupus. After discontinuation of the drug, symptoms and antibody titers decline usually over a period of weeks; however, the recovery can take more than a year (Vedove et al. 2009).

Drug-Drug Interactions

Relatively few important drug interactions occur between rheumatological and psychopharmacological agents. These are summarized in Table 14–2, with the exception of most chemotherapeutic agents (discussed in Chapter 8, "Oncology") and corticosteroids (discussed in Chapter 10, "Endocrine and Metabolic Disorders"). The most important possible interactions involve potential for increased gastrointestinal bleeding when nonsteroidal anti-inflammatory drugs are combined with serotonergic agents, particularly SSRIs, SNRIs, and tertiary-amine TCAs. The potential for synergistic myelosuppressive effects exists with the combination of immunosuppressive agents (sulfasalazine, azathioprine, chemotherapeutic agents) and psychotropics with this effect (e.g., clozapine, carbamazepine, valproate, mirtazapine). Gold, penicillamine, and leflunomide are relatively free of interactions.

Key Clinical Points

- Depression is highly prevalent among patients with rheumatological disorders.
- Randomized controlled trials have shown antidepressants to be effective for the treatment of depression in patients with rheumatoid arthritis.
- TCAs and SNRIs possess more analgesic potential than do SSRIs.
- Psychiatric drugs are uncommon causes of drug-induced lupus, with chlorpromazine and carbamazepine most common among those that do.
- Among the drugs used to treat rheumatological disorders, corticosteroids are the most likely to cause psychiatric side effects.

Table 14–2. Rheumatological drug–psychotropic drug interactions[a]

Medication	Interaction mechanism	Effects on psychotropic drugs and management
Azathioprine	Synergistic myelosuppression	Potential increased risk for blood dyscrasias with some psychotropics (e.g., clozapine, carbamazepine, valproate, mirtazapine)
NSAIDs	Additive anticoagulant effect	Increased risk of bleeding with SSRIs, SNRIs, and tertiary-amine TCAs
Sulfasalazine	Additive nausea	Increased nausea with some psychotropics (e.g., SSRIs, SNRIs, cholinesterase inhibitors, anticonvulsants, lithium)
	Synergistic myelosuppression	Potential increased risk for blood dyscrasias with some psychotropics (e.g., clozapine, carbamazepine, valproate, mirtazapine)
Tacrolimus	QT prolongation	Increased risk of cardiac arrhythmias with other QT-prolonging agents, including TCAs, typical antipsychotics, pimozide, risperidone, paliperidone, iloperidone, quetiapine, ziprasidone, and lithium

Note. NSAIDs=nonsteroidal anti-inflammatory drugs; SNRIs=serotonin-norepinephrine reuptake inhibitors; SSRIs=selective serotonin reuptake inhibitors; TCAs=tricyclic antidepressants.
[a]Drug interactions between chemotherapeutic agents used in rheumatology (e.g., cyclophosphamide, methotrexate, cyclosporine, tacrolimus) and psychotropic drugs are covered in Chapter 8, "Oncology."

References

Ash G, Dickens CM, Creed FH, et al: The effects of dothiepin on subjects with rheumatoid arthritis and depression. Rheumatology (Oxford) 38(10):959–967, 1999 10534546

Bird H, Broggini M: Paroxetine versus amitriptyline for treatment of depression associated with rheumatoid arthritis: a randomized, double blind, parallel group study. J Rheumatol 27(12):2791–2797, 2000 11128665

Cassis TB, Callen JP: Bupropion-induced subacute cutaneous lupus erythematosus. Australas J Dermatol 46(4):266–269, 2005 16197429

Chappell AS, Ossanna MJ, Liu-Seifert H, et al: Duloxetine, a centrally acting analgesic, in the treatment of patients with osteoarthritis knee pain: a 13-week, randomized, placebo-controlled trial. Pain 146(3):253–260, 2009 19625125

Dhavale HS, Gawande S, Bhagat V, et al: Evaluation of efficacy and tolerability of dothiepin hydrochloride in the management of major depression in patients suffering from rheumatoid arthritis. J Indian Med Assoc 103(5):291–294, 2005 16229336

Frakes EP, Risser RC, Ball TD, et al: Duloxetine added to oral nonsteroidal anti-inflammatory drugs for treatment of knee pain due to osteoarthritis: results of a randomized, double-blind, placebo-controlled trial. Curr Med Res Opin 27(12):2361–2372 (Erratum in Curr Med Res Opin 28[5]:822, 2012), 2011 22017192

Grace EM, Bellamy N, Kassam Y, Buchanan WW: Controlled, double-blind, randomized trial of amitriptyline in relieving articular pain and tenderness in patients with rheumatoid arthritis. Curr Med Res Opin 9(6):426–429, 1985 3886308

Hussain HM, Zakaria M: Drug-induced lupus secondary to sertraline. Aust N Z J Psychiatry 42(12):1074–1075, 2008 19031644

Joshi N, Khanna R, Shah RM: Relationship between depression and physical activity, disability, burden, and health-related quality of life among patients with arthritis. Popul Health Manag 18(2):104–114, 2015 25247246

Levenson JL, Dickens C, Irwin MR: Rheumatology, in The American Psychiatric Publishing Textbook of Psychosomatic Medicine: Psychiatric Care of the Medically Ill, 2nd Edition. Edited by Levenson JL. Arlington, VA, American Psychiatric Publishing, 2011, pp 571–591

Lim LS, Lefebvre A, Benseler S, Silverman ED: Longterm outcomes and damage accrual in patients with childhood systemic lupus erythematosus with psychosis and severe cognitive dysfunction. J Rheumatol 40(4):513–519, 2013 23457384

Lin EH, Katon W, Von Korff M, et al; IMPACT Investigators: Effect of improving depression care on pain and functional outcomes among older adults with arthritis: a randomized controlled trial. JAMA 290(18):2428–2429, 2003 14612479

Lin EH, Tang L, Katon W, et al: Arthritis pain and disability: response to collaborative depression care. Gen Hosp Psychiatry 28(6):482–486, 2006 17088163

Micca JL, Ruff D, Ahl J, Wohlreich MM: Safety and efficacy of duloxetine treatment in older and younger patients with osteoarthritis knee pain: a post hoc, subgroup analysis of two randomized, placebo-controlled trials. BMC Musculoskelet Disord 14:137, 2013 23590727

Parker JC, Smarr KL, Slaughter JR, et al: Management of depression in rheumatoid arthritis: a combined pharmacologic and cognitive-behavioral approach. Arthritis Rheum 49(6):766–777, 2003 14673962

Rathbun AM, Harrold LR, Reed GW: A description of patient- and rheumatologist-reported depression symptoms in an American rheumatoid arthritis registry population. Clin Exp Rheumatol 32(4):523–532, 2014 24984165

Slaughter JR, Parker JC, Martens MP, et al: Clinical outcomes following a trial of sertraline in rheumatoid arthritis. Psychosomatics 43(1):36–41, 2002 11927756

Tincani A, Brey R, Balestrieri G, et al: International survey on the management of patients with SLE, II: the results of a questionnaire regarding neuropsychiatric manifestations. Clin Exp Rheumatol 14 (suppl 16):S23–S29, 1996 9049450

Vedove CD, Del Giglio M, Schena D, Girolomoni G: Drug-induced lupus erythematosus. Arch Dermatol Res 301(1):99–105, 2009 18797892

Wohlreich MM, Sullivan MD, Mallinckrodt CH, et al: Duloxetine for the treatment of recurrent major depressive disorder in elderly patients: treatment outcomes in patients with comorbid arthritis. Psychosomatics 50(4):402–412, 2009 19687181

Yu B, Becnel J, Zerfaoui M, et al: Serotonin 5-hydroxytryptamine(2A) receptor activation suppresses tumor necrosis factor-alpha-induced inflammation with extraordinary potency. J Pharmacol Exp Ther 327(2):316–323, 2008 18708586

Zuniga Zambrano YC, Guevara Ramos JD, Penagos Vargas NE, et al: Risk factors for neuropsychiatric manifestations in children with systemic lupus erythematosus: case-control study. Pediatr Neurol 51(3):403–409, 2014 25160546

15

Surgery and Critical Care

James L. Levenson, M.D.

Stephen J. Ferrando, M.D.

James A. Owen, Ph.D.

The psychopharmacological treatment of patients in the critical care setting and perioperative period can be particularly challenging because of severe and multiorgan system disease, rapid shifts in clinical status, and the introduction of multiple medications such as anesthetics, analgesics, and antibiotics that may interact with psychotropic drugs. In this chapter, we address the prevention and treatment of delirium; management of psychotropic drugs in the perioperative period; psychopharmacological treatment of presurgical anxiety and acute and posttraumatic stress syndromes that are often seen in the wake of traumatic incidents, such as orthopedic trauma and burns; and drug-drug interactions that may be encountered in the critical care setting. The reader is referred to relevant chapters in this volume that address psychopharmacological treatment within specific organ system disease states.

Delirium

Delirium, characterized by disturbance in consciousness, attention and arousal, and cognition, is highly frequent in hospitalized patients who are medically ill. It causes lasting distress to patients and families and is an independent predictor of morbidity and mortality, particularly when persisting at hospital discharge (Inouye and Young 2006; McAvay et al. 2006). On admission to the general hospital, 14%–24% of patients have delirium, and during hospital admission, 6%–56% develop delirium, including as many as 87% of patients in intensive care units (ICUs; Inouye and Young 2006). Clinically, delirium has three subtypes: hypoactive, hyperactive, and mixed. The hypoactive form is often mistaken for depression, whereas the hyperactive form is associated with agitation, hallucinations, and delusions. Although management of behavioral disturbances of delirium accounts for approximately one-third of psychiatric consultation requests (Schellhorn et al. 2009), it remains underdiagnosed and undertreated.

The most common predisposing causes of delirium include age, central nervous system (CNS) and systemic disease, anticholinergic medications, and intoxication and withdrawal states from alcohol and pharmacological and toxic substances. The optimal management of delirium entails early assessment of patients at risk, identification and treatment of underlying causes (e.g., infection, dehydration, metabolic derangements), environmental interventions (i.e., optimizing level of stimulation, familiarizing with surroundings, frequent orientation), and psychopharmacology. It is important to review medications that may cause or exacerbate delirium, including benzodiazepines and other sedative-hypnotics, anticholinergics, antihistaminics, opioid analgesics, and corticosteroids.

Pharmacological approaches are but one component of delirium prevention. Numerous studies employing multimodal (i.e., combining delirium screening with nonpharmacological and pharmacological intervention) approaches to delirium prevention have documented reduced incidence and duration of delirium, as well as reductions in other important outcomes related to morbidity and care costs (Collinsworth et al. 2016), stressing the need for nonpharmacological interventions.

Psychopharmacological interventions for the treatment of delirium are aimed at correcting disturbances in one or more neurotransmitter systems (i.e., cholinergic, dopaminergic, noradrenergic, and serotonergic). Correction of sleep-wake cycle disturbance that is characteristic of delirium is targeted via anti-α_1-adrenergic, antihistaminic, and γ-aminobutyric acid (GABA) agonist properties. Psychopharmacology clinical trials in the published literature are aimed at the *prevention* of delirium in patients (mostly elderly) undergoing orthopedic, gastrointestinal, and cardiovascular surgeries and *treatment of delirium once diagnosed*. Medications studied in randomized controlled trials (RCTs) include haloperidol, olanzapine, risperidone, chlorpromazine, lorazepam, midazolam, propofol, donepezil, and dexmedetomidine. Quetiapine and aripiprazole have been studied only in open-label trials. The treatment of anticholinergic delirium requires specific psychopharmacological intervention and is covered separately later in this section. Delirium from alcohol withdrawal is covered in Chapter 18, "Substance Use Disorders."

Delirium Prevention Trials

A trial comparing haloperidol 5 mg/day given intravenously at 9 P.M. from the first to the fifth postoperative day after gastrointestinal surgery versus a similar volume of saline solution found a reduced incidence of delirium with haloperidol (10.5%) compared with saline (32.5%, P < 0.05) (Kaneko et al. 1999). The severity and duration of delirium, once developed, were also lower and shorter in the haloperidol group. No major adverse events were noted.

In an RCT comparing haloperidol with placebo in preventing delirium in elderly patients with hip fractures, haloperidol 0.5 mg or placebo was administered orally three times daily for 1–3 days before hip replacement surgery and was continued for 3 days postoperatively (Kalisvaart et al. 2005). The incidence of delirium did not differ between the haloperidol and placebo groups (15.1% vs. 16.5%, respectively). However, significant differences were seen between patients given haloperidol and those given placebo; those taking haloperidol had reduced severity of delirium (mean 4 points lower on the Delirium Rating Scale [DRS-98], $P < 0.001$), reduced duration of delirium (mean 6.4 days lower, P < 0.001), and reduced length of hospital stay (mean 5.5 days lower, $P < 0.001$). Importantly, no drug-related side effects, including extrapyramidal symptoms (EPS), were encountered. The low overall incidence of delirium was likely attributable, at least in part, to proactive assessment and follow-up, as observed by Marcantonio et al. (2001), with the effect of haloperidol being to reduce severity and shorten the duration of delirium once developed.

More recently, 457 patients 65 years or older who were admitted to the intensive care unit after noncardiac surgery were randomly assigned to receive haloperidol (0.5 mg intravenous bolus injection followed by continuous infusion at a rate of 0.1 mg/hour for 12 hours) versus placebo (Wang et al. 2012). The primary endpoint was delirium in the first 7 days, which was lower in the haloperidol patients (15.3% vs. 23.2%). Secondary outcomes were better in the haloperidol group as well, including longer mean time to onset of delirium, more delirium-free days, and shorter length of intensive care unit stay. There was no significant difference in all-cause 28-day mortality, and no drug-related side effects were documented.

One open-label RCT of haloperidol did not find any reduction in postoperative delirium (Fukata et al. 2014). Multisite prospective RCTs of haloperidol's ability to prevent delirium are currently under way (Schrijver et al. 2014; van den Boogaard et al. 2013).

Three small RCTs comparing donepezil with placebo did not yield significant differences between groups in the incidence of delirium (Liptzin et al. 2005; Marcantonio et al. 2011; Sampson et al. 2007).

Olanzapine 5 mg given orally preoperatively and immediately postoperatively was compared with placebo in a large RCT aimed at reducing the incidence of delirium in high-risk patients having joint replacement surgery (Larsen et al. 2010). The incidence of delirium was 15% in the olanzapine group compared with 41% in the placebo group ($P<0.001$). In addition, the olanzapine-treated group had lower Delirium Rating Scale—Revised–98 (DRS-R-98) scores during the first 5 postoperative days, required lower dosages of narcotics, and were more likely to be discharged to home (vs. a rehabilitation facility) compared with the placebo group.

Dexmedetomidine, an intravenously administered α_2-receptor agonist that decreases norepinephrine release centrally, was compared with midazolam and propofol in an open-label randomized trial for the prevention of delirium in patients undergoing valve replacement surgery (Maldonado et al. 2009). The incidence of delirium in the dexmedetomidine group was 10%, compared with 44% in both the midazolam and propofol groups, but dexmedetomidine patients received significantly lower amounts of opioid analgesia. Similar reductions in the incidence of agitated delirium have subsequently been documented in a number of RCTs comparing perioperative dexmedetomidine infusion with other anesthetic agents or sedatives (Pasin et al. 2014). However, other RCTs have found no preventive reduction in emergence delirium in pediatric patients when comparing dexmedetomidine with propofol or placebo (Bong et al. 2015) or with midazolam (Aydogan et al. 2013) and no reduction of postoperative delirium in adults (Shehabi et al. 2009).

In summary, there is limited evidence in adult and pediatric patients undergoing a variety of surgical procedures for pharmacological prophylaxis with antipsychotics or dexmedetomidine (Serafim et al. 2015). Adverse events, particularly EPS with antipsychotics, have been minimal in prevention trials, which is not surprising given the low doses used. Regardless of psychopharmacological strategy, there is an evidence base supporting multimodal interventions for prevention of delirium (Collinsworth et al. 2016).

Delirium Treatment Studies

The first pharmacological RCT in delirium compared haloperidol, chlorpromazine, and lorazepam (mean dosages 1.4 mg, 36 mg, and 4.6 mg orally per day, respectively) in patients with AIDS (Breitbart et al. 1996). Haloperidol and chlorpromazine were equally effective for both hyperactive and hypoactive variants, but lorazepam was ineffective and even worsened delirium in some patients, necessitating discontinuation. Notably, these patients had mild to moderate delirium symptoms, thus requiring only low dosages of medication, and the incidence of EPS was low.

More recent trials have produced mixed results, not surprising given the protean nature of delirium, the range of etiologies, and different treatment settings. A double-blind, placebo-controlled RCT in ICU patients found that haloperidol did not change the duration of delirium (Page et al. 2013). A prospective interventional cohort study in patients undergoing cardiac surgery found that protocol treatment with haloperidol compared with usual care found no difference in delirium incidence or duration, length of stay, or complication rate (Schrøder Pedersen et al. 2014). Only about a third of the delirious palliative care patients from 14 centers across four countries appeared to benefit from haloperidol (Crawford et al. 2013).

Small RCTs comparing haloperidol with atypical antipsychotics generally have not found significant differences in effectiveness and safety in treating delirium. Examples include a single-blind trial comparing haloperidol with risperidone (Han and Kim 2004); a study comparing haloperidol, risperidone, olanzapine, and quetiapine (Yoon et al. 2013); two RCTs comparing haloperidol and olanzapine (Maneeton et al. 2013; Skrobik et al. 2004); and a single-blind trial comparing haloperidol, olanzapine, and risperidone (Grover et al. 2011). None of these studies was placebo controlled.

Hu et al. (2004) compared olanzapine, parenteral haloperidol, and placebo in a heterogeneous group of delirious hospitalized patients. Improvement was greater with both drugs compared with placebo, with no endpoint difference between the two drugs.

There are a few placebo-controlled RCTs of atypical antipsychotics. Risperidone reduced the incidence of delirium in elderly patients who were experiencing subsyndromal delirium after on-pump cardiac surgery (Hakim et al. 2012). Two small studies found that delirium resolved more quickly with quetiapine (Devlin et al. 2010; Tahir et al. 2010).

As noted earlier in the subsection "Delirium Prevention Trials," there is some evidence that perioperative sedation with dexmedetomidine reduces the incidence of delirium compared with other sedatives. The only RCT of its efficacy in treating delirium found it superior to intravenous haloperidol (Reade et al. 2009).

In summary, although antipsychotics are widely used to treat delirium, the evidence base supporting their use remains very modest. A small number of small RCTs suggest similar efficacy of haloperidol (oral or parenteral), olanzapine, and risperidone for the treatment of delirium; however, the limited number of trials and the limitations and variability of the trial designs prevent firm conclusions about comparative efficacy or adverse effects. Patients treated with higher dosages of haloperidol (>4.5 mg/day by injection or >7.5–15 mg/day orally) may have a higher incidence of EPS compared with patients treated with olanzapine and risperidone administered orally at more modest equivalent dosages. Dexmedetomidine may be a promising agent for the prevention and treatment of delirium, and larger randomized double-blind comparison trials are indicated. There is no evidence that cholinesterase inhibitors are effective in treating delirium.

Currently, haloperidol remains the gold standard for the treatment of delirium, on the basis of consensus more than evidence (American Psychiatric Association 1999). Haloperidol has the advantage of being the only agent that can be given orally, intravenously (see next subsection), intramuscularly, and subcutaneously. A wealth of clinical experience supports the use of haloperidol over other agents in seriously medically ill patients. Until adequately designed comparative clinical trials suggest superior efficacy or side-effect profile for another agent, haloperidol should be the first-line treatment for delirium except in patients who are at elevated risk for EPS (e.g., those with Parkinson's disease) or who are allergic to haloperidol. In patients with preexisting significantly prolonged QTc, alternatives to QTc-prolonging antipsychotics (e.g., aripiprazole, benzodiazepines, propofol, dexmedetomidine) should be considered first.

High-Dose Intravenous Haloperidol

Intravenous haloperidol administered at high dosages, either by bolus or by continuous infusion, has been rarely used for the treatment of severely agitated patients in the critical care setting. Mean dosages of haloperidol have been reported to be as high as 100–480 mg/day in critically ill cancer patients (Adams et al. 1986) and to approach or exceed 1,000 mg/day for several days in agitated and difficult-to-wean ventilator patients (Riker et al. 1994), postcardiotomy patients (Sanders et al. 1991), and lung transplant patients (Levenson 1995).

That such high dosages of haloperidol did not cause significant EPS suggests that some patients with delirium are less vulnerable to EPS than, for example, patients with schizophrenia. Perhaps in patients with delirium, a reduction of CNS cholinergic function would be protective against EPS. Despite a widespread belief that antipsychotics cause less EPS when given intravenously than when administered intramuscularly or orally, no evidence supports this contention.

The primary concern with intravenous haloperidol is prolongation of the QTc interval and the potential for development of torsades de pointes (Beach et al. 2013; Hassaballa and Balk 2003; see also Chapter 2, "Severe Drug Reactions," and Chapter 6, "Cardiovascular Disorders"). In a review of 223 consecutive ICU patients treated with intravenous haloperidol, Sharma et al. (1998) found that 8 patients (3.6%) developed torsades de pointes, which was associated with high dosages (>35 mg), rapid infusion, and preexisting prolonged QTc (>500 ms in 84% of patients with torsades de pointes). A U.S. Food and Drug Administration (FDA) alert warned against the off-label use of intravenous haloperidol, particularly at higher than recommended dosages, citing "at least 28 case reports of QT prolongation and [torsades de pointes] in the medical literature, some with fatal outcome in the context of off-label intravenous use of haloperidol" (U.S. Food and Drug Administration 2007).

Higher dosages and intravenous administration of haloperidol appear to be associated with a higher risk of QT prolongation and torsades de pointes. The warning emphasizes the particular need for caution when using any formulation of haloperidol to treat patients who 1) have other QT-prolonging conditions, including electrolyte imbalance (particularly hypokalemia and hypomagnesemia); 2) have underlying cardiac abnormalities, hypothyroidism, or familial long QT syndrome; or 3) are taking drugs known to prolong the QT interval, including other antipsychotic medications, tricyclic antidepressants (TCAs), and lithium (for a listing, see CredibleMeds 2016). Continuous electrocardiographic monitoring is recommended if higher doses of haloperidol are given intravenously. Intravenous haloperidol normally should be given no faster than 1 mg/minute to reduce cardiovascular side effects, including torsades de pointes.

Dexmedetomidine Pharmacology

Dexmedetomidine, an α_2-receptor agonist that decreases sympathetic tone both centrally and peripherally, was approved by the FDA in 1999 for use in humans as a short-term medication (<24 hours) for analgesia and sedation in the ICU (Gertler et al. 2001). It has also been found to attenuate neuroendocrine and hemodynamic responses to anesthesia and surgery and to reduce anesthetic and opioid requirements. Furthermore, it has been shown to reduce neurocognitive impairment in the ICU and perioperatively compared with both placebo and comparator drugs (Li et al. 2015). Dexmedetomidine must be administered intravenously. It is rapidly and extensively distributed to tissues and rapidly eliminated almost entirely via cytochrome P450 2D6 (CYP2D6), with a half-life of 2–2.5 hours (Karol and Maze 2000). This rapid distribution and fast elimination allow adjustment of dosage and effects. Dexmedetomidine does not require dose adjustment in renal insufficiency; dose reduction in hepatic impairment is recommended by the manufacturer without specific dosing guidance. Infusion ranges of 0.2–0.7 μg/kg/hour have been reported in critically ill ICU patients, including those on ventilatory support and with organ failure (Maldonado et al. 2009; Reade et al. 2009). The most common side effects are hypotension, bradycardia, and respiratory suppression. The drug should be used cautiously in patients with heart and lung disease or in those taking vasodilators or β-blockers. It is a major substrate and inhibitor of CYP2D6 (see "Drug-Drug Interactions" later in this chapter).

Anticholinergic Delirium

Acetylcholine deficit is one of the critical pathogenetic mechanisms of delirium (Trzepacz 2000). Medications with antimuscarinic effects (e.g., benztropine, trihexyphenidyl, scopolamine, diphenhydramine, TCAs [especially tertiary-amine compounds]) cause delirium, and patients with impaired cholinergic neurotransmission (i.e., Alzheimer's disease) and other CNS insults (e.g., trauma, hypoxia, stroke) are highly susceptible to their effects. Anticholinergic delirium is addressed by removal of the offending agent, supportive measures, and, in severe refractory cases, treatment with physostigmine (adults 0.5–2 mg, children 0.01–0.03 mg/kg, given intravenously at ≤1 mg/minute every 20–30 minutes until symptoms resolve) (Moore et al. 2015).

Psychotropic Drugs in the Perioperative Period

The question whether to discontinue a psychiatric drug prior to surgery with general anesthesia is a common and complex one. In one survey of adults prior to elective surgery, 43% admitted to taking one or more psychotropic medications. Of these, 35% were taking antidepressants; 34% were taking benzodiazepines; 19% were taking combinations; and 11% were taking antipsychotics, lithium, or over-the-counter psychotropics such as melatonin (Scher and Anwar 1999). The potential risks of continuing a psychotropic drug before surgery include adverse interactions with anesthetic agents, interference with hemodynamic management (e.g., causing hypotension or hypertension), and postoperative complications (e.g., excessive sedation, ileus). Risks of discontinuing the drug include, at best, loss of therapeutic effect and, at worst, rebound exacerbation of the mental disorder and/or a withdrawal syndrome. The evidence base regarding these relative risks is scanty, composed mostly of case reports. Practical and ethical limitations make controlled trials unlikely.

A consensus of experts noted that the decision whether to stop a psychotropic drug prior to surgery should be individualized, taking into account the extent of surgery, the patient's condition (diagnosis, comorbidities, stability), the choice of anesthetic agents, the length of preoperative fasting, and the risks of discontinuation (withdrawal, relapse) (Huyse et al. 2006). They recommended that lithium, monoamine oxidase inhibitors (MAOIs), TCAs, and clozapine be discontinued prior to surgery; that selective serotonin reuptake inhibitors

(SSRIs) be continued in patients who are mentally and physical stable; and that for all other psychotropics, an individualized decision is required. Other experts caution against discontinuation, advising that the safest course of action for the vast majority of drug therapy is to continue the drug until the time of surgery, particularly drugs that can cause a withdrawal syndrome (Noble and Kehlet 2000; Smith et al. 1996).

Seemingly contradictory literature makes establishing clear guidelines difficult. For example, lithium and carbamazepine are reported both to cause resistance to neuromuscular blocking agents (Ostergaard et al. 1989) and to prolong their effects (Hill et al. 1977; Melton et al. 1993). Another difficulty in balancing risks is that some psychotropics may actually provide side benefits; for example, antipsychotics may enhance intraoperative hypothermia (Kudoh et al. 2004). In our opinion, the risks of discontinuation usually exceed the risks of continuing most psychotropic drugs. However, one possible exception is serotonergic antidepressants, which have in many but not all studies been associated with an increase in perioperative bleeding. A systematic review of 13 studies concluded that serotonergic antidepressants increased that risk, with odds ratios of 1.21–4.14 (Mahdanian et al. 2014). However, the absolute increase in risk and the magnitude of blood loss appear to be small, except in patients at high risk of bleeding (e.g., coagulopathy, thrombocytonia).

Even MAOIs can be continued with relative safety prior to surgery by use of specific "MAOI-safe" anesthetic techniques and/or substitution of reversible MAOIs (Smith et al. 1996). An exception is the cholinesterase inhibitors, which synergistically increase the effects of succinylcholine and similar neuromuscular blocking agents (Russell 2009) and may run the risk of causing or exacerbating postoperative delirium. Given the low risks of temporary cessation of therapy, cholinesterase inhibitors should be stopped prior to surgery.

In some cases, interruption of psychopharmacological therapy may be unavoidable, such as when a patient is unable to take oral medication postoperatively for a prolonged period. General strategies to cope with this possibility include 1) allowing patients to continue their usual drugs until the day of surgery when possible; 2) using alternatives to the oral route of administration if available (see Chapter 1, "Pharmacokinetics, Pharmacodynamics, and Principles of Drug-Drug Interactions"); 3) when alternative routes are not available, substituting an alternative drug of the same or different class, which can be administered by a non-oral route; and 4) returning gastrointestinal transit times to normal as soon as possible to restore reliable drug absorption from the gut (e.g., avoiding unnecessary gastrointestinal tubes and restrictions on oral intake and using non-opioid or opioid-reduced analgesia combined with early oral nutrition) (Noble and Kehlet 2000).

Treatment of Preoperative Anxiety

Preoperative anxiety is common in adults and children and has been treated with antianxiety medications, particularly benzodiazepines. Concerns have been expressed regarding whether preoperative sedating medication might delay discharge, especially because an increasing percentage of surgical procedures are being carried out on an outpatient basis. A Cochrane review of 17 studies found no evidence of a difference in time to discharge from hospital in adult patients who received anxiolytic premedication (Walker and Smith 2009).

Adults and Preoperative Anxiety

A number of randomized trials in adults have demonstrated the benefits of benzodiazepines, although the studies vary in type of surgery, patient demographics, dosage, and timing of medication. Compared with placebo, both oral diazepam (10 mg) in the evening before surgery and midazolam (1.5 mg) at least 15 minutes before surgery resulted in lower preoperative anxiety and a reduction in the usual postoperative increase in cortisol levels (Pekcan et al. 2005). In women undergoing abdominal hysterectomy, diazepam-treated patients showed lower postoperative anxiety and lower incidence of surgical wound infection up to 30 days after surgery compared with those given placebo (Levandovski et al. 2008). Another trial found that 50 mg clorazepate the evening before surgery prevented increases in anxiety and sympathoadrenal activity (Meybohm et al. 2007). However, a recent large placebo-controlled trial found that premedication with lorazepam did not improve the self-reported patient experience the day after surgery but was associated with a modest delay in extubation and a lower rate of early cognitive recovery (Maurice-Szamburski et al. 2015).

Alternative medications have also been found to be beneficial. A recent systematic review concluded that melatonin was superior to placebo and may be equally as effective as standard treatment with midazolam (Hansen et al. 2015). Premedication with 1,200 mg gabapentin improved (compared with placebo) preoperative anxiety, postoperative analgesia, and early knee mobilization after arthroscopic knee surgery (Ménigaux et al. 2005). Preoperative gabapentin may have other benefits in addition to anxiolysis, including postoperative analgesia; attenuation of the hemodynamic response to laryngoscopy and intubation; and prevention of chronic postsurgical pain, postoperative nausea and vomiting, and delirium (Kong and Irwin 2007). However, the data are not extensive, and another randomized trial found that although the similar drug pregabalin (75–300 mg administered orally) increased perioperative sedation, it failed to reduce preoperative state anxiety or postoperative pain or to improve the recovery process after minor elective surgery procedures (White et al. 2009). Finally, in a trial in moderate- and high-risk female gynecological surgery patients, Chen et al. (2008) reported that premedication with mirtazapine (30 mg) reduced the level of preoperative anxiety and the risk of postoperative nausea and vomiting.

Children and Preoperative Anxiety

Anxiety regarding impending surgery occurs in up to 60% of children. Preoperative anxiety in children has been associated with a number of problematic behaviors, both preoperatively (e.g., agitation, crying, enuresis, the need for physical restraint during anesthetic induction) and postoperatively (e.g., pain, sleeping disturbances, parent-child conflict, separation anxiety) (Wright et al. 2007). A variety of pharmacological and nondrug interventions have been studied, including benzodiazepines, clonidine, and hydroxyzine (Chaudhary et al. 2014; Dahmani et al. 2010).

As in adults, most drug trials in children have been of benzodiazepines. In a Cochrane review of studies of sedation for anxious children undergoing dental procedures, Lourenço-Matharu et al. (2012) were not able to reach any definitive conclusion regarding which was the most effective drug or method of sedation (except weak evidence for oral midazolam).

Alternative routes of administration are more often needed in young children than in older patients (see also Chapter 1). Sublingual midazolam 0.2 mg/kg was found to be as efficacious as oral midazolam 0.5 mg/kg (Kattoh et al. 2008). Adverse temporary cognitive effects may occur after receiving preoperative anxiolytics. A placebo-controlled trial of buccal midazolam (0.2 mg/kg) before anesthesia for multiple dental extractions in children found that midazolam impaired reaction times and psychomotor coordination at discharge, with recovery at 48 hours later. However, midazolam was also associated with significant postoperative anterograde amnesia (for information presented in the interval between premedication and surgery), which persisted at 48 hours (Millar et al. 2007).

Although midazolam is an effective anxiolytic for most children, a significant minority do not benefit from it (Kain et al. 2007). One study found preoperative clonidine or dexmedetomidine to have similar effects on anxiety and sedation postoperatively compared with midazolam; however, children given either clonidine or dexmedetomidine had less perioperative sympathetic stimulation and less postoperative pain than those given midazolam (Schmidt et al. 2007). Although melatonin has shown promise for preoperative anxiety in adults, studies in children have yielded more negative than positive results. In one trial, melatonin was as effective as midazolam in alleviating preoperative anxiety in children and was associated with a tendency toward faster recovery and a lower incidence of agitation and sleep disturbance postoperatively (Samarkandi et al. 2005). However, two subsequent studies found midazolam to be more effective than melatonin (Isik et al. 2008; Kain et al. 2009).

Acute and Posttraumatic Stress in the Critical Care Setting

Posttraumatic stress symptoms and disorders can occur as a result of traumatic physical injury, being in intensive care, and having major surgery (Bienvenu et al. 2013; Jackson et al. 2014). Although considerably less studied, acute stress disorder symptoms or early-onset posttraumatic stress disorder (PTSD) in the critical care setting are prevalent and appear to predict ongoing or later-onset PTSD and cognitive dysfunction (Davydow et al. 2013; McKibben et al. 2008).

Psychopharmacological treatment of PTSD in the months after a severe injury and/or ICU stay would be expected to follow usual treatment guidelines, with SSRIs being first-line treatment. However, no RCTs have been reported to guide treatment of patients with postsurgical or post-ICU PTSD.

Retrospective studies of PTSD prevention among soldiers who had sustained burns in combat and had at least one surgery revealed that intraoperative ketamine versus no ketamine (McGhee et al. 2008) was associated with a significant reduction in incident PTSD, but pre- and intraoperative midazolam (McGhee et al. 2009b) and propranolol (McGhee et al. 2009a) had no significant relationship to PTSD. In an RCT, intravenous ketamine produced rapid improvement in PTSD 24 hours later, but no studies of longer treatment are available (Feder et al. 2014). However, administration of ketamine immediately after a motor vehicle accident has also been found to *increase* PTSD incidence (Schönenberg et al. 2008), so further study is warranted. In a retrospective analysis of traumatic injury victims admitted to the hospital, higher morphine dosages in the week after injury were predictive of lower incidence of PTSD but not of major depression or other anxiety disorder, suggesting a beneficial effect of morphine on fear conditioning (Bryant et al. 2009). A pilot RCT investigating a 14-day prevention strategy for PTSD among hospitalized surgical trauma victims found no differences between propranolol, gabapentin, and placebo (Stein et al. 2007). A Cochrane review of pharmacological intervention to prevent PTSD, including studies in a variety of traumas that included surgery and septic shock, concluded that there was moderate quality evidence for the efficacy of hydrocortisone but no evidence to support the efficacy of propranolol, escitalopram, temazepam, and gabapentin (Amos et al. 2014). In an RCT in acute adult trauma inpatients, fewer PTSD symptoms were observed in patients undergoing a collaborative care intervention that included psychiatric medication when indicated than in patients receiving usual care (Zatzick et al. 2004).

In summary, data on PTSD prevention are sparse, with studies limited by small sample size and retrospective data. Findings that intraoperative ketamine, higher posttrauma morphine dosages, and stress corticosteroids after trauma and surgery are associated with lower rates of PTSD need to be corroborated by further prospective study with these agents, in addition to antidepressants, which are virtually unstudied.

Adverse Neuropsychiatric Effects of Critical Care and Surgical Drugs

Drugs used in surgery and critical care may have adverse neuropsychiatric effects. These drugs are summarized in Table 15–1 and discussed below.

Nitrous Oxide

Nitrous oxide anesthesia has been associated with reversible and irreversible cognitive impairment and psychotic symptoms; however, the causal nature of

Table 15–1. Psychiatric adverse effects of drugs used in surgery and critical care

Medication	Psychiatric adverse effects
Inhalational anesthetics	
Desflurane, enflurane, halothane, isoflurane, methoxyflurane, and sevoflurane	Malignant hyperthermia syndrome: delirium, autonomic instability, muscular rigidity, tremor
Neuromuscular blockers	
Succinylcholine	Malignant hyperthermia syndrome: delirium, autonomic instability, muscular rigidity, tremor
Nitrous oxide	Psychosis, reversible and irreversible cognitive impairment
Sympathomimetic agents	
Dobutamine, dopamine, epinephrine, isoproterenol, norepinephrine	Fear, anxiety, restlessness, tremor, insomnia, confusion, irritability, mania, psychosis
Vasodilators	
Amrinone, isosorbide, milrinone, nesiritide, nitroglycerin, and nitroprusside	Increased intracranial pressure, syncope
Intravenous sedative and anesthesia induction agents	
Etomidate, midazolam, and propofol	Excessive sedation, respiratory suppression, delirium (especially in combination with sedative-hypnotics and opioid analgesics)

these symptoms remains controversial because studies fail to account for multiple concurrent causal factors (Sanders et al. 2008). Potential mechanisms proposed include antagonism of the N-methyl-D-aspartic acid receptor and disruption of cortical methionine synthase, which may lead to B_{12} and folate deficiency. Women, young patients, and elderly patients with B_{12} deficiency appear to be most susceptible.

Inhalational Anesthetics and Succinylcholine

Inhalational anesthetics and succinylcholine may cause malignant hyperthermia, which is similar to neuroleptic malignant syndrome (see Chapter 2, "Severe Drug Reactions") in that it is characterized by delirium, autonomic instability, rigidity, and tremor. Antipsychotic medications have not been reported to predispose to this effect. Malignant hyperthermia is treated with dantrolene and supportive care.

Sympathomimetic Amines

Sympathomimetic amines include dopamine, dobutamine, and other drugs. Central effects of these medications include fear, anxiety, restlessness, tremor, insomnia, confusion, irritability, weakness, psychotic states, appetite reduction, nausea, and vomiting.

Vasodilator Hypotensive Agents

Vasodilator hypotensive agents include nitroglycerin and nitroprusside, among others. Increases in intracranial pressure can occur with central vasodilation. In patients whose intracranial pressure is already elevated, sodium nitroprusside should be used only with extreme caution.

Drug-Drug Interactions

Multiple potential drug-drug interactions are possible because of the use of psychopharmacological agents in the critical care and perisurgical arena (Table 15–2). Most of these potential interactions (e.g., for antibiotics, corticosteroids, analgesics, and cardiovascular medications) are covered in the relevant organ system disease chapters and in Chapter 1. The focus in this chapter is on anesthetic agents and intravenously administered agents used in the coronary care setting.

Inhalational Anesthetics

Pharmacodynamic effects of inhalational anesthetics (e.g., enflurane, halothane, isoflurane, methoxyflurane, desflurane, sevoflurane) include excessive sedation and respiratory suppression with sedating psychotropic drugs (sedative-hypnotics, barbiturates, drugs with antihistaminergic properties) and hy-

Table 15–2. Critical care and perisurgical drug–psychotropic drug interactions

Medication	Interaction mechanism	Effects on psychotropic drugs and management
Inhalational anesthetics		
Desflurane, enflurane, halothane, isoflurane, methoxyflurane, and sevoflurane	Additive sedation	Increased sedation with sedative-hypnotics and antihistaminic psychotropics (TCAs, antipsychotics).
	Additive hypotensive effect	Increased risk of hypotension with drugs that block α_1-adrenergic receptors (e.g., TCAs, MAOIs, typical and atypical antipsychotics).
	Halothane: sensitization of myocardium	Arrhythmias with sympathomimetic psychotropics (NRIs, SNRIs, TCAs, psychostimulants).
Nitrous oxide	Activation of supraspinal $GABA_A$ receptors	Sedative-hypnotics and propofol may block anesthetic activity of nitrous oxide.
	Potentiation of noradrenergic mechanisms	Additive analgesia with noradrenergic agents (SNRIs, NRIs, TCAs).
Nondepolarizing neuromuscular blocking agents		
Pancuronium and tubocurarine	Reversal of antinicotinic neuromuscular blockade	Cholinesterase inhibitors antagonize anesthesia because of these agents and should be stopped 2 weeks before surgery.
	Unknown mechanism	Lithium and carbamazepine have been found to both potentiate and inhibit neuromuscular blockade.

Table 15–2.   Critical care and perisurgical drug–psychotropic drug interactions *(continued)*

Medication	Interaction mechanism	Effects on psychotropic drugs and management
Depolarizing neuromuscular blocking agents		
Suxamethonium (succinylcholine)	Increasing acetylcholine-mediated neuromuscular depolarization	Cholinesterase inhibitors may prolong the duration of action of these agents.
	Blockade of depolarization	Psychotropics with anticholinergic properties (trihexyphenidyl, benztropine, TCAs, antipsychotics) may antagonize depolarization and reduce effectiveness.
Sedative-hypnotic induction agents		
Etomidate, midazolam, and propofol	Additive sedation	Increased sedation with sedative-hypnotics and antihistaminic psychotropics (TCAs, antipsychotics).
α_2-*Adrenergic sedative*		
Dexmedetomidine	Additive sedation	Increased sedation with sedative-hypnotics and antihistaminic psychotropics (TCAs, antipsychotics).
	Inhibition of CYP2D6	May inhibit the metabolism of psychotropics metabolized by this isozyme (e.g., TCAs, mirtazapine, venlafaxine, risperidone, opioids, atomoxetine) if given chronically (see Chapter 1), but there are no apparent interactions with short-term use.

Table 15–2. Critical care and perisurgical drug–psychotropic drug interactions *(continued)*

Medication	Interaction mechanism	Effects on psychotropic drugs and management
Sympathomimetic inotropic and pressor agents		
Dopamine, epinephrine, isoproterenol, and norepinephrine	MAO inhibition	Treatment with MAOIs 2–3 weeks prior to initiation of these agents may augment hypertensive effects and cause hypertensive crisis.
	Reversal of pressor effect	Risk of severe hypotension with coadministration of agents with β_2-agonist activity (epinephrine, isoproterenol) and drugs that block α_1-adrenergic receptors (e.g., TCAs, typical and atypical antipsychotics). Norepinephrine should be used as a pressor agent in this situation.
	Additive noradrenergic effects	With dopaminergic and noradrenergic psychotropics (e.g., bupropion, atomoxetine, duloxetine, TCAs), augmentation of hypertensive effects and CNS activation.
Dobutamine	Hypokalemia	Increased risk of cardiac arrhythmias with QT-prolonging agents, including TCAs, typical antipsychotics, pimozide, risperidone, paliperidone, iloperidone, quetiapine, ziprasidone, and lithium.

Table 15–2. Critical care and perisurgical drug–psychotropic drug interactions *(continued)*

Medication	Interaction mechanism	Effects on psychotropic drugs and management
Vasodilators		
Amrinone, isosorbide, milrinone, nesiritide, nitroglycerin, and nitroprusside	Additive hypotensive effects	Augmentation of hypotensive effects when combined with drugs that block α_1-adrenergic receptors (e.g., TCAs, MAOIs, typical and atypical antipsychotics) or with PDE5 inhibitors.

Note. CNS=central nervous system; CYP=cytochrome P450; GABA$_A$=γ-aminobutyric acid type A; MAO=monoamine oxidase; MAOIs=monoamine oxidase inhibitors; NRIs=norepinephrine reuptake inhibitors; PDE5=phosphodiesterase type 5; SNRIs=serotonin-norepinephrine reuptake inhibitors; TCAs=tricyclic antidepressants.

potensive effects with α_1-blocking psychotropics (e.g., TCAs, MAOIs, antipsychotics). Halothane in combination with sympathomimetic psychotropics (e.g., norepinephrine reuptake inhibitors [NRIs], serotonin-norepinephrine reuptake inhibitors [SNRIs], TCAs, psychostimulants) may cause arrhythmias secondary to halothane-induced myocardial sensitization to these agents. The mechanisms of neuroleptic malignant syndrome (see Chapter 2) and malignant hyperthermia are thought to be divergent, and there are no reports of antipsychotic treatment increasing the risk of malignant hyperthermia postoperatively.

Nitrous Oxide

The analgesic action of nitrous oxide is partially dependent on both the inhibition of supraspinal GABA type A (GABA$_A$) receptors and the activation of spinal GABA$_A$ receptors. Agents that activate the supraspinal GABA$_A$ receptor, such as midazolam and propofol, may interfere with nitrous oxide analgesia by inhibiting the activation of the descending inhibitory neurons (Sanders et al. 2008). Noradrenergic agents (e.g., TCAs, SNRIs, NRIs) and opioids may potentiate analgesia due to nitrous oxide via its activation of locus coeruleus and opioidergic neurons.

Nondepolarizing Neuromuscular Blocking Agents

Nondepolarizing neuromuscular blocking agents (e.g., tubocurarine, pancuronium) act by competitive inhibition at nicotinic cholinergic receptors, producing paralysis. Cholinesterase inhibitors may antagonize this type of neuromuscular blockade and, in fact, are used to reverse it. Cholinesterase inhibitors should be discontinued several weeks before surgery involving neuromuscular blocking agents (Russell 2009). Lithium and carbamazepine may both potentiate and inhibit neuromuscular blockade by these agents (Melton et al. 1993; Ostergaard et al. 1989).

Depolarizing Neuromuscular Blocking Agents

In contrast to the nondepolarizing agents, succinylcholine (suxamethonium) has acetylcholine-like actions; cholinesterase inhibitors prolong the duration of action of succinylcholine by inhibiting its plasma cholinesterase-mediated metabolism and increasing acetylcholine-mediated neuromuscular depolarization. Anticholinergic drugs may antagonize succinylcholine effects.

Sedative-Hypnotic Induction and Continuous Sedation Agents

Coadministration of sedative-hypnotic induction and continuous sedation agents (propofol, midazolam, etomidate) with CNS depressant psychotropics, including benzodiazepines, nonbenzodiazepine hypnotics, and antihistaminic drugs, may synergistically result in excessive sedation and respiratory suppression.

Dexmedetomidine

Because dexmedetomidine is a substrate and inhibitor of CYP2D6, pharmacokinetic interactions with some psychotropics might be expected, especially with prolonged infusion of this agent (see Chapter 1 for a listing of CYP2D6-interacting psychotropic drugs) (Karol and Maze 2000). With short-term use, dexmedetomidine does not appear to exhibit pharmacokinetic interactions. Dosage modifications of some concomitant medications (e.g., some anesthetics, sedatives, hypnotics, antihistaminic medications, opioids) may be needed primarily because of common pharmacodynamic actions of the two drugs.

Sympathomimetic Agents

Sympathomimetic agents (e.g., dopamine, dobutamine, epinephrine, norepinephrine, isoproterenol) are often used for vasoconstriction, bronchodilatation, combination with local anesthetics, and treatment of hypersensitizing reactions. Concurrent use of MAOIs (including tranylcypromine, phenelzine, moclobemide, and selegiline) with sympathomimetic agents may prolong and intensify cardiac stimulation and vasopressor effects because of increased release of catecholamines, which accumulate in intraneuronal storage sites during MAOI therapy. This interaction may result in headache, cardiac arrhythmias, vomiting, or sudden and severe hypertensive and/or hyperpyretic crises. For patients who have been receiving MAOIs within 2–3 weeks prior to administration of sympathomimetic agents, the initial dosage of dopamine should be reduced to no more than one-tenth of the usual dosage.

Dopamine may interact pharmacodynamically with noradrenergic agents, such as TCAs, NRIs, SNRIs, and psychostimulants, to cause a marked increase in heart rate and/or blood pressure. Patients with preexisting hypertension may have increased risk of an exaggerated pressor response with these drugs. Dobutamine may cause hypokalemia, so administration of this drug with QTc-prolonging psychotropic drugs requires close cardiac and serum potassium monitoring. Unlike dopamine, dobutamine does not appear to be an MAO substrate (Yan et al. 2002); however, absent substantial clinical data, caution is warranted when combining dobutamine with irreversible MAOIs.

Vasodilators

The principal pharmacological action of vasodilators (isosorbide dinitrate and mononitrate, nitroglycerin, nitroprusside, milrinone, amrinone, nesiritide) is relaxation of vascular smooth muscle and consequent dilatation of peripheral arteries and veins. Excessive hypotension may result through additive effects when vasodilators are used with psychotropics with α_1-antagonist properties, such as TCAs, MAOIs, and phenothiazines; atypical antipsychotics; and phosphodiesterase type 5 inhibitors, such as sildenafil, vardenafil, and tadalafil.

Key Clinical Points

Delirium

- The differential diagnosis of delirium is broad. Prevention and treatment require early assessment of patients at risk, identification and treatment of underlying causes (including, where possible, avoiding anticholinergic, sedative-hypnotic, antihistaminic, opioid analgesic, and corticosteroid drugs), environmental intervention, and psychopharmacology.
- For the prevention of delirium, a small number of RCTs in select patient populations undergoing surgery support the efficacy of olanzapine and dexmedetomidine in reducing the incidence of delirium and haloperidol in reducing the severity and duration of delirium.
- For the treatment of delirium not due to sedative or alcohol withdrawal, RCTs support the efficacy of haloperidol (oral or parenteral), chlorpromazine, olanzapine, risperidone, and dexmedetomidine, whereas benzodiazepines are less effective or are deleterious.

- Currently, haloperidol remains the gold standard treatment for delirium except in patients who have elevated risk for EPS, who are allergic, or who are being considered for intravenous administration and have a prolonged QTc interval.

Psychotropics in the Perioperative Period

- The decision to continue or stop a psychotropic drug in the perioperative period should be individualized, with consideration of the extent of surgery, the patient's medical condition, choice of anesthetic agents, length of preoperative fasting, and the risks of drug discontinuation (withdrawal or relapse of psychiatric disorder).
- The greatest perioperative risk exists with lithium, MAOIs, TCAs, and clozapine.

Preoperative Anxiety and Posttraumatic Stress Disorder

- For preoperative anxiety in adults and children, benzodiazepines are the most widely used agents; however, other agents such as gabapentin and α-adrenergic antagonist agents such as clonidine and dexmedetomidine may be viable alternatives.
- For PTSD secondary to illness or injury, evidence from small RCTs suggests efficacy of stress doses of hydrocortisone in reducing PTSD symptoms after cardiac surgery and septic shock. Evidence for other agents, such as propranolol, intraoperative ketamine, and opioid analgesics, is scant and inconclusive.

Drug Interactions

- There is significant potential for pharmacodynamic and pharmacokinetic interactions between psychotropic drugs and anesthetics and other agents used in the critical setting. In this setting, the prescription of psychotropic drugs should be done with caution, particularly because of the severity of medical comorbidity and the concurrent use of multiple medications.

References

Adams F, Fernandez F, Andersson BS: Emergency pharmacotherapy of delirium in the critically ill cancer patient. Psychosomatics 27(1)(suppl):33–38, 1986 3952253

American Psychiatric Association: Practice guideline for the treatment of patients with delirium. Am J Psychiatry 156(5)(suppl):1–20, 1999 10327941

Amos T, Stein DJ, Ipser JC: Pharmacological interventions for preventing post-traumatic stress disorder (PTSD). Cochrane Database of Systematic Reviews 2014, Issue 7. Art. No.: CD006239. DOI: 10.1002/14651858.CD006239.pub2 25001071

Aydogan MS, Korkmaz MF, Ozgül U, et al: Pain, fentanyl consumption, and delirium in adolescents after scoliosis surgery: dexmedetomidine vs midazolam. Paediatr Anaesth 23(5):446–452, 2013 23448434

Beach SR, Celano CM, Noseworthy PA, et al: QTc prolongation, torsades de pointes, and psychotropic medications. Psychosomatics 54(1):1–13, 2013 23295003

Bienvenu OJ, Gellar J, Althouse BM, et al: Post-traumatic stress disorder symptoms after acute lung injury: a 2-year prospective longitudinal study. Psychol Med 43(12):2657–2671, 2013 23438256

Bong CL, Lim E, Allen JC, et al: A comparison of single-dose dexmedetomidine or propofol on the incidence of emergence delirium in children undergoing general anaesthesia for magnetic resonance imaging. Anaesthesia 70(4):393–399, 2015 25311146

Breitbart W, Marotta R, Platt MM, et al: A double-blind trial of haloperidol, chlorpromazine, and lorazepam in the treatment of delirium in hospitalized AIDS patients. Am J Psychiatry 153(2):231–237, 1996 8561204

Bryant RA, Creamer M, O'Donnell M, et al: A study of the protective function of acute morphine administration on subsequent posttraumatic stress disorder. Biol Psychiatry 65(5):438–440, 2009 19058787

Chaudhary S, Jindal R, Girotra G, et al: Is midazolam superior to triclofos and hydroxyzine as premedicant in children? J Anaesthesiol Clin Pharmacol 30(1):53–58, 2014 24574594

Chen CC, Lin CS, Ko YP, et al: Premedication with mirtazapine reduces preoperative anxiety and postoperative nausea and vomiting. Anesth Analg 106(1):109–113, 2008 18165563

Collinsworth AW, Priest EL, Campbell CR, et al: A review of multifaceted care approaches for the prevention and mitigation of delirium in intensive care units. J Intensive Care Med 31(2):127–141, 2016 25348864

Crawford GB, Agar M M, Quinn SJ, et al: Pharmacovigilance in hospice/palliative care: net effect of haloperidol for delirium. J Palliat Med 16(11):1335–1341, 2013 24138282

CredibleMeds: Risk categories for drugs that prolong QT and induce torsades de pointes (TdP), June 15, 2016. Available at: https://crediblemeds.org. Accessed July 7, 2016.

Dahmani S, Brasher C, Stany I, et al: Premedication with clonidine is superior to benzodiazepines. A meta analysis of published studies. Acta Anaesthesiol Scand 54(4):397–402, 2010 20085541

Davydow DS, Zatzick D, Hough CL, Katon WJ: In-hospital acute stress symptoms are associated with impairment in cognition 1 year after intensive care unit admission. Ann Am Thorac Soc 10(5):450–457, 2013 23987665

Devlin JW, Roberts RJ, Fong JJ, et al: Efficacy and safety of quetiapine in critically ill patients with delirium: a prospective, multicenter, randomized, double-blind, placebo-controlled pilot study. Crit Care Med 38(2):419–427, 2010 19915454

Feder A, Parides MK, Murrough JW, et al: Efficacy of intravenous ketamine for treatment of chronic posttraumatic stress disorder: a randomized clinical trial. JAMA Psychiatry 71(6):681–688, 2014 24740528

Fukata S, Kawabata Y, Fujisiro K, et al: Haloperidol prophylaxis does not prevent postoperative delirium in elderly patients: a randomized, open-label prospective trial. Surg Today 44(12):2305–2313, 2014 24532143

Gertler R, Brown HC, Mitchell DH, Silvius EN: Dexmedetomidine: a novel sedative-analgesic agent. Proc Bayl Univ Med Cent 14(1):13–21, 2001 16369581

Grover S, Kumar V, Chakrabarti S: Comparative efficacy study of haloperidol, olanzapine and risperidone in delirium. J Psychosom Res 71(4):277–281, 2011 21911107

Hakim SM, Othman AI, Naoum DO: Early treatment with risperidone for subsyndromal delirium after on-pump cardiac surgery in the elderly: a randomized trial. Anesthesiology 116(5):987–997, 2012 22436797

Han CS, Kim YK: A double-blind trial of risperidone and haloperidol for the treatment of delirium. Psychosomatics 45(4):297–301, 2004 15232043

Hansen MV, Halladin NL, Rosenberg J, et al: Melatonin for pre- and postoperative anxiety in adults. Cochrane Database of Systematic Reviews 2015, Issue 4. Art. No.: CD009861. DOI: 10.1002/14651858.CD009861.pub2 25856551

Hassaballa HA, Balk RA: Torsade de pointes associated with the administration of intravenous haloperidol. Am J Ther 10(1):58–60, 2003 12522522

Hill GE, Wong KC, Hodges MR: Lithium carbonate and neuromuscular blocking agents. Anesthesiology 46(2):122–126, 1977 835845

Hu H, Deng W, Yang H, et al: A prospective random control study: comparison of olanzapine and haloperidol in senile delirium. Chongqing Medical Journal 8:1234–1237, 2004

Huyse FJ, Touw DJ, van Schijndel RS, et al: Psychotropic drugs and the perioperative period: a proposal for a guideline in elective surgery. Psychosomatics 47(1):8–22, 2006 16384803

Inouye SK, Young J: Delirium in older persons. N Engl J Med 354(11):1157–1165, 2006 16540616

Isik B, Baygin O, Bodur H: Premedication with melatonin vs midazolam in anxious children. Paediatr Anaesth 18(7):635–641, 2008 18616492

Jackson JC, Pandharipande PP, Girard TD, et al; Bringing to light the Risk Factors And Incidence of Neuropsychological dysfunction in ICU survivors (BRAIN-ICU) study investigators: Depression, post-traumatic stress disorder, and functional disability in survivors of critical illness in the BRAIN-ICU study: a longitudinal cohort study. Lancet Respir Med 2(5):369–379, 2014 24815803

Kain ZN, MacLaren J, McClain BC, et al: Effects of age and emotionality on the effectiveness of midazolam administered preoperatively to children. Anesthesiology 107(4):545–552, 2007 17893449

Kain ZN, MacLaren JE, Herrmann L, et al: Preoperative melatonin and its effects on induction and emergence in children undergoing anesthesia and surgery. Anesthesiology 111(1):44–49, 2009 19546692

Kalisvaart KJ, de Jonghe JF, Bogaards MJ, et al: Haloperidol prophylaxis for elderly hip-surgery patients at risk for delirium: a randomized placebo-controlled study. J Am Geriatr Soc 53(10):1658–1666, 2005 16181163

Kaneko T, Cai J, Ishikura T, et al: Prophylactic consecutive administration of haloperidol can reduce the occurrence of postoperative delirium in gastrointestinal surgery. Yonago Acta Med 42:179–184, 1999

Karol MD, Maze M: Pharmacokinetics and interaction pharmacodynamics of dexmedetomidine in humans. Baillieres Clin Anaesthesiol 14:261–269, 2000

Kattoh T, Katome K, Makino S, et al: Comparative study of sublingual midazolam with oral midazolam for premedication in pediatric anesthesia [in Japanese]. Masui 57(10):1227–1232, 2008 18975537

Kong VK, Irwin MG: Gabapentin: a multimodal perioperative drug? Br J Anaesth 99(6):775–786, 2007 18006529

Kudoh A, Takase H, Takazawa T: Chronic treatment with antipsychotics enhances intraoperative core hypothermia. Anesth Analg 98(1):111–115, 2004 14693598

Larsen KA, Kelly SE, Stern TA, et al: Administration of olanzapine to prevent postoperative delirium in elderly joint-replacement patients: a randomized, controlled trial. Psychosomatics 51(5):409–418, 2010 20833940

Levandovski R, Ferreira MB, Hidalgo MP, et al: Impact of preoperative anxiolytic on surgical site infection in patients undergoing abdominal hysterectomy. Am J Infect Control 36(10):718–726, 2008 18834731

Levenson JL: High-dose intravenous haloperidol for agitated delirium following lung transplantation. Psychosomatics 36(1):66–68, 1995 7871137

Li B, Wang H, Wu H, Gao C: Neurocognitive dysfunction risk alleviation with the use of dexmedetomidine in perioperative conditions or as ICU sedation: a meta-analysis. Medicine (Baltimore) 94(14):e597, 2015 25860207

Liptzin B, Laki A, Garb JL, et al: Donepezil in the prevention and treatment of post-surgical delirium. Am J Geriatr Psychiatry 13(12):1100–1106, 2005 16319303

Lourenço-Matharu L, Ashley PF, Furness S: Sedation of children undergoing dental treatment. Cochrane Database of Systematic Reviews 2012, Issue 3. Art. No.: CD003877. DOI: 10.1002/14651858.CD003877.pub4 22419289

Mahdanian AA, Rej S, Bacon SL, et al: Serotonergic antidepressants and perioperative bleeding risk: a systematic review. Expert Opin Drug Saf 13(6):695–704, 2014 24717049

Maldonado JR, Wysong A, van der Starre PJ, et al: Dexmedetomidine and the reduction of postoperative delirium after cardiac surgery. Psychosomatics 50(3):206–217, 2009 19567759

Maneeton B, Maneeton N, Srisurapanont M, Chittawatanarat K: Quetiapine versus haloperidol in the treatment of delirium: a double-blind, randomized, controlled trial. Drug Des Devel Ther 7(7):657–667, 2013 23926422

Marcantonio ER, Flacker JM, Wright RJ, Resnick NM: Reducing delirium after hip fracture: a randomized trial. J Am Geriatr Soc 49(5):516–522, 2001 11380742

Marcantonio ER, Palihnich K, Appleton P, Davis RB: Pilot randomized trial of donepezil hydrochloride for delirium after hip fracture. J Am Geriatr Soc 59 (suppl 2):S282–S288, 2011 22091574

Maurice-Szamburski A, Auquier P, Viarre-Oreal V, et al; PremedX Study Investigators: Effect of sedative premedication on patient experience after general anesthesia: a randomized clinical trials. JAMA 313(9):916–925, 2015 25734733

McAvay GJ, Van Ness PH, Bogardus ST Jr, et al: Older adults discharged from the hospital with delirium: 1-year outcomes. J Am Geriatr Soc 54(8):1245–1250, 2006 16913993

McGhee LL, Maani CV, Garza TH, et al: The correlation between ketamine and post-traumatic stress disorder in burned service members. J Trauma 64(2)(suppl):S195–S198, Discussion S197–S198, 2008 18376165

McGhee LL, Maani CV, Garza TH, et al: The effect of propranolol on posttraumatic stress disorder in burned service members. J Burn Care Res 30(1):92–97, 2009a 19060728

McGhee LL, Maani CV, Garza TH, et al: The relationship of intravenous midazolam and posttraumatic stress disorder development in burned soldiers. J Trauma 66(4)(suppl):S186–S190, 2009b 19359964

McKibben JB, Bresnick MG, Wiechman Askay SA, Fauerbach JA: Acute stress disorder and posttraumatic stress disorder: a prospective study of prevalence, course, and predictors in a sample with major burn injuries. J Burn Care Res 29(1):22–35, 2008 18182894

Melton AT, Antognini JF, Gronert GA: Prolonged duration of succinylcholine in patients receiving anticonvulsants: evidence for mild up-regulation of acetylcholine receptors? Can J Anaesth 40(10):939–942, 1993 8222033

Ménigaux C, Adam F, Guignard B, et al: Preoperative gabapentin decreases anxiety and improves early functional recovery from knee surgery. Anesth Analg 100(5):1394–1399, 2005 15845693

Meybohm P, Hanss R, Bein B, et al: Comparison of premedication regimes: a randomized, controlled trial [in German]. Anaesthesist 56:890–892, 894–896, 2007

Millar K, Asbury AJ, Bowman AW, et al: A randomised placebo-controlled trial of the effects of midazolam premedication on children's postoperative cognition. Anaesthesia 62(9):923–930, 2007 17697220

Moore PW, Rasimas JJ, Donovan JW: Physostigmine is the antidote for anticholinergic syndrome. J Med Toxicol 11(1):159–160, 2015 25339374

Noble DW, Kehlet H: Risks of interrupting drug treatment before surgery. BMJ 321(7263):719–720, 2000 10999886

Ostergaard D, Engbaek J, Viby-Mogensen J: Adverse reactions and interactions of the neuromuscular blocking drugs. Med Toxicol 4(5):351–368, 1989 2682131

Page VJ, Ely EW, Gates S, et al: Effect of intravenous haloperidol on the duration of delirium and coma in critically ill patients (Hope-ICU): a randomised, double-blind, placebo-controlled trial. Lancet Respir Med 1(7):515–523, 2013 24461612

Pasin L, Landoni G, Nardelli P, et al: Dexmedetomidine reduces the risk of delirium, agitation and confusion in critically Ill patients: a meta-analysis of randomized controlled trials. J Cardiothorac Vasc Anesth 28(6):1459–1466, 2014 25034724

Pekcan M, Celebioglu B, Demir B, et al: The effect of premedication on preoperative anxiety. Middle East J Anaesthesiol 18(2):421–433, 2005 16438017

Reade MC, O'Sullivan K, Bates S, et al: Dexmedetomidine vs haloperidol in delirious, agitated, intubated patients: a randomised open-label trial. Crit Care 13(3):R75, 2009 19454032

Riker RR, Fraser GL, Cox PM: Continuous infusion of haloperidol controls agitation in critically ill patients. Crit Care Med 22(3):433–440, 1994 8124994

Russell WJ: The impact of Alzheimer's disease medication on muscle relaxants. Anaesth Intensive Care 37(1):134–135, 2009 19160552

Samarkandi A, Naguib M, Riad W, et al: Melatonin vs. midazolam premedication in children: a double-blind, placebo-controlled study. Eur J Anaesthesiol 22(3):189–196, 2005 15852991

Sampson EL, Raven PR, Ndhlovu PN, et al: A randomized, double-blind, placebo-controlled trial of donepezil hydrochloride (Aricept) for reducing the incidence of postoperative delirium after elective total hip replacement. Int J Geriatr Psychiatry 22(4):343–349, 2007 17006875

Sanders KM, Murray GB, Cassem NH: High-dose intravenous haloperidol for agitated delirium in a cardiac patient on intra-aortic balloon pump. J Clin Psychopharmacol 11(2):146–147, 1991 2056143

Sanders RD, Weimann J, Maze M: Biologic effects of nitrous oxide: a mechanistic and toxicologic review. Anesthesiology 109(4):707–722, 2008 18813051

Schellhorn SE, Barnhill JW, Raiteri V, et al: A comparison of psychiatric consultation between geriatric and non-geriatric medical inpatients. Int J Geriatr Psychiatry 24(10):1054–1061, 2009 19326400

Scher CS, Anwar M: The self-reporting of psychiatric medications in patients scheduled for elective surgery. J Clin Anesth 11(8):619–621, 1999 10680101

Schmidt AP, Valinetti EA, Bandeira D, et al: Effects of preanesthetic administration of midazolam, clonidine, or dexmedetomidine on postoperative pain and anxiety in children. Paediatr Anaesth 17(7):667–674, 2007 17564649

Schönenberg M, Reichwald U, Domes G, et al: Ketamine aggravates symptoms of acute stress disorder in a naturalistic sample of accident victims. J Psychopharmacol 22(5):493–497, 2008 18208917

Schrijver EJ, de Vries OJ, Verburg A, et al: Efficacy and safety of haloperidol prophylaxis for delirium prevention in older medical and surgical at-risk patients acutely admitted to hospital through the emergency department: study protocol of a multicenter, randomized, double-blind, placebo-controlled clinical trial. BMC Geriatr 28(14):96, 2014

Schrøder Pedersen S, Kirkegaard T, Balslev Jørgensen M, Lind Jørgensen V: Effects of a screening and treatment protocol with haloperidol on post-cardiotomy delirium: a prospective cohort study. Interact Cardiovasc Thorac Surg 18(4):438–445, 2014 24357472

Serafim RB, Bozza FA, Soares M, et al: Pharmacologic prevention and treatment of delirium in intensive care patients: a systematic review. J Crit Care 30(4):799–807, 2015 25957498

Sharma ND, Rosman HS, Padhi ID, Tisdale JE: Torsades de pointes associated with intravenous haloperidol in critically ill patients. Am J Cardiol 81(2):238–240, 1998 9591913

Shehabi Y, Grant P, Wolfenden H, et al: Prevalence of delirium with dexmedetomidine compared with morphine based therapy after cardiac surgery: a randomized controlled trial (DEXmedetomidine COmpared to Morphine-DEXCOM Study). Anesthesiology 111(5):1075–1084, 2009 19786862

Skrobik YK, Bergeron N, Dumont M, Gottfried SB: Olanzapine vs haloperidol: treating delirium in a critical care setting. Intensive Care Med 30(3):444–449, 2004 14685663

Smith MS, Muir H, Hall R: Perioperative management of drug therapy, clinical considerations. Drugs 51(2):238–259, 1996 8808166

Stein MB, Kerridge C, Dimsdale JE, Hoyt DB: Pharmacotherapy to prevent PTSD: Results from a randomized controlled proof-of-concept trial in physically injured patients. J Trauma Stress 20(6):923–932, 2007 18157888

Tahir TA, Eeles E, Karapareddy V, et al: A randomized controlled trial of quetiapine versus placebo in the treatment of delirium. J Psychosom Res 69(5):485–490, 2010 20955868

Trzepacz PT: Is there a final common neural pathway in delirium? Focus on acetylcholine and dopamine. Semin Clin Neuropsychiatry 5(2):132–148, 2000 10837102

U.S. Food and Drug Administration: Information for healthcare professionals: haloperidol (marketed as Haldol, Haldol Decanoate and Haldol Lactate). 2007. Available at: http://www.fda.gov/Drugs/DrugSafety/PostmarketDrugSafetyInformationfor PatientsandProviders/DrugSafetyInformationforHeathcareProfessionals/ ucm085203.htm. Accessed April 28, 2016.

van den Boogaard M, Slooter AJ, Brüggemann RJ, et al: Prevention of ICU delirium and delirium-related outcome with haloperidol: a study protocol for a multi-center randomized controlled trial. Trials 21(14):400, 2013

Walker KJ, Smith AF: Premedication for anxiety in adult day surgery. Cochrane Database of Systematic Reviews 2009, Issue 4. Art. No.: CD002192. DOI: 10.1002/ 14651858.CD002192.pub2 19821294

Wang W, Li HL, Wang DX, et al: Haloperidol prophylaxis decreases delirium incidence in elderly patients after noncardiac surgery: a randomized controlled trial. Crit Care Med 40(3):731–739, 2012 22067628

White PF, Tufanogullari B, Taylor J, Klein K: The effect of pregabalin on preoperative anxiety and sedation levels: a dose-ranging study. Anesth Analg 108(4):1140–1145, 2009 19299776

Wright KD, Stewart SH, Finley GA, Buffett-Jerrott SE: Prevention and intervention strategies to alleviate preoperative anxiety in children: a critical review. Behav Modif 31(1):52–79, 2007 17179531

Yan M, Webster LT Jr, Blumer JL: Kinetic interactions of dopamine and dobutamine with human catechol-O-methyltransferase and monoamine oxidase in vitro. J Pharmacol Exp Ther 301(1):315–321, 2002 11907189

Yoon HJ, Park KM, Choi WJ, et al: Efficacy and safety of haloperidol versus atypical antipsychotic medications in the treatment of delirium. BMC Psychiatry 30(13):240, 2013

Zatzick D, Roy-Byrne P, Russo J, et al: A randomized effectiveness trial of stepped collaborative care for acutely injured trauma survivors. Arch Gen Psychiatry 61(5):498–506, 2004 15123495

16

Organ Transplantation

Marian Fireman, M.D.

Andrea F. DiMartini, M.D.

Catherine C. Crone, M.D.

Transplantation engenders many biopsychosocial stressors, resulting in rates of anxiety and mood symptoms, delirium, and cognitive disorders in transplant cohorts that are similar to or higher than rates in other medically ill populations. Untreated psychiatric disorders can have impacts on psychiatric as well as transplant medical outcomes and adherence to necessary posttransplant routines. Pharmacotherapy is an essential component of the psychiatric care of many transplant patients.

Organ disease alters many aspects of drug pharmacokinetics, changing the bioavailability and disposition of medications and both the intended therapeutic action and side effects. For a full review of pharmacokinetics of psychotropic drugs in general and in hepatic, renal, bowel, heart, and lung diseases in particular, the reader is referred to Chapter 1, "Pharmacokinetics, Pharmacodynamics, and Principles of Drug-Drug Interactions," and the respective chapters on these organ systems. Our primary focus for this chapter is on key points in the management of psychopathology in adult transplant patients. Topics include the physiological properties of the newly transplanted organ as this relates to drug pharmacokinetics, the psychopharmacological treatment of psychiatric illness that arises pretransplant to posttransplant, and the neuropsychiatric adverse effects and drug-drug interactions related to immunosuppressant medications. Considering these pharmacological issues and the wide interpatient variability, we provide guidelines for drug choice and dosing.

Posttransplant Pharmacological Considerations

Posttransplant Organ Functioning

For the majority of recipients, a newly transplanted organ functions immediately such that normal physiological parameters are quickly restored and pharmacokinetic abnormalities resolve. For patients with stable liver or kidney functioning within the first month following transplant, the clearance and steady-state volume of distribution of drugs have been shown to be similar to those of healthy volunteers (Hebert et al. 2003). Thus, most transplant recipients can be treated using normal therapeutic drug dosing, assuming that patients have recovered from the immediate postoperative complications (e.g., sedation, delirium, ileus) and are able to take oral medications.

For some recipients, however, the transplanted organ does not assume autonomous normal physiological functioning immediately, or the organ may assume normal functioning slowly over time. Posttransplant pharmacokinetic studies addressing these issues have been conducted mostly in liver and kidney recipients because of the importance of these organs in drug pharmacokinetics. Such studies have investigated only immunosuppressive medications because of the need to achieve and maintain stable immunosuppressant levels to prevent organ rejection, the ability to monitor serum levels, and the narrow therapeutic range of these drugs. These data can provide general guidance on psychotropic medication prescribing in specific types of posttransplant organ dysfunction.

Primary nonfunction, occurring in 3%–4% of liver and renal transplant recipients (Kemmer et al. 2007; U.S. Renal Data System 2008), is primary graft failure that results in death or retransplantation within 30 days of the transplant. For liver recipients with primary nonfunction, survival beyond the fifth postoperative day is uncommon, and life support until another organ becomes available is the focus of therapy. The intensive care unit team will often use intravenous benzodiazepines, propofol, dexmedetomidine, or narcotics for rapid sedation and pain management.

The most common allograft complication affecting pharmacokinetics in the immediate posttransplant period is delayed graft function (DGF). DGF occurs in 10%–50% of liver recipients (Angelico 2005). Such patients were shown to require half of the immunosuppressant dosage required by those without DGF, and these dosing requirements did not correlate with body weight. This finding suggests that in the early posttransplant period, metabolic capacity rather than volume of distribution is the critical factor in pharmacokinetics (Hebert et al. 2003; Lück et al. 2004).

DGF occurs in 25%–50% of renal transplant recipients and is defined as the recipient's requiring dialysis within the first week of transplant (Shoshes and Cecka 1998; U.S. Renal Data System 2008). Immunosuppressant pharmacokinetic studies show that DGF alters pharmacokinetics by mechanisms that increase the free fraction of parent drugs and renally excreted metabolites (Shaw et al. 1998). Delayed renal elimination of immunosuppressants for patients in severe or acute renal impairment posttransplant can result in levels three to six times higher than those in nonimpaired recipients for both renally excreted drugs and their metabolites (Bullingham et al. 1998; Shaw et al. 1998). DGF also affects the binding of drugs to plasma proteins even in the absence of hypoalbuminemia (Shaw et al. 1998).

Posttransplant Organ Rejection

Acute cellular rejection occurs in 20%–70% of liver transplant recipients, most often within the first 3 weeks posttransplant, and results in transient graft dysfunction. Delirium may be a clinical manifestation. Acute rejection is most commonly treated with high-dose steroids, effective in 65%–80% of cases. Alternative therapies, required in about 15% of cases, include antibody treatments, such as monoclonal therapy or antithymocyte globulin (Lake 2003). These agents, particularly high-dose steroids, can cause serious neuropsychiatric side effects (see the subsection "Neuropsychiatric Effects of Immunosuppressant Medications and Their Treatment" later in this chapter).

Chronic graft rejection, manifested by gradual obliteration of small bile ducts and microvascular changes, occurs in about 5%–10% of liver recipients and responds poorly to changes in immunosuppression. Patients may have jaundice and/or difficult-to-manage pruritus. Loss of liver synthetic function may not be evident until very late in the course (Lake 2003).

An estimated 20%–60% of kidney recipients will experience an episode of acute rejection, most often within the first 6 months after transplant. However, up to 25%–30% of recipients with stable or improving renal function will actually be in an undetected rejection episode (Rush et al. 1998; Shapiro et al. 2001). With treatment, acute rejection typically resolves quickly with restoration of prerejection renal function, whereas undetected subclinical rejection can result in gradually worsening renal function over time, with eventual graft loss (Rush et al. 1998).

Nearly 50% of heart transplant recipients will experience an episode of acute rejection (either humoral or cellular) within the first posttransplant year. Most episodes are treated with the addition of steroids to the baseline immunosuppressive regimen. Ischemic injury usually occurs in the early posttransplant period and can also cause allograft dysfunction (Michaels et al. 2003). Sinus node dysfunction or atrioventricular block requiring permanent pacing occurs in 5%–19% of heart transplant recipients and may be associated with rejection (Collins et al. 2003). Psychotropics, particularly those with the potential to prolong the QTc interval or cause conduction delay by other mechanisms, should be used with caution in these patients (see also Chapter 6, "Cardiovascular Disorders").

General Posttransplant Issues

In addition to overt DGF or rejection, some recipients will have transient physiological abnormalities in the weeks following transplant that could also affect pharmacokinetics (e.g., liver congestion and/or renal hypoperfusion in heart recipients, fluid overload in renal recipients, liver hypoperfusion and fluid overload in liver recipients). Liver transplant patients often develop pretransplant altered hemodynamics with fluid retention (i.e., ascites, peripheral edema, and pleural effusions) and/or hepatorenal syndrome. Generally, once normal hemodynamics are restored posttransplant, hepatorenal syndrome resolves. Nonetheless, up to 20% of patients may develop persisting fluid retention in the form of moderate to large pleural and peritoneal fluid collections, resulting in fluctuating drug volume of distribution. In addition, nearly 20% of liver recipients require postoperative dialysis in the days to weeks following transplant, mostly to treat resolving hepatorenal syndrome and volume overload (Contreras et al. 2002). Principles of psychotropic management during hemodialysis should be employed (see Chapter 5, "Renal and Urological Disorders").

In addition, underlying disease processes or other comorbid organ insufficiencies that are not corrected by organ transplant may have an impact on drug pharmacokinetics. For example, patients with cystic fibrosis who receive a lung transplant may continue to have delayed gastric emptying, pancreatic insufficiency with malabsorption, and altered liver metabolism and renal clearance that impair normal cyclosporine kinetics (Reynaud-Gaubert et al. 1997).

Chronic graft rejection is potentially reversible in the early stages but not once chronic dysfunction has set in, after which progressive graft failure may occur. Thus, for transplant recipients, adherence to lifelong immunosuppressants is critical. Unfortunately, for all organ types, immunosuppressant nonadherence is a major risk factor for rejection and may be responsible for up to 25%–30% of graft loss and late deaths after the initial recovery period (Bunzel and Laederach-Hofmann 2000; Schweizer et al. 1990). Attempts to identify and alleviate immunosuppressant side effects may improve adherence. Unfortunately, the treatment of most types of graft dysfunction (DGF or acute or chronic rejection) typically requires an increase in the dosage of the primary calcineurin-inhibiting medication and/or addition of other immunosuppressants, including monoclonal antibodies, steroids, mycophenolate, or sirolimus, which tend to create or exacerbate neuropsychiatric side effects (see the subsection "Neuropsychiatric Effects of Immunosuppressant Medications and Their Treatment" later in this chapter). Additionally, depression has been implicated in cases of nonadherence, and mood symptoms should be elicited and treated.

Finally, for all organ types, calcineurin-inhibiting immunosuppressants are nephrotoxic, and chronic use results in renal failure for 10%–20% of recipients by 5 years posttransplant (Ojo et al. 2003). Thus, the quality of renal function should always be considered, especially for long-term transplant recipients.

With the resumption of normal graft function, psychotropic medications that may have been prescribed in lower dosages pretransplant to account for diminished metabolism or elimination may need to be adjusted to higher dosages posttransplant. Another important consideration is pain management for patients taking chronic opioids pretransplant; higher than average dosages of narcotic analgesics may be required perioperatively. In one specific example, patients undergoing methadone maintenance therapy, for whom methadone was also used as their postoperative pain medication, required an average methadone dosage increase of 60% posttransplant, presumably to adjust for chronic downregulation of μ opiate pain receptors from chronic methadone exposure (Weinrieb et al. 2004) and improvement in metabolism posttransplant.

Living Organ Donation Issues: Recipients and Donors

Living donor liver transplant recipients make up only approximately 4% of liver transplant procedures in the United States (Health Resources and Services Administration Division of Transplantation 2006), but these recipients require special pharmacological consideration. Because living donor liver transplant recipients receive grafts that are 55%–60% of normal liver volume, they initially require smaller doses of medication. Pharmacokinetic studies with immunosuppressants suggest that medication doses should be reduced by 30% compared with doses given to deceased donor recipients to achieve similar therapeutic levels in the early postoperative period (Jain et al. 2008). In addition to the fact that a reduced-size liver clears drugs less readily, animal models suggest that glucuronide conjugation is impaired during the first several weeks of hepatic regeneration (Jain et al. 2008).

Living donor liver transplant recipients can experience an uncommon technical complication termed *small-for-size syndrome* (SFSS). SFSS occurs when a partial liver graft is unable to meet the functional demands of the recipient, resulting in a clinical syndrome characterized by postoperative liver dysfunction. The incidence of SFSS is reported to be in the 5%–10% range after partial liver transplant but may be higher depending on the status of the recipient and the type of graft used (Tucker and Heaton 2005). SFSS is characterized by prolonged cholestasis, elevated liver enzymes, and coagulopathy combined with manifestations of portal hypertension such as ascites. Without any intervention, approximately 50% of recipients with SFSS will die of sepsis within 4–6 weeks posttransplant (Dahm et al. 2005). Using psychotropics in these patients requires close attention to liver function, fluid status, and coagulopathy.

For living liver donors, little is known about the rate and extent of the restoration of hepatic function, especially following right lobe hepatectomy, a procedure involving more extensive removal of hepatic tissue (50%–60% of the liver mass). Existing literature suggests that the liver mass of donors can return to approximately 80%–100% of baseline by several weeks to months following donation, despite biochemical abnormalities persisting beyond 2 months (Emre 2001; Nadalin et al. 2004). One preliminary study of donor liver function showed that hepatic galactose elimination capacity, a measure of liver function, was only 50% by 10 days following hepatic resection despite rapid return of liver volume (Jochum et al. 2006). By 3 months, complete function was restored (Jochum et al. 2006).

Psychotropic considerations for live liver donors must take into account the time since donation and the potential for incomplete restoration of metabolic capacity. Long-term hepatic function in liver donors is unknown but is assumed to return to normal. Several studies of liver donors' psychological outcomes evaluated using specific psychiatric assessments found that substantial percentages of liver donors, 10%–14%, have symptoms that meet criteria for diagnosable depressive and/or anxiety disorders within the first year postdonation (Erim et al. 2006, 2007; Fukunishi et al. 2001).

Kidney donors lose half of their functional nephron mass with donor nephrectomy. In the year following nephrectomy, donor creatinine clearance can decrease by 30% compared with preoperative levels but still be within normal limits (Bieniasz et al. 2009). With long-term follow-up, kidney donors continue to have 72%–77% of predonation creatinine clearance and an incidence of proteinuria as high as 19%–31% (Najarian et al. 1992; Zafar et al. 2002). Although most donors experience a decrease in glomerular filtration rate immediately after donation, the risk of end-stage renal failure is low, approximately 0.2%–0.5% (Azar et al. 2007). In one study, after 1-year follow-up, 9.3% of donors were prescribed antidepressants for severe depression, suggesting a substantial need for psychotropics in donors (Azar et al. 2007).

Psychotropic Medications in Transplant Patients

Although no psychotropic medication is absolutely contraindicated for use in transplant patients, specific precautions and careful selection are necessary. Patients in end-stage organ failure are typically more sensitive to medication side effects. For example, patients with psychomotor retardation or cognitive impairment due to uremia, hypoxia, or hepatic encephalopathy often cannot tolerate psychotropics with significant sedating side effects (e.g., benzodiazepines, mirtazapine, paroxetine). Pharmacokinetic changes (e.g., delayed absorption, altered volume of distribution, impaired metabolism, reduced excretion) caused by organ failure will also require dosing adjustments. After transplant, drug-drug interactions become a greater concern because patients are maintained on a broad array of medications (e.g., immunosuppressants, antihypertensives, antibiotics, lipid-lowering agents, hypoglycemic drugs).

QTc interval prolongation is an important issue for patients prescribed psychotropic medications. Many psychotropics are known to prolong the QTc interval, and a number have been associated with torsades de pointes, a malignant ventricular arrhythmia. Many pretransplant patients may be taking other medications with known potential to cause QTc prolongation and/or torsades de pointes. Posttransplant, the immunosuppressant medications (e.g., cyclosporine, tacrolimus) are known to prolong QTc interval. Furthermore, posttransplant patients are frequently prescribed other medications with potential to prolong the QTc interval. Care must be taken when prescribing multiple medications known to prolong the QTc interval; frequent ECG monitoring and/or cardiology consultation may be necessary (Beach et al. 2013).

In the following subsections, we provide guidance by drug class regarding the selection of psychotropics with respect to specific side effects and organ disease. These guidelines apply both to pretransplant patients with organ failure and to posttransplant patients without complete restoration of organ function. Because few data are available specifically on transplant patients, information on nontransplant patients with advanced organ disease is included.

Antidepressants

The prevalence of depressive and anxiety disorders among transplant patients is high and contributes to increased morbidity and mortality if left untreated. Patients often do well with antidepressant therapy, and appropriate medication treatment should not be avoided because of concerns over organ disease. Antidepressants may provide additional benefits to the management of organ failure symptoms, such as nausea, anorexia, insomnia, pruritus, and intradialytic hypotension. Posttransplant, antidepressants can be helpful not only for primary psychiatric disorders but also for disorders that are secondary to immunosuppressants.

Selective Serotonin Reuptake Inhibitors

Selective serotonin reuptake inhibitors (SSRIs) are the primary choice for transplant patients because of their relative safety. Although relatively unstudied in posttransplant patients, citalopram, sertraline, paroxetine, and fluoxetine have been studied to varying degrees in patients with end-stage organ disease (Gottlieb et al. 2007; Kalender et al. 2007; Lacasse et al. 2004), with generally positive results; however, caution must be exercised because of the very limited number of randomized controlled trials.

SSRIs inhibit platelet activation and may prolong bleeding time. Although possibly beneficial for those patients with congestive heart failure who are prone to thromboembolism, SSRIs carry some risk for patients with cirrhosis, who are prone to bleeding due to varices, coagulopathy, and thrombocytopenia (Serebruany et al. 2003; Weinrieb et al. 2003). SSRIs should be used with caution in patients already taking drugs that increase bleeding risk (e.g., acetylsalicylic acid [aspirin] and other nonsteroidal anti-inflammatory drugs, antiplatelet agents) (Weinrieb et al. 2005). All of the SSRIs may cause some degree of QTc prolongation, although citalopram is the only agent that carries recommendations for dose limitation (Beach et al. 2013).

Among the SSRIs, citalopram and escitalopram have the fewest drug-drug interactions. U.S. Food and Drug Administration (FDA) recommendations call for limiting citalopram dosage to 40 mg/day; dosages not greater than 20 mg/day in patients with hepatic impairment or older than age 60 are suggested (Beach et al. 2013). Citalopram was effective for mild to moderate depression in depressed lung transplant recipients (Silvertooth et al. 2004).

Sertraline has the second fewest drug interactions of the SSRIs and is often the SSRI of choice because of issues of cost and decreased likelihood of QT prolongation as compared with citalopram. It significantly reduced itch scores in cholestatic jaundice patients, independent of effects on depression (Mayo et al. 2007). In dialysis patients, it lessened intradialytic hypotension, a common hemodialysis complication (Yalcin et al. 2002).

Paroxetine is generally associated with greater weight gain than other SSRIs, which may be beneficial for poor nutritional status, a common problem among patients with end-stage organ disease. In depressed patients with end-stage renal disease, paroxetine combined with psychotherapy reduced depression and improved nutritional status (e.g., serum albumin, predialysis blood urea nitrogen)

(Koo et al. 2005). Tolerability is a concern because of paroxetine's anticholinergic side effects and discontinuation syndrome.

Fluvoxamine is generally avoided in transplant patients because it is a strong inhibitor of multiple cytochrome P450 (CYP) isozymes. Use of this agent may result in adverse drug-drug interactions.

Vilazodone, approved by the FDA in 2011 for treatment of major depression, is both an SSRI and a partial serotonin type 1A (5-HT$_{1A}$) agonist. It does not appear to cause electrocardiogram changes. The metabolism of vilazodone may be inhibited by strong CYP3A4 inhibitors (Wang et al. 2015). Vortioxetine is an SSRI with additional agonist activity at 5-HT$_{1A}$ and 5-HT$_{1B}$ receptors and inhibitory activity at 5-HT$_3$, 5-HT$_7$, and 5-HT$_{1D}$ receptors. Levels of vortioxetine may be affected by CYP2D6 inhibitors (Garnock-Jones 2014). Vilazodone and vortioxetine are expensive as compared with other antidepressants, and there is little experience with use of these medications in patients with end-organ disease or with organ transplants.

Mirtazapine

Mirtazapine is a unique agent that preferentially blocks presynaptic α_2, histamine, and 5-hydroxytryptamine type 2 (5-HT$_2$) and type 3 (5-HT$_3$) receptors. By blocking 5-HT$_3$ receptors, mirtazapine provides antiemetic effects, a valuable feature for transplant patients with nausea from medications and organ failure (Kim et al. 2004). Mirtazapine may relieve persistent pruritus caused by uremia or cholestasis by blockade of histamine, 5-HT$_2$, and 5-HT$_3$ receptors (Davis et al. 2003). It may improve appetite and promote weight gain, which can be advantageous for some patients, but following transplant, mirtazapine may accentuate immunosuppressant-induced weight gain and hyperlipidemia (Kim et al. 2004; McIntyre et al. 2006). It may cause agranulocytosis, neutropenia, and other reductions in hematological parameters and should be used cautiously in patients taking drugs that can cause blood dyscrasias (e.g., immunosuppressants, interferon). Although rare, these events can be especially serious in immunocompromised patients. Because mirtazapine lacks inhibitory effects on CYP isozymes, there is little risk of drug-drug interactions (Crone and Gabriel 2004). Mirtazapine should not be combined with clonidine because these agents act in opposition at central α_2 receptors. Combination of these agents may result in loss of effectiveness of clonidine for treatment of hypertension (Abo-Zena et al. 2000).

Bupropion

Although the activating side effects associated with bupropion can be difficult for some patients to tolerate, activation and lack of sedation can be useful for transplant patients with persistent fatigue. Bupropion may also be useful for smoking cessation (Wagena et al. 2005). It can elevate blood pressure and should be used with caution in end-stage organ disease and posttransplant patients with preexisting and persistent hypertension associated with immunosuppressants. Although the risk of seizures is low at therapeutic doses, cautious use is required for patients at risk for seizures from other causes (e.g., hepatic encephalopathy, high-dose immunosuppression). Bupropion is a strong inhibitor of CYP2D6, so care must be exercised when it is combined with medications metabolized by this isozyme. Although most immunosuppressants are not metabolized by CYP2D6, other medications frequently prescribed to transplant patients (e.g., other psychotropics and β-blockers) are CYP2D6 substrates. In addition, use of lower doses is recommended in end-stage liver disease.

Serotonin-Norepinephrine Reuptake Inhibitors

Venlafaxine, desvenlafaxine, and duloxetine can elevate blood pressure, and caution should be exercised as with bupropion. Duloxetine has been reported to cause severe liver toxicity in rare cases (McIntyre et al. 2008; see also Chapter 4, "Gastrointestinal Disorders"). Levomilnacipran, the most recently approved medication in this class, is a more potent inhibitor of norepinephrine reuptake. This action may improve cognition but may also cause elevations in heart rate and blood pressure. Levels of levomilnacipran are affected by renal function, and doses must be decreased in moderate to severe renal impairment. Levels of levomilnacipran may be increased by strong CYP3A4 inhibitors (Scott 2014). Similar to other new agents, there is little known about the use of this drug in transplant patients.

Nefazodone

The risk of serious hepatotoxicity and CYP3A4 inhibition makes nefazodone an undesirable choice for transplant patients. There have been several cases of immunosuppressant toxicity due to nefazodone's inhibiting CYP3A4 (see the subsection "Drug-Drug Interactions" later in this chapter).

Trazodone

Trazodone is similar in action to nefazodone but lacks significant hepatotoxicity. The sedating side effects are helpful for persistent insomnia but may be intolerable for patients with psychomotor slowing or cognitive impairment, common among patients with end-stage organ disease and neuropsychiatric side effects from immunosuppressants. Care is needed in those heart disease patients who are more prone to its orthostatic and arrhythmogenic effects. Trazodone does not appear to have effects on the CYP isozymes.

Tricyclic Antidepressants

Tricyclic antidepressants (TCAs) are a secondary choice in the transplant population because of safety and tolerability issues. TCAs have significant effects on the cardiovascular system, producing quinidine-like (type 1A) antiarrhythmic activity, orthostatic hypotension, intraventricular conduction delay, QTc prolongation, and increased heart rate (Fusar-Poli et al. 2006). Weight gain, changes in lipid levels, and anticholinergic side effects may be undesirable for transplant patients (McIntyre et al. 2008). Secondary-amine TCAs (desipramine, nortriptyline) are preferred over tertiary-amine TCAs because of a less severe adverse-effect profile. Nortriptyline offers the advantage of established therapeutic drug levels and reports of safe use in some transplant recipients (Kay et al. 1991; Shapiro 1991).

Monoamine Oxidase Inhibitors

In general, monoamine oxidase inhibitors pose an excessive risk for safety and tolerability (e.g., drug-drug interactions, potential hypertensive crises) in transplant patients. Transdermal selegiline may be an option for those treatment-resistant patients who are unable to take oral medications or who lack adequate bowel absorption (Pae et al. 2007; see also Chapter 3, "Alternative Routes of Drug Administration").

Psychostimulants

Methylphenidate and dextroamphetamine are effective for short-term treatment of depressive symptoms in medically ill patients. Both offer the advantage of rapid onset of action and are useful in reducing apathy, fatigue, and cognitive dulling. Methylphenidate was markedly effective for at least four of eight liver transplant patients experiencing depression, apathy, and cognitive impairment (Plutchik et al. 1998). Although supraventricular tachycardia has been reported in a heart recipient treated with methylphenidate, stimulants have been used safely in patients with significant cardiac disease without marked changes in blood pressure or heart rate (Come and Shapiro 2005; Masand et al.

1991). Nevertheless, close monitoring for elevations in blood pressure or heart rate or for worsening congestive heart failure is necessary.

Modafinil has been used clinically in transplant patients; however, particularly at dosages of 400 mg/day or more, modafinil inhibits CYP2C9 and CYP2C19 and weakly induces CYP1A2 and CYP2B6. At higher doses, modafanil is a moderate to strong inducer of CYP3A4, which may be problematic in combination with immunosuppressants (see the subsection "Drug-Drug Interactions" later in this chapter). Armodafinil has metabolic interactions similar to those of modafinil.

Atomoxetine is a selective norepinephrine reuptake inhibitor used for the treatment of attention-deficit/hyperactivity disorder. It is not classified as a stimulant. No reports of atomoxetine use in transplant patients have been published. However, because of CYP2D6 inhibition and warnings regarding potential hepatotoxicity, other medications are preferred.

Benzodiazepines

Benzodiazepines are effective in providing anxiolysis to transplant patients but may worsen sedation, respiratory suppression, preexisting cognitive impairment, or encephalopathy in patients with end-stage organ disease. Lorazepam, oxazepam, and temazepam require only glucuronidation and may be a safer choice in patients with cirrhosis (Crone and Gabriel 2004) or impaired posttransplant hepatic function. Clonazepam has been successfully used to manage steroid-induced mania in transplant recipients (Viswanathan and Glickman 1989).

Buspirone

Buspirone, a serotonin partial agonist, is marketed for the treatment of generalized anxiety disorder. It is often ineffective for patients previously treated with benzodiazepines. It may be helpful in transplant patients with anxiety because it does not cause respiratory depression, but its metabolism may be affected by inhibitors of CYP3A4 and P-glycoprotein.

Antipsychotic Agents

Antipsychotics are commonly used for transplant patients to manage agitation and psychosis associated with acute delirium, mood disorders secondary to immunosuppressants (e.g., mania), and comorbid primary psychiatric disorders (e.g., bipolar disorder, schizophrenia). They can also be used for anxiolysis (e.g., in patients with advanced pulmonary disease or patients being weaned off ventilators). A concern is their risk of QTc prolongation, torsades de pointes, and sudden death (Beach et al. 2013; Haddad and Anderson 2002; Pacher and Kecskemeti 2004; see also Chapter 6). Transplant patients often have other risk factors for cardiac arrhythmia (e.g., electrolyte imbalance, renal or hepatic disease, heart failure, ventricular hypertrophy, other QTc-prolonging drugs) (Haddad and Anderson 2002; Zareba and Lin 2003).

Haloperidol

Haloperidol is the primary typical antipsychotic used in transplant patients because of its varied routes of administration, therapeutic efficacy, overall tolerability, and few side effects. It is an excellent choice for managing agitation and/or psychosis in delirious transplant patients (see also Chapter 15, "Surgery and Critical Care"). In rare cases, extremely high dosages of intravenous haloperidol (>1,000 mg/day) have been safely used to control severe agitation (Levenson 1995). Haloperidol can also treat psychosis from immunosuppressant neurotoxicity (see the subsection "Neuropsychiatric Effects of Immunosuppressant Medications and Their Treatment" later in this chapter) (Tripathi and Panzer 1993). Extrapyramidal side effects should be monitored in transplant patients with encephalopathy. QTc prolongation should be monitored closely in patients receiving haloperidol, particularly intravenous haloperidol (Beach et al. 2013).

Atypical Antipsychotics

Atypical antipsychotics may be employed for agitation, insomnia, anxiety, mania, and delirium associated with end-stage organ disease or posttransplant immunosuppressant reactions; however, no literature specific to transplant has been published. Atypical antipsychotics may cause weight gain, hyperlipidemia, and glucose intolerance, exacerbating the similar effects of immunosuppressant drugs. Olanzapine and quetiapine are often used in these patients for both their sedating side effects and lower risk of QTc prolongation. Aripiprazole may be a useful choice if sedation is not desired; it also has the lowest risk of QTc prolongation (Beach et al. 2013).

Mood Stabilizers

Lithium is complicated to use in patients awaiting transplant and those who are recent recipients because of problems with fluid imbalance. Other mood stabilizers pose more of a challenge after transplant because they interact with immunosuppressants, altering immunosuppressant drug levels. The choice of mood stabilizer for a transplant patient depends on the patient's history of symptoms and prior treatment and type of organ disease.

Lithium

Maintaining lithium levels within a narrow therapeutic window is complicated in transplant patients. In patients with dehydration, congestive heart failure, cirrhosis, nephrotic syndrome, or cystic fibrosis, sodium retention mechanisms are activated and lithium clearance is reduced (Thomsen and Schou 1999). Fluctuating fluid status from dehydration (due to fever, sweating, or decreased intake) or fluid overload (e.g., edema, ascites) can also make maintenance of stable nontoxic lithium levels difficult (Thomsen and Schou 1999). Cyclosporine, a common immunosuppressant, increases lithium levels by altering proximal tubular reabsorption (Vincent et al. 1987). Other drugs used before or after transplant (e.g., angiotensin-converting enzyme inhibitors, spironolactone, calcium channel blockers) can alter lithium levels. Lithium can cause renal tubular damage with loss of urine-concentrating ability (see Chapter 5). Posttransplant, these potential adverse effects of lithium must be carefully considered, especially when lithium is combined with nephrotoxic immunosuppressant therapy. Lithium can cause weight gain, cognitive slowing, and tremor, potentially aggravating common posttransplant problems (DasGupta and Jefferson 1990).

Valproic Acid

Valproic acid is a less desirable choice for patients with preexisting hepatic impairment, and its use for treatment of short-term immunosuppressant mood instability is not advisable given its potentially serious side effects (e.g., hepatotoxicity, thrombocytopenia, platelet dysfunction). Reduced serum albumin concentrations due to cirrhosis, renal disease, cachexia, other catabolic states and elevated free fatty acid concentrations in the setting of diabetes, hemodialysis, and hypertriglyceridemia can raise free valproic acid levels, resulting in an increased risk of sedation, cognitive slowing, and lethargy (Haroldson et al. 2000).

Carbamazepine and Oxcarbazepine

Carbamazepine may cause leukopenia and poses a rare risk of serious blood dyscrasias, including aplastic anemia and agranulocytosis, which are especially concerning for patients taking immunosuppressants or those who are immunocompromised because of end-stage organ disease (Schatzberg and DeBattista 2015). It may alter vitamin D levels and bone turnover, potentially increasing the risk for osteoporosis from immunosuppressant therapy (Mintzer et al. 2006). In patients with renal failure or cirrhosis, levels of carbamazepine and its pharmacologically active metabolite 10,11-epoxide should be closely monitored (Tutor-Crespo et al. 2008). Carbamazepine may induce CYP3A4, lowering tacrolimus and cyclosporine levels (see the subsection "Drug-Drug Interactions" later in this chapter). Oxcarbazepine, although not associated with blood dyscrasias, is a weak inducer of CYP3A4 and can reduce immunosuppressant levels (Rösche et al. 2001; Wang and Ketter 2002). Hyponatremia has been observed in up to 25%–50% of patients treated with oxcarbazepine, and oxcarbazepine use has also been associated with lower vitamin D levels and increased bone turnover (Asconapé 2002; Mintzer et al. 2006).

Gabapentin

Gabapentin can be used to treat anxiety disorders, neuropathic pain (e.g., immunosuppressant-induced neuropathy, postherpetic neuralgia), restless legs syndrome, and uremic pruritus (Colman and Stadel 1999; Molnar et al. 2006; Naini et al. 2007). These conditions are common in transplant patients, particularly those with renal failure. Because gabapentin is renally excreted rather than hepatically metabolized, the dosage must be reduced in proportion to the decline in creatinine clearance (Wong et al. 1995).

Topiramate

Topiramate is generally undesirable for transplant patients because of its tendency to cause cognitive impairment and possible metabolic acidosis (Schatzberg and DeBattista 2015). Cognitive side effects are especially problematic for patients with cognitive dysfunction due to end-stage organ disease or high-dose immunosuppressants.

Medications Used to Treat Substance Use Disorders

Medications to reduce cravings or block the effect of substances and potentially diminish relapse risk for alcohol, opioids, and tobacco have not been studied in transplant patients. Nevertheless, the known pharmacodynamics of these drugs can provide guidance for their use (see Chapter 18, "Substance Use Disorders").

For treating alcohol dependence, disulfiram is not advised in transplant patients because of possible serious side effects and significant interactions with drugs requiring CYP metabolism (e.g., posttransplant immunosuppressants) (Chick 1999; DiMartini et al. 2005; Krahn and DiMartini 2005). Acamprosate should be used cautiously because rare cases of cardiomyopathy, heart failure, and renal failure have occurred. In renal impairment (creatinine clearance 30–50 mL/min), half dose should be given; acamprosate is contraindicated for creatinine clearance of 30 mL/min or less (Overman et al. 2003; Saivin et al. 1998). Naltrexone, an opioid antagonist, is contraindicated in severe hepatic disease and may cause hepatotoxicity, particularly at dosages of 300 mg/day or more (Krahn and DiMartini 2005). Naltrexone may be helpful for short-term treatment of pruritus in severe liver disease (Parés 2014). Postoperative use is contraindicated because of antagonism of opioid analgesia. Patients surveyed following liver transplant were reluctant to use naltrexone because of potential hepatotoxicity (Weinrieb et al. 2001).

For nicotine dependence, nicotine replacement therapies are generally contraindicated in patients with serious heart disease because of the potential for increasing angina and heart rate and possibly exacerbating arrhythmias. Caution is advised, especially in heart transplant patients. Varenicline is renally excreted, and dose reductions are recommended in patients who have renal insufficiency or those undergoing dialysis. Side effects (e.g., nausea, vomiting) may be problematic in transplant patients.

Transplant patients undergoing methadone maintenance therapy for opioid dependence can be successfully managed, including through the provision of adequate postoperative analgesia. In patients with renal and hepatic failure, dose adjustment may be needed to minimize side effects and prevent worsening uremic or hepatic encephalopathy; however, higher doses may be required posttransplant because of resumption of normal metabolic capacity. Perioperatively, patients undergoing methadone maintenance therapy require careful attention to pain control. The dose can be increased for pain control or continued at a maintenance level with a different opioid added for acute postoperative pain. Sedation, respiratory depression, and other symptoms of opioid toxicity should be monitored (Jiao et al. 2010). Drug-drug interactions are common, particularly those mediated through CYP3A4 interactions. It is of note that methadone metabolism is not thought to be affected by cyclosporine (Indiana University Division of Clinical Pharmacology 2015; Meissner et al. 2014). A few cases of buprenorphine-induced hepatotoxicity in patients with known hepatitis C have been reported. Buprenorphine is metabolized by CYP3A4, and drug-drug interactions must be considered (Zuin et al. 2009), although these are less common than drug-drug interactions with methadone. Buprenorphine is not recommended perioperatively because it may precipitate withdrawal in patients taking opioids. Methadone has significant potential for QTc prolongation, whereas QTc prolongation with buprenorphine is minimal. If use of buprenorphine instead of methadone is possible, it may be a better choice in patients with end-organ disease and in posttransplant patients.

Drug-Specific Issues

Neuropsychiatric Effects of Immunosuppressant Medications and Their Treatment

Immunosuppressants commonly cause medical side effects (e.g., hyperglycemia, hypertension, nephrotoxicity, infections, increased risk for cancer), as well as neuropsychiatric side effects (see Table 16–1). Patients with neuropsychiatric symptoms often take combinations of immunosuppressants, making the contribution of any specific drug to the symptoms sometimes difficult to establish.

The mainstays of transplant immunosuppression are the calcineurin-inhibiting immunosuppressants (CNIs) cyclosporine and tacrolimus. Both drugs have similar neuropsychiatric side effects. Up to 40%–60% of transplant recipients experience mild symptoms, including tremulousness, headache, restlessness, insomnia, vivid dreams, photophobia, hyperesthesias or dysesthesias, anxiety, and agitation (Magee 2006; Tombazzi et al. 2006). Moderate to severe side effects—cognitive impairment, coma, seizures, focal neurological deficits, dysarthria, cortical blindness, and delirium—occur less often but can affect 21%–32% of patients during the early postoperative period (Bechstein 2000). Neuropsychiatric effects are more common with parenteral administration and early posttransplant, perhaps because of higher serum levels during this period.

CNIs have been associated with posterior reversible leukoencephalopathy syndrome, which produces a variety of symptoms depending on the location of the lesion(s). Symptoms may include headache, visual disturbances, seizures, focal neurological symptoms, decreased consciousness, and coma. Patients with

Table 16–1. Neuropsychiatric side effects of immunosuppressants

Medication	Neuropsychiatric side effects
Calcineurin inhibitors (cyclosporine/tacrolimus)	Fatigue, insomnia, anxiety, agitation, confusion, depression, hallucinations, cognitive impairment, seizures, neuropathy
Corticosteroids (e.g., prednisone)	Euphoria, depression, anxiety, agitation, insomnia, hallucinations, delusions, delirium, personality changes, cognitive impairment
Sirolimus	Pain, headache
Everolimus	Pain, headache, insomnia
Azathioprine	None described
Mycophenolate/mycophenolic acid	Pain, arthralgia, insomnia, tremor, headache, anxiety
Belatacept	Pain, headache, dizziness, tremor, insomnia, anxiety; associated with CNS posttransplant lymphoproliferative disorder
Monoclonal antibodies	
Basiliximab	Insomnia, fatigue, pain, headache, tremor
Alemtuzumab	Insomnia, anxiety
Rituximab	Anxiety, depression, delirium, hallucinations

Note. CNS=central nervous system.
Source. Alloway et al. 1998; Bajjoka and Anandan 2002; Bartynski and Boardman 2007; Bechstein 2000; DiMartini et al. 2008; Kershner and Wang-Cheng 1989; Magee 2006; National Library of Medicine 2015; Tombazzi et al. 2006.

moderate to serious symptoms should have a computed tomography scan or magnetic resonance imaging (MRI) of the brain to evaluate for characteristic cortical and subcortical white matter changes, typically involving the parietal or occipital lobes (Bartynski and Boardman 2007). Cases have been reported involving the anterior brain, cerebellum, and brain stem (Bartynski and Boardman 2007). Specific findings on fluid-attenuated inversion recovery MRI sequences and apparent diffusion coefficient mapping (sensitive to water diffusion) are especially useful in identifying the characteristic vasogenic edema seen in posterior reversible leukoencephalopathy syndrome (Ahn et al. 2003).

Neuropsychiatric adverse effects of high-dose corticosteroid treatment are reviewed in Chapter 10, "Endocrine and Metabolic Disorders."

Sirolimus, a non-CNI, appears to have relatively mild neuropsychiatric side effects, including tremor, insomnia, and headache. Azathioprine rarely causes neuropsychiatric side effects. Neuropsychiatric side effects with mycophenolate appear to be milder than those described with CNIs, but up to 20% of patients may complain of symptoms such as anxiety, depression, seizures, agitation, weakness, headache, insomnia, and tremor (Alloway et al. 1998; DiMartini et al. 2005). Everolimus also appears to have relatively mild neuropsychiatric side effects.

Belatacept, a T-cell costimulation blocker used primarily in renal transplant recipients, may cause headache. Belatacept and other immuosuppressants have been associated with CNS posttransplant lymphoproliferative disorder (Castellano-Sanchez et al. 2004; National Library of Medicine 2015).

Monoclonal antibodies, used for induction immunosuppression or adjunctive therapy, have generally mild and uncommon neuropsychiatric side effects. Muromonab-CD3 (Orthoclone OKT3) is an exception but is no longer used or available in the United States. Rituximab is associated with progressive multifocal leukoencephalopathy (Kranick et al. 2007).

Evaluation of posttransplant neuropsychiatric symptoms must include careful consideration of all possible etiologies, such as metabolic disturbances, infections, organ insufficiency, medication effects, and drug interactions. If side effects are believed to be secondary to CNIs, it may be necessary, if medically possible, to decrease the dose or switch to a different agent if symptoms are severe or life threatening. In general, symptoms resolve with reduction or discontinuation of the CNI. Anticonvulsants can successfully treat CNI-induced seizures and are not required long term. Seizures may also cease if CNI dosage reduction or discontinuation is possible. Corticosteroid-induced symptoms generally improve dramatically as the medication is tapered after transplant.

If treatment of neuropsychiatric symptoms is needed, it is important to choose medications with the fewest side effects, fewest active metabolites, least toxicity, and minimal side effects. Benzodiazepines may be used safely for a short term for sleep disturbances, anxiety, and agitation; long-term treatment with these agents is usually not advisable. SSRIs are generally considered first-line treatment for depressive and anxiety disorders (see subsection "Selective Serotonin Reuptake Inhibitors" earlier in this chapter). Haloperidol and other antipsychotics can be used for symptoms of delirium, hallucinations, delusions, mania, mood lability, irritability, and agitation.

Drug-Drug Interactions

Drug interactions commonly occur with immunosuppressants and other drugs frequently required by transplant patients (e.g., antihypertensives, antimicrobials, lipid-modifying agents, antiulcer drugs, analgesics, psychotropics). Most immunosuppressants have significant toxicities and narrow therapeutic indices. Glucocorticoids, CNIs, sirolimus, everolimus, and corticosteroids are all CYP3A4 substrates (Table 16–2). Inhibitors and inducers of CYP3A4 may cause clinically significant drug level changes, resulting in toxicity or inadequate immunosuppression. Glucocorticoids induce CYP3A4 and may decrease levels of drugs metabolized by CYP3A4 (e.g., quetiapine) (Indiana University Division of Clinical Pharmacology 2015; Pascussi et al. 2003).

Several drug interactions are particularly relevant to psychiatrists (see Tables 16–3 and 16–4). Among SSRIs, paroxetine is the most potent inhibitor of CYP2D6, which may increase the risk for drug-drug interactions. Fluoxetine has been well tolerated and successfully used in patients with cardiac disease and renal failure (Gottlieb et al. 2007; Kalender et al. 2007); however, its prolonged half-life and its potential for drug-drug interactions make it less desirable for the medically ill (Crone and Gabriel 2004). Both fluoxetine and its active metabolite, norfluoxetine, are inhibitors of CYP1A2, CYP2D6, CYP2C19, and CYP3A4. Because of its ability to inhibit CYP3A4, fluoxetine theoretically could prolong the metabolism of cyclosporine, tacrolimus, and sirolimus. However, a small study failed to detect significant changes in cyclosporine levels when fluoxetine was used (Strouse et al. 1996). No change in cyclosporine levels occurred in a small group of transplant recipients treated with citalopram (Liston et al. 2001). Sertraline inhibits CYP2D6 at dosages >200 mg/day and is a weak inhibitor of CYP3A4. One study reported that cyclosporine clearance was inhibited by sertraline (Lill et al. 2000), but another study failed to show any significant changes in cyclosporine levels for patients taking sertraline, paroxetine, or fluoxetine (Markowitz et al. 1998). Although there are no reports of elevated immunosuppressant levels with fluvoxamine, it is the least desirable choice among SSRIs because of its risk of drug-drug in-

Table 16–2.   Immunosuppressant metabolism and effects on metabolic systems

Immunosuppressant medication	Metabolized by	Inhibits	Induces
Corticosteroids	CYP3A4	CYP3A4 (high dose)	CYP3A4 (low dose)
Cyclosporine	CYP3A4 P-glycoprotein	CYP3A4 P-glycoprotein	—
Sirolimus	CYP3A4 P-glycoprotein	—	—
Everolimus	CYP3A4 P-glycoprotein	CYP3A4 P-glycoprotein	
Tacrolimus	CYP3A4 P-glycoprotein UGT	UGT	—

Note.   CYP=cytochrome P450; UGT=uridine 5′-diphosphate glucuronosyltransferase.
Source.   Augustine et al. 2007; Fireman et al. 2004; National Library of Medicine 2015; Warrington et al. 2004.

teractions (Crone and Gabriel 2004). It is a strong inhibitor of CYP1A2 and inhibits CYP2C9, CYP2C19, and CYP3A4. Nefazodone, a CYP3A4 inhibitor, has been implicated in several case reports of causing toxic CNI levels, leading in two cases to acute renal insufficiency and delirium and in two cases to elevated liver enzymes (Campo et al. 1998; Garton 2002; Helms-Smith et al. 1996; Wright et al. 1999). St. John's wort, a popular herbal remedy for depression, is an inducer of CYP3A4 and P-glycoprotein. Use of St. John's wort can result in reduced levels of CNIs and has resulted in transplant rejection (Fireman et al. 2004). In summary, it appears that only antidepressants that strongly inhibit or induce CYP3A4 may have clinically meaningful interactions with immunosuppressants (i.e., inhibitors nefazodone and perhaps fluvoxamine and inducer St. John's wort). In turn, CNIs may increase levels of psychotropics metabolized by CYP3A4, whereas glucocorticoids may decrease levels (Indiana University Division of Clinical Pharmacology 2015; Madhusoodanan et al. 2014).

Table 16–3.   Immunosuppressant drug–psychotropic drug interactions

Medication	Metabolic effect	Effects on psychotropic drug and management
Corticosteroids	Induces CYP3A4	Reduced levels and possibly subtherapeutic effect for pimozide, quetiapine, ziprasidone, iloperidone, fentanyl, meperidine, tramadol, buspirone, benzodiazepines (except oxazepam, lorazepam, and temazepam)
Cyclosporine	Inhibits CYP3A4	Increased levels and toxicities for pimozide, quetiapine, ziprasidone, iloperidone, fentanyl, meperidine, tramadol, buspirone, benzodiazepines (except oxazepam, lorazepam, and temazepam)
	Inhibits P-glycoprotein	Possible increase in bioavailability and toxicity for P-glycoprotein substrates, including carbamazepine, lamotrigine, phenytoin, paroxetine, venlafaxine, olanzapine, quetiapine, and risperidone
Tacrolimus	QT prolongation	Increased QT prolongation in combination with other QT-prolonging drugs such as TCAs, typical antipsychotics, pimozide, risperidone, paliperidone, iloperidone, quetiapine, ziprasidone, lithium

Note.   CYP = cytochrome P450; TCAs = tricyclic antidepressants.

In one case, a transplant recipient's cyclosporine level dropped 50% because of CYP3A4 induction by modafinil 200 mg/day (Cephalon 1998). Carbamazepine may lower drug levels of tacrolimus and cyclosporine by causing CYP3A4 induction (Baciewicz and Baciewicz 1989; Campana et al. 1996; Chabolla and Wszolek 2006), which can raise the risk of organ rejection due to inadequate immunosuppression.

Table 16–4.   Psychotropic drug–immunosuppressant drug interactions

Medication	Pharmacokinetic effect	Effects on immunosuppressant drug and management
Carbamazepine, oxcarbazepine, and phenytoin Armodafinil and modafinil	Induces CYP3A4	Increased metabolism and reduced exposure and therapeutic effect of CYP3A4 substrates, including corticosteroids, cyclosporine, tacrolimus, and sirolimus
St. John's wort	Induces CYP3A4 and P-gp	Reduced bioavailability and increased metabolism leading to reduced exposure and therapeutic effect of CYP3A4 or P-gp substrates, including corticosteroids, cyclosporine, tacrolimus, and sirolimus
Fluvoxamine and nefazodone	Inhibits CYP3A4	Reduced metabolism and increased exposure and toxicities of CYP3A4 substrates, including corticosteroids, cyclosporine, tacrolimus, and sirolimus

Note.   CYP = cytochrome P450; P-gp = P-glycoprotein.

The immunosuppressant drugs have important pharmacodynamic interactions. CNIs are nephrotoxic, and nephrotoxicity may be enhanced when CNIs are combined with aminoglycosides, amphotericin B, nonsteroidal anti-inflammatory drugs, vancomycin, and likely lithium (Alloway et al. 1998). Lithium should be used only when necessary in patients with end-organ failure and in posttransplant patients because side effects, drug-drug interactions, and changes in fluid status combined with the narrow therapeutic index of lithium make management quite complex. Frequent assessment of renal function, creatinine clearance, and lithium levels is necessary. In addition, immunosuppressants, psychotropics, and many other medications may prolong QT interval and have the potential to cause torsades de pointes; care must be taken when prescribing combinations of these medications.

Gastrointestinal symptoms (e.g., nausea, vomiting, diarrhea) are common adverse effects of immunosuppressant medications in more than 60% of patients undergoing combination therapy (Pescovitz and Navarro 2001). Gastrointestinal symptoms should always be evaluated, especially prior to administering psychotropics with similar adverse effects (e.g., SSRIs, venlafaxine).

Immunosuppressants have significant metabolic side effects (e.g., weight gain, glucose intolerance, hyperlipidemia) (Alloway et al. 1998; Augustine et al. 2007; Bajjoka and Anandan 2002). These side effects must be considered when psychotropic medications with similar effects, such as some of the atypical antipsychotics, are to be used. Psychotropic medications with minimal metabolic side effects should be considered (see drug choices in earlier section "Psychotropic Medications in Transplant Patients").

Conclusion

Transplantation is a challenging process for patients and medical professionals alike. Patients undergo acute and chronic pathophysiological changes and will be subjected to powerful medications with potentially serious side effects. In addition, psychiatric disorders are common in these patients, and the identification and prompt treatment of these disorders are important aspects of transplant care. We have reviewed the essential aspects of the transplant process relevant to pharmacotherapy. This review should provide the information necessary to deal with the psychotropic needs of this unique and complex patient population.

Key Clinical Points

- Psychiatric consultation can aid in the correct diagnosis and choice of proper medication.
- No psychotropic medications are absolutely contraindicated for use in transplant patients, but clinicians should carefully consider the type of organ disease, drug, dosage, potential for side effects, and possible drug-drug interactions.

- Patients should begin taking a psychotropic medication at a low dosage, and the dosage should be slowly titrated upward.
- Patients with organ disease often have some degree of cognitive impairment or encephalopathy and tend to be more sensitive to sedative and cognitive side effects of psychotropic medications.
- Selection of psychotropic medications should take into consideration other potential benefits a drug might provide to aid symptoms of organ disease (e.g., additionally treating pruritus, restless legs syndrome, nausea, anorexia, fatigue).
- Encephalopathy can be mistaken for depression, psychosis, mania, and anxiety disorders. Careful diagnosis is necessary to avoid use of psychotropic medications that may aggravate a patient's symptoms (e.g., worsen agitation or confusion).
- Psychotropic polypharmacy should be minimized if possible because transplant patients often take numerous drugs.
- Following transplantation, medications that inhibit or induce CYP3A4 should be avoided if possible because most immunosuppressants are CYP3A4 substrates.
- Immunosuppressants and many psychotropics may cause QTc prolongation, and care must be taken when prescribing these medications in combination.
- Although neuropsychiatric symptoms or changes in mental status may have many possible etiologies in the early posttransplant period, the possibility that symptoms reflect immunosuppressive medication side effects should always be entertained. Symptoms can diminish with a decrease in immunosuppressive medications.
- Drug-drug interactions should be carefully considered because patients may be taking a wide variety of medications in addition to immunosuppressants that may pose risk of significant interactions with psychotropics.

References

Abo-Zena RA, Bobek MB, Dweik RA: Hypertensive urgency induced by an interaction of mirtazapine and clonidine. Pharmacotherapy 20(4):476–478, 2000 10772378

Ahn KJ, Lee JW, Hahn ST, et al: Diffusion-weighted MRI and ADC mapping in FK506 neurotoxicity. Br J Radiol 76(912):916–919, 2003 14711782

Alloway RR, Holt C, Somerville KT: Solid organ transplant, in Pharmacotherapy Self-Assessment Program, 3rd Edition. Kansas City, KS, American College of Clinical Pharmacy, 1998, pp 219–272

Angelico M: Donor liver steatosis and graft selection for liver transplantation: a short review. Eur Rev Med Pharmacol Sci 9(5):295–297, 2005 16231593

Asconapé JJ: Some common issues in the use of antiepileptic drugs. Semin Neurol 22(1):27–39, 2002 12170391

Augustine JJ, Bodziak KA, Hricik DE: Use of sirolimus in solid organ transplantation. Drugs 67(3):369–391, 2007 17335296

Azar SA, Nakhjavani MR, Tarzamni MK, et al: Is living kidney donation really safe? Transplant Proc 39(4):822–823, 2007 17524822

Baciewicz AM, Baciewicz FA Jr: Cyclosporine pharmacokinetic drug interactions. Am J Surg 157(2):264–271, 1989 2644865

Bajjoka IE, Anandan JV: Liver transplantation, in Pharmacotherapy Self-Assessment Program, 4th Edition. Kansas City, KS, American College of Clinical Pharmacy, 2002, pp 169–202

Bartynski WS, Boardman JF: Distinct imaging patterns and lesion distribution in posterior reversible encephalopathy syndrome. AJNR Am J Neuroradiol 28(7):1320–1327, 2007 17698535

Beach SR, Celano CM, Noseworthy PA, et al: QTc prolongation, torsades de pointes, and psychotropic medications. Psychosomatics 54(1):1–13, 2013 23295003

Bechstein WO: Neurotoxicity of calcineurin inhibitors: impact and clinical management. Transpl Int 13(5):313–326, 2000 11052266

Bieniasz M, Domagala P, Kwiatkowski A, et al: The assessment of residual kidney function after living donor nephrectomy. Transplant Proc 41(1):91–92, 2009 19249485

Bullingham RE, Nicholls AJ, Kamm BR: Clinical pharmacokinetics of mycophenolate mofetil. Clin Pharmacokinet 34(6):429–455, 1998 9646007

Bunzel B, Laederach-Hofmann K: Solid organ transplantation: are there predictors for posttransplant noncompliance? A literature overview. Transplantation 70(5):711–716, 2000 11003346

Campana C, Regazzi MB, Buggia I, Molinaro M: Clinically significant drug interactions with cyclosporin. An update. Clin Pharmacokinet 30(2):141–179, 1996 8906896

Campo JV, Smith C, Perel JM: Tacrolimus toxic reaction associated with the use of nefazodone: paroxetine as an alternative agent. Arch Gen Psychiatry 55(11):1050–1052, 1998 9819077

Castellano-Sanchez AA, Li S, Qian J, et al: Primary central nervous system posttransplant lymphoproliferative disorders. Am J Clin Pathol 121(2):246–253, 2004 14983939

Cephalon: Provigil (modafinil) product information. Westchester, PA, Cephalon, 1998

Chabolla DR, Wszolek ZK: Pharmacologic management of seizures in organ transplant. Neurology 67(12) (suppl 4):S34–S38, 2006 17190920

Chick J: Safety issues concerning the use of disulfiram in treating alcohol dependence. Drug Saf 20(5):427–435, 1999 10348093

Colman E, Stadel BV: Gabapentin for postherpetic neuralgia. JAMA 282(2):134–135, 1999 10411191

Collins KK, Thiagarajan RR, Chin C, et al: Atrial tachyarrhythmias and permanent pacing after pediatric heart transplantation. J Heart Lung Transplant 22(10):1126–1133, 2003 14550822

Come CE, Shapiro PA: Supraventricular tachycardia associated with methylphenidate treatment in a heart transplant recipient. Psychosomatics 46(5):461–463, 2005 16145192

Contreras G, Garces G, Quartin AA, et al: An epidemiologic study of early renal replacement therapy after orthotopic liver transplantation. J Am Soc Nephrol 13(1):228–233, 2002 11752042

Crone CC, Gabriel GM: Treatment of anxiety and depression in transplant patients: pharmacokinetic considerations. Clin Pharmacokinet 43(6):361–394, 2004 15086275

Dahm F, Georgiev P, Clavien PA: Small-for-size syndrome after partial liver transplantation: definition, mechanisms of disease and clinical implications. Am J Transplant 5(11):2605–2610, 2005 16212618

DasGupta K, Jefferson JW: The use of lithium in the medically ill. Gen Hosp Psychiatry 12(2):83–97, 1990 2407615

Davis MP, Frandsen JL, Walsh D, et al: Mirtazapine for pruritus. J Pain Symptom Manage 25(3):288–291, 2003 12614964

DiMartini AF, Dew MA, Trzepacz PT: Organ transplantation, in The American Psychiatric Publishing Textbook of Psychosomatic Medicine. Edited by Levenson J. Washington, DC, American Psychiatric Publishing, 2005, pp 675–700

DiMartini A, Crone C, Fireman M, Dew MA: Psychiatric aspects of organ transplantation in critical care. Crit Care Clin 24(4):949–981, x, 2008 18929948

Emre S: Living donor liver transplantation: a critical review. Transplant Proc 33(7–8):3456–3457, 2001 11750479

Erim Y, Beckmann M, Valentin-Gamazo C, et al: Quality of life and psychiatric complications after adult living donor liver transplantation. Liver Transpl 12(12):1782–1790, 2006 17133566

Erim Y, Beckmann M, Kroencke S, et al: Psychological strain in urgent indications for living donor liver transplantation. Liver Transpl 13(6):886–895, 2007 17539009

Fireman M, DiMartini AF, Armstrong SC, Cozza KL: Immunosuppressants. Psychosomatics 45(4):354–360, 2004 15232051

Fukunishi I, Sugawara Y, Takayama T, et al: Psychiatric disorders before and after living-related transplantation. Psychosomatics 42(4):337–343, 2001 11496023

Fusar-Poli P, Picchioni M, Martinelli V, et al: Anti-depressive therapies after heart transplantation. J Heart Lung Transplant 25(7):785–793, 2006 16818121

Garnock-Jones KP: Vortioxetine: a review of its use in major depressive disorder. CNS Drugs 28(9):855–874, 2014 25145538

Garton T: Nefazodone and cyp450 3a4 interactions with cyclosporine and tacrolimus1. Transplantation 74(5):745, 2002 12352898

Gottlieb SS, Kop WJ, Thomas SA, et al: A double-blind placebo-controlled pilot study of controlled-release paroxetine on depression and quality of life in chronic heart failure. Am Heart J 153(5):868–873, 2007 17452166

Haddad PM, Anderson IM: Antipsychotic-related QTc prolongation, torsade de pointes and sudden death. Drugs 62(11):1649–1671, 2002 12109926

Haroldson JA, Kramer LE, Wolff DL, Lake KD: Elevated free fractions of valproic acid in a heart transplant patient with hypoalbuminemia. Ann Pharmacother 34(2):183–187, 2000 10676827

Health Resources and Services Administration Division of Transplantation: 2006 Annual Report of the U.S. Organ Procurement and Transplantation Network and the Scientific Registry of Transplant Recipients: Transplant Data 1996–2005. Rockville, MD, Health Resources and Services Administration, Healthcare Systems Bureau, Division of Transplantation, 2006. Available at: http://www.srtr.org/annual_reports/archives/2006/2006_Annual_Report/. Accessed July 14, 2016.

Hebert MF, Wacher VJ, Roberts JP, Benet LZ: Pharmacokinetics of cyclosporine pre- and post-liver transplantation. J Clin Pharmacol 43(1):38–42, 2003 12520626

Helms-Smith KM, Curtis SL, Hatton RC: Apparent interaction between nefazodone and cyclosporine (letter). Ann Intern Med 125(5):424, 1996 8702104

Indiana University Division of Clinical Pharmacology: P450 drug interaction table, 2015. Available at: http://medicine.iupui.edu/clinpharm/ddis/main-table. Accessed July 4, 2016.

Jain A, Venkataramanan R, Sharma R, et al: Pharmacokinetics of mycophenolic acid in live donor liver transplant patients vs deceased donor liver transplant patients. J Clin Pharmacol 48(5):547–552, 2008 18440919

Jiao M, Greanya ED, Haque M, et al: Methadone maintenance in liver transplantation. Prog Transplant 20(3):209–214, 2010 20929104

Jochum C, Beste M, Penndorf V, et al: Quantitative liver function tests in donors and recipients of living donor liver transplantation. Liver Transpl 12(4):544–549, 2006 16482561

Kalender B, Ozdemir AC, Yalug I, Dervisoglu E: Antidepressant treatment increases quality of life in patients with chronic renal failure. Ren Fail 29(7):817–822, 2007 17994449

Kay J, Bienenfeld D, Slomowitz M, et al: Use of tricyclic antidepressants in recipients of heart transplants. Psychosomatics 32(2):165–170, 1991 2027938

Kemmer N, Secic M, Zacharias V, et al: Long-term analysis of primary nonfunction in liver transplant recipients. Transplant Proc 39(5):1477–1480, 2007 17580166

Kershner P, Wang-Cheng R: Psychiatric side effects of steroid therapy. Psychosomatics 30(2):135–139, 1989 2652177

Kim J, Phongsamran P, Park S: Use of antidepressant drugs in transplant recipients. Prog Transplant 14(2):98–104, 2004 15264454

Koo JR, Yoon JY, Joo MH, et al: Treatment of depression and effect of antidepression treatment on nutritional status in chronic hemodialysis patients. Am J Med Sci 329(1):1–5, 2005 15654172

Krahn LE, DiMartini A: Psychiatric and psychosocial aspects of liver transplantation. Liver Transpl 11(10):1157–1168, 2005 16184540

Kranick SM, Mowry EM, Rosenfeld MR: Progressive multifocal leukoencephalopathy after rituximab in a case of non-Hodgkin lymphoma. Neurology 69(7):704–706, 2007 17698796

Lacasse Y, Beaudoin L, Rousseau L, Maltais F: Randomized trial of paroxetine in end-stage COPD. Monaldi Arch Chest Dis 61(3):140–147, 2004 15679006

Lake JR: Liver transplantation, in Current Diagnosis and Treatment in Gastroenterology, 2nd Edition. Edited by Friedman S. New York, McGraw-Hill, 2003, pp 813–834

Levenson JL: High-dose intravenous haloperidol for agitated delirium following lung transplantation. Psychosomatics 36(1):66–68, 1995 7871137

Lill J, Bauer LA, Horn JR, Hansten PD: Cyclosporine-drug interactions and the influence of patient age. Am J Health Syst Pharm 57(17):1579–1584, 2000 10984808

Liston HL, Markowitz JS, Hunt N, et al: Lack of citalopram effect on the pharmaco-kinetics of cyclosporine. Psychosomatics 42(4):370–372, 2001 11496034

Lück R, Böger J, Kuse E, et al: Achieving adequate cyclosporine exposure in liver transplant recipients: a novel strategy for monitoring and dosing using intravenous therapy. Liver Transpl 10(5):686–691, 2004 15108262

Madhusoodanan S, Velama U, Parmar J, et al: A current review of cytochrome P450 interactions of psychotropic drugs. Ann Clin Psychiatry 26(2):120–138, 2014 24812650

Magee CC: Pharmacology and side effects of cyclosporine and tacrolimus. March 29, 2006. Available at: http://www.uptodate.com/contents/pharmacology-and-side-effects-of-cyclosporine-and-tacrolimus?source=search_result&search=pharmacology+of+cyclosporine+and+tacrolimus&selectedTitle=1%7E150. Accessed April 29, 2016.

Markowitz JS, Gill HS, Hunt NM, et al: Lack of antidepressant-cyclosporine pharma-cokinetic interactions. J Clin Psychopharmacol 18(1):91–93, 1998 9472853

Masand P, Pickett P, Murray GB: Psychostimulants for secondary depression in medical illness. Psychosomatics 32(2):203–208, 1991 2027944

Mayo MJ, Handem I, Saldana S, et al: Sertraline as a first-line treatment for cholestatic pruritus. Hepatology 45(3):666–674, 2007 17326161

McIntyre RS, Soczynska JK, Konarski JZ, Kennedy SH: The effect of antidepressants on lipid homeostasis: a cardiac safety concern? Expert Opin Drug Saf 5(4):523–537, 2006 16774491

McIntyre RS, Panjwani ZD, Nguyen HT, et al: The hepatic safety profile of dulox-etine: a review. Expert Opin Drug Metab Toxicol 4(3):281–285, 2008 18363543

Meissner K, Blood J, Francis AM, et al: Cyclosporine-inhabitable cerebral drug transport does not influence clinical methadone pharmacodynamics. Anesthesiology 121:1281–1291, 2014

Michaels PJ, Espejo ML, Kobashigawa J, et al: Humoral rejection in cardiac transplantation: risk factors, hemodynamic consequences and relationship to transplant coronary artery disease. J Heart Lung Transplant 22(1):58–69, 2003 12531414

Mintzer S, Boppana P, Toguri J, DeSantis A: Vitamin D levels and bone turnover in epilepsy patients taking carbamazepine or oxcarbazepine. Epilepsia 47(3):510–515, 2006 16529614

Molnar MZ, Novak M, Mucsi I: Management of restless legs syndrome in patients on dialysis. Drugs 66(5):607–624, 2006 16620140

Nadalin S, Testa G, Malagó M, et al: Volumetric and functional recovery of the liver after right hepatectomy for living donation. Liver Transpl 10(8):1024–1029, 2004 15390329

Naini AE, Harandi AA, Khanbabapour S, et al: Gabapentin: a promising drug for the treatment of uremic pruritus. Saudi J Kidney Dis Transpl 18(3):378–381, 2007 17679749

Najarian JS, Chavers BM, McHugh LE, Matas AJ: 20 years or more of follow-up of living kidney donors. Lancet 340(8823):807–810, 1992 1357243

National Library of Medicine: DailyMed. Available at http://dailymed.nlm.nih.gov/dailymed/, 2015. Accessed July 4, 2016.

Ojo AO, Held PJ, Port FK, et al: Chronic renal failure after transplantation of a nonrenal organ. N Engl J Med 349(10):931–940, 2003 12954741

Overman GP, Teter CJ, Guthrie SK: Acamprosate for the adjunctive treatment of alcohol dependence. Ann Pharmacother 37(7-8):1090–1099, 2003 12841823

Pacher P, Kecskemeti V: Cardiovascular side effects of new antidepressants and antipsychotics: new drugs, old concerns? Curr Pharm Des 10(20):2463–2475, 2004 15320756

Pae CU, Lim HK, Han C, et al: Selegiline transdermal system: current awareness and promise. Prog Neuropsychopharmacol Biol Psychiatry 31(6):1153–1163, 2007 17614182

Parés A: Old and novel therapies for primary biliary cirrhosis. Semin Liver Dis 34(3):341–351, 2014 25057957

Pascussi JM, Gerbal-Chaloin S, Drocourt L, et al: The expression of CYP2B6, CYP2C9 and CYP3A4 genes: a tangle of networks of nuclear and steroid receptors. Biochim Biophys Acta 1619(3):243–253, 2003 12573484

Pescovitz MD, Navarro MT: Immunosuppressive therapy and post-transplantation diarrhea. Clin Transplant 15 (suppl 4):23–28, 2001 11778784

Plutchik L, Snyder S, Drooker M, et al: Methylphenidate in post liver transplant patients. Psychosomatics 39(2):118–123, 1998 9584537

Reynaud-Gaubert M, Viard L, Girault D, et al: Improved absorption and bioavailability of cyclosporine A from a microemulsion formulation in lung transplant recipients affected with cystic fibrosis. Transplant Proc 29(5):2450–2453, 1997 9270807

Rösche J, Fröscher W, Abendroth D, Liebel J: Possible oxcarbazepine interaction with cyclosporine serum levels: a single case study. Clin Neuropharmacol 24(2):113–116, 2001 11307049

Rush D, Nickerson P, Gough J, et al: Beneficial effects of treatment of early subclinical rejection: a randomized study. J Am Soc Nephrol 9(11):2129–2134, 1998 9808101

Saivin S, Hulot T, Chabac S, et al: Clinical pharmacokinetics of acamprosate. Clin Pharmacokinet 35(5):331–345, 1998 9839087

Schatzberg AF, DeBattista C: Manual of Clinical Psychopharmacology, 8th Edition. Washington, DC, American Psychiatric Publishing, 2015

Schweizer RT, Rovelli M, Palmeri D, et al: Noncompliance in organ transplant recipients. Transplantation 49(2):374–377, 1990 2305467

Scott LJ: Levomilnacipram extended-release: a review of its use in adult patients with major depressive disorder. CNS Drugs 28:1071–1082, 2014 25270036

Serebruany VL, Glassman AH, Malinin AI, et al: Selective serotonin reuptake inhibitors yield additional antiplatelet protection in patients with congestive heart failure treated with antecedent aspirin. Eur J Heart Fail 5(4):517–521, 2003 12921813

Shapiro PA: Nortriptyline treatment of depressed cardiac transplant recipients. Am J Psychiatry 148(3):371–373, 1991 1992842

Shapiro R, Randhawa P, Jordan ML, et al: An analysis of early renal transplant protocol biopsies—the high incidence of subclinical tubulitis. Am J Transplant 1(1):47–50, 2001 12095037

Shaw LM, Mick R, Nowak I, et al: Pharmacokinetics of mycophenolic acid in renal transplant patients with delayed graft function. J Clin Pharmacol 38(3):268–275, 1998 9549665

Shoskes DA, Cecka JM: Deleterious effects of delayed graft function in cadaveric renal transplant recipients independent of acute rejection. Transplantation 66(12):1697–1701, 1998 9884262

Silvertooth EJ, Doraiswamy PM, Clary GL, et al: Citalopram and quality of life in lung transplant recipients. Psychosomatics 45(3):271–272, 2004 15123855

Strouse TB, Fairbanks LA, Skotzko CE, Fawzy FI: Fluoxetine and cyclosporine in organ transplantation. Failure to detect significant drug interactions or adverse clinical events in depressed organ recipients. Psychosomatics 37(1):23–30, 1996 8600490

Thomsen K, Schou M: Avoidance of lithium intoxication: advice based on knowledge about the renal lithium clearance under various circumstances. Pharmacopsychiatry 32(3):83–86, 1999 10463373

Tombazzi CR, Waters B, Shokouh-Amiri MH, et al: Neuropsychiatric complications after liver transplantation: role of immunosuppression and hepatitis C. Dig Dis Sci 51(6):1079–1081, 2006 16865574

Tripathi A, Panzer MJ: Cyclosporine psychosis. Psychosomatics 34(1):101–102, 1993 8426884

Tucker ON, Heaton N: The 'small for size' liver syndrome. Curr Opin Crit Care 11(2):150–155, 2005 15758596

Tutor-Crespo MJ, Hermida J, Tutor JC: Relative proportions of serum carbamazepine and its pharmacologically active 10,11-epoxy derivative: effect of polytherapy and renal insufficiency. Ups J Med Sci 113(2):171–180, 2008 18509811

U.S. Renal Data System: USRDS 2008 annual data report: atlas of chronic kidney disease and end-stage renal disease in the United States. Bethesda, MD, National Institutes of Health, National Institute of Diabetes and Digestive and Kidney Diseases, 2008. Available at: https://www.usrds.org/atlas08.aspx. Accessed July 14, 2016.

Vincent HH, Wenting GJ, Schalekamp MA, et al: Impaired fractional excretion of lithium: a very early marker of cyclosporine nephrotoxicity. Transplant Proc 19(5):4147–4148, 1987 3314004

Viswanathan R, Glickman L: Clonazepam in the treatment of steroid-induced mania in a patient after renal transplantation. N Engl J Med 320(5):319–320, 1989 2643052

Wagena EJ, Knipschild PG, Huibers MJ, et al: Efficacy of bupropion and nortriptyline for smoking cessation among people at risk for or with chronic obstructive pulmonary disease. Arch Intern Med 165(19):2286–2292, 2005 16246996

Wang PW, Ketter TA: Pharmacokinetics of mood stabilizers and new anticonvulsants. Psychopharmacol Bull 36(1):44–66, 2002 12397847

Wang SM, Han C, Lee SJ, et al: Vilazodone for the treatment of major depressive disorder: focusing on its clinical studies and mechanism of action. Psychiatry Investig 12(2):155–163, 2015 25866514

Warrington JS, Greenblatt DJ, Von Moltke LL: Role of CYP3A enzymes in the biotransformation of triazolam in rat liver. Xenobiotica 34(5):463–471, 2004 15370962

Weinrieb RM, Van Horn DH, McLellan AT, et al: Alcoholism treatment after liver transplantation: lessons learned from a clinical trial that failed. Psychosomatics 42(2):110–116, 2001 11239123

Weinrieb RM, Auriacombe M, Lynch KG, et al: A critical review of selective serotonin reuptake inhibitor–associated bleeding: balancing the risk of treating hepatitis C–infected patients. J Clin Psychiatry 64(12):1502–1510, 2003 14728113

Weinrieb RM, Barnett R, Lynch KG, et al: A matched comparison study of medical and psychiatric complications and anesthesia and analgesia requirements in methadone-maintained liver transplant recipients. Liver Transpl 10(1):97–106, 2004 14755785

Weinrieb RM, Auriacombe M, Lynch KG, Lewis JD: Selective serotonin re-uptake inhibitors and the risk of bleeding. Expert Opin Drug Saf 4(2):337–344, 2005 15794724

Wong MO, Eldon MA, Keane WF, et al: Disposition of gabapentin in anuric subjects on hemodialysis. J Clin Pharmacol 35(6):622–626, 1995 7665723

Wright DH, Lake KD, Bruhn PS, Emery RW Jr: Nefazodone and cyclosporine drug-drug interaction. J Heart Lung Transplant 18(9):913–915, 1999 10528754

Yalcin AU, Sahin G, Erol M, Bal C: Sertraline hydrochloride treatment for patients with hemodialysis hypotension. Blood Purif 20(2):150–153, 2002 11818677

Zafar MN, Jawad F, Aziz T, et al: Donor follow-up in living-related renal transplantation. Transplant Proc 34(6):2443–2444, 2002 12270473

Zareba W, Lin DA: Antipsychotic drugs and QT interval prolongation. Psychiatr Q 74(3):291–306, 2003 12918603

Zuin M, Giorgini A, Selmi C, et al: Acute liver and renal failure during treatment with buprenorphine at therapeutic dose. Dig Liver Dis 41(7):e8–e10, 2009 18294936

17

Pain Management

Michael R. Clark, M.D., M.P.H., M.B.A.

J. Greg Hobelmann, M.D., M.P.H.

James L. Levenson, M.D.

Pain is the most common symptom for which people seek medical treatment (Cherry et al. 2003). According to a 2011 report from the Institute of Medicine, one in three Americans suffers from chronic pain, which is more than the total affected by cancer, heart disease, and diabetes combined (Institute of Medicine 2011). Both acute and chronic pain are associated with impairment in multiple quality-of-life and functional domains and are highly costly, making the treatment of pain a major personal and public health concern (O'Connor 2009).

In addition to opioids, a relatively small number of drug classes are employed in the treatment of chronic pain and especially neuropathic pain conditions (Moulin et al. 2007). Antidepressants and anticonvulsants remain the best studied and are first-line therapies, particularly for various painful polyneuropathies and postherpetic neuralgia (Dworkin et al. 2007; Johnson and

Rice 2014). Recent guidelines have been released for the multidisciplinary treatment of fibromyalgia, emphasizing evidence-based pharmacological therapies (Carville et al. 2008; Clauw 2014). Unfortunately, medications are generally underutilized and underdosed. In one study of patients with neuropathic pain, 73% complained of inadequate pain control, but 72% had never received anticonvulsants, 60% had never received tricyclic antidepressants (TCAs), 41% had never received opioids, and 25% had never received any of the above (Gilron et al. 2002). No algorithm can provide a simple, straightforward approach to the treatment of chronic pain. The disease itself may change over time such that treatment efficacy is altered, treatments may be selected on the basis of previous response, and drugs may be combined with the expectation of pharmacological synergies and minimized liabilities. Polypharmacy for the treatment of chronic pain also raises concerns of drug-drug interactions.

Psychiatric Comorbidity

Pain Disorder and Somatic Symptom Disorder

Although the actual diagnosis of somatic symptom disorder is rare in patients with chronic pain, multiple pain complaints are almost always present in somatizing patients. Patients in whom psychological factors play a dominant role in the perception of pain typically have more sites of pain, spread of pain beyond the area of original injury, more opioid and benzodiazepine use, and greater involvement with compensation and litigation (Streltzer et al. 2000). Somatization is often associated with "psychogenic" pain with no "real" cause, but this is a misconception addressed in the conceptualization of somatic symptom disorder in DSM-5 (American Psychiatric Association 2013), which eliminated basing diagnosis on the absence of a medical explanation of somatic symptoms. Psychological and physical domains interrelate and can cause significant decreases in quality of life regardless of the etiology of the pain (Rief and Martin 2014).

Substance Use

The prevalence of substance dependence or addiction in patients with chronic pain ranges from 3% to 48% depending on the population sampled (Morasco et al. 2011). The core criteria for a substance use disorder in patients with chronic pain include the loss of control in the use of the medication, excessive preoccupation with the medication despite adequate analgesia, and adverse consequences associated with its use (Compton et al. 1998). However, reliance on medications that provide pain relief can result in a number of stereotyped patient behaviors that can either represent or be mistaken for addiction. Persistent pain can lead to increased focus on opioid medications and measures to ensure an adequate medication supply even in the absence of addiction. Patients understandably fear the reemergence of pain and withdrawal symptoms if they run out of medication. Drug-seeking behavior may be the result of an anxious patient trying to maintain a previous level of pain control. These actions may represent pseudoaddiction that results from therapeutic dependence, as well as current or potential undertreatment, but not addiction (Kirsh et al. 2002).

Patients with substance use disorders have increased rates of chronic pain and are at the greatest risk for stigmatization and undertreatment with appropriate medications by health care practitioners (Rosenblum et al. 2003). Integrating care for chronic pain with innovative stepped-care models of substance abuse treatment would likely improve outcomes by tailoring the intensity of treatment to the individual patient's needs (Clark et al. 2008; Haibach et al. 2014).

Depression and Distress

Physical symptoms are common in patients with major depressive disorder. Approximately 60% of patients with depression report pain symptoms at diagnosis (Magni et al. 1985; von Knorring et al. 1983). Depression increases the risk of developing chronic pain (Von Korff et al. 1993), and chronic pain approximately doubles the incidence of depression (Patten 2001). Depressive symptoms, even without the categorical diagnosis of major depressive disorder, are an important comorbidity in patients with chronic pain and are associated with greater pain intensity; more pain persistence; and greater interference from pain, including more pain behaviors observed by others (Haythornthwaite et al. 1991), as well as with increased risk of suicidality and disability (Lerman et al. 2015; Tang and Crane 2006). Among the vegetative and somatic symptoms of depression, pain is second only to insomnia (Bras et al. 2010). Depression with comorbid pain is more resistant to treatment (Kroenke et al. 2008), but pain often subsides with improvement in depressive symptoms (Salerno et al. 2002). In addition to having greater efficacy for the treatment of neuropathic pain, serotonin-norepinephrine reuptake inhibitors (SNRIs) and TCAs are associated with faster rates of improvement and lower rates of relapse compared with selective serotonin reuptake inhibitors (SSRIs) (Cohen and Mao 2014; Rosenzweig-Lipson et al. 2007).

Anxiety, Fear, Catastrophizing, Anger, and Sleep

Patients with chronic pain syndromes have increased rates of both anxiety symptoms and anxiety disorders, such as generalized anxiety disorder, panic disorder, agoraphobia, and posttraumatic stress disorder (Outcalt et al. 2015). Fear of pain, movement, reinjury, and other negative consequences that result in the avoidance of activities promotes the transition to and sustaining of chronic pain and its associated disabilities, such as muscular reactivity, deconditioning, and guarded movement (Asmundson et al. 1999). This restriction of activities can result in physiological changes, such as weight gain and muscle atrophy, that can lead to functional deterioration. Pain-related cognitions such as catastrophizing and fear-avoidance beliefs are predictive of poor adjustment to chronic pain (Hasenbring et al. 2001). Anger has been reported by 70% of patients with chronic pain, with the anger directed at themselves (74%) and health care professionals (62%) (Okifuji et al. 1999). Posttraumatic stress disorder is increasingly recognized as a comorbid condition with significant consequences for patients with chronic pain disorders (Liebschutz et al. 2007).

There is also ample evidence that pain and poor sleep commonly occur together, although the direction of causality in their association remains unclear (Wong and Fielding 2012). However, sleep impairments have been shown to reliably predict exacerbations of chronic pain better than pain predicts sleep disturbances. It is likely that sleep disturbances adversely affect key processes in the development and maintenance of chronic pain, but further research is needed to better understand the underlying mechanisms (Finan et al. 2013). Treating the sleep disturbance may improve pain control (Alföldi et al. 2014).

Pain Description and Management

Acute Pain

Acute pain is usually the result of trauma from surgery, injury, or exacerbation of chronic disease, especially musculoskeletal conditions. Acute pain management is usually successful with straightforward strategies such as relaxation;

immobilization; analgesics, such as nonsteroidal anti-inflammatory drugs (NSAIDs), acetaminophen, and opioids; massage; and transcutaneous electrical nerve stimulation (Institute for Clinical Systems Improvement 2008). Acute pain management initiated as early as possible and focused on preventing the occurrence and reemergence of pain may allow for lower total doses of analgesics. The absence of signs consistent with acute pain, such as elevated heart rate, blood pressure, and diaphoresis, does not rule out the presence of pain.

Analgesics, especially opioids, should be prescribed only for pain relief (Manchikanti et al. 2012b). Although analgesia may produce other benefits, other symptoms commonly coinciding with acute pain, such as insomnia or anxiety, should be managed separately from pain. Sleep deprivation and anxiety may intensify the sensation of pain and increase requests for more medication. Reducing anxiety and insomnia often reduces analgesic requirements. In acute pain management, psychiatric consultation is requested when a patient requires more analgesia than expected or has a history of substance abuse. Patients with an active or recent history of opioid addiction and those receiving methadone maintenance therapy have increased tolerance to opioids and may require up to 50% higher doses of opioids. Although opioid use in these patients should be carefully monitored, adequate treatment of acute pain is a priority. Inadequate dosing is significantly more common than abuse or diversion. Dosage should be carefully individualized rather than based on preconceived expectations.

Selected Chronic Pain Conditions

Neuropathic Pain

Postherpetic neuralgia.   Postherpetic neuralgia is pain, often described as burning, stabbing, or throbbing, that persists or recurs at the site of shingles at least 3 months after an acute varicella zoster rash. Postherpetic neuralgia occurs in about 10% of patients with acute herpes zoster; occurs in more than 50% of patients older than age 65 who have shingles; and is more likely in individuals with cancer, diabetes, or immunosuppression. However, it occurs in less than 6% of immunocompetent persons (Johnson and Rice 2014). Approximately 15% of referrals to pain clinics are for the treatment of postherpetic neuralgia (Schmader 2002).

TCAs, anticonvulsants (e.g., carbamazepine, valproic acid, pregabalin, gabapentin), and opioids are the most common effective treatments for postherpetic neuralgia and may have potential for its prevention. Amitriptyline, gabapentin, or pregabalin provide pain relief in 50%–60% of patients with postherpetic neuralgia (Zin et al. 2008), and a 5% lidocaine patch is approved for postherpetic neuralgia. Unless otherwise contraindicated, TCAs should be the first choice for treating postherpetic neuralgia, followed by gabapentin or pregabalin (Moore et al. 2014).

Diabetic peripheral neuropathy pain.   Up to 90% of patients with diabetes mellitus will experience painful diabetic neuropathy, with duration of illness and poor glycemic control as contributing risk factors (Schreiber et al. 2015). This pain is described as burning that is either constant or episodic and is paroxysmal and lancinating in quality. It results from axonal degeneration and segmental demyelination (Mendell and Sahenk 2003). First-line pharmacological treatments for diabetic peripheral neuropathy pain include TCAs, SNRIs, and calcium channel–modulating anticonvulsants (Zin et al. 2008), which appear to be of comparable efficacy (Quilici et al. 2009; Snedecor et al. 2014). Other anticonvulsants have been shown to be effective in smaller studies. Experimental and clinical evidence has shown that opioids can be helpful in pain control as well if used as an adjuvant to first-line treatments (Schreiber et al. 2015).

Central poststroke pain and spinal cord injury.   Pain is common after stroke (8% of patients) or spinal cord trauma (60%–70% of patients) (Finnerup 2008; Ullrich 2007). Symptoms of spinal cord injury pain or central poststroke pain are often poorly localized, vary over time, and include allodynia (>50% of central poststroke pain patients), hyperalgesia, dysesthesias, lancinating pain, and muscle and visceral pain regardless of sensory deficits. Pain is described as burning, aching, lacerating, or pricking.

Central poststroke pain is difficult to treat; conventional analgesics and opiates have been shown to be ineffective. Randomized clinical trials have demonstrated efficacy for amitriptyline and for drugs that reduce neuronal hyperexcitability, including lidocaine (intravenous), mexiletine, lamotrigine, fluvoxamine, and gabapentin but not carbamazepine, phenytoin, or topiramate (Frese et al. 2006). Morphine is effective against allodynia but not other components of central pain syndromes (Nicholson 2004). Intravenous lidocaine may be the most efficacious agent, but the need for intravenous administration limits its use. Topical lidocaine may be beneficial for some patients (Hans et al. 2008). Magnetic stimulation and invasive electrical stimulation have also been shown to be effective in carefully selected individuals (Flaster et al. 2013).

Trigeminal neuralgia. Trigeminal neuralgia (tic douloureux) is a chronic pain syndrome with a prevalence of about 0.015% (Montano et al. 2015). It is characterized by severe, paroxysmal, recurrent, lancinating pain with a unilateral distribution of cranial nerve V, most commonly the mandibular division (Elias and Burchiel 2002). Sensory or motor deficits are not usually present. Less commonly, the facial or glossopharyngeal nerve is involved, with pain distribution to the ear, posterior pharynx, tongue, or larynx (Zakrzewska et al. 2005). Episodes of pain can be spontaneous or evoked by nonpainful stimuli to trigger zones, activities such as talking or chewing, or environmental conditions. Between episodes, patients are typically pain free. Uncontrolled pain with frequent or severe prolonged attacks increases the risk of insomnia, weight loss, social withdrawal, anxiety, panic attacks, and depression, including suicide (Montano et al. 2015).

Anticonvulsants are the mainstay of pharmacotherapy for trigeminal neuralgia. Placebo-controlled trials identify carbamazepine as first-line treatment (number needed to treat was 1.8). Trials also support the use of oxcarbazepine and lamotrigine. Evidence is insufficient to recommend clonazepam, gabapentin, phenytoin, tizanidine, topical capsaicin, or valproate (Cruccu et al. 2008). Given the pathophysiological similarities of trigeminal neuralgia with postherpetic neuralgia and painful peripheral neuropathies, other medications, such as the TCAs and SNRIs, would be appropriate pharmacological treatments to consider. Trigeminal neuralgia is often refractory to treatment, but advances in diagnostic imaging and invasive therapies such as gamma knife radiosurgery and neuromodulation are encouraging (Montano et al. 2015).

Complex regional pain syndrome. Complex regional pain syndrome (CRPS; formerly called reflex sympathetic dystrophy and causalgia) is an array of painful conditions characterized by ongoing spontaneous burning pain precipitated by a specific noxious trauma or cause of immobilization and often with hyperalgesia or allodynia to cutaneous stimuli. Pain is regional but not limited to a single peripheral nerve or dermatome. Often, there is evidence of edema, blood flow abnormalities, or sudomotor dysfunction in the pain region—usually an extremity. Motor changes, such as weakness, tremor, dystonia, and limitations in movement, are common (Harden et al. 2007). Sympathetically maintained pain is present in most, but not all, cases. Patients with sympathetically maintained pain often report hyperalgesia to cold stimuli. Sympathetically maintained pain is generally considered to respond to sympathetic blockade (Pontell 2008).

Patients with CRPS often exhibit affective (46%), anxiety (27%), and substance abuse (14%) disorders (Rommel et al. 2001), which are generally considered to be a consequence rather than a cause of chronic pain. Pharmacotherapy for CRPS has limited success, and few randomized controlled studies have been done to guide treatment selection. Symptoms often improve with NSAIDs or corticosteroids in the acute, or inflammatory, stage of the disease. Evidence suggests efficacy for gabapentin, pregabalin, carbamazepine, TCAs, and opioids. Increased risk for substance use disorders limits the use of opioids to prescribing contingent on functional improvement. Randomized controlled trials of calcitonin and bisphosphonates in patients with CRPS demonstrated reduced pain and improved joint mobility. Clinical trials of local anesthetic sympathetic blockade, once considered the gold standard therapy for CRPS, have proved inconclusive (Sharma et al. 2006). Other therapies include early intervention with reactivating physical therapies, electrical stimulation, and possibly even surgical sympathectomy (O'Connell et al. 2013). Invasive procedures should be limited to selected cases and considered only after psychosomatic assessment. If current recommendations are followed, prognosis is better than previously assumed (Birklein et al. 2015).

Phantom limb pain.   Feeling pain in a body part that has actually been removed occurs in 50%–80% of amputees within a year of the amputation. Phantom limb pain, considered to be neuropathic and described as stabbing, throbbing, burning, or cramping, is more intense in the distal portion of the phantom limb (Flor 2002; Niraj and Niraj 2014). Phantom pain is also common after mastectomy (Peuckmann et al. 2009). Although TCAs, gabapentin, and carbamazepine are considered first-line treatments for phantom pain, there is limited evidence to support their use. The benefit of these agents does not generally exceed the 30% placebo response observed in other pain studies. Newer antidepressants and anticonvulsants with generally fewer side effects may result in greater effectiveness if higher doses can be tolerated by patients. However, morphine, tramadol, gabapentin, calcitonin, intramuscular botulinum toxin, and ketamine have been shown to reduce phantom pain in controlled studies (Halbert et al. 2002; McCormick et al. 2014). Morphine, but not mexiletine, decreased postamputation pain of greater than 6 months' duration (Wu et al. 2008). Controlled trials have discredited anecdotal reports of the effectiveness of neural blockade (Manchikanti and Singh 2004). Studies evaluating cognitive-behavioral therapies and hypnotherapies have generally shown positive outcomes, but lack of randomized controlled trials makes it difficult to draw firm conclusions about their effectiveness (Niraj and Niraj 2014).

Headache

Migraine.   About 18% of women and 6% of men have migraines, with peak incidence between ages 30 and 40. Common migraine is a unilateral pulsatile headache, which may be associated with other symptoms such as nausea, vomiting, photophobia, and phonophobia. The classic form of migraine adds visual prodromal symptoms (Lipton et al. 2007). Placebo-controlled clinical trials suggest the use of NSAIDs and triptans for acute treatment of migraine attacks and propranolol, metoprolol, flunarizine, valproate, topiramate, and TCAs as prophylactic agents (Keskinbora and Aydinli 2008; Mulleners and Chronicle 2008). For chronic migraine (headache occurring on 15 or more days per month for more than 3 months), topiramate, amitriptyline, botulinum toxin type A, and cognitive-behavioral therapy have been shown to be effective (Carod-Artal 2014). In general, emphasis should be placed on prevention because chronic migraines are often complicated by medication-overuse headache due to excessive intake of acute medications (Ferrari et al. 2015).

Chronic daily headache.   Chronic daily headache affects about 5% of the population and is composed of constant (transformed) migraine, medication-overuse headache, chronic tension-type headaches, new-onset daily persistent headache, and hemicrania continua (Dodick 2006). Patients with chronic daily headache are more likely to overuse medication, leading to rebound headache; suffer psychiatric comorbidity such as depression and anxiety; report functional disability; and experience stress-related headache exacerbations (Lake 2001). Chronic daily headache is difficult to manage and is often unresponsive to medications (Halker et al. 2011). Placebo-controlled clinical trials are few but support the use of amitriptyline, gabapentin, topiramate, and botulinum toxin type A (Dodick 2006), but placebo response rates have sometimes been high (Couch and Amitriptyline Versus Placebo Study Group

2011). As with other chronic pain syndromes, empirical support exists for treating patients with other agents such as the SNRIs, TCAs, and anticonvulsants. Combined medication and cognitive-behavioral psychotherapy is more effective than either treatment alone (Lipchik and Nash 2002).

Fibromyalgia

Fibromyalgia is a chronic pain syndrome characterized by widespread musculoskeletal pain in all four limbs and trunk, stiffness, and exaggerated tenderness. These symptoms are usually accompanied by poor sleep and fatigue. Fibromyalgia is diagnosed in 3.4% of women and 0.5% of men and is clustered in families (Arnold et al. 2004). Current research suggests that fibromyalgia may be a syndrome of dysfunctional central pain processing influenced by a variety of processes, including infection, physical trauma, psychological traits, and psychopathology (Abeles et al. 2007). Historically, there has been doubt about the organic basis for fibromyalgia. There is no irrefutable evidence from diagnostic techniques, such as brain imaging, that the condition has strong biological underpinnings (Clauw 2015). Guidelines for fibromyalgia treatment are available (Carville et al. 2008; Clauw 2014). Placebo-controlled trials suggest pain reduction with cyclobenzaprine (Tofferi et al. 2004), milnacipran (Mease et al. 2009), gabapentin (Moore et al. 2014), pregabalin (Arnold et al. 2008), duloxetine (in females but not males), and tramadol (Crofford 2008). Although there is no evidence that SSRIs are more effective than placebo in treating pain, fatigue, and sleep problems in patients with fibromyalgia, they can be considered for treating comorbid depression (Walitt et al. 2015).

Pain in Sickle Cell Anemia

Pain is the hallmark of sickle cell disease. Sickle cell pain is mainly nociceptive, resulting from tissue ischemia and microcirculatory vaso-occlusion by sickled or less malleable red blood cells. It may be acute or chronic, with acute painful episodes most often affecting long bones and joints and the lower back (Ballas 2005). Placebo-controlled trials demonstrate efficacy of NSAIDs in acute pain (Dunlop and Bennett 2014: article withdrawn; update being prepared). Chronic pain and acute painful episodes not controlled by NSAIDs are best managed with a combination of long-acting opioids and short-acting opioids for breakthrough pain. The benefits of long-term opioids must be balanced against the risks of addiction. Chronic therapy with hydroxyurea, which increases the concentration of fetal hemoglobin, also reduces pain (Yawn et al. 2014). There is limited evidence for the benefits of psychological treatments (Anie and Green 2015).

Nociceptive Pain

Tissue injury and inflammation trigger the release of local mediators of pain and inflammation, including prostaglandins, serotonin, bradykinin, adenosine, and cytokines. These substances sensitize tissue nociceptors and produce the sensation of pain. Somatic (musculoskeletal) pain and visceral pain are generally nociceptive in origin but may also have neuropathic elements. Somatic pain is a localized stabbing or sharp pain, whereas visceral pain is diffuse, with aching, pressure, colicky, or sharp qualities. Musculoskeletal pain includes soft tissue injuries, intra-articular disorders, bone pain, muscle pain syndromes, and neck and lower-back conditions. Mild to moderate nociceptive pain generally responds to NSAIDs, but severe pain may require opioids. Expert consensus guidelines recommend topical NSAIDs, capsaicin cream, and intra-articular corticosteroids for osteoarthritis pain (Zhang et al. 2008). In an open-label trial of lidocaine patch 5%, significant pain improvement was reported in patients with osteoarthritis (Gammaitoni et al. 2004). In addition, duloxetine has been shown to be well tolerated and effective in treating osteoarthritis knee pain in both younger and older adults (Micca et al. 2013; Risser et al. 2013).

Malignant Pain

One-third of newly diagnosed oncology patients and 65%–85% of those with advanced disease report significant pain (Skaer 2004). Management of malignancy-related pain is often suboptimal; many patients receive subtherapeutic doses of analgesics in spite of published guidelines for cancer pain management (National Cancer Institute 2015). Cancer pain may have both nociceptive and neuropathic components. Neuropathic pain is often managed with anticonvulsants, TCAs, SNRIs, or opioids. Mild nociceptive pain can be managed with acetaminophen or NSAIDs, but most patients with malignancies experience moderate to severe pain, generally treated with opioids. Short-acting opioids are used for initiation of therapy, for pain that is highly variable, or in medically unstable patients. Once analgesic requirements become stable, patients should be switched to long-half-life or sustained-release forms. Inadequate opioid dosing often results because of fear of addiction or respiratory depression. Patients become opioid tolerant with long-term dosing and may need dosage increases to maintain pain control (Fielding et al. 2013). Particular nociceptive pain syndromes may respond to specific treatments. For example, in clinical trials, bisphosphonates reduced pain from bone metastases (Shaiova 2006).

Pharmacological Treatment

Various medications are commonly used to treat pain. A summary of some of these drugs, including demonstrated pain benefits, is provided in Table 17–1.

Opioids

Opioids reduce the sensory and affective components of pain by interacting with μ, δ, and κ opioid receptors located on the peripheral nerves in the central nervous system modulating pain transmission. Opioids are potent analgesics for all types of neuropathic and nociceptive pain. Controversy surrounds the long-term use of opioids for chronic nonmalignant pain (Noble et al. 2008). Evidence for the efficacy of opioids in chronic pain is considered weak and supports a dose-dependent risk for serious adverse effects (Chou et al. 2015). Studies are generally less than 18 months in duration and are complicated by high rates of discontinuation due to adverse events or insufficient pain relief. Opioids should be slowly tapered and discontinued if the burdens (side effects, toxicities, aberrant drug-related behaviors) outweigh the objective benefits (analgesia, functional improvement).

Successful treatment with opioids requires the assessment and documentation of improvements in function and analgesia without accompanying adverse side effects and aberrant behaviors. Guidelines have been established for the use of opioids for treating chronic pain to help balance the beneficial effects of opioid use with undesirable adverse effects (Manchikanti et al. 2012a, 2012b; Stein et al. 2010). Suitable patients are those with moderate or severe pain persisting for more than 3 months and adversely affecting function or quality of life.

Before opioid therapy is initiated, additional factors, such as the patient's specific pain syndrome, response to other therapies, and potential for aberrant drug-related behaviors (misuse, abuse, addiction, diversion), should be considered (Ballantyne and LaForge 2007; see also Chapter 18, "Substance Use

Table 17–1.   Examples of research efficacy for medications in treating chronic pain, by medication class

Class or agent	Conditions for which research evidence of efficacy exists
TCAs	Painful peripheral neuropathy, headache, migraine, trigeminal neuralgia, PHN, central pain, poststroke pain, orofacial pain, postmastectomy pain, irritable bowel syndrome
SSRIs	Somatic symptom disorder, irritable bowel syndrome, headache, diabetic peripheral neuropathy, fibromyalgia, pain in rheumatoid arthritis
SNRIs	Diabetic peripheral neuropathy, fibromyalgia, migraine prophylaxis, pain in osteoarthritis
Atypical antidepressants	Neuropathic pain, tension-type headache
Anticonvulsants	Trigeminal neuralgia, diabetic peripheral neuropathy, PHN, migraine, postamputation pain, Guillain-Barré syndrome, HIV neuropathy, central poststroke pain, central pain/spinal cord injury pain, lower back pain, radicular pain, cluster headache
Opioids	Acute pain, breakthrough pain, mixed efficacy in numerous chronic nociceptive pain syndromes (e.g., lower back) and neuropathic pain syndromes (e.g., PHN, peripheral neuropathies)
Antipsychotics	Diabetic neuropathy, PHN, trigeminal neuralgia, headache, facial pain, HIV/AIDS pain, cancer, musculoskeletal pain

Note.   PHN=postherpetic neuralgia;   SNRIs=serotonin-norepinephrine reuptake inhibitors;   SSRIs=selective serotonin reuptake inhibitors;   TCAs=tricyclic antidepressants.

Disorders"). A patient's suitability for chronic opioid therapy can be assessed with standardized questionnaires (Chou et al. 2009). Commonly used instruments include the Opioid Risk Tool (ORT); the Diagnosis, Intractability, Risk, Efficacy (DIRE) screening scale; and the Screener and Opioid Assessment for Patients in Pain (SOAPP) (all three are available for download at www.opioidrisk.com/node/1209). Treatment outcomes, including analgesia, activities of daily living, adverse events, and potential aberrant drug-related behaviors, can be assessed with the Pain Assessment and Documentation Tool (available for download at www.practiceadvisor.org/docs/default-source//Documents/Pain_Assessment_and_Documentation_Tool). The presence of aberrant drug-related behaviors should always be evaluated. The Current Opioid Misuse Measure (COMM; available for download at www.opiodprescribing.com/documents/09-comm_inflexxion.pdf) is used to evaluate patients who are taking opioids for concurrent signs or symptoms of intoxication, emotional volatility, poor response to medication, addiction, health care use patterns, and problematic medication behaviors (Sehgal et al. 2012).

Clinically available opioids include naturally occurring compounds (morphine, codeine), semisynthetic derivatives (hydromorphone, oxymorphone, hydrocodone, oxycodone, dihydrocodeine, buprenorphine), and synthetic opioid analgesics (fentanyl, meperidine, methadone, tramadol, pentazocine, propoxyphene). *Morphine,* because of its hydrophilicity, has poor oral bioavailability (22%–48%) and delayed central nervous system access and onset of action. This delay prolongs the analgesic effect of morphine relative to its plasma half-life, which decreases the potential for accumulation and toxicity. Morphine is a more effective epidural or spinal analgesic than oxycodone. *Codeine* is a prodrug that is active only once it is metabolized to morphine. *Oxycodone* is an opioid analgesic with high oral bioavailability (>60%), a faster onset of action, and more predictable plasma levels than morphine. In comparison with morphine, oxycodone has similar analgesic efficacy, releases less histamine, and causes fewer hallucinations (Riley et al. 2008). *Hydrocodone* is similar to oxycodone, with rapid oral absorption and onset of analgesia. Hydrocodone is metabolized by N-demethylation to hydromorphone, which has properties similar to those of morphine, except lower rates of side effects. *Fentanyl* is highly lipophilic, with affinity for neuronal tissues and the potential for transdermal or transmucosal delivery. The duration of action of transdermal preparations is up to 72 hours, with considerable interindividual variability.

Meperidine can cause seizures and an agitated delirium, believed to be caused by accumulation of the active metabolite normeperidine, which has anticholinergic properties. This is particularly a concern in patients with renal insufficiency because normeperidine is eliminated by the kidneys. *Tramadol* is a "semi-opioid" that weakly binds to μ opioid receptors and weakly inhibits the reuptake of serotonin and norepinephrine. There is a risk for serotonin syndrome when tramadol is used in conjunction with other agents that inhibit the reuptake of serotonin.

Methadone warrants special consideration in the treatment of chronic pain because of its low cost, high bioavailability, rapid onset of action, slow hepatic clearance, multiple receptor affinities, lack of neurotoxic metabolites, and incomplete cross-tolerance with other opioids. However, compared with other opioids, methadone has significantly greater risk of inadvertent overdose due to longer time for adaptation with oral use and greater variation in plasma half-life (15–120 hours) (Sandoval et al. 2005). Extensive tissue distribution and prolonged half-life prevent withdrawal symptoms when methadone is dosed once a day. However, elimination is biphasic, and the more rapid elimination phase equates with analgesia that is limited to approximately 6 hours. Repeated dosing, with accumulation in tissue, may increase analgesia duration to 8–12 hours. Therefore, methadone should usually be given twice daily. Methadone was shown to be effective for chronic pain in a study of 100 patients, with a mean duration of treatment of 11 months (Peng et al. 2008). It is also associated with QTc prolongation and torsades de pointes, especially when given intravenously or at high doses, as well as increased rates of all-cause mortality at all doses (Ray et al. 2015).

The most common side effect of chronic opioid therapy is decreased gastrointestinal motility, causing constipation, vomiting, and abdominal pain. Oral opioids differ in their propensity to cause symptoms of gastrointestinal dysmotility (Heiskanen and Kalso 1997). An often unrecognized side effect of opioids is a paradoxical development of chronic abdominal pain called *narcotic bowel syndrome*. It can cause worsening pain despite increasing doses of the opioid used to treat the pain (Drossman and Szigethy 2014). Transdermal opioids (fentanyl, buprenorphine) have fewer gastrointestinal side effects than oral opioids (Tassinari et al. 2008). Meperidine is not preferred in patients with acute pancreatitis because all opioids are equally likely to cause spasm of the sphincter of Oddi (Thompson 2001).

Long-term opioid administration may result in analgesic tolerance or opioid-induced hyperalgesia, which may be due to alterations in psychophysiological pathways (Mitra 2008; Wachholtz et al. 2015). When tolerance develops, coadministration of other analgesics, opioid rotation to a more potent agonist, or intermittent cessation of certain agents may restore analgesic effect (Mercadante 1999; Vorobeychik et al. 2008). Opioid rotation from morphine or hydromorphone may be beneficial because the 3-glucuronide metabolites of either drug can accumulate within the cerebrospinal fluid and produce neuroexcitatory effects, such as allodynia, myoclonus, delirium, and seizures (Smith 2000). Rotation to mixed agonist-antagonist opioids (buprenorphine, pentazocine) may precipitate withdrawal symptoms in patients undergoing chronic opioid therapy.

As the supply of opioids has increased over the past two decades in an effort to better treat pain, the number of deaths associated with prescription opioids has increased dramatically. Several factors have been associated with this increase, including too high doses for naïve patients, too rapid titration of doses, insufficient patient monitoring, and insufficient knowledge of drug metabolism and drug interactions (Agarin et al. 2015). There are several guidelines available for the prescription of opioids that can help limit fatalities (Manchikanti et al. 2012a, 2012b).

Antidepressants

The analgesic properties of antidepressants are underappreciated (Barkin and Fawcett 2000). The neurobiology of pain suggests that all antidepressants might be effective for treatment of chronic pain (McCleane 2008). The TCAs and SNRIs, in particular, are prescribed for many chronic pain syndromes, including diabetic neuropathy, postherpetic neuralgia, central pain, poststroke pain, tension-type headache, migraine, and oral-facial pain (Saarto and Wiffen 2007). The analgesic effect of antidepressants is independent of their antidepressant effect and is thought to be mediated primarily by the blockade of reuptake of norepinephrine and serotonin, increasing their levels and enhancing the activation of descending inhibitory neurons in the dorsal horn of the spinal cord (Micó et al. 2006). Antidepressants may also produce antinociceptive effects by other mechanisms. For example, TCAs block a subtype of sodium channel implicated in neuropathic pain (Dick et al. 2007).

Tricyclic Antidepressants

Meta-analyses and systematic reviews of randomized controlled trials concluded that TCAs have the best evidence base for the treatment of neuropathic pain and are effective for headache syndromes (Derry et al. 2015; Finnerup et al. 2015; Moulin et al. 2014). TCAs have been shown in controlled trials to effectively treat central poststroke pain, postherpetic neuralgia, painful diabetic and nondiabetic polyneuropathy, and postmastectomy pain syndrome but not spinal cord injury pain, phantom limb pain, or pain in HIV neuropathy. TCA agents are equally effective for pain, but secondary-amine TCAs (e.g., nortriptyline) are better tolerated than tertiary agents (e.g., amitriptyline) (Dworkin et al. 2007; Finnerup et al. 2005). Antidepressants generally produce analgesia at lower dosages and with earlier onset of action than expected for the treatment of depression (Rojas-Corrales et al. 2003). However, lack of analgesic effect—for example, in spinal cord injury pain—may be due to inadequate dosing. Chronic pain of postherpetic neuralgia and diabetic peripheral neuropathy has been successfully treated with TCAs at average dosages of 100–250 mg/day (Onghena and Van Houdenhove 1992). In contrast, a study of a U.S. health insurance claims database found that the average dosage of TCAs for the treatment of neuropathic pain in patients ages 65 and older was only 23 mg/day (Berger et al. 2006), suggesting unrealized potential for additional pain relief. Advantages of TCAs include low cost and the ability to monitor optimal titration with serum levels to ensure adequate trials and avoidance of toxicity.

Serotonin-Norepinephrine Reuptake Inhibitors

Duloxetine, venlafaxine, desvenlafaxine, and milnacipran inhibit the presynaptic reuptake of serotonin, norepinephrine, and, to a lesser extent, dopamine. They are associated with fewer side effects than TCAs and can be titrated more quickly, but titration cannot be monitored by serum levels.

In placebo-controlled trials, venlafaxine significantly reduced neuropathic pain following breast cancer treatment (Tasmuth et al. 2002) and decreased allodynia and hyperalgesia associated with neuropathic pain (Yucel et al. 2005). Studies also suggest that venlafaxine is effective for atypical facial pain, migraine prophylaxis, and fibromyalgia (Forssell et al. 2004; Ozyalcin et al. 2005; VanderWeide et al. 2015). Response increases with increasing dosage; venlafaxine 150–225 mg/day produced a greater percentage of reduction in pain than

75 mg/day (50% vs. 32%) in a placebo-controlled study of painful diabetic neuropathy (Rowbotham et al. 2004). Duloxetine possesses analgesic efficacy in preclinical models and in clinical populations such as those with fibromyalgia and painful diabetic neuropathy (Arnold et al. 2005; Wernicke et al. 2006). Guidelines for the treatment of neuropathic pain recommend duloxetine at adequate doses as an effective treatment (Argoff et al. 2006; Lunn et al. 2014). The efficacy of duloxetine in painful diabetic neuropathy increases with increasing pain but is not related to the severity of diabetes or neuropathy (Ziegler et al. 2007). Milnacipran significantly improved symptoms of fibromyalgia, including pain, physical functioning, and patient global impression of change in a large placebo-controlled trial (Mease et al. 2009). Duloxetine has been shown to be well tolerated and effective in treating osteoarthritis knee pain in both younger and older adults (Micca et al. 2013; Risser et al. 2013).

Selective Serotonin Reuptake Inhibitors

In clinical trials, the efficacy of SSRIs in chronic pain syndromes has been inconsistent and disappointing, especially in the treatment of neuropathic pain (Finnerup et al. 2005). In a Cochrane review, Banzi et al. (2015) found SSRIs to be no more efficacious than placebo for migraine and less efficacious than TCAs for tension-type headache. Fluoxetine improved outcome measures in women with fibromyalgia (Rani et al. 1996) and was comparable to amitriptyline at significantly reducing rheumatoid arthritis pain (Arnold et al. 2002). Citalopram improved irritable bowel syndrome symptoms independent of effects on anxiety and depression (Tack et al. 2006). Patients with pain disorder experienced significant analgesic effects, independent of changes in depression, with citalopram but not with the noradrenergic reuptake inhibitor reboxetine (Aragona et al. 2005). Paroxetine and citalopram, but not fluoxetine, have shown benefit for painful diabetic peripheral neuropathy in controlled studies (Goodnick 2001). Despite better efficacy, TCAs increase catecholamines, which likely diminish insulin sensitivity and may exacerbate glucose intolerance (Mumoli et al. 2014). In contrast, increased serotonergic function improves sensitivity to insulin, making SSRIs an alternative for some patients with diabetes. One comparison study of gabapentin, paroxetine, and citalopram for painful diabetic peripheral neuropathy found better acceptability, adherence, and mood with SSRIs, with similar efficacy for pain (Giannopoulos et al. 2007). Overall, although not recommended as a first-line therapy for chronic pain, SSRIs may be worth considering when comorbid depression is present and the pain symptoms coincide with it.

Novel Antidepressants

Few controlled trials have examined the efficacy of novel antidepressants such as mirtazapine and bupropion in treating pain syndromes. Mirtazapine decreased the duration and intensity of chronic tension-type headache in a controlled trial with patients with treatment-refractory headaches (Bendtsen and Jensen 2004). In a controlled trial of patients with neuropathic pain, sustained-release bupropion decreased pain intensity and interference of pain with quality of life (Semenchuk et al. 2001). Although several reports suggest efficacy for trazodone in treating chronic pain, controlled studies do not support its use in patients with chronic pain (Goodkin et al. 1990). Vortioxetine and vilazodone are fairly new antidepressants that selectively inhibit serotonin reuptake and also have action at serotonin type 3 and 1A receptors. They have been shown to be effective antidepressants, but their efficacy in treating pain has not yet been studied.

Anticonvulsants

Anticonvulsants are effective for treating a variety of neuropathic pain syndromes, including trigeminal neuralgia, diabetic neuropathy, postherpetic neuralgia, and migraine prophylaxis (Seidel et al. 2013; Tremont-Lukats et al. 2000). They reduce pain by inhibiting excessive neuronal activity. The number needed to treat ranges from <2 to 4 for anticonvulsants, with better compliance when compared with TCAs because of fewer adverse effects (Finnerup et al. 2005).

First-Generation Anticonvulsants

Phenytoin was first reported as a successful treatment for trigeminal neuralgia in 1942 (Bergouignan 1942). Carbamazepine is the most widely studied first-generation anticonvulsant effective for neuropathic pain (Wiffen et al. 2014a). Valproic acid is most commonly used in the prophylaxis of migraine but is also effective for neuropathic pain (Gill et al. 2011; Jensen et al. 1994). Valproate was effective as a prophylactic treatment in more than two-thirds of patients with migraine and almost 75% of those with cluster headache (Gallagher et al. 2002). Improvement occurred in frequency of headache, duration or headache-days per month, intensity of headache, use of other medications for acute treatment of headache, the patient's opinion of treatment, and ratings of depression and anxiety (Kaniecki 1997; Klapper 1997; Rothrock 1997).

Second-Generation Anticonvulsants

Newer anticonvulsants were developed to target novel pharmacological mechanisms for the suppression of nociceptive processes. Gabapentin demonstrated analgesic efficacy in placebo-controlled trials of diabetic peripheral neuropathy pain, postherpetic neuralgia, fibromyalgia, and postamputation phantom limb pain (Chandra et al. 2006; Moore et al. 2014). A retrospective analysis found patients with chronic pain were more likely to respond to gabapentin if allodynia was a feature of their neuropathic pain (Gustorff et al. 2002). Gabapentin significantly decreased the pain associated with Guillain-Barré syndrome as well as the concomitant consumption of fentanyl (Pandey et al. 2002).

Pregabalin, a gabapentin analogue with rapid onset of action and better bioavailability, is effective for the treatment of painful diabetic neuropathy, postherpetic neuralgia, and central neuropathic pain associated with spinal cord injury (Siddall et al. 2006; Sonnett et al. 2006; van Seventer et al. 2006). In patients with postherpetic neuralgia, flexible dosing strategies resulted in fewer discontinuations, higher final dosage, and slightly better pain relief compared with fixed-dose schedules (Stacey et al. 2008). The most common side effects include sedation, peripheral edema, dizziness, and dry mouth (Toth 2014). Pregabalin has been shown to reduce postoperative pain but with the disadvantages of increased sedation and visual disturbances (Mishriky et al. 2015). Gabapentin and pregabalin are entirely renally excreted, so the dose must be lowered in patients with impaired renal function. In patients on chronic hemodialysis, a single dose of the drug is given three times a week after dialysis (Atalay et al. 2013).

In a meta-analysis of controlled trials, Wiffen and Rees (2013) found that lamotrigine produced positive but disappointing results for pain associated with HIV-related neuropathy and central poststroke pain and had no significant effect on diabetic neuropathy pain, trigeminal neuralgia, or intractable neuropathic pain.

Next-Generation Anticonvulsants

Topiramate offers the advantages of minimal hepatic metabolism and unchanged renal excretion, few drug interactions, a long half-life, and the unusual side effect of weight loss. Topiramate is effective for migraine prophylaxis (Silberstein et al. 2006). There is some evidence of its effectiveness for reducing pain from chronic low-back pain, lumbar radiculopathy, and diabetic neuropathy (Khoromi et al. 2005; Muehlbacher et al. 2006), but its benefits are not clearly established (Wiffen et al. 2013a). A randomized placebo-controlled trial of oxcarbazepine for painful diabetic neuropathy found that about 35% of patients treated with oxcarbazepine experienced > 50% improvement in their pain compared with 18% of patients given placebo (Dogra et al. 2005). Tiagabine, vigabatrin, retigabine, levetiracetam, lacosamide, and zonisamide are new anticonvulsants with a spectrum of pharmacological actions and antinociceptive effects in animal models, but few clinical studies exist to support their use as a first-line therapy for patients with chronic pain (Wiffen et al. 2013b, 2014b). Although variable, these agents can cause significant cognitive impairment. In an open-label trial with various chronic pain conditions, tiagabine was found to be similar to gabapentin in pain reduction but to result in greater improvement in sleep quality (Todorov et al. 2005). Zonisamide was not effective in a controlled trial for diabetic neuropathy pain, and the drug was poorly tolerated (Atli and Dogra 2005).

Combinations of anticonvulsants with complementary mechanisms of action may increase effectiveness and decrease adverse effects of treatment. Patients with multiple sclerosis or trigeminal neuralgia who could not continue with carbamazepine or lamotrigine at therapeutic dosages because of intolerable side effects were given gabapentin as an augmentation agent (Solaro et al. 2000). Gabapentin was titrated to pain relief with no new side effects up to a maximum dosage of 1,200 mg/day, at which time either carbamazepine or lamotrigine was tapered until side effects were no longer present. When anticonvulsants were combined with tramadol, synergistic effects were found for inhibiting allodynia and blocking nociception (Codd et al. 2008).

Benzodiazepines

Benzodiazepines are commonly prescribed for insomnia, anxiety, and occasionally spasticity in patients with chronic pain, but no studies demonstrate any benefit for these target symptoms, and the drugs may be counterproductive in these patients (Taricco et al. 2000). Benzodiazepines decreased pain in only a limited number of chronic pain conditions, such as trigeminal neuralgia, tension headache, and temporomandibular disorders (Dellemijn and

Fields 1994). Clonazepam may provide long-term relief for the episodic lancinating variety of phantom limb pain (Bartusch et al. 1996) as well as cancer-related neuropathic pain (Howard et al. 2014). In a study of patients with acute sciatica, those who received diazepam had worse outcomes in terms of pain than those who received placebo (Brötz et al. 2010). Benzodiazepines can cause sedation and cognitive impairment, especially in elderly patients (Buffett-Jerrott and Stewart 2002). In patients with chronic pain, the use of benzodiazepines, but not opioids, was associated with decreased activity levels, higher rates of health care visits, increased domestic instability, depression, and more disability days (Ciccone et al. 2000). Combining benzodiazepines with opioids may be countertherapeutic and potentially dangerous. Studies of methadone-related mortality found high rates of benzodiazepine use, with the cause of death being attributed to a combination of drug effects, especially in patients receiving methadone for chronic pain (Caplehorn and Drummer 2002). However, antihyperalgesic (reduction of increased sensitivity to pain) properties have been confirmed in healthy patients (Howard et al. 2014).

Antipsychotics

Antipsychotics have been studied in a variety of chronic pain conditions, including diabetic neuropathy, postherpetic neuralgia, headache, facial pain, pain associated with AIDS and cancer, and musculoskeletal pain. Compared with typical antipsychotics, atypical antipsychotics offer a broader therapeutic spectrum and have lower rates of extrapyramidal effects. However, they are associated with metabolic disruptions, such as weight gain and new-onset diabetes, which somewhat offset their benefits.

A meta-analysis of 11 controlled trials suggests that some antipsychotics have analgesic efficacy in headache (haloperidol) and trigeminal neuralgia (pimozide), but antipsychotics' role in chronic pain is mainly as add-on therapy to other agents (Seidel et al. 2013). In an open-label study, the addition of quetiapine to patients' existing but ineffective fibromyalgia treatment regimen did not decrease pain but produced significant improvements on the Fibromyalgia Impact Questionnaire and quality-of-life measures (Hidalgo et al. 2007). Studies of ziprasidone and olanzapine showed beneficial effects but low response rates and poor tolerability (Calandre et al. 2007; Rico-Villademoros et al. 2005). Results are difficult to interpret because comorbid depressive, anxiety, and sleep disorders in patients with fibromyalgia might respond to treatment with atypical antipsychotics.

Local Anesthetics

Local anesthetic agents act as membrane stabilizers in hyperactive neurons carrying nociceptive information. Topical lidocaine has been approved for the treatment of postherpetic neuralgia and does not produce significant serum levels (Khaliq et al. 2007). Individual studies indicate that it is effective for the treatment of neuropathic pain (Derry et al. 2014). Results are mixed in studies treating HIV neuropathy pain (Cheville et al. 2009; Estanislao et al. 2004). Oral mexiletine is an effective treatment for neuropathic pain in patients with painful diabetic neuropathy, peripheral nerve injury, alcoholic neuropathy, and phantom limb pain, but not in patients with cancer-related pain (Jarvis and Coukell 1998; Kalso et al. 1998; Nishiyama and Sakuta 1995). Mexiletine decreased not only reports of pain but also the accompanying paresthesias and dysesthesias (Dejgard et al. 1988). Mexiletine decreased pain and sleep disturbances associated with painful diabetic neuropathy (Oskarsson et al. 1997). Analgesic effect did not correlate with plasma mexiletine levels.

Calcium Channel Blockers

The most commonly prescribed calcium channel blocker for chronic pain is verapamil, which has proved effective in the treatment of migraine and cluster headaches (Lewis and Solomon 1996; Markley 1991). Intrathecal ziconotide, a neuron-specific calcium channel blocker that is derived from the toxin of the cone snail (*Conus magnus*), has been approved for intrathecal use for the treatment of refractory pain of cancer or AIDS. It has potent analgesic, antihyperesthetic, and antiallodynic activity, as well as synergistic analgesic effects when administered with morphine, without producing tolerance (Christo and Mazloomdoost 2008).

Capsaicin

Topically applied capsaicin has moderate to poor efficacy in the treatment of chronic musculoskeletal or neuropathic pain but is clearly more effective at high doses if tolerated (Smith and Brooks 2014). However, capsaicin may be useful as an adjunct or a sole therapy for a small number of patients who are unresponsive to or intolerant of other treatments (Mason et al. 2004).

Drug-Drug Interactions

In this section, we review only drug interactions between psychotropic drugs and opioids, triptans, NSAIDs, and local anesthetics. (Selected interactions are listed in Table 17–2.) Most pharmacokinetic interactions between pain drugs and psychotropic drugs result from psychotropic drug–mediated inhibition or induction of cytochrome P450 (CYP)–mediated drug metabolism. Many opioids are metabolized by CYP2D6, an enzyme significantly inhibited by fluoxetine, paroxetine, moclobemide, and bupropion. The triptan antimigraine medications rizatriptan, sumatriptan, and zolmitriptan undergo metabolism by monoamine oxidase type A. Monoamine oxidase inhibitors (MAOIs) increase the levels of these drugs and possibly their toxicity. Mexiletine, a CYP1A2 inhibitor, may inhibit metabolism of olanzapine and clozapine. NSAIDs, including cyclooxygenase isoenzyme 2 inhibitors but not acetylsalicylic acid (aspirin), may precipitate lithium toxicity by reducing its excretion (Hersh et al. 2007). Valproate inhibition of glucuronidation increases lamotrigine levels severalfold and may cause toxicities unless lamotrigine dosage is reduced by at least 50% (Gidal et al. 2003). See Chapter 1, "Pharmacokinetics, Pharmacodynamics, and Principles of Drug-Drug Interactions," for a general discussion of drug interactions.

Pharmacodynamic interactions also occur between pain medications and psychotropic agents. The phenylpiperidine series opioids, meperidine (pethidine), fentanyl, tramadol, methadone, dextromethorphan, and propoxyphene are weak serotonin reuptake inhibitors and may precipitate serotonin syndrome in combination with MAOIs (including some fatalities) (Choong and Ghiculescu 2008; Gillman 2005) and SSRIs (Ailawadhi et al. 2007; Rang et al. 2008). Morphine, codeine, oxycodone, and buprenorphine are less likely to precipitate serotonin toxicity with MAOIs, TCAs, SSRIs, or SNRIs. The constipating effects of opioids are additive in combination with drugs possessing anticholinergic activity, including TCAs and anticholinergic agents used to treat extrapyramidal symptoms (e.g., trihexyphenidyl, benztropine). Methadone is associated with prolonged QTc (Ehret et al. 2007), which is exacerbated in the presence of CYP3A4 inhibitors (e.g., fluvoxamine, fluoxetine, nefazodone) and other QT-prolonging agents (e.g., TCAs, typical and atypical antipsychotics). A 2006 U.S. Food and Drug Administration alert warns of possible serotonin syndrome precipitated by the combined use of SSRIs or SNRIs and triptan antimigraine medications (Evans 2007).

Table 17–2. Pain drug–psychotropic drug interactions

Pain drug	Mechanism of interaction	Clinical effects and management
Opioids		
Dextromethorphan, fentanyl, meperidine (pethidine), methadone, propoxyphene, and tramadol	Increased serotonin activity (have serotonin reuptake inhibitor activity)	Possible serotonin syndrome or hyperpyrexia when combined with SSRIs, SNRIs, MAOIs, or TCAs. Avoid concurrent use; discontinue offending opioid. Consider morphine for pain management.
Methadone	Prolonged QT interval	Potentiates QT prolongation induced by TCAs or antipsychotics (typical and atypical). May lead to cardiac arrhythmias or torsades de pointes. Avoid concurrent use. Consider other opioid analgesic.
NSAIDs		
Celecoxib (and other COX-2 inhibitors), ibuprofen, and naproxen	Reduced renal blood flow	Reduced lithium elimination, leading to lithium toxicity. Monitor lithium levels; reduce lithium dose. Consider ASA.
Antimigraine agents		
Almotriptan, eletriptan, frovatriptan, naratriptan, rizatriptan, sumatriptan, and zolmitriptan	Serotonin agonist activity	Possible serotonin syndrome in combination with SSRIs, SNRIs, MAOIs, or TCAs. Use with caution. Instruct patient about symptoms.

Table 17–2.   Pain drug–psychotropic drug interactions *(continued)*

Pain drug	Mechanism of interaction	Clinical effects and management
Local anesthetic		
Mexiletine	Inhibition of CYP1A2	Increased levels of olanzapine or clozapine, possibly increasing toxicity. Avoid concurrent use. Reduce antipsychotic dose.

Note.   ASA=acetylsalicylic acid (aspirin); COX-2=cyclooxygenase isoenzyme 2; CYP=cytochrome P450; MAOIs=monoamine oxidase inhibitors; NSAIDs=nonsteroidal anti-inflammatory drugs; SNRIs=serotonin-norepinephrine reuptake inhibitors; SSRIs=selective serotonin reuptake inhibitors; TCAs=tricyclic antidepressants.

Key Clinical Points

Medication Selection

- Functional outcomes should be determined prior to initiating therapy.
- SNRIs and TCAs are first-line therapies.
- Anticonvulsants are second-line therapies.
- Atypical antipsychotics and opioids are third-line therapies.
- If possible, serum levels should be optimized.

Medication Combinations

- The following medication combinations may increase analgesic effect:
  - SNRI+anticonvulsant
  - SNRI+antidepressant
  - SNRI+anticonvulsant+opioid
  - Antidepressant+atypical antipsychotic
  - Antidepressant+anticonvulsant 1+anticonvulsant 2 with a different mechanism
  - Antidepressant+mood-stabilizing anticonvulsant

Cautions

- Major depressive disorder is underdiagnosed and under-treated, so patients should be treated aggressively if disabling pain persists.
- Opioids should be avoided in the presence of major depressive disorder.
- Short-acting pain medications should be avoided in the presence of major depressive disorder.
- The dosage of opioids should not be increased if two successive increases provide no benefit.
- SSRIs have utility in pain management; they should not be avoided.

Drug Interactions

- Serum levels can provide useful insights into real-world interactions.
- Gabapentin, pregabalin, and topiramate are primarily renally excreted.
- Caution is needed when combining valproate and lamotrigine; the lamotrigine dosage should be reduced by ≥50%.
- CYP2D6 inhibitors, including several antidepressants, inhibit opioid metabolism.

References

Abeles AM, Pillinger MH, Solitar BM, Abeles M: Narrative review: the pathophysiology of fibromyalgia. Ann Intern Med 146(10):726–734, 2007 17502633

Agarin T, Trescot AM, Agarin A, et al: Reducing opioid analgesic deaths in America: what health providers can do. Pain Physician 18(3):E307–E322, 2015 26000678

Ailawadhi S, Sung KW, Carlson LA, Baer MR: Serotonin syndrome caused by interaction between citalopram and fentanyl. J Clin Pharm Ther 32(2):199–202, 2007 17381671

Alföldi P, Wiklund T, Gerdle B: Comorbid insomnia in patients with chronic pain: a study based on the Swedish quality registry for pain rehabilitation (SQRP). Disabil Rehabil 36(20):1661–1669, 2014 24320022

American Psychiatric Association: Diagnostic and Statistical Manual of Mental Disorders, 5th Edition. Arlington, VA, American Psychiatric Association, 2013

Anie KA, Green J: Psychological therapies for sickle cell disease and pain. Cochrane Database of Systematic Reviews 2015, Issue 5. Art. No.: CD001916. DOI: 10.1002/14651858.CD001916.pub3 25966336

Aragona M, Bancheri L, Perinelli D, et al: Randomized double-blind comparison of serotonergic (citalopram) versus noradrenergic (reboxetine) reuptake inhibitors in outpatients with somatoform, DSM-IV-TR pain disorder. Eur J Pain 9(1):33–38, 2005 15629872

Argoff CE, Backonja MM, Belgrade MJ, et al: Consensus guidelines: treatment planning and options. Diabetic peripheral neuropathic pain. Mayo Clin Proc 81(4)(suppl): S12–S25, 2006 16608049

Arnold LM, Hess EV, Hudson JI, et al: A randomized, placebo-controlled, double-blind, flexible-dose study of fluoxetine in the treatment of women with fibromyalgia. Am J Med 112(3):191–197, 2002 11893345

Arnold LM, Hudson JI, Hess EV, et al: Family study of fibromyalgia. Arthritis Rheum 50(3):944–952, 2004 15022338

Arnold LM, Rosen A, Pritchett YL, et al: A randomized, double-blind, placebo-controlled trial of duloxetine in the treatment of women with fibromyalgia with or without major depressive disorder. Pain 119(1-3):5–15, 2005 16298061

Arnold LM, Russell IJ, Diri EW, et al: A 14-week, randomized, double-blinded, placebo-controlled monotherapy trial of pregabalin in patients with fibromyalgia. J Pain 9(9):792–805, 2008 18524684

Asmundson GJ, Norton PJ, Norton GR: Beyond pain: the role of fear and avoidance in chronicity. Clin Psychol Rev 19(1):97–119, 1999 9987586

Atalay H, Solak Y, Biyik Z, et al: Cross-over, open-label trial of the effects of gabapentin versus pregabalin on painful peripheral neuropathy and health-related quality of life in haemodialysis patients. Clin Drug Investig 33(6):401–408, 2013 23572323

Atli A, Dogra S: Zonisamide in the treatment of painful diabetic neuropathy: a randomized, double-blind, placebo-controlled pilot study. Pain Med 6(3):225–234, 2005 15972086

Ballantyne JC, LaForge KS: Opioid dependence and addiction during opioid treatment of chronic pain. Pain 129(3):235–255, 2007 17482363

Ballas SK: Pain management of sickle cell disease. Hematol Oncol Clin North Am 19(5):785–802, 2005 16214644

Banzi R, Cusi C, Randazzo C, et al: Selective serotonin reuptake inhibitors (SSRIs) and serotonin-norepinephrine reuptake inhibitors (SNRIs) for the prevention of tension-type headache in adults. Cochrane Database of Systematic Reviews 2015, Issue 5. Art. No.: CD011681. DOI: 10.1002/14651858.CD011681 25931277

Barkin RL, Fawcett J: The management challenges of chronic pain: the role of antidepressants. Am J Ther 7(1):31–47, 2000 11319571

Bartusch SL, Sanders BJ, D'Alessio JG, Jernigan JR: Clonazepam for the treatment of lancinating phantom limb pain. Clin J Pain 12(1):59–62, 1996 8722737

Bendtsen L, Jensen R: Mirtazapine is effective in the prophylactic treatment of chronic tension-type headache. Neurology 62(10):1706–1711, 2004 15159466

Berger A, Dukes EM, Edelsberg J, et al: Use of tricyclic antidepressants in older patients with painful neuropathies. Eur J Clin Pharmacol 62(9):757–764, 2006 16802165

Bergouignan M: Successful cures of essential facial neuralgias by sodium diphenylhydantoinate [in French]. Rev Laryngol Otol Rhinol (Bord) 63:34–41, 1942

Birklein F, O'Neill D, Schlereth T: Complex regional pain syndrome: an optimistic perspective. Neurology 84(1):89–96, 2015 25471395

Bras M, Dordević V, Gregurek R, Bulajić M: Neurobiological and clinical relationship between psychiatric disorders and chronic pain. Psychiatr Danub 22(2):221–226, 2010 20562750

Brötz D, Maschke E, Burkard S, et al: Is there a role for benzodiazepines in the management of lumbar disc prolapse with acute sciatica? Pain 149(3):470–475, 2010 20362397

Buffett-Jerrott SE, Stewart SH: Cognitive and sedative effects of benzodiazepine use. Curr Pharm Des 8(1):45–58, 2002 11812249

Calandre EP, Hidalgo J, Rico-Villademoros F: Use of ziprasidone in patients with fibromyalgia: a case series. Rheumatol Int 27(5):473–476, 2007 17039363

Caplehorn JR, Drummer OH: Fatal methadone toxicity: signs and circumstances, and the role of benzodiazepines. Aust N Z J Public Health 26(4):358–362, discussion 362–363, 2002 12233958

Carod-Artal FJ: Tackling chronic migraine: current perspectives. J Pain Res 7:185–194, 2014 24748814

Carville SF, Arendt-Nielsen L, Bliddal H, et al; EULAR: EULAR evidence-based recommendations for the management of fibromyalgia syndrome. Ann Rheum Dis 67(4):536–541, 2008 17644548

Chandra K, Shafiq N, Pandhi P, et al: Gabapentin versus nortriptyline in post-herpetic neuralgia patients: a randomized, double-blind clinical trial—the GONIP Trial. Int J Clin Pharmacol Ther 44(8):358–363, 2006 16961166

Cherry DK, Burt CW, Woodwell DA: National Ambulatory Medical Care Survey: 2001 summary. Adv Data (337):1–44, 2003 12924075

Cheville AL, Sloan JA, Northfelt DW, et al: Use of a lidocaine patch in the management of postsurgical neuropathic pain in patients with cancer: a phase III double-blind crossover study (N01CB). Support Care Cancer 17(4):451–460, 2009 19142669

Choong K, Ghiculescu RA: Iatrogenic neuropsychiatric syndromes. Aust Fam Physician 37(8):627–629, 2008 18704211

Chou R, Fanciullo GJ, Fine PG, et al: Opioids for chronic noncancer pain: prediction and identification of aberrant drug-related behaviors: a review of the evidence for an American Pain Society and American Academy of Pain Medicine clinical practice guideline. J Pain 10(2):131–146, 2009 19187890

Chou R, Turner JA, Devine EB, et al: The effectiveness and risks of long-term opioid therapy for chronic pain: a systematic review for a National Institutes of Health Pathways to Prevention Workshop. Ann Intern Med 162(4):276–286, 2015 25581257

Christo PJ, Mazloomdoost D: Interventional pain treatments for cancer pain. Ann N Y Acad Sci 1138:299–328, 2008 18837908

Ciccone DS, Just N, Bandilla EB, et al: Psychological correlates of opioid use in patients with chronic nonmalignant pain: a preliminary test of the downhill spiral hypothesis. J Pain Symptom Manage 20(3):180–192, 2000 11018336

Clark MR, Stoller KB, Brooner RK: Assessment and management of chronic pain in individuals seeking treatment for opioid dependence disorder. Can J Psychiatry 53(8):496–508, 2008 18801211

Clauw DJ: Fibromyalgia: a clinical review. JAMA 311(15):1547–1555, 2014 24737367

Clauw DJ: Fibromyalgia and related conditions. Mayo Clin Proc 90(5):680–692, 2015 25939940

Codd EE, Martinez RP, Molino L, et al: Tramadol and several anticonvulsants synergize in attenuating nerve injury–induced allodynia. Pain 134(3):254–262, 2008 17532139

Cohen SP, Mao J: Neuropathic pain: mechanisms and their clinical implications. BMJ 348:f7656, 2014 24500412

Compton P, Darakjian J, Miotto K: Screening for addiction in patients with chronic pain and "problematic" substance use: evaluation of a pilot assessment tool. J Pain Symptom Manage 16(6):355–363, 1998 9879160

Couch JR; Amitriptyline Versus Placebo Study Group: Amitriptyline in the prophylactic treatment of migraine and chronic daily headache. Headache 51(1):33–51, 2011 21070231

Crofford LJ: Pain management in fibromyalgia. Curr Opin Rheumatol 20(3):246–250, 2008 18388513

Cruccu G, Gronseth G, Alksne J, et al; American Academy of Neurology Society; European Federation of Neurological Society: AAN-EFNS guidelines on trigeminal neuralgia management. Eur J Neurol 15(10):1013–1028, 2008 18721143

Dejgard A, Petersen P, Kastrup J: Mexiletine for treatment of chronic painful diabetic neuropathy. Lancet 1(8575-6):9–11, 1988 2891940

Dellemijn PL, Fields HL: Do benzodiazepines have a role in chronic pain management? Pain 57(2):137–152, 1994 8090510

Derry S, Wiffen PJ, Moore RA, Quinlan J: Topical lidocaine for neuropathic pain in adults. Cochrane Database of Systematic Reviews 2014, Issue 7. Art. No.: CD010958. DOI: 10.1002/14651858.CD010958.pub2 25058164

Derry S, Wiffen PJ, Aldington D, Moore RA: Nortriptyline for neuropathic pain in adults. Cochrane Database of Systematic Reviews 2015, Issue 1. Art. No.: CD011209. DOI: 10.1002/14651858.CD011209.pub2 25569864

Dick IE, Brochu RM, Purohit Y, et al: Sodium channel blockade may contribute to the analgesic efficacy of antidepressants. J Pain 8(4):315–324, 2007 17175203

Dodick DW: Clinical practice. Chronic daily headache. N Engl J Med 354(2):158–165, 2006 16407511

Dogra S, Beydoun S, Mazzola J, et al: Oxcarbazepine in painful diabetic neuropathy: a randomized, placebo-controlled study. Eur J Pain 9(5):543–554, 2005 16139183

Drossman D, Szigethy E: The narcotic bowel syndrome: a recent update. Am J Gastroenterol 2(1):22–30, 2014 25207609

Dunlop R, Bennett KC: WITHDRAWN: Pain management for sickle cell disease in children and adults. Cochrane Database of Systematic Reviews 2014, Issue 4. Art. No.: CD003350. DOI: 10.1002/14651858.CD003350.pub3 24711059

Dworkin RH, O'Connor AB, Backonja M, et al: Pharmacologic management of neuropathic pain: evidence-based recommendations. Pain 132(3):237–251, 2007 17920770

Ehret GB, Desmeules JA, Broers B: Methadone-associated long QT syndrome: improving pharmacotherapy for dependence on illegal opioids and lessons learned for pharmacology. Expert Opin Drug Saf 6(3):289–303, 2007 17480178

Elias WJ, Burchiel KJ: Trigeminal neuralgia and other neuropathic pain syndromes of the head and face. Curr Pain Headache Rep 6(2):115–124, 2002 11872182

Estanislao L, Carter K, McArthur J, et al; Lidoderm-HIV Neuropathy Group: A randomized controlled trial of 5% lidocaine gel for HIV-associated distal symmetric polyneuropathy. J Acquir Immune Defic Syndr 37(5):1584–1586, 2004 15577414

Evans RW: The FDA alert on serotonin syndrome with combined use of SSRIs or SNRIs and triptans: an analysis of the 29 case reports. MedGenMed 9(3):48, 2007 18092054

Ferrari A, Baraldi C, Sternieri E: Medication overuse and chronic migraine: a critical review according to clinical pharmacology. Expert Opin Drug Metab Toxicol 11(7):1127–1144, 2015 26027878

Fielding F, Sanford TM, Davis MP: Achieving effective control in cancer pain: a review of current guidelines. Int J Palliat Nurs 19(12):584–591, 2013 24356502

Finan PH, Goodin BR, Smith MT: The association of sleep and pain: an update and a path forward. J Pain 14(12):1539–1552, 2013 24290442

Finnerup NB: A review of central neuropathic pain states. Curr Opin Anaesthesiol 21(5):586–589, 2008 18784483

Finnerup NB, Otto M, McQuay HJ, et al: Algorithm for neuropathic pain treatment: an evidence based proposal. Pain 118(3):289–305, 2005 16213659

Finnerup NB, Attal N, Haroutounian S, et al: Pharmacotherapy for neuropathic pain in adults: a systematic review and meta-analysis. Lancet Neurol 14(2):162–173, 2015 25575710

Flaster M, Meresh E, Rao M, Biller J: Central poststroke pain: current diagnosis and treatment. Top Stroke Rehabil 20(2):116–123, 2013 23611852

Flor H: Phantom-limb pain: characteristics, causes, and treatment. Lancet Neurol 1(3):182–189, 2002 12849487

Forssell H, Tasmuth T, Tenovuo O, et al: Venlafaxine in the treatment of atypical facial pain: a randomized controlled trial. J Orofac Pain 18(2):131–137, 2004 15250433

Frese A, Husstedt IW, Ringelstein EB, Evers S: Pharmacologic treatment of central post-stroke pain. Clin J Pain 22(3):252–260, 2006 16514325

Gallagher RM, Mueller LL, Freitag FG: Divalproex sodium in the treatment of migraine and cluster headaches. J Am Osteopath Assoc 102(2):92–94, 2002 11866398

Gammaitoni AR, Galer BS, Onawola R, et al: Lidocaine patch 5% and its positive impact on pain qualities in osteoarthritis: results of a pilot 2-week, open-label study using the Neuropathic Pain Scale. Curr Med Res Opin 20 (suppl 2):S13–S19, 2004 15563742

Giannopoulos S, Kosmidou M, Sarmas I, et al: Patient compliance with SSRIs and gabapentin in painful diabetic neuropathy. Clin J Pain 23(3):267–269, 2007 17314587

Gidal BE, Sheth R, Parnell J, et al: Evaluation of VPA dose and concentration effects on lamotrigine pharmacokinetics: implications for conversion to lamotrigine monotherapy. Epilepsy Res 57(2-3):85–93, 2003 15013050

Gill D, Derry S, Wiffen PJ, Moore RA: Valproic acid and sodium valproate for neuropathic pain and fibromyalgia in adults. Cochrane Database of Systematic Reviews 2011, Issue 10. Art. No.: CD009183. DOI: 10.1002/14651858.CD009183.pub2 21975791

Gillman PK: Monoamine oxidase inhibitors, opioid analgesics and serotonin toxicity. Br J Anaesth 95(4):434–441, 2005 16051647

Gilron I, Bailey J, Weaver DF, Houlden RL: Patients' attitudes and prior treatments in neuropathic pain: a pilot study. Pain Res Manag 7(4):199–203, 2002 12518177

Goodkin K, Gullion CM, Agras WS: A randomized, double-blind, placebo-controlled trial of trazodone hydrochloride in chronic low back pain syndrome. J Clin Psychopharmacol 10(4):269–278, 1990 2149565

Goodnick PJ: Use of antidepressants in treatment of comorbid diabetes mellitus and depression as well as in diabetic neuropathy. Ann Clin Psychiatry 13(1):31–41, 2001 11465683

Gustorff B, Nahlik G, Spacek A, Kress HG: Gabapentin in the treatment of chronic intractable pain [in German]. Schmerz 16(1):9–14, 2002 11845336

Haibach JP, Beehler GP, Dollar KM, Finnell DS: Moving toward integrated behavioral intervention for treating multimorbidity among chronic pain, depression, and substance-use disorders in primary care. Med Care 52(4):322–327, 2014 24556895

Halbert J, Crotty M, Cameron ID: Evidence for the optimal management of acute and chronic phantom pain: a systematic review. Clin J Pain 18(2):84–92, 2002 11882771

Halker RB, Hastriter EV, Dodick DW: Chronic daily headache: an evidence-based and systematic approach to a challenging problem. Neurology 76(7) (suppl 2):S37–S43, 2011 21321350

Hans GH, Robert DN, Van Maldeghem KN: Treatment of an acute severe central neuropathic pain syndrome by topical application of lidocaine 5% patch: a case report. Spinal Cord 46(4):311–313, 2008 17607309

Harden RN, Bruehl S, Stanton-Hicks M, Wilson PR: Proposed new diagnostic criteria for complex regional pain syndrome. Pain Med 8(4):326–331, 2007 17610454

Hasenbring M, Hallner D, Klasen B: Psychological mechanisms in the transition from acute to chronic pain: over- or underrated? [in German]. Schmerz 15(6):442–447, 2001 11793149

Haythornthwaite JA, Sieber WJ, Kerns RD: Depression and the chronic pain experience. Pain 46(2):177–184, 1991 1749640

Heiskanen T, Kalso E: Controlled-release oxycodone and morphine in cancer related pain. Pain 73(1):37–45, 1997 9414055

Hersh EV, Pinto A, Moore PA: Adverse drug interactions involving common prescription and over-the-counter analgesic agents. Clin Ther 29(suppl):2477–2497, 2007 18164916

Hidalgo J, Rico-Villademoros F, Calandre EP: An open-label study of quetiapine in the treatment of fibromyalgia. Prog Neuropsychopharmacol Biol Psychiatry 31(1):71–77, 2007 16889882

Howard P, Twycross R, Shuster J, et al: Benzodiazepines. J Pain Symptom Manage 47(5):955–964, 2014 24681184

Institute for Clinical Systems Improvement: Assessment and management of acute pain. March 2008. Available at: http://www.icsi.org. Accessed December 1, 2009.

Institute of Medicine: Relieving Pain in America: A Blueprint for Transforming Prevention, Care, Education and Research. Report from the Committee on Advancing Pain Research, Care and Education. Washington, DC, National Academies Press, 2011. Available at: http://books.nap.edu/openbook.php?record_id=13172. Accessed July 7, 2016.

Jarvis B, Coukell AJ: Mexiletine: a review of its therapeutic use in painful diabetic neuropathy. Drugs 56(4):691–707, 1998 9806111

Jensen R, Brinck T, Olesen J: Sodium valproate has a prophylactic effect in migraine without aura: a triple-blind, placebo-controlled crossover study. Neurology 44(4):647–651, 1994 8164818

Johnson RW, Rice AS: Clinical practice: postherpetic neuralgia. N Engl J Med 371(16):1526–1533, 2014 25317872

Kalso E, Tramèr MR, McQuay HJ, Moore RA: Systemic local-anaesthetic-type drugs in chronic pain: a systematic review. Eur J Pain 2(1):3–14, 1998 10700296

Kaniecki RG: A comparison of divalproex with propranolol and placebo for the prophylaxis of migraine without aura. Arch Neurol 54(9):1141–1145, 1997 9311358

Keskinbora K, Aydinli I: A double-blind randomized controlled trial of topiramate and amitriptyline either alone or in combination for the prevention of migraine. Clin Neurol Neurosurg 110(10):979–984, 2008 18620801

Khaliq W, Alam S, Puri N: Topical lidocaine for the treatment of postherpetic neuralgia. Cochrane Database of Systematic Reviews 2007, Issue 2. Art. No.: CD004846. DOI: 10.1002/14651858.CD004846.pub3 17443559

Khoromi S, Patsalides A, Parada S, et al: Topiramate in chronic lumbar radicular pain. J Pain 6(12):829–836, 2005 16326371

Kirsh KL, Whitcomb LA, Donaghy K, Passik SD: Abuse and addiction issues in medically ill patients with pain: attempts at clarification of terms and empirical study. Clin J Pain 18(4)(suppl):S52–S60, 2002 12479254

Klapper J: Divalproex sodium in migraine prophylaxis: a dose-controlled study. Cephalalgia 17(2):103–108, 1997 9137847

Kroenke K, Shen J, Oxman TE, et al: Impact of pain on the outcomes of depression treatment: results from the RESPECT trial. Pain 134(1-2):209–215, 2008 18022319

Lake AE III: Behavioral and nonpharmacologic treatments of headache. Med Clin North Am 85(4):1055–1075, 2001 11480258

Lerman SF, Rudich Z, Brill S, et al: Longitudinal associations between depression, anxiety, pain, and pain-related disability in chronic pain patients. Psychosom Med 77(3):333–341, 2015 25849129

Lewis TA, Solomon GD: Advances in cluster headache management. Cleve Clin J Med 63(4):237–244, 1996 8764694

Liebschutz J, Saitz R, Brower V, et al: PTSD in urban primary care: high prevalence and low physician recognition. J Gen Intern Med 22(6):719–726, 2007 17503105

Lipchik GL, Nash JM: Cognitive-behavioral issues in the treatment and management of chronic daily headache. Curr Pain Headache Rep 6(6):473–479, 2002 12413406

Lipton RB, Bigal ME, Diamond M, et al; AMPP Advisory Group: Migraine prevalence, disease burden, and the need for preventive therapy. Neurology 68(5):343–349, 2007 17261680

Lunn MP, Hughes RA, Wiffen PJ: Duloxetine for treating painful neuropathy, chronic pain or fibromyalgia. Cochrane Database of Systematic Reviews 2014, Issue 1. Art. No.: CD007115. DOI: 10.1002/14651858.CD007115.pub3 24385423

Magni G, Schifano F, De Leo D: Pain as a symptom in elderly depressed patients. Relationship to diagnostic subgroups. Eur Arch Psychiatry Neurol Sci 235(3):143–145, 1985 4092711

Manchikanti L, Singh V: Managing phantom pain. Pain Physician 7(3):365–375, 2004 16858476

Manchikanti L, Abdi S, Atluri S, et al; American Society of Interventional Pain Physicians: American Society of Interventional Pain Physicians (ASIPP) guidelines for responsible opioid prescribing in chronic non-cancer pain: part I—evidence assessment. Pain Physician 15(3)(suppl):S1–S65, 2012a 22786448

Manchikanti L, Abdi S, Atluri S, et al; American Society of Interventional Pain Physicians: American Society of Interventional Pain Physicians (ASIPP) guidelines for responsible opioid prescribing in chronic non-cancer pain: Part 2—guidance. Pain Physician 15(3)(suppl):S67–S116, 2012b 22786449

Markley HG: Verapamil and migraine prophylaxis: mechanisms and efficacy. Am J Med 90(5A):48S–53S, 1991 2039020

Mason L, Moore RA, Derry S, et al: Systematic review of topical capsaicin for the treatment of chronic pain. BMJ 328(7446):991, 2004 15033881

McCleane G: Antidepressants as analgesics. CNS Drugs 22(2):139–156, 2008 18193925

McCormick Z, Chang-Chien G, Marshall B, et al: Phantom limb pain: a systematic neuroanatomical-based review of pharmacologic treatment. Pain Med 15(2):292–305, 2014 24224475

Mease PJ, Clauw DJ, Gendreau RM, et al: The efficacy and safety of milnacipran for treatment of fibromyalgia. a randomized, double-blind, placebo-controlled trial. J Rheumatol 36(2):398–409, 2009 19132781

Mendell JR, Sahenk Z: Clinical practice: painful sensory neuropathy. N Engl J Med 348(13):1243–1255, 2003 12660389

Mercadante S: Opioid rotation for cancer pain: rationale and clinical aspects. Cancer 86(9):1856–1866, 1999 10547561

Micca JL, Ruff D, Ahl J, Wohlreich MM: Safety and efficacy of duloxetine treatment in older and younger patients with osteoarthritis knee pain: a post hoc, subgroup analysis of two randomized, placebo-controlled trials. BMC Musculoskelet Disord 14:137, 2013 23590727

Micó JA, Ardid D, Berrocoso E, Eschalier A: Antidepressants and pain. Trends Pharmacol Sci 27(7):348–354, 2006 16762426

Mishriky BM, Waldron NH, Habib AS: Impact of pregabalin on acute and persistent postoperative pain: a systematic review and meta-analysis. Br J Anaesth 114(1):10–31, 2015 25209095

Mitra S: Opioid-induced hyperalgesia: pathophysiology and clinical implications. J Opioid Manag 4(3):123–130, 2008 18717507

Montano N, Conforti G, Di Bonaventura R, et al: Advances in diagnosis and treatment of trigeminal neuralgia. Ther Clin Risk Manag 11:289–299, 2015 25750533

Moore RA, Wiffen PJ, Derry S, et al: Gabapentin for chronic neuropathic pain and fibromyalgia in adults. Cochrane Database of Systematic Reviews 2014, Issue 4. Art. No.: CD007938. DOI: 10.1002/14651858.CD007938.pub3 24771480

Morasco BJ, Gritzner S, Lewis L, et al: Systematic review of prevalence, correlates, and treatment outcomes for chronic non-cancer pain in patients with comorbid substance use disorder. Pain 152(3):488–497, 2011 21185119

Moulin DE, Clark AJ, Gilron I, et al; Canadian Pain Society: Pharmacological management of chronic neuropathic pain—consensus statement and guidelines from the Canadian Pain Society. Pain Res Manag 12(1):13–21, 2007 17372630

Moulin D, Boulanger A, Clark AJ, et al; Canadian Pain Society: Pharmacological management of chronic neuropathic pain: revised consensus statement from the Canadian Pain Society. Pain Res Manag 19(6):328–335, 2014 25479151

Muehlbacher M, Nickel MK, Kettler C, et al: Topiramate in treatment of patients with chronic low back pain: a randomized, double-blind, placebo-controlled study. Clin J Pain 22(6):526–531, 2006 16788338

Mulleners WM, Chronicle EP: Anticonvulsants in migraine prophylaxis: a Cochrane review. Cephalalgia 28(6):585–597, 2008 18454787

Mumoli N, Cocciolo M, Vitale J, et al: Diabetes mellitus associated with clomipramine treatment: a retrospective analysis. Acta Diabetol 51(1):167–168, 2014 23824324

National Cancer Institute: PDQ Cancer Information Summaries: Pain. Available at: http://www.cancer.gov/cancertopics/pdq/supportivecare/pain/healthprofessional/allpages. Updated May 21, 2015. Accessed June 17, 2015.

Nicholson BD: Evaluation and treatment of central pain syndromes. Neurology 62(5)(suppl 2):S30–S36, 2004 15007162

Niraj S, Niraj G: Phantom limb pain and its psychologic management: a critical review. Pain Manag Nurs 15(1):349–364, 2014 24602439

Nishiyama K, Sakuta M: Mexiletine for painful alcoholic neuropathy. Intern Med 34(6):577–579, 1995 7549147

Noble M, Tregear SJ, Treadwell JR, Schoelles K: Long-term opioid therapy for chronic noncancer pain: a systematic review and meta-analysis of efficacy and safety. J Pain Symptom Manage 35(2):214–228, 2008 18178367

O'Connell NE, Wand BM, McAuley J, et al: Interventions for treating pain and disability in adults with complex regional pain syndrome. Cochrane Database of Systematic Reviews 2013, Issue 4. Art. No.: CD009416. DOI: 10.1002/14651858.CD009416.pub2 23633371

O'Connor AB: Neuropathic pain: quality-of-life impact, costs and cost effectiveness of therapy. Pharmacoeconomics 27(2):95–112, 2009 19254044

Okifuji A, Turk DC, Curran SL: Anger in chronic pain: investigations of anger targets and intensity. J Psychosom Res 47(1):1–12, 1999 10511417

Onghena P, Van Houdenhove B: Antidepressant-induced analgesia in chronic nonmalignant pain: a meta-analysis of 39 placebo-controlled studies. Pain 49(2):205–219, 1992 1535121

Oskarsson P, Ljunggren JG, Lins PE; The Mexiletine Study Group: Efficacy and safety of mexiletine in the treatment of painful diabetic neuropathy. Diabetes Care 20(10):1594–1597, 1997 9314641

Outcalt SD, Kroenke K, Krebs EE, et al: Chronic pain and comorbid mental health conditions: independent associations of posttraumatic stress disorder and depression with pain, disability, and quality of life. J Behav Med 38(3):535–543, 2015 25786741

Ozyalcin SN, Talu GK, Kiziltan E, et al: The efficacy and safety of venlafaxine in the prophylaxis of migraine. Headache 45(2):144–152, 2005 15705120

Pandey CK, Bose N, Garg G, et al: Gabapentin for the treatment of pain in Guillain-Barré syndrome: a double-blinded, placebo-controlled, crossover study. Anesth Analg 95(6):1719–1723, 2002 12456446

Patten SB: Long-term medical conditions and major depression in a Canadian population study at waves 1 and 2. J Affect Disord 63(1-3):35–41, 2001 11246078

Peng P, Tumber P, Stafford M, et al: Experience of methadone therapy in 100 consecutive chronic pain patients in a multidisciplinary pain center. Pain Med 9(7):786–794, 2008 18564997

Peuckmann V, Ekholm O, Rasmussen NK, et al: Chronic pain and other sequelae in long-term breast cancer survivors: nationwide survey in Denmark. Eur J Pain 13(5):478–485, 2009 18635381

Pontell D: A clinical approach to complex regional pain syndrome. Clin Podiatr Med Surg 25(3):361–380, vi, 2008 18486850

Quilici S, Chancellor J, Löthgren M, et al: Meta-analysis of duloxetine vs pregabalin and gabapentin in the treatment of diabetic peripheral neuropathic pain. BMC Neurol 9:6, 2009 19208243

Rang ST, Field J, Irving C: Serotonin toxicity caused by an interaction between fentanyl and paroxetine. Can J Anaesth 55(8):521–525, 2008 18676387

Rani PU, Naidu MU, Prasad VB, et al: An evaluation of antidepressants in rheumatic pain conditions. Anesth Analg 83(2):371–375, 1996 8694321

Ray WA, Chung CP, Murray KT, et al: Out-of-hospital mortality among patients receiving methadone for noncancer pain. JAMA Intern Med 175(3):420–427, 2015 25599329

Rico-Villademoros F, Hidalgo J, Dominguez I, et al: Atypical antipsychotics in the treatment of fibromyalgia: a case series with olanzapine. Prog Neuropsychopharmacol Biol Psychiatry 29(1):161–164, 2005 15610961

Rief W, Martin A: How to use the new DSM-5 somatic symptom disorder diagnosis in research and practice: a critical evaluation and a proposal for modifications. Annu Rev Clin Psychol 10:339–367, 2014 24387234

Riley J, Eisenberg E, Müller-Schwefe G, et al: Oxycodone: a review of its use in the management of pain. Curr Med Res Opin 24(1):175–192, 2008 18039433

Risser RC, Hochberg MC, Gaynor PJ, et al: Responsiveness of the Intermittent and Constant Osteoarthritis Pain (ICOAP) scale in a trial of duloxetine for treatment of osteoarthritis knee pain. Osteoarthritis Cartilage 21(5):691–694, 2013 23485934

Rojas-Corrales MO, Casas J, Moreno-Brea MR, et al: Antinociceptive effects of tricyclic antidepressants and their noradrenergic metabolites. Eur Neuropsychopharmacol 13(5):355–363, 2003 12957334

Rommel O, Malin JP, Zenz M, Jänig W: Quantitative sensory testing, neurophysiological and psychological examination in patients with complex regional pain syndrome and hemisensory deficits. Pain 93(3):279–293, 2001 11514087

Rosenblum A, Joseph H, Fong C, et al: Prevalence and characteristics of chronic pain among chemically dependent patients in methadone maintenance and residential treatment facilities. JAMA 289(18):2370–2378, 2003 12746360

Rosenzweig-Lipson S, Beyer CE, Hughes ZA, et al: Differentiating antidepressants of the future: efficacy and safety. Pharmacol Ther 113(1):134–153, 2007 17010443

Rothrock JF: Clinical studies of valproate for migraine prophylaxis. Cephalalgia 17(2):81–83, 1997 9137842

Rowbotham MC, Goli V, Kunz NR, Lei D: Venlafaxine extended release in the treatment of painful diabetic neuropathy: a double-blind, placebo-controlled study. Pain 110(3):697–706, 2004 15288411

Saarto T, Wiffen PJ: Antidepressants for neuropathic pain. Cochrane Database of Systematic Reviews 2007, Issue 4. Art. No.: CD005454. DOI: 10.1002/14651858. CD005454.pub2 17943857

Salerno SM, Browning R, Jackson JL: The effect of antidepressant treatment on chronic back pain: a meta-analysis. Arch Intern Med 162(1):19–24, 2002 11784215

Sandoval JA, Furlan AD, Mailis-Gagnon A: Oral methadone for chronic noncancer pain: a systematic literature review of reasons for administration, prescription patterns, effectiveness, and side effects. Clin J Pain 21(6):503–512, 2005 16215336

Schmader KE: Epidemiology and impact on quality of life of postherpetic neuralgia and painful diabetic neuropathy. Clin J Pain 18(6):350–354, 2002 12441828

Schreiber AK, Nones CF, Reis RC, et al: Diabetic neuropathic pain: physiopathology and treatment. World J Diabetes 6(3):432–444, 2015 25897354

Sehgal N, Manchikanti L, Smith HS: Prescription opioid abuse in chronic pain: a review of opioid abuse predictors and strategies to curb opioid abuse. Pain Physician 15(3)(suppl):ES67–ES92, 2012 22786463

Seidel S, Aigner M, Ossege M, et al: Antipsychotics for acute and chronic pain in adults. Cochrane Database of Systematic Reviews 2013, Issue 8. Art. No.: CD004844. DOI: 10.1002/14651858.CD004844.pub3 23990266

Semenchuk MR, Sherman S, Davis B: Double-blind, randomized trial of bupropion SR for the treatment of neuropathic pain. Neurology 57(9):1583–1588, 2001 11706096

Shaiova L: Difficult pain syndromes: bone pain, visceral pain, and neuropathic pain. Cancer J 12(5):330–340, 2006 17034669

Sharma A, Williams K, Raja SN: Advances in treatment of complex regional pain syndrome: recent insights on a perplexing disease. Curr Opin Anaesthesiol 19(5):566–572, 2006 16960493

Siddall PJ, Cousins MJ, Otte A, et al: Pregabalin in central neuropathic pain associated with spinal cord injury: a placebo-controlled trial. Neurology 67(10):1792–1800, 2006 17130411

Silberstein SD, Hulihan J, Karim MR, et al: Efficacy and tolerability of topiramate 200 mg/d in the prevention of migraine with/without aura in adults: a randomized, placebo-controlled, double-blind, 12-week pilot study. Clin Ther 28(7):1002–1011, 2006 16990078

Skaer TL: Practice guidelines for transdermal opioids in malignant pain. Drugs 64(23):2629–2638, 2004 15537367

Smith H, Brooks JR: Capsaicin-based therapies for pain control. Prog Drug Res 68:129–146, 2014 24941667

Smith MT: Neuroexcitatory effects of morphine and hydromorphone: evidence implicating the 3-glucuronide metabolites. Clin Exp Pharmacol Physiol 27(7):524–528, 2000 10874511

Snedecor SJ, Sudharshan L, Cappelleri JC, et al: Systematic review and meta-analysis of pharmacological therapies for painful diabetic peripheral neuropathy. Pain Pract 14(2):167–184, 2014 23534696

Solaro C, Messmer Uccelli M, Uccelli A, et al: Low-dose gabapentin combined with either lamotrigine or carbamazepine can be useful therapies for trigeminal neuralgia in multiple sclerosis. Eur Neurol 44(1):45–48, 2000 10894995

Sonnett TE, Setter SM, Campbell RK: Pregabalin for the treatment of painful neuropathy. Expert Rev Neurother 6(11):1629–1635, 2006 17144773

Stacey BR, Barrett JA, Whalen E, et al: Pregabalin for postherpetic neuralgia: placebo-controlled trial of fixed and flexible dosing regimens on allodynia and time to onset of pain relief. J Pain 9(11):1006–1017, 2008 18640074

Stein C, Reinecke H, Sorgatz H: Opioid use in chronic noncancer pain: guidelines revisited. Curr Opin Anaesthesiol 23(5):598–601, 2010 20585244

Streltzer J, Eliashof BA, Kline AE, Goebert D: Chronic pain disorder following physical injury. Psychosomatics 41(3):227–234, 2000 10849455

Tack J, Broekaert D, Fischler B, et al: A controlled crossover study of the selective serotonin reuptake inhibitor citalopram in irritable bowel syndrome. Gut 55(8):1095–1103, 2006 16401691

Tang NK, Crane C: Suicidality in chronic pain: a review of the prevalence, risk factors and psychological links. Psychol Med 36(5):575–586, 2006 16420727

Taricco M, Adone R, Pagliacci C, Telaro E: Pharmacological interventions for spasticity following spinal cord injury. Cochrane Database of Systematic Reviews 2000, Issue 2. Art. No.: CD001131. DOI: 10.1002/14651858.CD001131 10796750

Tasmuth T, Härtel B, Kalso E: Venlafaxine in neuropathic pain following treatment of breast cancer. Eur J Pain 6(1):17–24, 2002 11888224

Tassinari D, Sartori S, Tamburini E, et al: Adverse effects of transdermal opiates treating moderate-severe cancer pain in comparison to long-acting morphine: a meta-analysis and systematic review of the literature. J Palliat Med 11(3):492–501, 2008 18363493

Thompson DR: Narcotic analgesic effects on the sphincter of Oddi: a review of the data and therapeutic implications in treating pancreatitis. Am J Gastroenterol 96(4):1266–1272, 2001 11316181

Todorov AA, Kolchev CB, Todorov AB: Tiagabine and gabapentin for the management of chronic pain. Clin J Pain 21(4):358–361, 2005 15951655

Tofferi JK, Jackson JL, O'Malley PG: Treatment of fibromyalgia with cyclobenzaprine: a meta-analysis. Arthritis Rheum 51(1):9–13, 2004 14872449

Toth C: Pregabalin: latest safety evidence and clinical implications for the management of neuropathic pain. Ther Adv Drug Saf 5(1):38–56, 2014 25083261

Tremont-Lukats IW, Megeff C, Backonja MM: Anticonvulsants for neuropathic pain syndromes: mechanisms of action and place in therapy. Drugs 60(5):1029–1052, 2000 11129121

Ullrich PM: Pain following spinal cord injury. Phys Med Rehabil Clin N Am 18(2):217–233, vi, 2007 17543770

van Seventer R, Feister HA, Young JP Jr, et al: Efficacy and tolerability of twice-daily pregabalin for treating pain and related sleep interference in postherpetic neuralgia: a 13-week, randomized trial. Curr Med Res Opin 22(2):375–384, 2006 16466610

von Knorring L, Perris C, Eisemann M, et al: Pain as a symptom in depressive disorders, II: relationship to personality traits as assessed by means of KSP. Pain 17(4):377–384, 1983 6664683

Von Korff M, Le Resche L, Dworkin SF: First onset of common pain symptoms: a prospective study of depression as a risk factor. Pain 55(2):251–258, 1993 8309712

VanderWeide LA, Smith SM, Trinkley KE: A systematic review of the efficacy of venlafaxine for the treatment of fibromyalgia. J Clin Pharm Ther 40(1):1–6, 2015 25294655

Vorobeychik Y, Chen L, Bush MC, Mao J: Improved opioid analgesic effect following opioid dose reduction. Pain Med 9(6):724–727, 2008 18816332

Wachholtz A, Foster S, Cheatle M: Psychophysiology of pain and opioid use: implications for managing pain in patients with an opioid use disorder. Drug Alcohol Depend 146:1–6, 2015 25468815

Walitt B, Urrútia G, Nishishinya MB, et al: Selective serotonin reuptake inhibitors for fibromyalgia syndrome. Cochrane Database of Systematic Reviews 2015, Issue 6. Art. No.: CD011735. DOI: 10.1002/14651858.CD011735 26046493

Wernicke JF, Pritchett YL, D'Souza DN, et al: A randomized controlled trial of duloxetine in diabetic peripheral neuropathic pain. Neurology 67(8):1411–1420, 2006 17060567

Wiffen PJ, Rees J: Lamotrigine for chronic neuropathic pan and fibromyalgia in adults. Cochrane Database of Systematic Reviews 2013, Issue 12. Art. No.: CD006044. DOI: 10.1002/14651858.CD006044.pub4 24297457

Wiffen PJ, Derry S, Lunn MP, Moore RA: Topiramate for neuropathic pain and fibromyalgia in adults. Cochrane Database of Systematic Reviews 2013a, Issue 8. Art. No.: CD008314. DOI: 10.1002/14651858.CD008314.pub3 23996081

Wiffen PJ, Derry S, Moore RA, et al: Antiepileptic drugs for neuropathic pain and fibromyalgia—an overview of Cochrane reviews. Cochrane Database of Systematic Reviews 2013b, Issue 11. Art. No.: CD010567. DOI: 10.1002/14651858.CD010567.pub2 24217986

Wiffen PJ, Derry S, Moore RA, Kalso EA: Carbamazepine for chronic neuropathic pain and fibromyalgia in adults. Cochrane Database of Systematic Reviews 2014a, Issue 4. Art. No.: CD005451. DOI: 10.1002/14651858.CD005451.pub3 24719027

Wiffen PJ, Derry S, Moore RA, Lunn MP: Levetiracetam for neuropathic pain in adults. Cochrane Database of Systematic Reviews 2014b, Issue 7. Art. No.: CD010943. DOI: 10.1002/14651858.CD010943.pub2 25000215

Wong WS, Fielding R: The co-morbidity of chronic pain, insomnia, and fatigue in the general adult population of Hong Kong: prevalence and associated factors. J Psychosom Res 73(1):28–34, 2012 22691556

Wu CL, Agarwal S, Tella PK, et al: Morphine versus mexiletine for treatment of post-amputation pain: a randomized, placebo-controlled, crossover trial. Anesthesiology 109(2):289–296, 2008 18648238

Yawn BP, Buchanan GR, Afenyi-Annan AN, et al: Management of sickle cell disease: summary of the 2014 evidence-based report by expert panel members. JAMA 312(10):1033–1048, 2014 25203083

Yucel A, Ozyalcin S, Koknel Talu G, et al: The effect of venlafaxine on ongoing and experimentally induced pain in neuropathic pain patients: a double blind, placebo controlled study. Eur J Pain 9(4):407–416, 2005 15979021

Zakrzewska JM, Forssell H, Glenny AM: Interventions for the treatment of burning mouth syndrome. Cochrane Database of Systematic Reviews 2005, Issue 1. Art. No.: CD002779. DOI: 10.1002/14651858.CD002779.pub2 15674897

Zhang W, Moskowitz RW, Nuki G, et al: OARSI recommendations for the management of hip and knee osteoarthritis, Part II: OARSI evidence-based, expert consensus guidelines. Osteoarthritis Cartilage 16(2):137–162, 2008 18279766

Ziegler D, Pritchett YL, Wang F, et al: Impact of disease characteristics on the efficacy of duloxetine in diabetic peripheral neuropathic pain. Diabetes Care 30(3):664–669, 2007 17327338

Zin CS, Nissen LM, Smith MT, et al: An update on the pharmacological management of post-herpetic neuralgia and painful diabetic neuropathy. CNS Drugs 22(5):417–442, 2008 18399710

18

Substance Use Disorders

Jozef Bledowski, M.D.

The substance use disorders are present in a significant proportion of the population, with a disproportionate representation in the medically ill. It is well known that substance use disorders increase the risk for accidental and intentional injury, precipitation of acute and chronic medical illness, and extended hospital stays and delayed recovery. Hence, it is not surprising that the substance use disorders are very commonly encountered in both inpatient and outpatient medical settings. With regard to substance use in the United States, the 2013 National Survey on Drug Use and Health (Substance Abuse and Mental Health Services Administration 2014) found that among individuals ages 12 years and older, 25.5% use tobacco; 22.9% engage in binge drinking; 6.5% engage in heavy alcohol use (defined as binge drinking on at least 5 days out of a month); and 9.4% use illicit drugs (with marijuana being the most commonly used), which includes 2.5% who engage in the nonmedical use of prescription medications, mostly opioids (two-thirds of the 2.5%). It is estimated that approximately 15%–30% of hospitalized patients and up to 36% of medically hospitalized patients receiving psychiatric consultation are found to have at least one comorbid substance use disorder (Katz et al. 2008; Schellhorn et al. 2009). The adverse impact of substance intoxication, overdose, withdrawal, and chronic use is frequently encountered in the medically ill. Although alcohol and tobacco remain the most commonly used substances, misuse of prescription medications (particularly opioids) trails close behind and is quickly reaching epidemic proportions. Furthermore, with the legalization of marijuana in several states, the emergence of so-called designer drugs (e.g., 3,4-methylenedioxymethamphetamine [MDMA], synthetic cannabinoids, bath salts), and the rising incidence of recreational over-the-counter drug use (e.g., dextromethorphan, pseudoephedrine), the playing field is quickly changing.

In this chapter, I discuss pharmacological management of select intoxication syndromes, withdrawal syndromes, and management of abstinence and craving in select substance use disorders, with special emphasis on the medically ill. Within each section, pharmacological management of substance use disorders in pregnancy is discussed. I conclude with reference tables for potential neuropsychiatric effects and drug-drug interactions of these pharmacological agents.

Substance Intoxication

Severe intoxication can be life threatening, but few antidotes exist to reverse most intoxication syndromes. The major exception is opioid overdose. Deaths due to opioid overdose have now surpassed motor vehicle collisions as the most common cause of unintentional death in the United States (Warner et al. 2011).

Naloxone is an opioid receptor antagonist with particularly high affinity for μ opioid receptors, hence making it the drug of choice in managing acute opioid intoxication and overdose, for which it is approved by the U.S. Food and Drug Administration. Given its extensive first-pass hepatic metabolism and low bioavailability when given orally, naloxone's bioavailability is much greater when the drug is administered via parenteral or inhalation routes. Although naloxone is rapidly effective in reversing the effects of most opioids, administration in buprenorphine intoxication, given that buprenorphine has a considerably high affinity for and slower rate of association with and dissociation from the μ opioid receptor, often requires higher doses of naloxone and results in a delay in its effectiveness (Kim and Nelson 2015).

Naloxone is generally safe to use in the medically ill and is without absolute contraindications. In addition to acute agitation, the most common and potentially adverse consequence of naloxone administration is the precipitation of acute opioid withdrawal. More commonly seen in chronic opioid users (including chronic pain patients), acute opioid withdrawal precipitated by naloxone can cause sympathetic hyperactivity resulting in malignant hypertension, arrhythmias, and seizures (Kim and Nelson 2015). Nevertheless, the benefit of using naloxone clearly outweighs any potential risk, particularly when opioid intoxication results in life-threatening respiratory compromise. In fact, recent programs have actually encouraged ready availability of naloxone in high-risk populations, even going so far as to provide family members and friends of opioid-addicted individuals with prescriptions for naloxone (Kim et al. 2009). For this very reason, in 2014, the U.S. Food and Drug Administration (FDA) approved a naloxone autoinjector that can be easily administered (intramuscularly or subcutaneously) by a family member or caregiver.

Naloxone is listed as pregnancy category C because of a lack of well-controlled studies in humans. Furthermore, its use in pregnancy can precipitate severe withdrawal in the mother and fetus, which can then result in fetal distress and preterm labor (ACOG Committee on Health Care for Underserved Women and American Society of Addiction Medicine 2012; Zelner et al. 2015). There is a potential risk of precipitating hypertensive crisis with naloxone use in women during labor (Schoenfeld et al. 1987). As with most category C drugs, its use should be reserved for cases in which there is clear potential for reduction in morbidity and/or mortality.

Benzodiazepine overdoses, either alone or in combination with other substances, are commonplace. Flumazenil, an imidazobenzodiazepine, functions as a competitive antagonist at the central benzodiazepine receptor and is FDA approved as an antidote in the management of benzodiazepine intoxication (both therapeutic or iatrogenic, such as in conscious sedation or anesthesia, and secondary to recreational or suicidal overdose). Flumazenil has a fairly low bioavailability when given by mouth; hence, it is primarily administered parenterally. However, it can be administered orally and even rectally, albeit at higher doses, when necessary for long-term management and prevention of resedation, particularly in comatose patients (Weinbroum et al. 1997). Its rapid onset of action makes it quite effective in managing acute benzodiazepine overdose.

Flumazenil can also be used to reverse general anesthesia and promote quicker recovery as well as manage overdose with nonbenzodiazepine sedative-hypnotics (i.e., zolpidem, zaleplon, and eszopiclone). Despite its utility, flumazenil carries a significant potential for adverse effects. The most common side effects include acute agitation, dizziness, nausea, and vomiting. Serious and potentially life-threatening adverse effects include seizures, bradycardia, hypotension, and ventricular arrhythmias (Longmire and Seger 1993). Despite this, flumazenil does not typically produce significant hemodynamic changes with appropriate administration (Weinbroum et al. 1997). The risk of seizures with flumazenil use is higher in patients with seizure disorders and head injury, as well as in habitual or chronic sedative-hypnotic users. Of particular concern is the use of flumezanil in combined benzodiazepine and proarrhythmic/proconvulsant drug ingestions (e.g., tricyclic antidepressants, carbamazepine, phenothiazines, isoniazid, theophylline, clozapine), which may significantly increase the risk for treatment-emergent seizures and ventricular arrhythmias (Seger 2004; Weinbroum et al. 2003). Such risks are reduced by starting with low-dose flumazenil via slow infusion and titration (Weinbroum et al. 1997).

Flumazenil is listed as pregnancy category C because of a relative lack of controlled studies in humans. The consensus is that its use in pregnancy should be reserved for cases in which there is clear risk of morbidity or mortality in the mother and/or fetus and supportive measures are either inadequate or impractical (Zelner et al. 2015).

Substance Use Disorders

There are a number of pharmacological options for the treatment of withdrawal states, as well as for the maintenance of abstinence via management of craving or by blocking the central effects of certain substances. Nevertheless, there are limited data on the use of these agents in the medically ill. Hence, discussion of the pharmacological properties and potential adverse effects requires extrapolation to the medically ill. Of particular focus in this chapter will be alcohol, opioids, nicotine, and stimulants, along with some additional information on more novel substances of abuse.

Alcohol Use Disorder

Alcohol use disorder is one of the most commonly encountered substance use disorders in the medically ill. It has been estimated that 21%–42% of patients admitted to general medical wards and 30%–40% of those admitted to intensive care units have signs and symptoms that meet diagnostic criteria for alcohol use disorder (de Wit et al. 2010). In fact, close to 50% of all trauma patients have detectable serum alcohol levels at the time of admission (de Wit et al. 2010). Heavy alcohol use can cause hypoglycemia; electrolyte imbalances (hyponatremia, hypokalemia, hypomagnesemia, and hypophosphatemia); deficiency of thiamine, folate, and other B vitamins; bone marrow suppression leading to pancytopenia; cardiotoxicity resulting in arrhythmias and left ventricular dysfunction; acute and chronic hepatic failure (cirrhosis); renal insufficiency or failure; pancreatitis; increased risk for bleeding; and increased risk for nosocomial infections and sepsis. These effects result in increased requirement for critical care services, longer hospital length of stay, delayed rehabilitation, and a twofold increase in mortality (de Wit et al. 2010; Moss and Burnham 2006; O'Brien et al. 2007).

Alcohol Withdrawal Syndrome

Alcohol withdrawal syndrome (AWS) is characterized by a constellation of symptoms, including autonomic hyperarousal and neurological dysfunction, that can lead to potentially life-threatening sequelae. AWS typically occurs approximately 6–24 hours following a steep drop in blood alcohol levels or complete cessation in alcohol consumption. Uncomplicated AWS typically peaks in 48–72 hours and subsides in 5–7 days, although residual sequelae, such as anxiety, insomnia, and autonomic hyperarousal, can last much longer. Common symptoms of AWS include anxiety, insomnia, irritability, nausea and vomiting, tremulousness, perceptual disturbances (visual, auditory, tactile), diaphoresis, tachycardia, and hypertension. This can then progress to delirium tremens with severe autonomic instability, with extreme fluctuations in heart rate and blood pressure, hyperthermia, arrhythmias, clouding of sensorium, delirium, psychosis, grand mal seizures, coma, and even death.

Although more than 50% of patients with alcohol use disorder will experience some degree of withdrawal, the majority experience only mild symptoms without further progression (Mirijello et al. 2015). Contrary to long-held beliefs, most individuals with alcohol use disorder will not develop severe alcohol withdrawal symptoms. In fact, the prevalence of severe withdrawal leading to delirium tremens in patients admitted for AWS is between 3% and 5% (Schuckit 2014). Delirium tremens carries a mortality risk of between 1% and

4% in otherwise uncomplicated inpatients and can be as high as 20% in the hospitalized medically ill (Maldonado et al. 2014; Schuckit 2014). Less severe withdrawal symptoms can still be dangerous in more vulnerable patients. For example, less severe increases in heart rate and blood pressure may precipitate myocardial infarction in a patient with marginal coronary reserve.

The risk for added morbidity, extended length of stay, delayed rehabilitation, and potential long-term cognitive sequelae as a direct result of complicated withdrawal underscores the importance of early identification and treatment of medically ill patients at risk for developing severe AWS. The most commonly used instrument for measuring AWS severity, the revised Clinical Institute Withdrawal Assessment for Alcohol (CIWA-Ar), was standardized primarily in an uncomplicated alcohol-dependent population (Sullivan et al. 1989). Screening instruments for alcohol use disorder, such as the Alcohol Use Disorders Identification Test (AUDIT) and its revised version (AUDIT-PC), have been studied in medically ill patients but have not been validated for use in the medically ill and have not been studied in the critically ill (Bohn et al. 1995; Pecoraro et al. 2014). To rectify this, Maldonado and colleagues (2014) have piloted a screening instrument, the Prediction of Alcohol Withdrawal Severity Scale (PAWSS), to identify medically ill patients who may be at greatest risk for developing severe alcohol withdrawal by looking at factors such as prior history of alcohol withdrawal, history of withdrawal seizures or delirium tremens, concomitant use of sedative-hypnotics, recent drinking history, blood alcohol level on admission, and physical evidence of autonomic hyperactivity. Early identification of at-risk medically ill patients before they develop withdrawal symptoms would facilitate decisions to initiate pharmacological prophylactic measures.

The effective management of alcohol withdrawal in the medically ill involves implementation of vigilant monitoring parameters and correction of associated and comorbid physiological insults, including the correction of electrolyte imbalances (particularly magnesium, potassium, and calcium), as well as adequate nutritional supplementation. Of greatest concern is the propensity, particularly for medically ill patients with alcohol use disorder, to develop thiamine (vitamin B_1) deficiency, which can then lead to the development of Wernicke's encephalopathy and, if left untreated, Korsakoff's syndrome. Thiamine should be administered parenterally (preferably intravenously, so as to establish an adequate concentration gradient to promote passive diffusion across the blood-brain barrier) and before giving glucose to prevent depletion of existing thiamine stores. Whereas current guidelines in the United States (Isenberg-Grzeda et al. 2014; Kleber et al. 2006) call for supplementing with 100 mg of thiamine daily (preferably administered parenterally, although most often given orally), newer guidelines in the United Kingdom (Thomson et al. 2002), implemented by the Royal College of Physicians, call for higher doses of thiamine in patients who may be at risk for or are already developing signs or symptoms of Wernicke's encephalopathy (i.e., confusion, ataxia, ophthalmoplegia): parenteral thiamine 500 mg three times daily for the first 3 days, followed by 250 mg daily for 5 additional days or longer, depending on clinical response (Isenberg-Grzeda et al. 2014; Thomson et al. 2002). Although no general consensus regarding thiamine dosing strategies exists, recent evidence has suggested that, at least in the United States, practitioners have been underdosing thiamine, particularly in the population most at risk for Wernicke's encephalopathy (Isenberg-Grzeda et al. 2014). Furthermore, it is important to remember that thiamine deficiency also occurs in severely medically ill patients without alcohol use disorder (e.g., hyperemesis gravidarum, anorexia nervosa, AIDS and cancer-related cachexia, prolonged stays in the intensive care unit). High-dose thiamine supplementation is urgently indicated when AWS occurs alongside one of these other conditions.

Although supportive measures are most often sufficient to manage mild AWS in medically ill patients, more intensive interventions are required to manage moderate to severe AWS. Pharmacological prophylaxis and management of alcohol withdrawal is accomplished primarily by administration of γ-aminobutyric acid (GABA) agonists (typically benzodiazepines and less often barbiturates). Benzodiazepines are the most frequently utilized and most proven pharmacological agents for effectively managing AWS. However, benzodiazepines can have unintended consequences, such as delirium, respiratory depression, and paradoxical disinhibition, particularly in medically ill or vulnerable patients (e.g., elderly; patients with history of head injury or preexisting neurocognitive disorder, respiratory insufficiency, or sleep apnea). Benzodiazepines are major risk factors for the development of delirium in intensive care patients (Pandharipande et al. 2006, 2008). Benzodiazepines and other sedative-hypnotics can also contribute to the development of hepatic encephalopathy. However, because of the potential life-threating sequelae of advanced AWS, one cannot fail to treat this condition. Hence, caution must be used when identifying patients at risk for developing AWS, given that there are significant risks in both undermedicating and overmedicating with benzodiazepines in medically vulnerable patients.

Benzodiazepines are considered the most effective agents in halting the progression of AWS, preventing and treating withdrawal-related seizures, and treating delirium tremens (Mirijello et al. 2015). Decisions regarding the choice of which benzodiazepine to use in managing AWS should be individualized to each patient. Specifically, factors impacting drug metabolism and clearance, such as the patient's age and the presence of hepatic impairment, should be considered when choosing a benzodiazepine. The most commonly used long-acting benzodiazepines for AWS, chlordiazepoxide and diazepam, initially undergo hepatic oxidation (phase I hepatic metabolism), thereby producing active metabolites, which allows for less frequent dosing and a smoother taper, hence making them favored agents in fixed-dose and loading-dose strategies. However, these pharmacokinetic properties can result in the accumulation of active metabolites in individuals with reduced hepatic clearance, such as the elderly; hepatic congestion due to heart failure; or cirrhosis. This can result in respiratory depression and delirium. Hence, in patients with impaired hepatic function, the shorter-acting agents lorazepam and oxazepam are favored for managing AWS. Both lorazepam and oxazepam bypass hepatic oxidation and undergo clearance via glucuronidation (phase II hepatic metabolism), thereby not producing active metabolites. Even with these agents, caution is warranted in severe hepatic and renal impairment. Of the most commonly used benzodiazepines in the management of AWS, lorazepam, chlordiazepoxide, and diazepam are available in both parenteral and oral formulations; oxazepam is available only in an oral formulation, hence limiting its use in the critically ill (Mirijello et al. 2015). There is a particular concern with high-dose lorazepam infusions, particularly in critically ill patients, because they can cause propylene glycol toxicity, resulting in metabolic acidosis, acute tubular necrosis, seizures, and arrhythmias (Horinek et al. 2009).

Most benzodiazepines are pregnancy category D, primarily because of reported associations with congenital malformations (cleft lip or palate, cardiovascular malformations, and duodenal atresia) with their use in the first trimester. However, a recent systematic review of the studies on which this association is based did not support a link between benzodiazepines in the first trimester and major congenital malformations (Bellantuono et al. 2013). Benzodiazepine use in pregnancy has also been associated with preterm labor and fetal distress. Hence, decisions regarding the use of benzodiazepines must take into account the potential risks of untreated AWS in pregnancy, which, in and of itself, can result in fetal distress and precipitation of preterm labor, not to mention the previously outlined inherent risks to the mother (DeVido et al. 2015).

Both standing (fixed-dose and loading-dose) and symptom-triggered dosing strategies exist for benzodiazepines in the management of AWS. Earlier studies have shown that symptom-triggered benzodiazepine administration in AWS can reduce total benzodiazepine requirement and duration of treatment, but this is contingent on the careful systematic execution of such protocols in well-controlled settings (DeCarolis et al. 2007; Saitz et al. 1994). More recent studies suggest that although symptom-triggered dosing strategies have their advantages, both loading-dose and fixed-dose strategies appear to be equally efficacious and may be preferred in cases of severe alcohol withdrawal, especially given evidence of more rapid improvement when such strategies are used in the early stages (Maldonado et al. 2012).

Although benzodiazepines remain the gold standard in the management of AWS, other pharmacological agents have been shown to have potential utility as monotherapies and adjunctive therapies in select patient populations. Alternative agents for the management of AWS include barbiturates (e.g., phenobarbital), propofol, baclofen, anticonvulsants (e.g., carbamazepine, gabapentin, valproic acid, topiramate), α_2 agonists (e.g., clonidine, dexmedetomidine), and β-blockers (e.g., propranolol). Barbiturates, like benzodiazepines, are GABA agonists and, although no longer as commonly used because of their significant drug-drug interactions and narrow therapeutic index, still have potential utility as monotherapy or adjunctive therapy in managing treatment-refractory AWS, particularly in the emergency or critical care setting (Mirijello et al. 2015; Rosenson et al. 2013). Phenobarbital, a long-acting barbiturate, is the most commonly used barbiturate in treating AWS. It carries higher risk in the elderly and those with hepatic impairment, primarily because of the potential for accumulation of active metabolites, which can then cause oversedation, respiratory depression, and delirium. Phenobarbital is an inducer of cytochrome P450 (CYP) enzymes; hence, significant drug-drug interactions may preclude its use in patients who are following complex pharmacological regimens. Propofol is a parenteral (intravenous) sedative that is used for induction and maintenance of anesthesia exclusively in the emergency, critical care, and procedural settings. It is a GABA agonist as well as an N-methyl-D-aspartate (NMDA) receptor antagonist, has a short half-life, and is highly lipophilic. Propofol has been shown in case series to be quite effective in managing benzodiazepine-refractory delirium tremens in the intensive care unit (McCowan and Marik 2000). Baclofen, a $GABA_B$ receptor agonist, appeared to be comparable to diazepam in managing AWS in one very small randomized controlled trial (Addolorato et al. 2006). Because baclofen is primarily renally excreted with only minimal hepatic metabolism, it can be considered as an option for AWS in patients with severe hepatic impairment.

Phenobarbital and baclofen are pregnancy category D and C, respectively, and should be used with extreme caution in pregnancy. Propofol is pregnancy category B and can be used safely in pregnancy.

Anticonvulsants have also been advocated for managing AWS; however, their role is mainly adjunctive, and they are most effective in the management of withdrawal seizures. A Cochrane review of 56 studies of anticonvulsants for alcohol withdrawal did not show a statistically significant difference in CIWA-Ar scores or major outcomes (delirium tremens, life-threatening adverse events) between anticonvulsants and placebo or anticonvulsants compared with each other; however, anticonvulsants did show a protective benefit against seizures (Minozzi et al. 2010). In this particular review, carbamazepine was the only anticonvulsant associated with a statistically significant reduction in alcohol withdrawal symptoms when compared with benzodiazepines (Minozzi et al. 2010). Of the anticonvulsants, carbamazepine and oxcarbazepine, valproate, gabapentin and pregabalin, and topiramate have been studied in AWS and shown to have some potential utility as adjunctive therapies in treating AWS (Hammond et al. 2015). Carbamazepine and gabapentin seem to have the most evidence supporting their use in mild to moderate AWS, and valproate seems mostly useful as an adjunctive treatment in managing AWS (Hammond et al. 2015).

Anticonvulsants exert their effects via inhibition of voltage-gated sodium channels (carbamazepine, oxcarbazepine, valproate, and topiramate) or voltage-gated calcium channels (gabapentin and pregabalin), ultimately resulting in GABAergic agonism. Carbamazepine is a known CYP inducer (primarily CYP3A4), and valproate (including valproic acid and divalproex sodium) is a CYP inhibitor. Gabapentin and pregabalin do not undergo hepatic metabolism and are excreted via the kidney unchanged. Topiramate is also predominantly renally excreted without significant hepatic metabolism (Asconape 2014). It is also a carbonic anhydrase inhibitor, thus increasing the risk for development of metabolic acidosis and formation of renal calculi. Furthermore, topiramate often causes cognitive dysfunction or blunting and paresthesias.

Use of most anticonvulsants in the first trimester of pregnancy should be exercised with extreme caution. Gabapentin (and pregabalin) and oxcarbazepine are listed as pregnancy category C. Valproate, carbamazepine, and topiramate are pregnancy category D. Of the anticonvulsants, valproate carries the highest risk of teratogenicity (neural tube defects), which appears to be dose-dependent (Tomson et al. 2015).

The sympatholytic drugs (primarily α_2 agonists) have been shown in some studies to be useful in the management of AWS, particularly as adjunctive agents. Specifically, these agents may assist in tempering the autonomic hyperactivity associated with AWS. β-Blockers have not been widely studied and seem to have limited utility in AWS. Clonidine and dexmedetomidine, both α_2 agonists, have been studied and found effective primarily as adjunctive agents in AWS (Muzyk et al. 2011). Dexmedetomidine is a centrally acting α_2 agonist used exclusively in the critical care setting, principally as an alternative to standard sedation protocols and to assist in managing agitation or delirium in mechanically ventilated patients (Pandharipande et al. 2007). It has recently garnered attention as a potentially useful agent in managing treatment-refractory and severe AWS in critically ill patients, particularly by nature of its benzodiazepine-sparing effect (Frazee et al. 2014; Mueller et al. 2014). This benzodiazepine-sparing effect is particularly beneficial in critically ill patients because reduced benzodiazepine burden can help in decreasing the risk for delirium. When used long term, clonidine does have a potential for rebound tachycardia and hypertension with discontinuation. Both clonidine and dexmedetomidine have been associated with significant hypotension and bradycardia. Although monotherapy is not recommended at this time, use of α_2 agonists (particularly dexmedetomidine) as adjuncts in severe or refractory AWS should be strongly considered, especially in the critically ill population.

Both clonidine and dexmedetomidine are pregnancy category C, and their use in pregnancy and lactation should involve careful consideration of potential risk versus benefit. Use of β-blockers in AWS should be reserved as adjunctive while recognizing that these agents can mask sympathetic symptoms associated with AWS, often falsely lowering CIWA-Ar scores. β-Blockers (particularly nonselective ones) are contraindicated in patients with asthma, chronic obstructive pulmonary disease (COPD), hypoglycemia, and some cardiac conduction abnormalities (e.g., second- and third-degree heart block).

Antipsychotics are not specifically indicated for managing AWS but can be beneficial as adjunctive therapies for managing associated agitation and delirium. Haloperidol, in particular, has been extensively and safely used in the medically ill. Its availability in multiple dosage formulations (intramuscular, intravenous, oral, and rectal) further adds to its versatility, particularly in critical care settings. Alternatively, sedating atypical antipsychotics (particularly olanzapine and quetiapine) can be used and may be more effective adjuncts in promoting sleep-wake cycle restoration and managing agitation in patients with delirium tremens. Caution should be exercised when using antipsychotics in patients with AWS, particularly because of the drugs' potential for lowering seizure threshold and inducing cardiac arrhythmias. Antipsychotics for delirium are discussed in more detail in Chapter 15, "Surgery and Critical Care."

Finally, although intravenous ethanol infusions have been used historically to manage AWS, this practice has fallen out of favor, primarily because of the narrow therapeutic index, inability to safely dose, and potential for multiorgan toxicity. Furthermore, a randomized controlled trial in critically ill patients did not support the use of intravenous ethanol infusion over diazepam in AWS prophylaxis (Weinberg et al. 2008).

Alcohol Abstinence and Craving

The main drugs that are FDA approved for the maintenance of abstinence in alcohol use disorder are disulfiram, naltrexone (both a daily oral formulation and an intramuscular monthly formulation), and acamprosate. Disulfiram is an agent that functions via aversive conditioning, primarily exerting its effects by inhibition of the hepatic enzyme aldehyde dehydrogenase, resulting in the accumulation of toxic acetaldehyde. This precipitates an acute reaction resulting in nausea, vomiting, flushing, hypotension, dizziness, diaphoresis, headache, and anxiety or panic symptoms. In fact, patients who are taking disulfiram and providers who are caring for these patients should be cautioned against using products containing alcohol (e.g., mouthwash, medications such as cough syrup and certain intravenous solutions, foods cooked in alcohol, hand sanitizer, alcohol swabs) because some patients are so sensitive that even slight contact (topical or olfactory) can precipitate this violent reaction. Disulfiram is the oldest and longest studied of the FDA-approved medications for alcohol use disorder, but the evidence for its efficacy is rather weak (Fuller et al. 1986). A challenge with using disulfiram, possibly more so than with drugs that function by reducing cravings, is the significant potential for noncompliance. Indeed, the best setting for disulfiram use is supervised, which reduces the risk for noncompliance but also limits its use to patients with intact psychosocial support and strong motivation to achieve sobriety and to those in intensive outpatient or residential settings. Disulfiram is available only in an oral formulation; it relies exclusively on enteral absorption and hepatic metabolism. Disulfiram is potentially hepatotoxic, has precipitated fulminant hepatic failure, and is contraindicated in patients with end-stage liver disease. It is also potentially cardiotoxic and can precipitate arrhythmias and congestive heart failure, particularly in patients with cardiovascular risk factors. Furthermore, severe disulfiram toxicity can precipitate both sensorimotor and cognitive adverse effects (e.g., peripheral neuropathy, visual disturbances, weakness, fatigue, confusion, florid delirium). Disulfiram is pregnancy category C, and its use should generally be avoided in pregnancy.

Naltrexone functions primarily as a competitive antagonist at the μ opioid receptor and to a lesser extent at the κ and δ opioid receptors. The once-daily oral formulation was approved for treating alcohol use disorder by the FDA in 1994, and the monthly depot formulation was approved in 2006. Naltrexone promotes abstinence by blocking critical pathways in the reward center of the brain that are responsible for the reinforcing effects of alcohol, as well as reducing cravings for alcohol. Administering naltrexone to a patient who is taking or has recently taken opioids can rapidly precipitate opioid withdrawal (Quigley and Boyce 2001). Patients who have recently used opioids should typically wait at least 7–10 days before starting naltrexone to avoid precipitation of acute withdrawal. It is recommended that patients taking oral naltrexone stop the medication at least 3 days before scheduled procedures that may require the use of centrally acting opioid agonists. Those taking the monthly depot formulation of naltrexone present a greater challenge and should forgo opioid agonist therapy (i.e., scheduled surgeries or procedures) for at least 3 weeks following the administration of naltrexone. Although administration of opioids in the fourth week following depot naltrexone administration is possible, it often requires use of much larger doses of opioids to provide adequate analgesia (Curatolo and Trinh 2014). However, because of opioid receptor up-regulation and increased receptor sensitivity, patients are at a significantly increased risk for respiratory depression and autonomic instability with administration of opioids during the fourth week following depot naltrexone administration, thereby necessitating close monitoring (Curatolo and Trinh 2014).

Oral naltrexone is heavily hepatically metabolized, whereas the depot formulation bypasses first-pass hepatic oxidation. Both formulations carry the risk of hepatotoxicity and should be used with caution in patients with liver impairment (Garbutt 2010). Guidelines recommend avoiding use of naltrexone in patients when transaminases are elevated to three times the normal range and in patients with end-stage liver disease (Ross and Peselow 2009). Naltrexone is pregnancy category C.

Acamprosate is the third FDA-approved medication for alcohol use disorder, gaining formal approval in 2004. It has a fairly complex mechanism of action, exerting influence primarily via modulation of glutamatergic (NMDA) and GABAergic receptors (Plosker 2015). Like naltrexone, acamprosate functions by reducing cravings; in contrast to naltrexone, however, acamprosate functions primarily by inhibiting negative reinforcement (Ross and Peselow 2009). Acamprosate is fairly well tolerated, with the most common side effect being mild to moderate gastrointestinal distress (primarily diarrhea; possibly nausea or vomiting, flatulence, and anorexia) (Plosker 2015). Although there have been reports of increased anxiety, depression, and suicidality with acamprosate use, these adverse effects are relatively rare (Plosker 2015). In a recent meta-analysis, both acamprosate and naltrexone were found to reduce propensity for return to drinking, and no statistically significant difference was found between the two (Jonas et al. 2014). Acamprosate does not undergo hepatic metabolism and is excreted unchanged by the kidney. It does not cause any significant CYP drug-drug interactions and can be used safely in individuals with hepatic impairment. Caution should be exercised in patients with reduced glomerular filtration rate (i.e., the elderly and patients with renal insufficiency), and it should generally be avoided in end-stage renal disease (Plosker 2015). Acamprosate is listed as pregnancy category C.

Other agents that may have abstinence-promoting utility in alcohol use disorder have also been studied, with the most evidence for anticonvulsants, particularly topiramate and gabapentin (Hammond et al. 2015; Leung et al. 2015; Shinn and Greenfield 2010). Other agents with potential utility include baclofen, serotonergic agents (e.g., selective serotonin reuptake inhibitors [SSRIs] and ondansetron), and aripiprazole (Edwards et al. 2011). Although not currently being used for alcohol use disorder in the United States, nalmefene and sodium oxybate are being used in other countries and hold promise as effective agents (Keating 2014; Paille and Martini 2014). Nalmefene, an opioid antagonist, has a longer half-life and less propensity for inducing hepatotoxicity than naltrexone (Ross and Peselow 2009). Because hepatic impairment is common in patients with alcohol use disorder, abstinence-promoting medications that do not require hepatic metabolism would be desirable. Baclofen, gabapentin, and topiramate should be considered if acamprosate is not feasible in such patients. However, the evidence base is not strong enough to make specific recommendations regarding their use.

Sedative-, Hypnotic-, or Anxiolytic-Related Disorders

Sedative, hypnotic, and anxiolytic medications are commonly prescribed and quite readily abused. Benzodiazepines, barbiturates, and GABAergic sleep aids (i.e., zolpidem, eszopiclone, and zaleplon) fall into this category. Benzodiazepines with a short half-life, particularly alprazolam, have the highest potential for abuse and dependence. In contrast to AWS, withdrawal from benzodiazepines may have a delayed onset (particularly with benzodiazepines that have a long half-life) and more protracted course.

Sedative, hypnotic, and anxiolytic withdrawal can be more severe than withdrawal from other substances, including alcohol. The management of such withdrawal is similar to that of AWS, which is discussed in the subsection "Alcohol Use Disorder" earlier in this chapter. Management typically involves utilization of a GABAergic agent, as most have fairly good cross-reactivity. The exception is alprazolam, which has a novel chemical structure with a triazole ring that seems to have higher binding affinity for a certain subgroup of the benzodiazepine receptor as compared with other benzodiazepines (Browne and Hauge 1986; Sachdev et al. 2014). As a result, alprazolam withdrawal can often be difficult to manage and refractory to treatment with the most commonly utilized benzodiazepines (i.e., lorazepam, chlordiazepoxide, oxazepam) and barbiturates (i.e., phenobarbital) used in managing AWS. In fact, alprazolam withdrawal often requires the use of alprazolam or clonazepam, which has been shown to be a potentially effective alternative in managing alprazolam withdrawal (Sachdev et al. 2014).

Opioid Use Disorder

Opioid use disorder is among the most frequently encountered substance use disorders in the medically ill. Opioid use disorder is highly comorbid with chronic pain and blood-borne infectious diseases (particularly hepatitis C and HIV/AIDS). Now reaching epidemic proportions, opioid use disorders and resultant withdrawal states are commonplace in general medical wards and intensive care units.

Opioid Withdrawal Syndrome

Opioid withdrawal is characterized by autonomic hyperactivity, which results in restlessness, diaphoresis, yawning, rhinorrhea, lacrimation, piloerection, mydriasis, myalgias, and gastrointestinal distress (e.g., cramps, nausea, vomiting, and diarrhea). Although opioid withdrawal is not typically considered to be life threatening, there have been reported fatalities and significant morbidity with ultrarapid detoxification methods, such as those utilizing naltrexone implants (Hamilton et al. 2002). Opioid withdrawal still has a significant impact on the medically ill, often protracting hospital stays and increasing the risk for complications.

Methadone, a synthetic opioid, functions as an agonist at the μ opioid receptor. Its long half-life and high receptor binding affinity made it the traditional choice agent for the management of opioid withdrawal as well as promoting abstinence and reducing opioid craving (discussed in the next subsection). Methadone can be given orally and intravenously. It is primarily hepatically metabolized and is a substrate of CYP3A4; hence, significant drug-drug interactions exist (see Table 18–2 later in this chapter). Of particular importance is the potential for certain antiretrovirals (e.g., efavirenz, darunavir, nevirapine), rifampin, St. John's wort, carbamazepine, phenytoin, and phenobarbital to reduce plasma levels of methadone and effectively precipitate opioid withdrawal (Meemken et al. 2015; Tetrault and Fiellin 2012). Common side effects include sedation, constipation, diaphoresis, urinary retention, and decreased libido. Of greatest concern is the potential for methadone to cause QTc prolongation, which ultimately resulted in a black box warning issued by the FDA in 2006. This risk is further increased when methadone is used intravenously, when it is used concomitantly with other QTc-prolonging agents, or when it is combined with drugs that inhibit the CYP3A4 such as ritonavir, quetiapine, fluoxetine, fluconazole, and ciprofloxacin (Kleber 2007; Meemken et al. 2015; Mujtaba et al. 2013; Tetrault and Fiellin 2012).

Methadone is a pregnancy category C drug and readily crosses the placenta. Given the high prevalence of HIV/AIDS and hepatitis C virus (HCV) infection in intravenous opioid users, such potential drug-drug interactions are of significant importance. No significant drug-drug interactions exist between methadone and antiretrovirals commonly used to treat HCV infection (Meemken et al. 2015). Regarding methadone use in pregnancy, serum levels of methadone may be decreased because of increased clearance. Adverse effects in pregnancy and lactation, which are mostly limited to central nervous system (CNS)/respiratory depression and neonatal abstinence syndrome, should be weighed against the potential benefit of reducing the possible risk of maternal-fetal distress associated with opioid withdrawal that can precipitate preterm labor and other complications (Minozzi et al. 2013).

Buprenorphine, a partial agonist at the μ opioid receptor and potent antagonist at the κ opioid receptor, was approved by the FDA in 2002 for the management of opioid dependence. It has become a viable, and often preferential, alternative to methadone for management of opioid withdrawal, particularly in the medically ill. This is especially because of its decreased risk of QTc prolongation, as well as its partial agonist and antagonist properties, which impart a ceiling effect that minimizes respiratory depression with dose escalation (Ciraulo et al. 2006; Fareed et al. 2013; Wedam et al. 2007). Furthermore, buprenorphine, although also a substrate of CYP3A4, has fewer significant drug-drug interactions, particularly with antiretrovirals used to treat HIV, as compared with methadone (Meemken et al. 2015). The exceptions are the antiretroviral drugs atazanavir and ritonavir, which inhibit CYP3A4 and can significantly increase serum levels of buprenorphine and its active metabolite, norbuprenorphine (Meemken et al. 2015). Much as with methadone, there are no significant drug-drug interactions between buprenorphine and antivirals used in the treatment of HCV infection (Meemken et al. 2015).

Buprenorphine is typically administered sublingually either alone or in combination with naloxone. This is largely because of its extensive first-pass metabolism and low bioavailability when administered orally (Ciraulo et al. 2006). Buprenorphine has also been successfully used intravenously in managing acute opioid withdrawal in medically ill patients (Welsh et al. 2002). Caution should be exercised when using buprenorphine in patients with hepatic impairment, particularly those with severe impairment. Buprenorphine, as well as the buprenorphine-naloxone combination, is relatively contraindicated for use in end-stage liver disease. Use in patients undergoing chronic opioid therapy or in those requiring acute opioid-analgesic therapy, such as in the postoperative setting, is relatively contraindicated given the propensity for buprenorphine to occupy μ and κ opioid receptor sites with high binding affinity, thus blocking analgesia and potentially precipitating withdrawal. However, given its partial agonist properties, buprenorphine can be used as an alternative monotherapy for patients with coexisting opioid use disorder and chronic pain, reducing the risk of fatal respiratory depression.

Whereas methadone is the most commonly used medication for detoxification in pregnancy, buprenorphine has been shown to have similar outcomes and safety profile in pregnancy and lactation (Jones et al. 2012). Buprenorphine both alone and in combination with naloxone is pregnancy category C. The combination, although less studied, appears to have similar maternal and fetal outcomes and has been shown to be safe in pregnant women; however, further prospective studies are necessary to investigate potential impacts on fetal development (Debelak et al. 2013; Lund et al. 2013). In addition, buprenorphine alone and in combination with naloxone has the added benefits of decreased frequency and severity of neonatal abstinence syndrome and shorter duration of neonatal hospitalization as compared with methadone (Jones et al. 2010; Lund et al. 2013; Meyer et al. 2015; Wiegand et al. 2015).

Clonidine is used as an alternative, often second- or third-line, agent in the management of acute opioid withdrawal symptoms. It may be preferred in medically complicated patients with end-stage liver disease and/or cardiac conduction abnormalities, which may preclude use of buprenorphine and methadone, respectively. The pharmacological properties and use of clonidine were discussed earlier in the subsection "Alcohol Use Disorder."

Opioid Abstinence and Craving

Methadone and buprenorphine (particularly the formulation with naloxone) are the most commonly utilized pharmacological agents for reducing craving and promoting abstinence in individuals with opioid use disorder. In moderate to high doses, both methadone and buprenorphine are found to be equally efficacious and have similar side effect profiles when used as maintenance treatment of opioid use disorder (Mattick et al. 2014). Although less commonly used, naltrexone is also used in reducing cravings and relapse prevention in opioid use disorder. Finally, levomethadyl acetate (LAAM), a synthetic opioid and potent agonist at the μ opioid receptor, was approved for use in 1993 and subsequently was taken off the market by the FDA in 2003 because of a significant risk for lethal arrhythmias due to QTc prolongation (Deamer et al. 2001; Wedam et al. 2007; Wieneke et al. 2009). Given its significantly longer half-life, LAAM can be dosed less frequently than methadone, which gives LAAM an advantage with regard to treatment retention. There has been a resurgence of interest in reevaluating the use and safety profile of LAAM (Gryczynski et al. 2012; Wolstein et al. 2009).

Tobacco Use Disorder

Tobacco, particularly cigarette, use is the leading cause of preventable illness and death in the United States (Jamal et al. 2014; U.S. Department of Health and Human Services 2014). Cigarette smoking has been associated with the development of multiple acute and chronic illnesses, including adenocarcinoma of the lung, hepatocellular carcinoma, colorectal cancer, COPD, cardiovascular disease, congenital malformations (cleft lip or palate), ectopic pregnancy, spontaneous abortion, macular degeneration, and diabetes, among others (U.S. Department of Health and Human Services 2014). A comprehensive discussion of the implications of tobacco use in the medically ill is beyond the scope of this chapter. Nevertheless, pharmacological treatment strategies exist to prevent and ameliorate withdrawal symptoms as well as promote abstinence by reducing cravings associated with nicotine.

Tobacco Withdrawal

Tobacco withdrawal can result in severe anxiety, irritability, restlessness, dysphoria, insomnia, and appetite stimulation. Such symptoms can obviously complicate medical treatment. The psychoactive substance nicotine is primarily responsible for the highly addictive nature of tobacco. Nicotine replacement therapy (NRT) remains the mainstay in the prevention and management of nicotine withdrawal in medical settings (Rigotti et al. 2008). NRT is available as a transdermal patch, a lozenge, gum, a nasal spray, and an inhaler. NRT is safe to use in most medically ill patients, but caution should be exercised in patients with recent coronary events, especially given nicotine's potential for myocardial excitability (e.g., tachycardia, hypertension, increased cardiac work/demand, precipitation of arrhythmias) (Sobieraj et al. 2013; Woolf et al. 2012). NRT has been proven safe in long-term studies, with no significant adverse outcomes in a recent study during which it was used for up to 52 weeks (Schnoll et al. 2015). NRT use in pregnancy is deemed relatively safe, with a recent review of existing studies concluding that there is no significant risk for major congenital malformations in children born to mothers receiving NRT (Dhalwani et al. 2015).

Tobacco Abstinence and Craving

The primary agents used in maintaining tobacco abstinence function by either direct nicotine replacement or reduction of cravings by alternative mechanisms. NRT, bupropion, and varenicline are the mainstays of treatment. Bupropion, a norepinephrine-dopamine reuptake inhibitor, is thought to exert its effects on nicotine craving by enhancement of dopaminergic pathways in reward centers of the brain. It can be used safely in medically ill patients, with caution in patients with a history of seizures and in those whose seizure threshold may be decreased (e.g., because of a recent cerebrovascular accident or traumatic brain injury, withdrawal from alcohol or sedatives, or medications that are known to lower seizure threshold). Seizure risk is significant with bupropion doses >450 mg and with use of the immediate-release formulation. Furthermore, because bupropion is a potent CYP2D6 inhibitor, drug-drug interactions can occur. The most common side effects of bupropion include insomnia, anxiety, dry mouth, and appetite suppression. Bupropion is pregnancy category C given the relative lack of well-designed studies.

Varenicline was approved by the FDA in 2006 for smoking cessation. It is a partial agonist at nicotinic acetylcholine receptors, functioning to reduce nicotine cravings and promote abstinence. The most common adverse effect associated with varenicline is nausea. Among the most serious adverse effects are precipitation of mood instability, hostility, severe depression, and suicidality, which prompted the FDA to issue a black box warning. Despite this, a recent meta-analysis did not show any statistically significant risk of adverse neuropsychiatric symptoms with varenicline (Cahill et al. 2013). Furthermore, although earlier studies raised concerns about potential cardiovascular risk with varenicline, the studies were methodologically flawed, and meta-analysis did not support such a risk (Cahill et al. 2013). Varenicline is primarily renally excreted and is without significant drug-drug interactions. Caution should be exercised when using in patients with renal impairment.

Varenicline is a category C drug because it has not been adequately studied in pregnancy. Nevertheless, use of varenicline is not recommended in pregnancy, primarily because of potential risk of adverse neuropsychiatric sequelae that can affect mother and fetus.

Cocaine and Other Stimulant-Related Disorders

Cocaine and methamphetamine are among the most pervasive and commonly abused stimulants in the medically ill. Cocaine use in particular is linked to serious cardiac sequelae, including malignant hypertension, myocardial infarction, arrhythmias, dilated cardiomyopathy, and resultant heart failure (Phillips et al. 2009). Caution should be exercised when using certain medications otherwise commonly administered to cardiac patients. Historically, β-blockers were considered to be contraindicated, primarily because of the theoretical risk for unopposed α_1 receptor agonism, which can cause coronary vasoconstriction in cocaine intoxication. Hence, use of medications such as labetalol that have mixed α and β receptor antagonist properties may be preferred. In addition, partially as a result of the cardiovascular effects of cocaine (e.g., vasoconstriction, rhabdomyolysis), acute kidney injury is not uncommon (Goel et al. 2014). Both cocaine and other psychostimulants (e.g., methamphetamine) are known to be associated with increased risk for stroke, seizures, movement disorders (e.g., dyskinesias, tics, early-onset Parkinson's disease with chronic use), and hypothalamic dysregulation resulting in hyperpyrexia (Sanchez-Ramos 2015; Westover et al. 2007). Hypothalamic temperature dysregulation coupled with rhabdomyolysis and relative dopamine depletion (often seen with cocaine toxicity and in chronic use) can increase risk for (or mimic) neuroleptic malignant syndrome (NMS). Hence, caution should be exercised when using antipsychotics (or other dopamine antagonists) for managing acute agitation associated with psychostimulant intoxication, primarily because of the risk for precipitating NMS. As a result, benzodiazepines are preferred as first-line agents.

Stimulant withdrawal typically results in prominent central nervous system depression and most often presents with fatigue, sluggishness, hypersomnolence, hyperphagia, irritability, and dysphoria. There are no medications specifically approved for the management of stimulant withdrawal, but a number of medications have been studied for the management of cravings associated with stimulant use. These include dopaminergic agents (e.g., amphetamines, disulfiram by virtue of its function as a dopamine β-hydroxylase inhibitor), GABAergic agents (particularly topiramate), serotonergic agents (e.g., ondansetron, SSRIs), and agents with multimodal, glutamatergic mechanisms such as modafanil (Karila et al. 2008; Ross and Peselow 2009). A recent Cochrane review did not support the use of psychostimulats (i.e., dexamphetamine, bupropion, methylphenidate, and modafanil) in managing stimulant use disorders (Pérez-Mañá et al. 2013). Topiramate may have some potential utility in managing cocaine and other stimulant use disorders; however, well-designed larger-scale studies are needed (Shinn and Greenfield 2010).

Cannabis and Synthetic Cannabinoids

Cannabis is the most commonly used illicit drug, with more widespread use expected pending legislation legalizing both the medicinal and recreational use of marijuana in various states (Substance Abuse and Mental Health Services Administration 2014). The debate as to the safety and utility of cannabis in treating various medical conditions (e.g., glaucoma, chronic intractable cancer-related pain, spasticity associated with multiple sclerosis, anorexia/cachexia associated with HIV/AIDS and cancer) is beyond the scope of this chapter and is reviewed elsewhere (Aggarwal et al. 2009; Whiting et al. 2015). Cannabis use is known to be associated with short-term memory deficits, inattention, executive dysfunction, somnolence, hyperphagia, increased anxiety, euphoria, and perceptual disturbances (Hoch et al. 2015). In addition, use of cannabis has been associated with the precipitation of frank psychosis, which can range in severity from mild paranoia to schizophrenia spectrum disorder in vulnerable individuals (Moore et al. 2007).

Synthetic cannabinoids (e.g., K2, Spice) represent a wide array of cannabinoid receptor agonists that appear to have more potent binding affinity at the CB_1 receptor, which is thought to contribute to increased toxicity when compared with naturally occurring cannabis (Castaneto et al. 2014). Symptoms associated with synthetic cannabinoid intoxication range from anxiety, blurred vision, diaphoresis, myoclonic jerks, tremors, tachycardia, and hypertension to frank affective disturbances, aggression or hostility, seizures, psychosis, and delirium (Castaneto et al. 2014; Pourmand et al. 2014).

Withdrawal from cannabinoids (both natural and synthetic) can cause symptoms that are often mild but are nonetheless distressing, including anxiety, agitation, irritability, insomnia, and mood lability (Macfarlane and Christie 2015). Management of cannabinoid withdrawal is typically supportive in nature. There is no approved medication for treating cannabis use disorder; however, studies are under way examining the role of CB receptor agonists (e.g., dronabinol), which may have some utility in this regard. Furthermore, gabapentin and N-acetylcysteine have been shown in recent placebo-controlled trials to have some utility in promoting abstinence (Balter et al. 2014).

Other Substance Use Disorders

There are a number of other substances with multimodal mechanisms of action that impact monoamine, opioid, and/or glutamatergic pathways. These substances include novel agents that seem to have exploded onto the scene within the past decade. Some are extracted from naturally occurring plants, whereas others are synthetic analogues. An extensive discussion of each of these substances is beyond the scope of this chapter; however, discussion of some common agents, key clinical findings, and specific management recommendations is warranted.

The hallucinogens include both naturally occurring and synthetic compounds. Examples of common hallucinogens include phencyclidine (PCP, "angel dust"), lysergic acid diethylamide (LSD, "acid"), dimethyltryptamine, ketamine ("special K"), dextromethorphan (DXM, "skittles," "robo"), psilocybin ("magic mushrooms," "shrooms"), mescaline, and Salvia divinorum. Hallucinogens commonly precipitate perceptual disturbances and contribute to an altered sense of self, time, and space. There may also be frank dissociation, euphoria, and emotional as well as physical numbing. Some degree of sympathetic activation resulting in tachycardia and hypertension is common.

PCP, ketamine, and DXM are dissociative agents (Passie and Halpern 2014). PCP intoxication can be quite dramatic, often resulting in significant disinhibition and agitation or hostility, accompanied by prominent sympathomimetic and cholinergic (e.g., bronchospasm, sialorrhea, flushing, miosis) signs and symptoms (Passie and Halpern 2014). Vertical and/or horizontal nystagmus is often present, and patients can become floridly delirious or even comatose (Dominici et al. 2015). There is also evidence of increased muscle tone, which can precipitate dystonic reactions and rhabdomyolysis (Passie and Halpern 2014). Complications can include cardiac conduction abnormalities, arrhythmias, renal failure (due to rhabdomyolysis), hypertensive crisis, intracranial hemorrhage, and increased risk for NMS. As a result, benzodiazepines are preferred first-line agents in managing agitation due to PCP intoxication, given that antipsychotics can contribute to muscle rigidity and temperature dysregulation or hyperthermia and increase risk for NMS. Ketamine has similar properties to PCP; however, its effects are much less profound in comparison (Passie and Halpern 2014). Methoxetamine ("M-ket"), a newer drug that has surfaced in the United States, is a PCP analogue. Methoxetamine intoxication and adverse effects are similar to those of PCP and may include respiratory depression and pulmonary edema (Pourmand et al. 2014).

MDMA (Ecstasy, "Molly") is an analogue of methamphetamine with some similarities to the hallucinogens. It is more serotonergic, hence contributing to the vivid experiences and "connection" that individuals feel to others and to their environment when they are under its influence. MDMA causes sympathetic activation and can result in an increase in cardiac workload, malignant hypertension that predisposes the individual to stroke and acute myocardial infarction, and disseminated intravascular coagulation (Pourmand et al. 2014). Tremors and muscle rigidity can also be seen, which may cause rhabdomyolysis and predispose the individual to renal failure. Because of MDMA's serotonergic properties, bruxism, vivid dreams, and gastrointestinal distress are also seen. Caution should be taken with using serotonergic agents given the potential for precipitating serotonin syndrome. Like SSRIs, MDMA stimulates release of antidiuretic hormone, which can result in hyponatremia (Pourmand et al. 2014). As with PCP, MDMA intoxication can be managed by supportive measures (hydration, reassurance, redirection, correction of metabolic or electrolyte abnormalities) followed by use of benzodiazepines to manage agitation if necessary.

The cathinone derivatives, more commonly known as "bath salts," have properties similar to those of MDMA. They typically cause sympathomimetic effects and also have some hallucinogenic as well as serotonergic properties. Presenting signs may include tachycardia, hypertension, hyperthermia, diaphoresis, muscle rigidity, and rhabdomyolysis, resulting in renal failure, adverse cardiovascular effects, agitation, psychosis, florid delirium, and seizures (Miotto et al. 2013). Given the prominent serotonergic properties of the cathinone derivatives, individuals using these substances are at risk for serotonin syndrome. Temperature dysregulation, coupled with muscle breakdown or rigidity along with dehydration, can predispose patients to NMS. Recommended treatment is supportive measures and benzodiazepines for agitation. As with MDMA, antipsychotics and other dopamine antagonists and serotonergic agents should be used with extreme caution.

The opioid receptor agonists kratom (a plant alkyloid) and desomorphine ("krokodil," an opioid derivative of codeine) have recently made an appearance in the United States, coming from Southeast Asia and eastern Europe, respectively (Pourmand et al. 2014). Both tend to cause significant CNS/respiratory depression, but kratom tends to have some stimulant properties at lower doses (Pourmand et al. 2014). Krokodil, on the other hand, is injected and often causes significant local necrosis at the injection site, which can spread and evolve into gangrene. As with opioids, naloxone can be used to reverse severe CNS/respiratory depression associated with the intoxication.

Last, concomitant with the spread of prescription drug abuse, over-the-counter medications such as DXM (present in cough syrup and cold remedies) and pseudoephedrine (present in allergy and cold medications) have become quite popular, particularly among adolescents and teenagers. This seems to be primarily due to ease of access and has prompted stricter monitoring guidelines regarding their purchase in most states. DXM has a multimodal mechanism of action that involves serotonergic and glutamatergic pathways. Intoxication produces a dissociative reaction, similar to that seen with other hallucinogens. Pseudoephedrine has stimulant properties and is converted into methamphetamine and methcathinone. Clinical findings and management of DXM and pseudoephedrine toxicity are analogous to those for hallucinogens (as well as MDMA) and stimulants, respectively.

Neuropsychiatric Effects of Drugs Used for Substance-Related Disorders

Table 18–1 lists the more common neuropsychiatric adverse effects with drugs used for managing substance-related disorders.

Drug-Drug Interactions

Acamprosate and varenicline are without significant drug-drug interactions. Furthermore, baclofen, gabapentin, pregabalin, and topiramate are primarily renally excreted and thereby have minimal drug-drug interactions. Table 18–2 lists some of the more common drug-drug interactions between medications used for substance-related disorders.

Table 18–1.   Neuropsychiatric adverse effects of drugs that treat substance abuse–related disorders

Medication	Neuropsychiatric adverse effects
Acamprosate	Common: anxiety, insomnia, anorexia Serious: suicidality, clinical depression
α₂ Agonists (e.g., clonidine, dexmedetomidine)	Common: drowsiness, sedation, nervousness, agitation, sexual dysfunction Serious: clinical depression
Anticonvulsants (e.g., carbamazepine, valproic acid, topiramate, gabapentin)	Common: sedation, confusion, fatigue, appetite or weight changes, psychomotor slowing, cognitive blunting Serious: paresthesias (with topiramate), clinical depression, seizure exacerbation, suicidality, psychosis, delirium
Baclofen	Common: sedation, psychomotor slowing, fatigue, cognitive blunting Serious: respiratory depression, withdrawal with discontinuation, seizures, delirium
Barbiturates (e.g., phenobarbital)	Common: somnolence, psychomotor slowing, amnesia Serious: dependence, withdrawal seizures, suicidality, clinical depression, respiratory depression, delirium
Benzodiazepines (e.g., lorazepam, diazepam)	Common: somnolence, lethargy, psychomotor slowing, amnesia Serious: dependence, withdrawal seizures, clinical depression, delirium, amnesia
β-Blockers (e.g., propranolol)	Common: fatigue, sexual dysfunction, psychomotor slowing Serious: no serious neuropsychiatric adverse effects
Buprenorphine	Common: sedation, insomnia, depression Serious: withdrawal, seizures, respiratory depression, delirium
Bupropion	Common: anxiety, insomnia, appetite suppression Serious: seizures, suicidality, agitation, hallucinations, paranoia, delirium

Table 18–1. Neuropsychiatric adverse effects of drugs that treat substance abuse–related disorders *(continued)*

Medication	Neuropsychiatric adverse effects
Disulfiram	Common: alcohol-disulfiram reaction, drowsiness, anxiety or panic symptoms Serious: optic neuritis and other multiple sclerosis–like symptoms, psychosis, respiratory depression, seizures
Flumazenil	Common: agitation, anxiety, fatigue, confusion Serious: seizures, resedation (due to short half-life), iatrogenic precipitation of benzodiazepine withdrawal syndrome
Methadone	Common: somnolence or sedation, psychomotor slowing, cognitive blunting Serious: respiratory depression or arrest, withdrawal, seizures, delirium, coma
Naltrexone	Common: insomnia, anxiety, fatigue, somnolence Serious: suicidality, clinical depression, iatrogenic precipitation of opioid withdrawal syndrome
Propofol	Common: sedation, cognitive impairment Serious: respiratory depression or arrest, propofol infusion syndrome, opisthotonus, delirium, coma
Varenicline	Common: insomnia, abnormal dreams, appetite suppression, somnolence Serious: suicidality, severe clinical depression, agitation or hostility, behavioral disturbances, exacerbation of underlying psychiatric disorder, seizures, hallucinations

Source. McEvoy 2008.

Table 18–2.   Psychotropic drug–drugs for substance abuse interactions

Medication	Interaction mechanism	Effects on psychotropic drugs and management
Buprenorphine	See methadone below	Similar drug interaction profile to methadone (see below), although generally attenuated effects, particularly less concomitant sedation and QT prolongation.
	Opioid antagonism	May induce withdrawal in patients taking opioid analgesics and methadone.
Clonidine	Additive hypotensive effect	Increased risk of hypotensive effects with antipsychotics, TCAs, and MAOIs; increased risk of dry mouth and eyes with TCAs and antipsychotics.
	Inhibits norepinephrine release	May decrease the therapeutic effect of TCAs and NRIs, including atomoxetine. Similarly, TCAs and NRIs may decrease the effects of clonidine.
Disulfiram	Inhibits CYP2E1, CYP1A2, and possibly other CYP enzymes	Increased levels and toxicity of phenytoin (and possibly mephenytoin and fosphenytoin), olanzapine, and risperidone.
	Inhibits acetaldehyde metabolism	Many oral medications in liquid form and some intravenous infusions contain small amounts of alcohol, which would provoke a disulfiram reaction.
	Inhibits dopamine β-hydroxylase	Increased seizure potential with illicit cocaine use.
Flumazenil	GABA antagonism	Contraindicated in patients receiving a benzodiazepine for control of intracranial pressure or status epilepticus or in cases of TCA overdose.

Table 18–2. Psychotropic drug–drugs for substance abuse interactions *(continued)*

Medication	Interaction mechanism	Effects on psychotropic drugs and management
Methadone	Opioid antagonism	Decreased methadone effect and possibly withdrawal in combination with naloxone, naltrexone, pentazocine, nalbuphine, butorphanol, and buprenorphine.
	Induces CYP3A4	Decreased serum levels of methadone and possible withdrawal in combination with phenytoin, St. John's wort, phenobarbital, carbamazepine, rifampin, and some antiretroviral medications (see Chapter 12, "Infectious Diseases").
	Inhibits CYP3A4	Increased serum levels of methadone and potential excessive sedation and respiratory suppression with CYP3A4 inhibitors such as fluvoxamine and nefazodone.
	Potentiation of opioid sedation	Coadministration with benzodiazepines or strong antihistamines (e.g., tertiary-amine TCAs, quetiapine, diphenhydramine) can potentiate opioid sedation.
	QT prolongation	Additive risk for QT prolongation and electrolyte disturbances with psychotropics that increase QT interval, including TCAs, typical antipsychotics, pimozide, risperidone, paliperidone, iloperidone, quetiapine, ziprasidone, and lithium (see also Chapter 6, "Cardiovascular Disorders").
Naltrexone	Opioid antagonism	Blocks the effect of opioids administered for pain, cough, and diarrhea. Use should be avoided in patients dependent on opioids for control of severe pain.
	Unknown	Increases area under the plasma concentration–time curve of acamprosate by 25%.[a]

Note. CYP=cytochrome P450; GABA=γ-aminobutyric acid; MAOIs=monoamine oxidase inhibitors; NRIs=norepinephrine reuptake inhibitors; TCAs=tricyclic antidepressants

[a]Acamprosate product monograph (Mason et al. 2003).

Key Clinical Points

- Substance use disorders are overwhelmingly represented in the medically ill.
- Opioid overdose has surpassed motor vehicle accidents as the most common cause of unintentional deaths in the United States.
- Whereas only 3%–5% of patients admitted for alcohol withdrawal syndrome (AWS) will progress to delirium tremens, mortality rates due to delirium tremens can be as high as 20% in the medically ill.
- Despite evidence suggesting a possible adjunctive role for anticonvulsants and α_2 agonists, benzodiazepines remain the gold standard in the management of moderate and severe AWS.
- High-dose thiamine should be administered parenterally to high-risk patients with a history of heavy alcohol use who are presenting with altered mental status, patients with drastic weight loss and malnutrition, and patients with poor oral intake and/or prominent evidence of cachexia.
- Methadone can significantly prolong the QTc interval and should be used with extreme caution in cardiac patients.
- Significant drug-drug interactions exist between methadone and antivirals.
- By virtue of its partial agonism, buprenorphine has less risk of respiratory depression with dosage escalation as compared with methadone.
- Although pharmacological agents for tobacco use disorder exist, the most effective strategies involve the concomitant implementation of psychosocial interventions.
- Cocaine and amphetamine-like agents carry significant risks for cardiovascular and neurological sequelae, even in younger patients without other risk factors.

- Further studies are necessary to elucidate the safety of long-term cannabis use in the medically ill.
- Over the past few decades, newer substances of abuse have surfaced. This creates challenges when caring for the medically ill, which are further complicated by the fact that many of these substances do not show up on standard toxicology assays. Hence, early identification of clinical signs and prompt implementation of supportive measures is imperative.

References

ACOG Committee on Health Care for Underserved Women; American Society of Addiction Medicine: ACOG Committee Opinion No. 524: Opioid abuse, dependence, and addiction in pregnancy. Obstet Gynecol 119(5):1070–1076, 2012 22525931

Addolorato G, Leggio L, Abenavoli L, et al: Baclofen in the treatment of alcohol withdrawal syndrome: a comparative study vs diazepam. Am J Med 119(3):276.e13–18, 2006 16490478

Aggarwal SK, Carter GT, Sullivan MD, et al: Medicinal use of cannabis in the United States: historical perspectives, current trends, and future directions. J Opioid Manag 5(3):153–168, 2009 19662925

Asconape JJ: Use of antiepileptic drugs in hepatic and renal disease, in Handbook of Clinical Neurology: Neurologic Aspects of Systemic Disease, Part I. Edited by Biller J, Ferro J. Amsterdam, Elsevier, 2014, pp 417–432

Balter RE, Cooper ZD, Haney M: Novel pharmacologic approaches to treating cannabis use disorder. Curr Addict Rep 1(2):137–143, 2014 24955304

Bellantuono C, Tofani S, Di Sciascio G, Santone G: Benzodiazepine exposure in pregnancy and risk of major malformations: a critical overview. Gen Hosp Psychiatry 35(1):3–8, 2013 23044244

Bohn MJ, Babor TF, Kranzler HR: The Alcohol Use Disorders Identification Test (AUDIT): validation of a screening instrument for use in medical settings. J Stud Alcohol 56(4):423–432, 1995 7674678

Browne JL, Hauge KJ: A review of alprazolam withdrawal. Drug Intell Clin Pharm 20(11):837–841, 1986 3536383

Cahill K, Stevens S, Perera R, Lancaster T: Pharmacological interventions for smoking cessation: an overview and network meta-analysis. Cochrane Database of Systematic Reviews 2013, Issue 5. Art. No.: CD009329. DOI: 10.1002/14651858. CD009329.pub2 23728690

Castaneto MS, Gorelick DA, Desrosiers NA, et al: Synthetic cannabinoids: epidemiology, pharmacodynamics, and clinical implications. Drug Alcohol Depend 144:12–41, 2014 25220897

Ciraulo DA, Hitzemann RJ, Somoza E, et al: Pharmacokinetics and pharmacodynamics of multiple sublingual buprenorphine tablets in dose-escalation trials. J Clin Pharmacol 46(2):179–192, 2006 16432270

Curatolo C, Trinh M: Challenges in the perioperative management of the patient receiving extended-release naltrexone. A A Case Rep 3(11):142–144, 2014 25612099

Deamer RL, Wilson DR, Clark DS, Prichard JG: Torsades de pointes associated with high dose levomethadyl acetate (ORLAAM). J Addict Dis 20(4):7–14, 2001 11760927

Debelak K, Morrone WR, O'Grady KE, Jones HE: Buprenorphine + naloxone in the treatment of opioid dependence during pregnancy—initial patient care and outcome data. Am J Addict 22(3):252–254, 2013 23617867

DeCarolis DD, Rice KL, Ho L, et al: Symptom-driven lorazepam protocol for treatment of severe alcohol withdrawal delirium in the intensive care unit. Pharmacotherapy 27(4):510–518, 2007 17381377

DeVido J, Bogunovic O, Weiss RD: Alcohol use disorders in pregnancy. Harv Rev Psychiatry 23(2):112–121, 2015 25747924

de Wit M, Jones DG, Sessler CN, et al: Alcohol-use disorders in the critically ill patient. Chest 138(4):994–1003, 2010 20923804

Dhalwani NN, Szatkowski L, Coleman T, et al: Nicotine replacement therapy in pregnancy and major congenital anomalies in offspring. Pediatrics 135(5):859–867, 2015 25847803

Dominici P, Kopec K, Manur R, et al: Phencyclidine Intoxication Case Series Study. J Med Toxicol 11(3):321–325, 2015 25502414

Edwards S, Kenna GA, Swift RM, Leggio L: Current and promising pharmacotherapies, and novel research target areas in the treatment of alcohol dependence: a review. Curr Pharm Des 17(14):1323–1332, 2011 21524263

Fareed A, Patil D, Scheinberg K, et al: Comparison of QTc interval prolongation for patients in methadone versus buprenorphine maintenance treatment: a 5-year follow-up. J Addict Dis 32(3):244–251, 2013 24074190

Frazee EN, Personett HA, Leung JG, et al: Influence of dexmedetomidine therapy on the management of severe alcohol withdrawal syndrome in critically ill patients. J Crit Care 29(2):298–302, 2014 24360597

Fuller RK, Branchey L, Brightwell DR, et al: Disulfiram treatment of alcoholism: a Veterans Administration cooperative study. JAMA 256(11):1449–1455, 1986 3528541

Garbutt JC: Efficacy and tolerability of naltrexone in the management of alcohol dependence. Curr Pharm Des 16(19):2091–2097, 2010 20482515

Goel N, Pullman JM, Coco M: Cocaine and kidney injury: a kaleidoscope of pathology. Clin Kidney J 7(6):513–517, 2014 25859366

Gryczynski J, Kinlock TW, Kelly SM, et al: Opioid agonist maintenance for probationers: patient-level predictors of treatment retention, drug use, and crime. Subst Abus 33(1):30–39, 2012 22263711

Hamilton RJ, Olmedo RE, Shah S, et al: Complications of ultrarapid opioid detoxification with subcutaneous naltrexone pellets. Acad Emerg Med 9(1):63–68, 2002 11772672

Hammond CJ, Niciu MJ, Drew S, Arias AJ: Anticonvulsants for the treatment of alcohol withdrawal syndrome and alcohol use disorders. CNS Drugs 29(4):293–311, 2015 25895020

Hoch E, Bonnetn U, Thomasius R, et al: Risks associated with the non-medicinal use of cannabis. Dtsch Arztebl Int 112(16):271–278, 2015 25939318

Horinek EL, Kiser TH, Fish DN, MacLaren R: Propylene glycol accumulation in critically ill patients receiving continuous intravenous lorazepam infusions. Ann Pharmacother 43(12):1964–1971, 2009 19920159

Isenberg-Grzeda E, Chabon B, Nicolson SE: Prescribing thiamine to inpatients with alcohol use disorders: how well are we doing? J Addict Med 8(1):1–5, 2014 24343128

Jamal A, Agaku IT, O'Connor E, et al; Centers for Disease Control and Prevention (CDC): Current cigarette smoking among adults—United States, 2005–2013. MMWR Morb Mortal Wkly Rep 63(47):1108–1112, 2014 25426653

Jonas DE, Amick HR, Feltner C, et al: Pharmacotherapy for adults with alcohol use disorders in outpatient settings: a systematic review and meta-analysis. JAMA 311(18):1889–1900, 2014 24825644

Jones HE, Kaltenbach K, Heil SH, et al: Neonatal abstinence syndrome after methadone or buprenorphine exposure. N Engl J Med 363(24):2320–2331, 2010 21142534

Jones HE, Heil SH, Baewert A, et al: Buprenorphine treatment of opioid-dependent pregnant women: a comprehensive review. Addiction 1071995 7674678 (suppl 1):5–27, 2012 23106923

Karila L, Gorelick D, Weinstein A, et al: New treatments for cocaine dependence: a focused review. Int J Neuropsychopharmacol 11(3):425–438, 2008 17927843

Katz G, Durst R, Shufman E, et al: Substance abuse in hospitalized psychiatric patients. Isr Med Assoc J 10(10):672–675, 2008 19009943

Keating GM: Sodium oxybate: a review of its use in alcohol withdrawal syndrome and in the maintenance of abstinence in alcohol dependence. Clin Drug Investig 34(1):63–80, 2014 24307430

Kim D, Irwin KS, Khoshnood K: Expanded access to naloxone: options for critical response to the epidemic of opioid overdose mortality. Am J Public Health 99(3):402–407, 2009 19150908

Kim HK, Nelson LS: Reducing the harm of opioid overdose with the safe use of naloxone: a pharmacologic review. Expert Opin Drug Saf 14(7):1137–1146, 2015 25865597

Kleber HD: Pharmacologic treatments for opioid dependence: detoxification and maintenance options. Dialogues Clin Neurosci 9(4):455–470, 2007 18286804

Kleber HD, Weiss RD, Anton RF: Practice Guideline for the Treatment of Patients With Substance Use Disorders, 2nd Edition. Arlington, VA, American Psychiatric Publishing, 2014

Leung JG, Hall-Flavin D, Nelson S, et al: The role of gabapentin in the management of alcohol withdrawal and dependence. Ann Pharmacother 49(8):897–906, 2015 25969570

Longmire AW, Seger DL: Topics in clinical pharmacology: flumazenil, a benzodiazepine antagonist. Am J Med Sci 306(1):49–52, 1993 8101045

Lund IO, Fischer G, Welle-Strand GK, et al: A comparison of buprenorphine + naloxone to buprenorphine and methadone in the treatment of opioid dependence during pregnancy: maternal and neonatal outcomes. Subst Abuse 7:61–74, 2013 23531704

Macfarlane V, Christie G: Synthetic cannabinoid withdrawal: a new demand on detoxification services. Drug Alcohol Rev 34(2):147–153, 2015 25588420

Maldonado JR, Nguyen LH, Schader EM, Brooks JO III: Benzodiazepine loading versus symptom-triggered treatment of alcohol withdrawal: a prospective, randomized clinical trial. Gen Hosp Psychiatry 34(6):611–617, 2012 22898443

Maldonado JR, Sher Y, Ashouri JF, et al: The "Prediction of Alcohol Withdrawal Severity Scale" (PAWSS): systematic literature review and pilot study of a new scale for the prediction of complicated alcohol withdrawal syndrome. Alcohol 48(4):375–390, 2014 24657098

Mason BJ, Goodman AM, Dixon RM, et al: A pharmacokinetic and pharmacodynamic drug interaction study of acamprosate and naltrexone. Neuropsychopharmacology 27(4):596–606, 2003 12377396

Mattick RP, Breen C, Kimber J, Davoli M: Buprenorphine maintenance versus placebo or methadone maintenance for opioid dependence. Cochrane Database of Systematic Reviews 2014, Issue 2. Art. No.: CD002207. DOI: 10.1002/14651858. CD002207.pub4 24500948

McCowan C, Marik P: Refractory delirium tremens treated with propofol: a case series. Crit Care Med 28(6):1781–1784, 2000 10890619

McEvoy GK: American Hospital Formulary Service (AHFS) Drug Information 2008. Bethesda, MD, American Society of Health-System Pharmacists, 2008.

Meemken L, Hanhoff N, Tseng A, et al: Drug-drug interactions with antiviral agents in people who inject drugs (PWID) requiring substitution therapy. Ann Pharmacother 49(7):796–807, 2015 25902733

Meyer MC, Johnston AM, Crocker AM, Heil SH: Methadone and buprenorphine for opioid dependence during pregnancy: a retrospective cohort study. J Addict Med 9(2):81–86, 2015 25622120

Minozzi S, Amato L, Vecchi S, Davoli M: Anticonvulsants for alcohol withdrawal. Cochrane Database of Systematic Reviews 2010, Issue 3. Art. No.: CD005064. DOI: 10.1002/14651858.CD005064.pub3 20238337

Minozzi S, Amato L, Bellisario C, et al: Maintenance agonist treatments for opiate-dependent pregnant women. Cochrane Database of Systematic Reviews 2013, Issue 12. Art. No.: CD006318. DOI: 10.1002/14651858.CD006318.pub3 24366859

Miotto K, Striebel J, Cho AK, Wang C: Clinical and pharmacological aspects of bath salt use: a review of the literature and case reports. Drug Alcohol Depend 132(1–2):1–12, 2013 23916320

Mirijello A, D'Angelo C, Ferrulli A, et al: Identification and management of alcohol withdrawal syndrome. Drugs 75(4):353–365, 2015 25666543

Moore THM, Zammit S, Lingford-Hughes A, et al: Cannabis use and risk of psychotic or affective mental health outcomes: a systematic review. Lancet 370(9584):319–328, 2007 17662880

Moss M, Burnham EL: Alcohol abuse in the critically ill patient. Lancet 368(9554):2231–2242, 2006 17189035

Mueller SW, Preslaski CR, Kiser TH, et al: A randomized, double-blind, placebo-controlled dose range study of dexmedetomidine as adjunctive therapy for alcohol withdrawal. Crit Care Med 42(5):1131–1139, 2014 24351375

Mujtaba S, Romero J, Taub CC: Methadone, QTc prolongation and torsades de pointes: current concepts, management and a hidden twist in the tale? J Cardiovasc Dis Res 4(4):229–235, 2013 24653586

Muzyk AJ, Fowler JA, Norwood DK, Chilipko A: Role of α2-agonists in the treatment of acute alcohol withdrawal. Ann Pharmacother 45(5):649–657, 2011 21521867

O'Brien JMJr, Lu B, Ali NA, et al: Alcohol dependence is independently associated with sepsis, septic shock, and hospital mortality among adult intensive care unit patients. Crit Care Med 35(2):345–350, 2007 17205003

Paille F, Martini H: Nalmefene: a new approach to the treatment of alcohol dependence. Subst Abuse Rehabil 5:87–94, 2014 25187751

Pandharipande P, Shintani A, Peterson J, et al: Lorazepam is an independent risk factor for transitioning to delirium in intensive care unit patients. Anesthesiology 104(1):21–26, 2006 16394685

Pandharipande PP, Pun BT, Herr DL, et al: Effect of sedation with dexmedetomidine vs lorazepam on acute brain dysfunction in mechanically ventilated patients: the MENDS randomized controlled trial. JAMA 298(22):2644–2653, 2007 18073360

Pandharipande P, Cotton BA, Shintani A, et al: Prevalence and risk factors for development of delirium in surgical and trauma intensive care unit patients. J Trauma 65(1):34–41, 2008 18580517

Passie T, Halpern JH: Hallucinogens and related drugs, in Clinical Manual of Addiction Psychopharmacology, 2nd Edition. Edited by Kranzler HR, Ciraulo DA, Zindel LR. Washington, DC, American Psychiatric Publishing, 2014, pp 261–320

Pecoraro A, Ewen E, Horton T, et al: Using the AUDIT-PC to predict alcohol withdrawal in hospitalized patients. J Gen Intern Med 29(1):34–40, 2014 23959745

Pérez-Mañá C, Castells X, Torrens M, et al: Efficacy of psychostimulant drugs for amphetamine abuse or dependence. Cochrane Database of Systematic Reviews 2013, Issue 9. Art. No.: CD009695. DOI: 10.1002/14651858.CD009695.pub2 23996457

Phillips K, Luk A, Soor GS, et al: Cocaine cardiotoxicity: a review of the pathophysiology, pathology, and treatment options. Am J Cardiovasc Drugs 9(3):177–196, 2009 19463023

Plosker GL: Acamprosate: a review of its use in alcohol dependence. Drugs 75(11):1255–1268, 2015 26084940

Pourmand A, Armstrong P, Mazer-Amirshahi M, Shokoohi H: The evolving high: new designer drugs of abuse. Hum Exp Toxicol 33(10):993–999, 2014 24501103

Quigley MA, Boyce SH: Unintentional rapid opioid detoxification. Emerg Med J 18(6):494–495, 2001 11696513

Rigotti NA, Munafo MR, Stead LF: Smoking cessation interventions for hospitalized smokers: a systematic review. Arch Intern Med 168(18):1950–1960, 2008 18852395

Rosenson J, Clements C, Simon B, et al: Phenobarbital for acute alcohol withdrawal: a prospective randomized double-blind placebo-controlled study. J Emerg Med 44(3):592–598.e2, 2013 22999778

Ross S, Peselow E: Pharmacotherapy of addictive disorders. Clin Neuropharmacol 32(5):277–289, 2009 19834993

Sachdev G, Gesin G, Christmas AB, Sing RF: Failure of lorazepam to treat alprazolam withdrawal in a critically ill patient. World J Crit Care Med 3(1):42–44, 2014 24834401

Saitz R, Mayo-Smith MF, Roberts MS, et al: Individualized treatment for alcohol withdrawal: a randomized double-blind controlled trial. JAMA 272(7):519–523, 1994 8046805

Sanchez-Ramos J: Neurologic complications of psychomotor stimulant abuse. Int Rev Neurobiol 120:131–160, 2015 26070756

Schellhorn SE, Barnhill JW, Raiteri V, et al: A comparison of psychiatric consultation between geriatric and non-geriatric medical inpatients. Int J Geriatr Psychiatry 24(10):1054–1061, 2009 19326400

Schnoll RA, Goelz PM, Veluz-Wilkins A, et al: Long-term nicotine replacement therapy: a randomized clinical trial. JAMA Intern Med 175(4):504–511, 2015 25705872

Schoenfeld A, Friedman S, Stein LB, et al: Severe hypertensive reaction after naloxone injection during labor. Arch Gynecol 240(1):45–47, 1987 3827314

Schuckit MA: Recognition and management of withdrawal delirium (delirium tremens). N Engl J Med 371(22):2109–2113, 2014 25427113

Seger DL: Flumazenil—treatment or toxin. J Toxicol Clin Toxicol 42(2):209–216, 2004 15214628

Shinn AK, Greenfield SF: Topiramate in the treatment of substance-related disorders: a critical review of the literature. J Clin Psychiatry 71(5):634–648, 2010 20361908

Sobieraj DM, White WB, Baker WL: Cardiovascular effects of pharmacologic therapies for smoking cessation. J Am Soc Hypertens 7(1):61–67, 2013 23266101

Substance Abuse and Mental Health Services Administration: Results from the 2013 National Survey on Drug Use and Health: Summary of National Findings. 2014. Available at: http://www.samhsa.gov/data/sites/default/files/NSDUHresults PDFWHTML2013/Web/NSDUHresults2013.pdf. Accessed April 20, 2015.

Sullivan JT, Sykora K, Schneiderman J, et al: Assessment of alcohol withdrawal: the revised clinical institute withdrawal assessment for alcohol scale (CIWA-Ar). Br J Addict 84(11):1353–1357, 1989 2597811

Tetrault JM, Fiellin DA: Current and potential pharmacological treatment options for maintenance therapy in opioid-dependent individuals. Drugs 72(2):217–228, 2012 22235870

Thomson AD, Cook CCH, Touquet R, Henry JA; Royal College of Physicians, London: The Royal College of Physicians report on alcohol: guidelines for managing Wernicke's encephalopathy in the accident and emergency department. Alcohol Alcohol 37(6):513–521, 2002 12414541

Tomson T, Xue H, Battino D: Major congenital malformations in children of women with epilepsy. Seizure 28:46–50, 2015 25777785

U.S. Department of Health and Human Services: The health consequences of smoking—50 years of progress: a report of the Surgeon General. Atlanta, GA, U.S. Department of Health and Human Services, CDC, 2014. Available at http://www.surgeongeneral.gov/library/reports/50-years-of-progress/full-report.pdf. Accessed June 22, 2015.

Warner M, Chen LH, Makuc DM, et al: Drug poisoning deaths in the United States, 1980–2008. NCHS Data Brief 81(81):1–8, 2011 22617462

Wedam EF, Bigelow GE, Johnson RE, et al: QT-interval effects of methadone, levomethadyl, and buprenorphine in a randomized trial. Arch Intern Med 167(22):2469–2475, 2007 18071169

Weinberg JA, Magnotti LJ, Fischer PE, et al: Comparison of intravenous ethanol versus diazepam for alcohol withdrawal prophylaxis in the trauma ICU: results of a randomized trial. J Trauma 64(1):99–104, 2008 18188105

Weinbroum AA, Flaishon R, Sorkine P, et al: A risk-benefit assessment of flumazenil in the management of benzodiazepine overdose. Drug Saf 17(3):181–196, 1997 9306053

Weinbroum AA, Glick A, Belhassen B: Flumazenil is innocuous in a paroxysmal supraventricular tachycardia and radiofrequency ablation: a paediatric case report and review of the literature. Paediatr Anaesth 13(4):349–354, 2003 12753451

Welsh CJ, Suman M, Cohen A, et al: The use of intravenous buprenorphine for the treatment of opioid withdrawal in medically ill hospitalized patients. Am J Addict 11(2):135–140, 2002 12028743

Westover AN, McBride S, Haley RW: Stroke in young adults who abuse amphetamines or cocaine: a population-based study of hospitalized patients. Arch Gen Psychiatry 64(4):495–502, 2007 17404126

Whiting PF, Wolff RF, Deshpande S, et al: Cannabinoids for medical use: a systematic review and meta-analysis. JAMA 313(24):2456–2473, 2015 26103030

Wiegand SL, Stringer EM, Stuebe AM, et al: Buprenorphine and naloxone compared with methadone treatment in pregnancy. Obstet Gynecol 125(2):363–368, 2015 25569005

Wieneke H, Conrads H, Wolstein J, et al: Levo-alpha-acetylmethadol (LAAM) induced QTc-prolongation—results from a controlled clinical trial. Eur J Med Res 14(1):7–12, 2009 19258204

Wolstein J, Gastpar M, Finkbeiner T, et al: A randomized, open-label trial comparing methadone and Levo-Alpha-Acetylmethadol (LAAM) in maintenance treatment of opioid addiction. Pharmacopsychiatry 42(1):1–8, 2009 19153939

Woolf KJ, Zabad MN, Post JM, et al: Effect of nicotine replacement therapy on cardiovascular outcomes after acute coronary syndromes. Am J Cardiol 110(7):968–970, 2012 22727182

Zelner I, Matlow J, Hutson JR, et al; Toxicology Investigators Consortium (ToxIC): Acute poisoning during pregnancy: observations from the Toxicology Investigators Consortium. J Med Toxicol 11(3):301–308, 2015 25783189

Index

Page numbers printed in **boldface** *type refer to tables or figures.*